Public Health in the Arab World

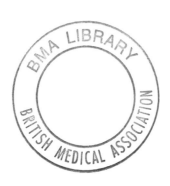

Public Health in the Arab World

Edited by

Samer Jabbour
Senior Lecturer, Faculty of Health Sciences, American University of Beirut, Lebanon

Rita Giacaman
Professor of Public Health, Institute of Community and Public Health, Birzeit University, West Bank, Occupied Palestinian Territory

Marwan Khawaja
Chief, Social Statistics Section, UN Economic and Social Commission for Western Asia (UN ESCWA), Beirut, Lebanon

Iman Nuwayhid
Professor and Dean, Faculty of Health Sciences, American University of Beirut, Lebanon

Associate Editor

Rouham Yamout
Research Associate, Faculty of Health Sciences, American University of Beirut, Lebanon

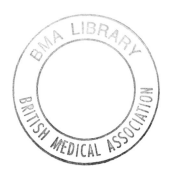

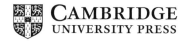
CAMBRIDGE
UNIVERSITY PRESS

CAMBRIDGE UNIVERSITY PRESS
Cambridge, New York, Melbourne, Madrid, Cape Town,
Singapore, São Paulo, Delhi, Mexico City

Cambridge University Press
The Edinburgh Building, Cambridge CB2 8RU, UK

Published in the United States of America
by Cambridge University Press, New York

www.cambridge.org
Information on this title: www.cambridge.org/9780521516747

First published 2012

Printed in the United Kingdom at the University Press, Cambridge

*A catalogue record for this publication is available from the
British Library*

Library of Congress Cataloging-in-Publication Data

Public health in the Arab world / editors, Samer Jabbour ... [et al.] ;
associate editor, Rouham Yamout.
    p. ; cm.
  Includes bibliographical references and index.
  ISBN 978-0-521-51674-7 (Hardback)
  I. Jabbour, Samer.   II. Yamout, Rouham.
  [DNLM: 1. Arab World–Middle East.   2. Public Health–Middle
East.   3. Health Services–Middle East.   4. Healthcare Disparities–
Middle East.   WA 540 JA2]
    362.10956–dc23

                                                                    2011035581

ISBN 978-0-521-51674-7 Hardback

For Huda Zurayk
Who has brought us together
The Editors

Table of Contents

Some chapters refer to a Web Appendix. This can be found at: www.cambridge.org/9780521516747

Foreword

As a wave of uprisings spread from Tunisia to Egypt to Bahrain to Yemen to Libya and to Saudi Arabia in early 2011, France's Special Representative to the United Nations, Gerard Araud, wrote that, after all, "there is an international community. The world is changing and I think it is changing for the better." To those of us living outside of the Arab world the signs were strong that some kind of permanent political change was indeed taking place. The demand for democracy and liberty seemed to be ushering in a new era of solidarity among a truly global civil society. Was this assessment reliable? Or should one perhaps be cautious about interpretations of even the most promising of events, especially when those interpretations come from former colonial powers.

For what is taking place in the local contexts of Arab countries – in towns and villages, among rural and urban communities, and within families and networks of friends – is surely more complex. Revolution should be put in its proper place. The reality of lives lived under the political regimes of the Arab world should give us reason to pause before we judge what we see on our television screens or read in our newspapers.

At the same time as the 2011 Arab uprisings were taking place, I sat in a classroom at the Institute of Community and Public Health at Birzeit University in the occupied Palestinian territory. Twenty-five students at the Institute were describing what they saw as obstacles to achieving health in their land. The students had diverse backgrounds: pharmacists, junior officials from the Ministry of Health (and Education), a physiotherapist, laboratory technicians, nurses, a UNRWA worker, a dentist, and a statistician. Each was allowed to identify only one obstacle. We looked for connections among their concerns, put together broad themes, and finally voted on what mattered most to this group of students at a specific place and time – Birzeit, March 3, 2011.

In order of votes, here is what these students identified as urgent priorities. The first, by a considerable margin, was a set of predicaments facing young people. We might call this group of technical concerns "adolescent health". But what these students had to say went much further than the term "adolescent health" can ever imply. They wanted to join health among young people to issues of agency and opportunity in their society. Young women and men were crucial assets to Palestinian society, they said, assets that were being neglected, even wasted.

Next came a group of issues that were judged equally important to one another: the conditions for Palestinians living in the vicinity of Israeli settlements, the ongoing violence against Palestinians in East Jerusalem, and maternal health. Finally, a smaller number of votes were cast for an array of highly diverse matters: medical errors, shortages of medicines, weak regulation of health professionals, lack of universal health care, the inequity of health conditions between those living in Gaza and those in the West Bank and East Jerusalem, the impact of price inflation on health, child health, violence against children in schools, and the effects of migration on urban health.

Amid this much more detailed report card on the health predicaments facing Palestinians, revolution, and the lessons that needed to be learned from revolution, entered, but didn't dominate, our discussion. We were, from time to time, drawn back to what one student called the "Arab context". What did those words mean? At their most elemental level, they meant "realising the right to achieve our needs". But those needs were far thicker than were being described by the now supposedly legitimised "international community". The uprisings had cast fresh light on often despotic or dynastic political regimes. This particular reading of the "Arab context" was one that suited many Western observers. It allowed them to put much of the blame for the problems faced by Arab peoples on Arab societies themselves. It cleansed the West of responsibility. But a deeper analysis of the "Arab context", as shown in microcosm by the students at Birzeit, revealed a far more disquieting assessment. The fabric of Arab health today is woven from coarse historical and political threads, threads drawn from old European colonial powers, remnants of the Cold War, and newer hegemonic, notably American, interests.

In the broad movement that is public health today, the reach of concern for human wellbeing has grown in unprecedented ways. The geographically widened moral commitment made by scientists engaged in health research has been one of the most striking shifts in science since the Enlightenment. The problems of poverty and human development are now central concerns for all scientific communities. But even with this new sense of global identity in science, some parts of the world still seem to exist on the margins of our concern. Africa, Asia, and Latin America receive appropriately large attention. But what is strange is the relatively muted interest in the Arab world within mainstream public and global health.

Public Health in the Arab World is the most important corrective intervention to this pervasive bias since Western powers divided Arab lands – and betrayed Arab peoples – over half a century ago. This volume is an extraordinary collaboration between 86 public health scientists, over two-thirds of whom are living in Arab countries today, with many others having been born and raised in Arab lands. The peoples of Lebanon, Egypt, the Occupied Palestinian Territory, Morocco, Syria, Tunisia, United Arab Emirates, Qatar, Saudi Arabia, Bahrain, Kuwait, Sudan, and Jordan are all directly represented here. The collaboration extends to a broad diaspora across the United States, United Kingdom, Canada, Belgium, France, and Australia. The World Health Organisation has also played an important part through the contributions of its scientific staff in WHO's Geneva Headquarters and Eastern Mediterranean Regional and Country Offices. It is a book whose ideas and conclusions are driven by data. This fact is recognition that the very best platform for political advocacy is reliable information (the role of Marwan Khawaja, Chief of Social Statistics at UN ESCWA in Beirut and a co-editor of this work, is indicative of a commitment to assembling the best available evidence to underpin policy).

But when one looks closely at the origins of these writers, one cannot escape the special contributions made by two centres – the American University of Beirut (AUB) and Birzeit University. One fifth of the authors of *Public Health in the Arab World* come from the Faculty of Health Sciences at AUB, an extraordinary tribute to the long and successful leadership of Professor Huda Zurayk, currently Director of the Faculty's Center for Research on Population and Health. The book is justly dedicated to her. The Faculty's present Dean, Professor Iman Nuwayhid, is a co-editor of this volume, as is Samer Jabbour, a Senior Lecturer in the Faculty.

Each year, the Institute of Community and Public Health at Birzeit University hosts a writers' workshop for researchers working in the occupied Palestinian territory. The meeting gathers together public health scientists from not only within the occupied territory, but also from outside – from Norway, Canada, the United States, and Britain, all with the support of the charity, Medical Aid for Palestinians. The purpose is to create a forum that supports the study and analysis of the conditions shaping health under occupation. It provides a place where the voice of Palestinians can be heard outside of the region (peer-reviewed abstracts from the meeting are published on *The Lancet*'s Website). This international collaboration, led by Professors Rita Giacaman (also a co-editor of the current volume) and Rana Khatib, began in 2007 and resulted in a series of five papers in *The Lancet* in 2009, entitled "Health in the occupied Palestinian territory." Two subsequent workshops have produced two volumes of abstracts. The Institute has been a remarkable and inspiring catalyst for mobilising generations of young health researchers to join the cause of science in the service of social change in the Arab World.

Scrawled on the Separation Wall at the Kalandia checkpoint between Jerusalem and Ramallah are the words: "This wall doesn't limit freedom of the mind." *Public Health in the Arab World* proves that this is so. This book offers the clearest voice yet heard from Arab public health scientists (indeed, perhaps from Arab scientists and scholars of all kinds). It is an indispensable statement of possibility, a passionate analysis that creates an astonishing opportunity for action. It is a manifesto for justice.

Richard Horton FRCP FMedSci
The Lancet
32 Jamestown Road
London
UK
richard.horton@lancet.com
December 22, 2011

Acknowledgments

The original idea behind this volume was to publish the proceedings and papers presented during the 50th Anniversary International Conference of the Faculty of Health Sciences (FHS) at the American University of Beirut (AUB), held in Beirut, December 2004. However, the editors recognized the need for a larger volume on public health in the Arab world. The Ford Foundation, which had supported the Conference and provided funds for publishing its proceedings and papers, extended a grant to support the work to develop the volume. This has happened thanks to Montasser Kamal, Officer for Reproductive Health at the Foundation's Cairo office, who understood the importance of the work and was enthusiastic to have the Foundation support it. For that, we are truly grateful. The FHS and AUB have also extended considerable support, starting during the tenure of Huda Zurayk as dean, for faculty time and logistics to support the editorial work. The Center for Research on Population and Health at FHS also provided valuable support. This effort could not have proceeded without this institutional support.

The cover illustration is designed by Rana Barazi Tabbara, MD, MPH. With a background career in Family Medicine, a recent MPH from the Faculty of Health Sciences at the American University of Beirut, and a long-practiced hobby in mixed-media arts, Barazi Tabbara is a firm believer in health promotion through artistic expression. The art work on the cover illustration consists of a series of hand-painted tiles, each 5×5 cm, inspired by some of the themes and concepts highlighted in this book.

Many people have contributed to the development of this volume. A small but committed advisory group provided useful comments and guidance, especially in the initial stages. We appreciate the input of Ross Brownson, Jocelyn DeJong, Nabil Kronfol, David McCoy, Belgacem Sabri, David Sanders, and Huda Zurayk. Norbert Hirschhorn carried out English- and style-editing of many chapters and provided insightful comments on others. Aida Farha at AUB's Saab Medical Library provided very helpful library services throughout the project. Hilda Nassar, medical librarian at AUB, Aida Farha and Maya Abou Saad helped develop the index. Nadine Haddad carried out literature searches on various topics while an MPH student at FHS/AUB. Suzanne El Khechen and Joyce Haddad in the Dean's Office at FHS/AUB kindly provided administrative assistance to the editorial team. Amr Awad, Dima Bteddini, Taghreed Elhajj, Zeina Ghantous, Nadine Haddad, Doris Jaalouk, Alena Mack, and Mohamed Salem, all graduate students or research assistants at FHS at the time, volunteered time to take and transcribe minutes of the two meetings that brought together editors and lead authors. Joseph Azar, Chadi Barbour, and Hala Dimechkie at FHS; Nada Sbaiti El-Zein at AUB's Computing and Networking Services; and Farihan Hamdan, an independent consultant, provided valuable IT services. Leila Roumani and Racha Fadlallah helped correct the book proofs.

Our first editor at Cambridge University Press, Marc Strauss, saw the potential value of the volume when the proposal was first presented to him. We thank him for giving us the opportunity. However, for much of the time that it took to complete the volume, we worked with editors Richard Marley, Joanna Chamberlin and Emma Walker. They were supportive of the work, insightful in giving advice, and quick to respond to inquiries. We thank them for their patience and dedication.

Many authors in this volume have provided internal peer reviews for other chapters. In addition, all chapters have undergone external peer review. Sameh El-Saharty and Salman Rawaf kindly reviewed and provided valuable perspectives about several chapters in Section 6 (Health Systems). The editors are grateful for the contribution of both internal and external reviewers and would like to acknowledge the following external reviewers:

Hanan Abdul Rahim (Qatar), Carla Abou-Zahr (Switzerland), Houssain Abouzaid (Lebanon), Raeda Abu Al Rub (Jordan), Abdulrazzak Abyad (Lebanon), Mustafa Afifi (UAE), Narjis Ajeel (Iraq), Kamel Ajlouni (Jordan), Kristine Ajrouch (USA), Naira Al Awqati (Jordan), William Aldis (Thailand), Aysa Al-Riyami (Oman), Ricardo Araya (UK), Haroutune Armenian (USA), Elsheikh Badr (Sudan), Guitelle Baghdadi-Sabeti (Switzerland), Arwa Baidar (Yemen), Seifeddin G. Ballal (Saudi Arabia), Brian K. Barber (USA), Alaka Basu (USA), Malek Batal (Canada), David Bishai (USA), Thomas Bossert (USA), Sofiane Bouhdiba (Tunisia), Derick Brinkerhoff (USA), Melani Cammett (USA), Guy Carrin (Switzerland), Monique Chaaya (Lebanon), Sir Iain Chalmers (UK), Mario Dal Poz (Switzerland), Nadia Dalloul (Lebanon), Ivan Dimov Ivanov (Switzerland), Azza El Nouman (Egypt), Sameh el-Saharty (USA), Heba Elgazzar (USA), Eltigani Eltigani (Saudi Arabia), Sameera El-Tuwaijri (USA), Ibtihal Fadhil (Egypt), Ali Fakhro (Bahrain), Laila Farhood (Lebanon), Mahmoud Fathalla (Egypt), Stephen Fawcett (USA), Osman Galal (USA), Michele Ruth Gamburd (USA), Muntaha Garaibeh (Jordan), Richard Garfield (USA), Buthaina Ghanem (Jordan), Farha Ghannam (USA), Hassen Ghannem (Tunisia), Jen'nan Ghazal Read (USA), Richard Gosselin (USA), Emily Grundy (UK), Hani Guend (Canada), Jean RD Guimarães (Brazil), Omran Habib (Iraq), Nadim Haddad (Lebanon), Gail Harrison (USA), Allan Hill (USA), Norbert Hirschhorn (UK), Dennis Hogan (USA), Marcia Inhorn (USA), Tushar K. Joshi (India), Miloud Kaddar (Switzerland), Montasser Kamal (Egypt), Zeina Kanafani (Lebanon), Khaled Khatab (Germany), Nadir Kheir (Qatar), Eberhard Kienle (Egypt), Judith Kulig (Canada), Adam Leive (USA), Socrates Litsios (Switzerland), Frederick M. Burkle (USA), Chowra Makarermi (Canada), Jihad Makhoul (Lebanon), Bernard Manyena (UK), Theodor Marmor (USA), José Carlos Martines (Switzerland), Abdel Aziz Mousa Thabet (Occupied Palestinian Territory), Alok Mukhopadhyay (India), Mona Nabulsi (Lebanon), Marion Nestle (USA), Olcay Neyzi (Turkey), Peter Pellett (USA), Guénaël Rodier (Denmark), Najib Saab (Lebanon), Ritu Sadana (Switzerland), Shadi Saleh (Lebanon), Monica Schoch-Spana (USA), Zohair Sebai (Saudi Arabia), Ravi Shankar (Nepal), Hania Sholkamy (Egypt), Katherine Smith (UK), Nicholas Spencer (UK), Devi Sridhar (UK), Mayssun Sukarieh (Lebanon), Derek Summerfield (UK), Simon Szreter (UK), Yoke van der Meulen-Rabaia (Occupied Palestinian Territory), Tony Waterston (UK), Sheldon Watts (Egypt), Johanna Wyn (Australia), Hassan Zaky (Egypt), Nicolas Zdanowicz (Belgium), Zachary Zimmer (USA).

Contributors

Ynesse Abdul-Malak, RN, MPH
Research Scientist, Psychiatry and Behavioral Sciences, Upstate Medical University, Syracuse, New York, USA

Sawsan Abdulrahim, PhD
Assistant Professor, Faculty of Health Sciences, American University of Beirut, Beirut, Lebanon

Rima Afifi, PhD
Professor and Associate Dean, Faculty of Health Sciences, American University of Beirut, Beirut, Lebanon

Ala Alwan, MD
Assistant Director-General, Noncommunicable Diseases and Mental Health, World Health Organization, Geneva, Switzerland

Nisreen Alwan, MBChB, MPH, MSc
Clinical Research Fellow and Specialist Registrar in Public Health, Nutritional Epidemiology Group, University of Leeds, Leeds, UK

Mohammad Assai, MBBS, MPH
Regional Adviser, Community-based Initiatives, World Health Organization Regional Office for the Eastern Mediterranean, Cairo, Egypt

Amr A. Awad, MD, MS
Monitoring and Evaluation Advisor, Center for Leadership and Management, Management Sciences for Health, Aswan, Egypt

Peter Barss, MD, ScD, MPH
Medical Health Officer, Interior Health Authority, Salmon Arm, BC; Clinical Professor, University of British Columbia, Vancouver, BC, Canada

Hyam Bashour, MD, PhD
Professor, Faculty of Medicine, Damascus University, Damascus, Syria

Manal Benkirane, MD, MPH
Program Officer, Association de Lutte contre le SIDA, Morocco

Habiba Ben Romdhane, MD
Professor and Director, Department of Cardiovascular Disease Epidemiology and Prevention, Faculty of Medicine, University of Tunis, Tunis, Tunisia.

Krishna Bose, PhD, MPH
Scientist, Department of Child and Adolescent Health and Development, World Health Organization, Geneva, Switzerland

Rayana Bou-Haka, MD, MPH
Medical Officer, Emergency and Humanitarian Action, World Health Organization Regional Office for the Eastern Mediterranean, Cairo, Egypt

Sylvia Chiffoleau, PhD
Chargée de Recherche CNRS, Chercheuse à l'Institut Français du Proche Orient, Beirut, Lebanon

Jocelyn DeJong, PhD
Associate Professor, Faculty of Health Sciences, American University of Beirut, Beirut, Lebanon

Omar Dewachi, MBChB, PhD
Assistant Professor, Faculty of Health Sciences, American University of Beirut, Beirut, Lebanon

Driss Zine-Eddine El-Idrissi, PhD
Senior Health Economist, the World Bank, Washington, DC, USA

Fadi El-Jardali, PhD
Associate Professor, Faculty of Health Sciences, American University of Beirut, Beirut, Lebanon

Abbas El-Zein, PhD
Associate Professor, School of Civil Engineering, University of Sydney, Sydney, Australia

Fadi A. Fathallah, PhD
Professor and Director, Occupational Biomechanics Laboratory, University of California, Davis, CA, USA

Rim Fayad, MS
Project Manager, Department of Policy & Strategy, The Executive Council, Government of Dubai, Dubai, United Arab Emirates

Hala Ghattas, MSc, PhD
Assistant Professor, Faculty of Agriculture and Food Sciences, American University of Beirut, Beirut, Lebanon

Rita Giacaman, PharmD, MPhil
Professor, Research and Program Coordinator, Institute of Community and Public Health, Birzeit University, Birzeit, Occupied Palestinian Territory

Rima R. Habib, PhD
Associate Professor, Faculty of Health Sciences, American University of Beirut, Beirut, Lebanon

Rana A. Hajjeh, MD
Director, Division of Bacterial Diseases, National Center for Immunizations and Respiratory Diseases, Centers for Disease Control and Prevention, Atlanta, GA, USA

Samia Halileh, MD, PhD
Assistant Professor, Institute of Community and Public Health, Birzeit University, Birzeit, Occupied Palestinian Territory

Abdelmonem S. Hassan, MS, PhD
Associate Professor, Department of Health Sciences, Qatar University, Doha, Qatar

Jamil Hilal, MLitt
Sociologist and Senior Research Fellow, Birzeit University, Ramallah, Occupied Palestinian Territory

Abdullatif Husseini, PhD, MPH, MS
Associate Professor, Institute of Community and Public Health, Birzeit University, Birzeit, Occupied Palestinian Territory

Ghena A. Ismail, PsyD, C. Psych
Psychologist, Correctional Service Canada, Regional Treatment Center, Kingston, ON, Canada

Doris Jaalouk, PhD, MPH
Assistant Professor, Faculty of Nursing and Health Sciences, Notre Dame University-Louaize, Zouk Mosbeh, Lebanon

Samer Jabbour, MD, MPH
Senior Lecturer, Faculty of Health Sciences, American University of Beirut, Beirut, Lebanon

Diana Jamal, MPH
Research Assistant, Faculty of Health Sciences, American University of Beirut, Beirut, Lebanon

Aisha O. Jumaan, PhD
Team Lead, Division of Public Health Systems and Workforce Development, Center for Global Health, Centers for Disease Control and Prevention, Atlanta, GA, USA

Mey Jurdi, PhD
Professor and Chair, Environmental Health Department, Faculty of Health Sciences, American University of Beirut, Beirut, Lebanon

Afamia Kaddour, MSc, PhD Candidate
Research fellow, INSERM and Université Paris-Sud XI, Paris, France

Elie G. Karam, MD
Professor and Head, Department of Psychiatry and Clinical Psychology, Faculty of Medicine, Balamand University; Executive Director, Institute for Development Research Advocacy and Applied Care (IDRAAC), Beirut, Lebanon

Zeinab Khadr, PhD
Research Professor, Social Research Center, American University in Cairo, Cairo, Egypt

Mohamad Hassan Khalil, MD
Cardiology Consultant, Health Insurance Organization; Coordinator, Committee for Defending People's Right to Health, Cairo, Egypt

Rana Khatib, PhD
Associate Professor and Director, Institute of Community and Public Health, Birzeit University, Birzeit, Occupied Palestinian Territory

Marwan Khawaja, PhD
Chief, Social Statistics Section, United Nations Economic and Social Commission for Western Asia, Beirut, Lebanon

Nabil M. Kronfol, MD, DrPH
President, Lebanese HealthCare Management
Association, Beirut, Lebanon

Natalia Linos, MS, PhD Candidate
Harvard School of Public Health, Harvard
University, USA

Elisabeth Longuenesse, PhD
Researcher, CNRS, Paris, France; Director, Institut
Français du Proche Orient, Beirut, Lebanon

Ahmed Mandil, MBChB, DrPH
Professor, High Institute of Public Health, University
of Alexandria, Alexandria, Egypt; Coordinator, Saudi
Board of Community Medicine, College of Medicine,
King Saud University, Saudi Arabia

Awad Mataria, PhD
Technical Officer, Health Economics and Health Care
Financing Unit, World Health Organization Regional
Office for the Eastern Mediterranean, Cairo, Egypt

Zafar Mirza, MD, MPH
Coordinator, Department of Public Health, Innovation
and Intellectual Property, Director General's Office,
World Health Organization, Geneva, Switzerland

Driss Moussaoui, MD
Professor and Chairman, Ibn Rushd University
Psychiatric Centre, Casablanca, Morocco; President,
World Association for Social Psychiatry

Hani Mowafi, MD, MPH
Assistant Professor, Department of Emergency
Medicine, Boston University School of Medicine,
Boston, MA, USA; Associate Faculty, Harvard
Humanitarian Initiative, Cambridge, MA, USA

Mona Mowafi, ScD, MHS
Research Fellow, Harvard School of Public Health,
Boston, MA, USA

Abdulrahman O. Musaiger, MPH, DrPH
Director, Arab Center for Nutrition, & Professor of
Nutrition, University of Bahrain, Manama, Bahrain

Cynthia Myntti, MPH, PhD, MArch
Professor, Faculty of Health Sciences & Project Leader,
The Neighborhood Initiative, President's Office,
American University of Beirut, Beirut, Lebanon

Mayssa T. Nehlawi, MPH, CHES
Health Writer and Editor, Editorwrites, USA

Adib Nehmeh, DEA,
Regional Advisor on MDGs, United Nations
Economic and Social Commission for Western Asia,
Beirut, Lebanon

Iman Nuwayhid, MD, DrPH
Professor and Dean, Faculty of Health Sciences,
American University of Beirut, Beirut, Lebanon

Omar Obeid, PhD
Professor, Faculty of Agriculture and Food Sciences,
American University of Beirut, Beirut, Lebanon

Hoda Rashad, PhD
Research Professor and Director, Social Research
Center, American University in Cairo, Cairo, Egypt

David Rawaf, BSc
Medical Student, St George's University of London,
London, UK

Salman Rawaf, MD, PhD
Professor of Public Health, Director, World Health
Organization Collaborating Centre, Faculty of
Medicine, Imperial College, London, UK

Belgacem Sabri, MD, MPA, MA
Director, Health Systems and Services Development
Division, World Health Organization Regional Office
for the Eastern Mediterranean, Cairo, Egypt

Mariana M. Salamoun, BS, MA
Research Associate, Institute for Development
Research Advocacy and Applied Care (IDRAAC),
Beirut, Lebanon

Mohamed E. Salem, MD, MPH
Researcher, Social Research Center, American
University in Cairo, Cairo, Egypt

Tanya Salem, BSN, MPH
Associate, the Advisory Group, Kuwait, Kuwait

Bruno Schoumaker, PhD
Professor, Centre de Recherche en Démographie et
Sociétés, Université Catholique de Louvain, Belgium

Olivia Shabb, BA, PsyD
Candidate PGSP-Stanford PsyD Consortium, Palo
Alto, California, USA

Sherine Shawky MD, DrPH
Research Professor, Social Research Center,
American University in Cairo, Cairo, Egypt

Alaa Shukrallah, MBBCh, MSc
Chairperson, Association for Health and Environmental Development; Member of the Executive Committee, Committee for Defending People's Right to Health, Cairo, Egypt; Senior consultant at Development Support Centre, Egypt

Abla Mehio Sibai, PhD
Professor, Faculty of Health Sciences, American University of Beirut; Director, Center for Studies on Aging, Beirut, Lebanon

Sameen Siddiqi, MD, MSc, DrMed
Coordinator, Health Systems Development, World Health Organization Regional Office for the Eastern Mediterranean, Cairo, Egypt

Dominique Tabutin, PhD
Professeur, Centre de Recherche en Démographie et Sociétés, Université Catholique de Louvain, Belgium

Maha Talaat, MD, DrPH
Head, Infection Control Unit, Global Disease Detection and Response Program, US Naval Medical Research Unit No. 3, Cairo, Egypt

Rania A. Tohme, MD, MPH
Epidemic Intelligence Service Officer, Centers for Disease Control & Prevention, Atlanta, GA, USA

Susan Watts, PhD
Social Scientist, World Health Organization Regional Office for the Eastern Mediterranean, Cairo, Egypt

Livia Wick, PhD
Assistant Professor, Faculty of Arts and Sciences, American University of Beirut, Beirut, Lebanon

Rouham Yamout, MD, MPH
Research Associate, Faculty of Health Sciences, American University of Beirut, Beirut, Lebanon

Nasser Yassin, PhD
Assistant Professor and Director, Outreach and Practice Unit, Faculty of Health Sciences, American University of Beirut, Beirut, Lebanon

Kathryn M. Yount, PhD
Associate Professor, Hubert Department of Global Health and Department of Sociology, Emory University, Atlanta, GA, USA

Huda Zurayk, PhD
Professor and Director, Center for Research on Population and Health, Faculty of Health Sciences, American University of Beirut, Beirut, Lebanon

Contributors of Boxes in Chapters

Gamal Khalafalla Mohamed Ali, PhD
Secretary General, Federal Pharmacy and Poisons Board, Khartoum, Sudan (Chapter 32)

Norbert Hirschhorn, MD
Lecturer, Yale University School of Public Health, New Haven, CT, USA (Chapter 17)

Nour Kibbi, BA
Medical Student, Yale University School of Medicine, New Haven, CT, USA (Chapter 6)

Contributors whose work is reproduced in the volume

Chadi S. Cortas, MD
Department of Medicine, Brigham & Women's Hospital and Harvard Medical School, Boston, USA (Chapter 26)

Tony Laurance, MA
WHO West Bank and Gaza Strip, Jerusalem, Occupied Palestinian Territory (Chapter 24)

Asad Ramlawi, MD
Palestinian Ministry of Health, Ramallah, Occupied Palestinian Territory (Chapter 24)

Guido Sabatinelli, MD
United Nations Relief and Works Agency for Palestine Refugees in the Near East, Amman, Jordan (Chapter 24)

Luay Shabaneh, PhD
Palestinian Central Bureau of Statistics, Ramallah, Occupied Palestinian Territory (Chapter 24)

Note: The views expressed herein are those of the authors and do not necessarily reflect the views of the United Nations.

Introduction

Samer Jabbour, Rita Giacaman, Marwan Khawaja,
Iman Nuwayhid, and Rouham Yamout

This edited book brings the voice of a diverse and multidisciplinary group of academics and practitioners who have lived and worked in the Arab world to regional and international audiences, emphasizing context and lived experiences. It aims to stimulate discussions about health in light of the demographic, epidemiological, economic, social, and political changes taking place. The editors hope that the book fills some of the gaps in an otherwise growing body of literature on public health in the region.

The book primarily targets academics, researchers, and students of public health, medicine, other health professions, and Arab/Middle Eastern studies. However, public health practitioners, health policy makers, and program managers are also likely to find the book useful because of its relevance to policy and practice. Personnel working with regional and international organizations involved in population health, development, and/or humanitarian aid will also recognize its benefits to their own work. Finally, this book is likely to interest general readers concerned with the Arab world; especially because public health in this region has not received the attention it deserves from scholars.

The Arab World and Public Health

Different and overlapping terms are used to refer to this region of the world. The "Middle East" is most commonly used in the media and political literature to describe the Mashreq countries (Iraq, Jordan, Lebanon, Occupied Palestinian Territory, and Syria) and Arab peninsula/Gulf states, in addition to Egypt, Turkey, Iran, and Israel. The "Middle East and North Africa" is commonly used by the World Bank and other development agencies, and includes additionally the Arab states north of the Sahara desert. The "Eastern Mediterranean region," used by the World Health Organization

(WHO) covers a wider area that includes 19 Arab countries (but not Algeria, Mauritania, and Comoros) in addition to Afghanistan, Iran, and Pakistan. Other UN agencies use additional terms and each includes a different set of Arab states. ESCWA and UNIFEM use "Western Asia" to refer to its 14 members, all Arab states. UNFPA, UNDP, UNICEF and UNESCO use "Arab states" to refer to almost all countries of the region.

This muddled representation of our region is perhaps a reflection of the way in which the Arab world has been defined for different purposes at different periods by different actors. This is precisely why we have opted to use the term "Arab World." This term, preferred by many people in the region, recognizes linguistic, political, historical, and socio-cultural links among the Arab countries, and among both the Arab and non-Arab populations in these countries.

The "Arab world" includes the 22 member states of the League of Arab States. The League was founded in 1945 and includes Palestine, officially recognized in the UN literature as "Occupied Palestinian Territory (OPT)." Countries joined the League at different periods (see Web Appendix) with Comoros the last to join in 1993.

It is worth noting that, even though the different communities of the Arab world share a set of common features justifying their perception as a unity, the region is not homogenous. Diversity, in terms of culture, religion, ethnicity, economy, and political systems, are the defining features. This book attempts to expose both the commonality and diversity, especially in relation to public health, among Arab countries as much as possible.

The book addresses major political and social issues affecting health, as well as overall contextual developments in the region. Chapters discuss a range of problems of importance to public health such as foreign interventionism, war and occupation, the challenges of globalization, autocratic governance,

Public Health in the Arab World, ed. Samer Jabbour et al. Published by Cambridge University Press. © Samer Jabbour et al., 2012.

tyranny and corruption, deteriorating economies, and weak social protection. This book was written before revolutions and protests broke out in several Arab countries forcing significant political changes including the bringing down of long-term presidents in Tunisia, Egypt and Libya. Chapters 2, 28, and 37 were modified at the time of submission to include perspectives related to these historic developments.

Values and Frameworks

There is agreement among the authors and editors of this book on the values that underpin this work. The starting point is seeing health as a right engraved in social contracts between the state and its citizens. Social solidarity, engagement of the public, and mobilization of community capacity are considered the most important mechanisms to promote health. Health promotion is seen within the context of work toward equity, social justice, and broader social change. Although these values do not emerge explicitly from every chapter, they form the basis for this collective endeavor.

At the outset, we had hoped that authors would agree on and utilize a common conceptual framework. However, it became clear during the writing process that this could not be achieved for various reasons. Different authors have different ways of conceptualizing social realities and, therefore, public health theory and practice. Quite often, there is indeed a need to resort to more than one framework and use more than one approach to suit the purpose and the intended messages of a given chapter. Some themes are better served by reporting quantitative materials, others require qualitative analyses, and yet others focus on theoretical discussions, reviews, or case studies. As things have evolved, we have become more aware of how contrasting views of public health may enrich scholarship. Although a range of approaches guided the writing of chapters, the book as a whole can be seen as presenting a population health perspective, where health is broadly conceptualized and where its social determinants take a central role in analysis.

Scope of Work

The book covers some of the basic themes of modern public health, such as social determinants and population groups, and explores topics of emerging interest, such as community resilience, participatory interventions, human security and health, and social change. This book is introductory and is by no means exhaustive as it omits or covers briefly other important topics because of the constraints of space and the unavailability of data and/or suitable authors. Some of these topics have been addressed across chapters. For example, tobacco use, of great interest to public health in the region, is discussed in several chapters rather than as the subject of a dedicated chapter. With more space, many topics would have received more attention because of their relevance to public health, such as public health ethics, the health of ethnic groups, consanguinity, and genetics. The book does not address issues related to two populations of interest that might be of interest to some readers: the Palestinian Arab population of historic Palestine, which is now part of Israel, and the Diaspora from Arab countries around the world.

Perhaps the greatest challenge that author teams have faced stems from the limited availability of high quality evidence or published work on key public health issues from a population health perspective. Gray literature is not easily accessible, and its quality is variable at best. Many regional health and development datasets are not available to authors or to the public. Comparability of data from different settings and years is questionable. This reflects the suboptimal quality of administrative registers and health information systems especially with regard to exposing inequalities.

Section/Chapter Contents

Section I of this book is devoted to the context of public health and describes the factors that have shaped health conditions, health systems, and public health. Chapter 1 presents a historical perspective. Longuenesse, Chiffoleau, Kronfol, and Dewachi discuss the influences of colonialism, independence, and the state-building project on the rise of the medical profession and the development of public health. They find that post-colonial Arab states with different political orientations have developed state welfare programs that have had a favorable influence on health. In Chapter 2, Jabbour, Yamout, Hilal, and Nehmeh examine the political, social, and economic determinants and conditions, and development patterns important to health and well-being. They find that factors such as poverty, unemployment, especially among the youth, and social, economic, and political exclusion not only underlie public health problems but can also help explain the emergence of the revolutions and popular protests beginning in January 2011 in the region.

In Chapter 3, Tabutin and Schoumaker examine the remarkable demographic transitions since 1950 with falling mortality leading to increasing life expectancy but persistent population growth due to slower rates of fertility decline. They point to demographic phenomena of particular importance in this region, including population growth, ageing, large youth segments, and large-scale population displacement and migration. Such changes have important implications for health and health services. One of the most pressing issues related to population growth is the widespread environmental degradation and dwindling resources explored by Jurdi, Fayad, and El-Zein in Chapter 4. While some natural resources, such as oil and gas, are abundant, the region is the most water-insecure in the world. Diverse drivers impact environmental change through three main processes: resource depletion, rising consumerism, and conflict. Although environmental action is gaining strength, much remains to be done to slow and reverse environmental degradation.

Whereas Section 1 explores the broad determinants of health, Section 2 focuses on specific determinants. In Chapter 5, Khadr, Rashad, Watts, and Salem present evidence for health inequities using classical stratifiers, such as wealth, and consider less visible inequities related to clustering of disadvantage as well as less common stratifiers such as deprivation. Khadr et al present an original analysis of official health policy documents and find limited attention to health equity. In Chapter 6, Khawaja, Mowafi, and Linos introduce a framework that includes economic capital, social capital, and cultural capital to understand the relation between assets and health. They discuss methods for measuring social capital used in two large studies in Lebanon and the Occupied Palestinian Territory. The authors review evidence from the region linking different assets and health and conclude with a discussion of research and policy implications.

In Chapter 7, Yount examines gender disparities in health through the lifespan. Among children under 5, mortality rates and access to education, nutrition, and health care favor boys. Among adults, she finds more over-weight and obesity and more mental health problems among women. She reviews studies on gender-based violence affecting both women and men. In Chapter 8, Rashad and Khadr wrap up Section II by proposing an agenda for research and action on social determinants. Acknowledging that health equity is not yet a priority in Arab countries, they stress the need for research and action to prioritize equity. There is a need for more research to improve the identification and monitoring of inequities. They propose policy reforms to frame health equity as a corporate responsibility of governments and discuss how to move from research into policy and action through, for example, learning from the experiences of development work.

The determinants discussed in Sections 1 and 2 are reflected in health outcomes, such as avoidable conditions, the focus of Section 3, and the health of population groups, the focus of Section 4. In Chapter 9, Myntti and Giacaman introduce Section 3 by suggesting that the standard approach of counting mortality and morbidity is insufficient to understanding health and disease. This approach does not incorporate non-professional sources of knowledge or insights into health as a positive construct. The authors stress the need to explore local meanings and practices of health and call for incorporating subjective approaches, such as self-rated health and quality of life measures, which include people's view of their own health, into assessments.

In Chapter 10, Musaiger, Ghattas, Hassan, and Obeid discuss nutrition and food security. Various Arab countries are at different states of the nutrition transition and shoulder a double nutritional burden with both under-nutrition and over-nutrition becoming important public health issues. Food insecurity, already a serious challenge especially in countries in conflict, promises to worsen over the ensuing decades due to shrinking land and water resources and inadequate investments in agriculture. In Chapter 11, Hajjeh, Talaat, and Jumaan discuss the unfinished agenda of infectious diseases, including those of epidemic potential such as tuberculosis and vaccine-preventable diseases such as polio and measles. They also discuss emerging threats such as HIV/AIDS and health care-associated infections. They propose an agenda for action that includes addressing the social determinants of infectious diseases, health system strengthening, surveillance, and human capacity building.

In Chapter 12, Alwan, Alwan, and Jabbour review the increasing burden of non-communicable diseases (NCDs): 5 of the top 10 killers in the region are NCDs.

The public health response in Arab countries has been inadequate. Considering that the top NCDs share common determinants and risk factors such as tobacco use, Alwan et al propose an integrated approach to NCD prevention and control that builds on local evidence and international experiences as part of a global strategy for NCD prevention and control. In Chapter 13, Ben Romdhane, Husseini, and Jabbour expand the discussion through focusing on the NCD associated with the highest burden, cardiovascular disease (CVD). They show important inequalities in CVD and its risks. They also explore the thorny issue of appropriate care for CVD and its risk factors, identifying missed opportunities for prevention. They highlight data showing over-utilization of invasive approaches in CVD diagnosis and treatment fueled by the oversupply of technology.

In Chapter 14, Karam, Salamoun, Jaalouk, Shabb, and Moussaoui carry out an epidemiologic review of mental disorders, including in different age groups, their determinants, and assess the situation of mental health services. They identify problems faced in the management of mental disorders. They contrast the high prevalence rates with the "limited mobilization and policy laziness" in addressing mental disorders as reflected in the limited resources devoted to mental health. In Chapter 15, Ismail argues for the need for an alternative framework in approaching and addressing mental health, especially in the context of conflict where aid agencies and NGOs rush to provide mental health interventions based on Western models and diagnoses. Such a framework should consider context, avoid pathologizing suffering and medicalization, and examine conditions that increase the resilience of people and communities.

In Chapter 16, Barss concludes Section 3 by focusing on injuries. Intentional injuries form a major burden in conflict situations, whereas road traffic injuries are the most important in non-conflict settings. Barss' review includes conditions such as torture and gender-based violence. Advocating a broad public health framework, Barss stresses the need for multidisciplinary and multisectoral approaches to injury prevention, building and expanding on the classical Haddon matrix of injury.

Section 4 focuses on the health of population groups. In Chapter 17, Shawky, Yamout, Halileh, and Salem review child health. Taking a social-determinants-of-health framework, they examine disparities, intermediate determinants (such as child feeding practices), and

structural determinants (such as conflict). They also review health services, such as immunization, and child health systems. They propose a way forward that stresses primary health care, work on determinants, and coordinated policy. In Chapter 18, Afifi, DeJong, Bose, Salem, Awad, and Benkirane focus on youth, a group they note has recently received world attention. They discuss factors such as the youth "bulge," high unemployment, and globalization as presenting unique challenges. They review health status, risk factors and types of behaviors, protective factors, and health determinants, realizing that health issues among young people have not received due attention. They convey messages using the voices of youth themselves and review promising youth programs.

In Chapter 19, DeJong, Bashour, and Kaddour focus on women. They warn of generalizations about women's health across the diverse region. They review measurement issues and specific health conditions such as maternal and reproductive health and then proceed to examine the links between women's health, social practices, and the social roles of women. A particular feature of this chapter is a review of health policies and services for women and the rising civil society activism on women's health. In Chapter 20, Sibai, Tohme, Yamout, Yount, and Kronfol examine the health of older people. They emphasize the need to see this group within the cultural context of Arab societies where older people have traditionally had a special status. Changes such as urbanization, nuclearization of the family and economic stresses have threatened this status and, consequently, the resources and care available for older people. State security and care systems have not kept up with these changes.

Chapters 21 and 22 discuss two population groups not defined by age or sex but where age and gender dynamics are also important. Both chapters focus on workers, albeit from different perspectives. In Chapter 21, Abdulrahim and Abdul Malak address female migrant domestic workers, the largest group of unprotected workers in the region. There is limited literature on the health of this group but their social conditions point to adversity. They share the results of in-depth interviews with a group of such workers in Lebanon about their health care choices. The authors stress the importance of human agency in the lives of these workers. In Chapter 22, Habib, Fathallah, and Nuwayhid examine the broader category of workers' health. They distinguish between a narrow focus on occupational health and safety, which is still neglected by policy makers, and a broader perspective that considers determinants such as the legal framework, social exclusions, unemployment, and globalization. They examine health issues in selected groups such as agricultural workers and conclude by proposing expanded research and emphasis on workers' health as a social agenda.

Section 5 explores a major issue in this region, public health in war and violent conflict, using country examples. In Chapter 23, Mowafi and BuHaka introduce the section by reviewing the key issues concerning conflict and health with emphasis on insecurity. They examine the characteristics of humanitarian emergencies and explore how conflict, displacement, and health are related. They review direct and indirect impacts of conflict on health and the challenge of measuring these impacts and advocate for building community capacity to address the impact of conflict. In Chapter 24, reproduced from the 2009 *Lancet* series on health in the Occupied Palestinian Territory, Giacaman, Khatib, Shabaneh, Ramlawi, Sabri, Sabatinelli, Khawaja, and Laurance describe health status and health services under Israeli occupation. Over 50% of the population is under the national poverty line. The authors use both conventional and subjective measures to describe health status. They find disjointed and inadequate public-health and health-service response to pervasive health challenges.

In Chapter 25, Rawaf and Rawaf describe the health conditions and suffering in Iraq over three decades due to wars and sanctions. They show the progressive decline and destruction of the health system across time and different eras, including most recently during the US-led invasion and subsequent occupation in 2003. They review recent efforts to rebuild this system and propose a public health framework that focuses on policy and organizational development along with reform of financing, services, and regulation. In Chapter 26, published with permission from *Global Public Health*, Nuwayhid, Zurayk, Yamout, and Cortas discuss community resilience observed among displaced Lebanese people during the summer 2006 war. They add to prior literature by linking community resilience with political, historical, cultural, ideological, and religious factors. They propose a framework of analysis and discuss how public health needs to learn from such experiences.

Section 6 provides an entry to understanding the complexity of health systems. In Chapter 27, Jabbour and Rawaf introduce the section by asking questions and pointing to major problems in system set-ups. For example, they wonder whether what we have can be described as "systems" in light of the disjointed nature of its parts, and whether the widespread primary care network can be inaccurately described as primary *health* care in the Alma Ata spirit. In Chapter 28, Siddiqi and Jabbour focus on health system governance (HSG) and policy making, situating these within the broader governance in the region. They discuss a framework for analyzing HSG developed regionally and used in a six-country study and reflect on the results. The authors examine the response of Arab countries to governance challenges such as trade in health service and contracting and conclude with a set of recommendations to strengthen HSG.

In Chapter 29, Sabri, El-Idrissi, and Mataria discuss health system financing and link it at the outset to the struggle for the right to health. They note inadequate spending on health in many countries, inequitable structures of health care expenditures, and poor social health protection. They propose financing arrangements according to national income category. Moving forward requires generating evidence, increasing health investments, designing sustainable financing arrangements, and building capacity. In Chapter 30, El-Jardali, Longuenesse, Jamal, and Kronfol examine the health workforce. There are limited data on the public health workforce, as compared to the biomedical workforce. The region has the second lowest health workforce density after Sub-Saharan Africa. There are disparities in the distribution of this workforce by national income, physicians, and urban areas. Major challenges include planning, development of appropriate policies and coordination among ministries, management, and education.

In Chapter 31, Kronfol and Jabbour discuss healthcare delivery. They emphasize diversity of delivery systems and progress made in expanding delivery networks but see challenges in ambulatory and hospital care, such as inequalities, quality of care, patient satisfaction, and inefficiencies. They identify governance/policy, health system, and social/structural barriers to access and utilization. They discuss delivery reform initiatives and identify actionable priorities, foremost of which being ensuring equitable access. In Chapter 32, Khatib, Mirza, and Mataria discuss the challenge of ensuring access to essential medicines. They examine and find major deficits in four key areas: rational selection and use of medicines, affordable prices, sustainable financing, and reliable health and supply systems. They review case studies from several countries noting important experiences on which the region can build. They stress the need for regional collaboration, for example in procurement.

Section 7 wraps up the book by providing an outlook for public health seen within the larger social agenda for equitable development and change. In Chapter 33, Zurayk, Giacaman, and Mandil propose a vision for graduate education in public health that is based on the comprehensive approach to population health. They review regional programs and use case studies of three institutions to discuss the progress made toward the comprehensive approach. They advocate for the model of independent schools of public health. They discuss challenges facing universities and health system constraints facing public health education and call for collective action. In Chapter 34, Afifi, Nuwayhid, Nehlawi and Assai discuss participatory community interventions emphasizing that these are grounded in equity, mutual respect, and trust. They review the literature on the conceptual basis of these interventions and what they can or cannot offer. They review case studies in communities in Egypt, Syria, Lebanon, and Morocco and provide a critical analysis of lessons learned and the ethical and political ramifications. They conclude with a discussion of the way forward.

Chapters 35 and 36 discuss approaches to health within the wider social and political scope. In Chapter 35, Wick argues that scholarship on health in the region constructs not only its own interpretation of health but also of what the Arab world means. She reviews articles on health in the region that have appeared in *Social Science and Medicine* since its inception and finds that only a few articles have explored critically the political and socio-economic causes of ill-health and inequality representing a "de-politicization" of scholarship.

In Chapter 36, Dewachi, Jabbour, Yassin, Nuwayhid, and Giacaman provide a regional perspective on health and human security. They discuss that this concept features prominently in the international development literature but there is limited attention to its public health dimensions or applications in the region. The authors trace the shift from national to human security, review ways of defining and measuring human security, and examine the relevance of human security to understanding public health.

Chapters 37 and 38 discuss mobilization for change. In Chapter 37, Shukrallah and Khalil link the health care crisis in Egypt with the broader societal crises perpetuated by the regimes of Sadat and Mubarak. With the support of international financial institutions, the government pushed liberalization and privatization reforms. They describe civil society mobilization that opposed the neoliberal reforms and managed to block the passage of ministerial decrees that would have changed the face of health care in Egypt. In Chapter 38, reproduced from a 2006 special issue of the *British Medical Journal* on the Middle East, Jabbour, El-Zein, Nuwayhid, and Giacaman advocate that action in the health arena can contribute to political and social reform. While acknowledging limited public debate on health in the region, they see opportunities for action. They describe examples of successful initiatives and stress that health professionals advocating change must start from within the health sector but push for broader mobilization.

In the Postscript, the editors discuss the implication of the protests and revolutions unfolding in several Arab countries beginning in the winter of 2010–2011 for public health, as this book was written before the onset of these events.

Note: The views expressed herein are those of the authors and do not necessarily reflect the views of the United Nations.

Public Health, the Medical Profession, and State Building: A Historical Perspective

Elisabeth Longuenesse, Sylvia Chiffoleau, Nabil M. Kronfol, and Omar Dewachi

As the opening chapter in this volume, it is perhaps appropriate to look at history, as this can provide insights about the progress that public health has made, the challenges that it still faces today, and the options for future action. This chapter traces the main contributions to the development and evolution of public health policies in the Arab world. In so doing, several key themes, among many others, emerge: the impact of colonialism and encounter with Western medicine, the relation of public health to the state building and modernization project, the role of the medical profession, and changing policies in relation to changing political and economic realities. We intend to develop these themes and show their complex interactions in laying the foundations for modern public health.

We will argue that public health was a principal tool in the modernization project (seen as an ideological and socio-political project) which emerged in the late Ottoman period, and later subjected to the interests of colonial powers. The newly independent Arab states relied on promoting social "progress" and providing access to benefits of development, with health at the heart, as a foundation of legitimacy. This is translated in health system financing and organization and education, regulation, and large scale employment of health professionals. We focus on the medical profession, as it played a central role in both the public health and modernization projects. As champions of health, physicians have gained immense prestige commensurate with their responsibilities and their relation to the state and its political choices.

Approach

Health and disease are socially constructed concepts that vary in time and place based on the experiences, practices, and representations of social and professional groups, including physicians (Becker et al 1961; Freidson

1970; Boltanski 1971) Such concepts are useful in observing social change (Augé and Herzlich 1983). In many industrialized countries, research has examined the representation of health and disease, health systems organization, hospital management, medical practice, and the inter-relationships among health professionals, patients, and governments. Foucault's work demonstrated medicine's role in society, disciplining the body as an instrument of power.

In the Arab world, research on the history and sociology of health and medicine remains limited. While medieval Arab medicine has long interested historians of science, the history of modern public health in the region has received less attention. Researchers have examined epidemics (Watts 1999) and changes in medical practice during the nineteenth century (Gallagher 1983; Jagailloux 1986), colonial times (Turin 1971), and in the twentieth century (Chiffoleau 1997). Several other volumes and research studies, referenced throughout this chapter, have attempted to fill the gaps. This chapter builds on prior works to provide a socio-historical perspective of the social, economic, and political processes that have greatly influenced health, and the development of public health, in the Arab world. This has led us to recognize several distinct, but overlapping rather than discontinuous, eras and corresponding processes.

Historians might argue, perhaps rightly, that in the Arab world, like other regions and cultures, modern public health has old historical seeds (Watts 2003). Obviously, this would depend on what we assign to the definition of public health. For example, management of disasters of public health proportion was done well early in the Arab-Islamic civilization. Health systems, including hospitals for the mentally ill (bimaristans), and healthy administration of public space were reasonably developed in the peak of the Arab-Islamic empire. The principles of social justice and the right of all to protection are enshrined in religious principles and organizational set-ups in the region.

While recognizing the importance of these historical seeds, our analysis is grounded in seeing public health as a modern development, emerging principally in reaction to health problems associated with urbanization and industrialization in nineteenth century Europe, and thus rooted in social reform movements and emergence of modern states. Public health in the Arab world developed in relation to, and sometimes in conflict with, European powers and their public health.

The latter, argues Camau et al (1990), "as a system of distinct roles is a feature of the modern state." Medicine and the medical profession were central to the emerging public health. The French Revolution placed medicine at the service of its utopian vision to eradicate human ills produced by an unjust society. This led, Foucault observes, to "the birth of two great myths: the myth of a nationalized medical profession, organized as clergy; and the myth of a total disappearance of diseases" with society "amended back to its original health" (Foucault 2003 p. 36 [first published in 1963]). Therefore, there was a political dimension to the tasks of physicians.

Later in the nineteenth century, poor environmental conditions and rising poverty in urban areas forced governments to intervene to prevent epidemics and ameliorate health conditions through sanitation and urban planning measures. Public health was variably defined as *environmental sanitation*, *preventive medical science*, and *the promotion of positive health* (Suchman 1963). The state entrusted health teams, predominantly physicians but also other professionals, such as labor inspectors and engineers (Gaudin 1987), to implement measures to protect public health while serving multiple goals: economic (maintaining a healthy workforce), political (preserving the urban order), social (promoting well-being), and imperial (controlling the colonies). The latter goal, as we will discuss later, was an important feature of the Arab counter with Western colonialism and a defining aspect of public health development in the region.

A note of caution is worthwhile here. Although Arab countries share broad trends of relationships among state projects, citizens' expectations and behaviors, and professional interests, each country has marked its own specific path. We will not deal with all Arab countries but seek instead to show, through examples based on available data, how these relationships have evolved.

Health and Medicine in the Nineteenth Century Reforms

Both the Ottoman Empire and Egypt under the reign of Muhammad Ali faced the economic and imperial penetration of European powers; aware of their "backwardness," they tried to catch up through top-down reform policies borrowing the techniques of Western modern science. In the field of health and medicine, the introduction of European medicine did not lead to an abrupt break with established traditions as both Arabic and European medicine shared the same ancestry of ancient Greek medicine. Representations of the body and disease in the Arab world in the early nineteenth century were based on the theory of "tempers," hardly different from those prevailing in *Ancien Régime* (defined as the old socio-political regime before eighteenth and nineteenth century revolutions in Europe and the establishment of the modern nation state). Europe. Arab populations had a multitude of healthcare options, the dominant one being traditional medicine, a modified form of classical Arabic medicine. Patients had freedom of choice and autonomy but illness and health care were considered private matters. Therefore, the state's increasing involvement in health and healing must have appeared as a radical novelty.

Ottoman and Egyptian authorities did not initially plan to provide broad population health services (despite their importance in the Islamic tradition, hospitals had become mere charitable institutions rather than dedicated to the art of healing). Instead they first focused on sanitary reforms and quarantines to protect armies from epidemics. Establishment of medical schools in Cairo and Istanbul (1827), whose graduates were mainly absorbed into the army, supported this system. The Egyptian army's demobilization after defeat in Syria in 1840 led Muhammad Ali to appoint military doctors to civilian institutions, thus extending the benefits of modern medicine. Clot-Bey, a French doctor residing in Egypt for nearly 40 years, established a provisional health care system whereby health officer graduates from the medical school in Cairo worked in hospitals of major regional cities and disseminated rules of environmental hygiene and smallpox vaccination, often with the help of barbers.

During the reign of the Ottoman Sultan Abdul Hamid II (1876–1909), the authorities expanded medical care and public health measures in the Arab provinces, for example, increased the number of municipal hospitals and multiplied the posts of civilian sanitary doctors and stations to ward off cholera and other infectious epidemics from overseas ships.

During the last third of the nineteenth century, community hospitals initiated by Christian missionaries emerged, significantly enhancing health care provision, especially in the southern Levant (Bourmaud 2008; Chiffoleau forthcoming). The Mashreq presents thus the originality of having introduced modern medicine and public health without the pressure of external force.

Fighting epidemics coming from abroad remained a priority. Plague had disappeared from Europe but was everywhere in the East until the mid-nineteenth century. Cholera was not endemic but the region witnessed many outbreaks due to international trade with the East since 1831. It was above all to try to stop the ravages of cholera that Ottoman *Tanzimat* (Turkish for "organization") and Muhammad Ali established a network of "lazarets" and sanitary offices managed by indigenous officials and consular representatives of Western powers. Quarantine measures for pilgrims were also used extensively by the British in Iraq and the Gulf until the early twentieth century. Those institutions were called the Health Administration of Alexandria and the Health Council of Constantinople (Panzac 1985). But since these local quarantine measures hindered trade and navigation, Western powers launched international sanitary conferences to redirect health systems to their advantage. Twelve such conferences were convened from 1851 to 1938 and can be considered the first attempt at a coordinated international health policy. At the turn of the twentieth century, the progressive elaboration of an international health legislation led to the disappearance of quarantine measures in Europe. The global spread of epidemic cholera that started in the pilgrimage of Mecca in 1865 reversed the earlier liberal emphasis of these conferences in the direction of more severe measures against the "risk group": religious pilgrims. In the East, a large health control operation was built up with the Ottoman and Egyptian authorities fully participating through the joint Health Councils of Alexandria and Constantinople.

Colonial Health Policies and Medicalization of the Society

Western colonialism of the Arab region occurred over a long period. It started much earlier and lasted longer in North Africa, especially in Algeria (occupied in 1832), but came later and was shorter in the Levant and Mesopotamia, which came under "mandates" imposed by the League of Nations. Independence granted by Britain to Egypt (1922) and Iraq (1932) did not free these countries from foreign domination, although it resulted in a reorientation in social and health policies (see Box 1 and Chapter 25). The effects of colonial orders were quite different in different Arab regions and countries, depending on pre-colonial experiences of modernization and the nature and policies of colonial powers. But everywhere, social and health policies were determined above all by the interests of the colonizers, for whom trade and export of agricultural products were priorities. These policies were implemented in authoritarian ways. Sanitation became a means of controlling a population considered backward, ignorant, and dangerous (Camau et al 1990; Arnold 1993; Rivet 1995; Mitchell 2002).

> **Box 1.** Mandatory Inoculations and the Cholera Epidemic in Iraq, 1923
>
> On August 3, 1923, three cases of cholera were reported among Indian workers living in a secluded camp of the British India Steam Navigation Company on Shat-el-Arab River below Basra. Within days, deaths spear outside the Basra municipal area leading the Health Directorate in Baghdad to cordon off affected areas and halt travel from Basrah to prevent the spread of infection by road or river, but these measures were too late. Within weeks, cholera spread to all provinces south of Baghdad. Sanitation and quarantine strategies were no match against the rapidity of circulation and mobility of both people and the bacterium. The rapid spread of the epidemic was a symptom of the developments in Iraq under the British mandate (1920–1932).
>
> The mandate authorities carried out were major urban development and transportation projects. As both a state-building and empire-building project, the railway expanded between Basra and Baghdad along the Euphrates, with extensions to other areas. The railway played an important role in connecting different territories of the new Iraqi state, facilitating the mobility of goods and people, as well as linking the territories with other parts of the empire. The British were most interested in securing the movement of military supplies, creating a network for the circulation of goods (especially grains) for export and within different regions of Iraq, and facilitating the movement of pilgrims to religious sites in Karbala,

Box 1. (*cont.*)

Najaf, and Samara – a major source of economic income to the state, the Holy Cities, and the British-controlled railway company. During the 1920s, both road and river traffic increased substantially. Iraq was on a rapid track toward commercial and economic development, which Iraqi and British officials saw as crucial to the creation of the state. Ironically, the very geographic realities that seemed to promise a successful state were the nightmare that haunted the newly established Health Services.

In the past, local epidemic outbreaks were more easily contained through closing off infected areas from road and river routes. However, with the rapid mobility of people and products and connections with the other parts of the British Empire, vectors and carriers of diseases were also being offered an express ride. Cholera, which was endemic in India, arrived in Iraq much faster through ships and newly developed pilgrim routes. In case of plague epidemics, which usually hit the major cities of Baghdad and Basra, it was train cars stocked with grain, which offered rats a comfortable ride between different cities and aided in the spread of the epidemic. According to one health report, epidemics threatened the economic order of things in the new state:

"The solution to prevent the spread of infectious disease by complete closure of traffic routes was suitable to the Turkish administration, but can no longer be employed in a country which is rapidly developing and whose commerce, the motive power of its development, depends so vitally on the freedom of its traffic routes".

The need to preserve the economic vitality of the new state became pronounced during the cholera epidemic of 1923. By September of that year, anxiety was widespread among Health Services officials as this was the time when thousands of Shi'a pilgrims flock into the Holy City of Karbala. The thought of thousands of people moving from all over the country, as well as neighboring Iran, into the heart of the epidemic south of Iraq was apocalyptic. This was a true test for the Iraqi government and the British civil administration. The Iraqi government had decided earlier that year to delegate control of local dispensaries and hospitals to provincial authorities, despite objections from British officials and the Ministry of Interior. The epidemic forced the suspension of the decentralization process and put these dispensaries under the control of the central government and the central Health Directorate.

At first, health authorities made a futile proposition to the government to forbid the Shi'a pilgrimage to Karbala that year. Officials were very reluctant to do so for fear of a backlash from the Shi'a community, especially with the recent memory of uprising and unrest in 1920, which had put the British political administration under scrutiny by the public, both in Iraq and Britain. As a compromise, the Iraqi government gave the Directorate a carte blanche to "adopt any measure of prevention, short of stopping the pilgrimage." A massive door-to-door campaign was ordered to inoculate all the inhabitants of Karbala and Najaf. Inspections and inoculation posts were established on all bridges crossing the Euphrates at cities and towns of Twairij, Musayib, and Najaf. Inoculated persons were given a certificate. Every traveler between Baghdad and the Holy Cities passing any of these stations was inoculated if he/she could not produce a certificate. About 90,000 people made the pilgrimage that year; only a small percentage escaped inoculation. Roughly 300,00 inoculations were performed by the health services.

At first authorities had to request the vaccine from India because of the need for such large quantities. They quickly realized that, with the extension of the epidemic, there would still be a shortage of vaccine. Steps were taken to begin manufacturing the cholera vaccine on a large scale in the small Central Laboratory at Baghdad. Strains were flown in from Cairo, and isolated locally. Vaccine production started at 2,000 doses a day and reached 10,000 to 12,000 doses a day within weeks. Along with the supply from India, this was enough to meet the needs.

The management of the cholera epidemic in Iraq in 1923 sheds an important light on the complex process of nation and state building under the mandate. For the first time, a massive invasive medical intervention was introduced in epidemic management and pilgrimage, going beyond roadblocks, quarantine, and isolation. With absence of census and accurate vital statistics, health cards, death rates, and registrations became a technology, through which the new state created the conditions for its sustainability and legitimacy. The beginning of house-to-house inoculations exemplifies how, in addition to its health benefits, public health was a tool of the political project, closely associated with the management of population mobility and security, sustaining economic circulation, and legitimizing rapid urbanization.

Box 2. Lebanon: The Development of Public Health Over One and a Half Centuries

The first information on public health services in Lebanon dates from 1864, when the country adopted the "Mutassarifieh" regime for Mount Lebanon, imposed by European military interventions to end the interconfessional disturbances of 1860–1864. In 1864, Baabda, then the capital, had a public health team comprising an Italian physician-in-chief assisted by two Lebanese physicians and another Italian physician. The team provided treatment to security forces and their dependants as well as to prisoners, inoculation campaigns against smallpox, distribution of quinine tablets against malaria, and treatment of venereal diseases. Medications were prepared in a central pharmacy. The team licensed the few pharmacists and midwives and signed health-related legal documents. Two small hospitals were built, financed through a tax on emigrants (Khoury 2010). Health care in Beirut was delegated to the municipality. In 1875, efforts were expanded to develop the water distribution system from Dbayeh (through a concession to the privately owned Companie des Eaux).

During World War I, a smallpox epidemic ravaged the country threatening the Ottoman and German armies based in Lebanon. A new physician (Dr Husni Mohieddine) was assigned the task of organizing the health sector in 1916. This was done by designating 23 district health authorities covering Mount Lebanon, with one physician in charge of each district. These physicians combated smallpox, malaria, and cholera and established public baths to disinfect clothes in order to stem the tide of typhus that, together with the famine, decimated large numbers of citizens.

Under the French mandate from 1920, a directorate of health was established within the Ministry of Interior, and a health council was appointed to formulate health legislation. In 1932, the health services for the capital (now Beirut) were delegated to the municipality and became for a long time afterwards independent from the Ministry of Health, a situation that lasted well into Independence (Ministry of Health and Assistance, 1921–23).

This period witnessed the establishment of several hospitals, principally those related to universities such as that of the American University of Beirut and the Hotel Dieu de France (Université Saint Joseph), as well as large community hospitals (Saint Georges, Makassed, Bhannes, Asfourieh) owned by philanthropic and religious groups. In addition, small private hospitals, patterned on the French model "cliniques" were established between 1920 and 1969 by private physicians returning from specialization training abroad (mainly from France at that time) (Ministry of Health and Assistance, 1925–26).

At Independence in 1943, the Ministry of Health, titled the Ministry of Health and Assistance (is'af), had three directorates: Technical Affairs, Quarantine, and Administration, reflecting the scope of its work. However, the Lebanese government stressed the need for educating its public servants in public health. Through fellowships provided by the Rockefeller Foundation, most health directors in Lebanon and Syria were sent to the Harvard School of Public Health to receive the Diploma of Public Health (DPH). These officials returned and initiated the development of the Ministry of Health. Hospitals were built in the main cities of the provinces (regional) and smaller facilities in the districts (qada), thus initiating a prototype referral system. These public hospitals were mainly tasked to serve the indigent population and treat patients suffering from then-prevalent infectious diseases. One could detect a plan for decentralization in the offing as qada physicians were also appointed. The Ministry of Health also developed water and sewage systems, activated spraying, eliminated ponds all in order to stem the tide of malaria, diarrhea, and other communicable diseases.

In 1946, legislation was passed to establish the Order of Physicians and to initiate the licensure of health professionals through an exam, the colloquium. The formal decree establishing the Ministry of Health was legislated in 1961, and except for minor revisions remains the same today.

In the early 1960s, after the civil disturbances of 1958, and the election of a new President (President Fuad Chehab), major reforms were implemented across all sectors. In health affairs, the National Social Security Fund was established in 1964 (The Maternity and Illness branch was implemented in 1971); the Office of Social Development (now the Ministry of Social Affairs) which was developed in 1959, epitomizes the principles of Primary Health Care; the "Magnet Centers" were traced in 1964 to formulate the plans for social and economic development. However the onset of the civil war in 1975 curtailed many of these reforms (Kronfol and Mroueh, 1985).

Poverty, Death, and Disease: Suffering Exacerbated by Colonialism

Health conditions were miserable in conquered populations. Diseases varied from one region to another, but suffering was universal; everywhere one could find both endemic diseases due to malnutrition and poor hygiene and epidemics. But the conditions were not uniform. For example, compared with the North African region, health conditions in Egypt were better thanks to public health developments under Mohammad Ali and his successors. By the second half of the nineteenth century, epidemics were diminishing, although common diseases – diarrhea, pneumonia – caused by under-nutrition and poverty persisted (Panzac 1982).

Colonization made things worse for many countries. In addition to deaths and disabilities due to direct violence, many colonial policies, e.g., confiscation of peasant land and re-organizing the local economies in service of global economic and colonial interests, had dire consequences. Rural economies suffered turmoil; many inhabitants were pushed to displace to precarious urban living. British policies to increase cotton crops in Egypt, such as irrigation approaches ignorant of age-old practices for proper drainage, brought new health problems, as these approaches favored breeding of mosquitoes, and with it malaria (Mitchell 2002). In the absence of serious preventive measures, "development" projects, such as roads (Rivet 2002; Box 1), led to more epidemic challenges. Toward the end of the nineteenth century and turn of the twentieth century, British policies neglected public health to a large degree, reflecting policies at the empire's home.

Algeria demonstrates the most painful case. Two decades after French occupation (when the so-called "pacification" was completed), health conditions were deplorable: smallpox, cholera, typhus, syphilis and eye diseases decimated the population. The violence of pacification and expropriation of peasant lands led to famine and drought with consequent weakening of resistance and spread of epidemics.

The Policies of Medicalization

While colonialism was largely responsible for further deterioration of already poor health conditions, colonialist powers took certain measures to ameliorate conditions thought to be most threatening to the colonial project, i.e., epidemics. These measures were based on moralizing policies related to hygiene and medicalization. The discovery in the 1870s, and onward, of germs established the rationale for epidemic control. The case of Egypt is illustrative. By killing Egyptians in large numbers, epidemics threatened the

economy. The British were not interested in upgrading social services and preferred repressive control aimed at identifying risks and addressing threats of epidemics. However, common and pervasive illnesses – gastrointestinal, respiratory, and parasitic diseases – were thoroughly ignored (Chiffoleau 1997).

But medicine was more than an instrument of epidemic control. Medicine was considered a leading vehicle of civilizing the population, even to a greater extent than education. The contradictions of colonization appeared all too obvious in this role assigned to medicine. The contemptuous image of the indigenes held by the colonizers exaggerated the disciplinary character of sanitary measures imposed on local populations: "Civilization is injected as a vaccine" (Rivet 2002: 129). Local populations resisted mass immunization and other prevention measures associated with the hated political and military control but quickly adopted individual treatments and recognized the abilities of colonial physicians to heal, showing selectivity and pragmatism in dealing with what the colonialist offered.

In Egypt, smallpox immunization campaigns were associated with the ill-perceived conscription program. Its preventive nature was poorly understood. Similarly, the French colonialists in Algeria forced its own vision of health measures soon after occupation. Public health measures included old tools: hygiene, isolation, quarantine, and smallpox vaccination. A vaccination campaign launched in 1847 was interrupted a decade later, due to insufficient French government funding and local non-cooperation. Larger-scale vaccination campaigns resumed in the 1870s after French colonizers succeeded in suppressing uprisings. In Iraq, as in many Arab countries, public health was placed primarily under the auspices of the Ministry of the Interior, meaning the association of health actions with security (see Box 1). It was with the independence of Iraq and the creation of a Ministry of Health and Social Affairs in the 1930s that the promotion of population health became a major government concern (Dewachi 2008).

In addition to public health measures, Western-style curative care was introduced on various scales, aiming at gaining the hearts and minds of the locals (Turin 1971). Egyptians and Algerians did not hesitate to acquire Western drugs seen as effective against malaria crises or ophthalmia. Curative practices remained marginal due to a pervasive shortage of health care exacerbated by lack of physicians.

The Birth of a Medical Profession

Under colonialism, physicians were regarded as agents of civilization. However, the establishment of an indigenous medical profession quickly led to confrontation with colonial rules and practices and revealed, although differently in different countries, the close links of medicine, public health, and the national project.

In the early nineteenth century, while medical practices in Europe and in the Ottoman Empire were rather similar, their conceptual bases were diverging. European physicians relied on experimental methods to analyze the causes of diseases, while Muslim ones focused on empirical observations (Gallagher 1983). European physicians, introduced to Ottoman courts starting in the eighteenth century, represented Western interests, especially those of merchants, advocating the importance of health for the development of trade.

In the Maghreb, modern medicine long remained the province of European physicians. The first medical school in Algiers was founded in 1857. Only a handful of locals were given the privilege of attending this school, and only toward the end of nineteenth century. In contrast, institutions of medical training were established before the colonial era in the Mashreq. In addition to the medical school of Muhammad Ali in Cairo, the Ottomans established a medical school in Damascus in 1903. In parallel, two medical schools were established in Lebanon as part of concurrent missionary projects: Americans established the Syrian Protestant College (later American University of Beirut) in 1866 and French Jesuits established the *Université Saint-Joseph* in 1883. Graduates from those two schools worked not only in Syria and Lebanon but also in Anatolia, Palestine, Egypt, and even Mesopotamia, usually in private clinics but sometimes in small private hospitals. The role of missionaries was essential in establishing hospitals in the region. In 1920, Damascus had an Italian and a French hospital (Hanna 1996). In Bahrain and Oman, American missionaries opened the first two modern hospitals in the first few years of the twentieth century.

Upon occupying Egypt in 1881, the British reorganized the school of medicine, introducing access fees and numerous strict curricular reforms and imposed the use of English. Recruitment was limited to the needs of minimal governmental action. Local physicians were confined to the role of medical officers while senior and prestigious functions were reserved for foreigners. In Iraq, where the British lacked confidence in Ottoman medicine represented by a small number of modern-trained physicians, large numbers of military doctors from the Empire, of British and Indian origins, were recruited. The first medical school was founded in 1925, and education was delivered from the outset in English, despite the objection of nationalists.

The choice of the language of medical education was a national issue and has had long lasting implications. The Damascus School of Medicine gave up Turkish in favor of Arabic in the 1920s, but the Cairo University medical school, which had gradually Arabized its curriculum during the nineteenth century, was forced to implement English language in medical training after the English occupation. This remains the case today. The School of Medicine of the Syrian Protestant College, having used Arabic for two decades, shifted to English in 1882 (Dodge 1958 p. 22). Marwa Elshakry (forthcoming) gives an account of this transition to English and shows how the inclusion of Darwin's theory in curricula, the so-called "Darwin Crisis," led to the resignation of many Arabic-speaking teachers. At the *Université Saint-Joseph* medical school in Beirut, medicine has always been taught in French. The choice of the education language determined, and still does now, where the brightest graduates go to acquire specialty training.

In Egypt and other Arab countries under mandate, "local" physicians relegated to inferior positions were frustrated and tirelessly asserted their competence. Their sentiments became part of the national struggle. Remarkably, in Egypt, local physicians succeeded in developing a different perspective whereby public health attention was directed toward endemic diseases rather than against epidemics as proposed by colonial medicine. The first professional associations created in the 1920s in Egypt and Iraq revealed the tension between submission to the British model and the policies of the allied monarchies and aspirations to nationalist interests. Involvement of physicians in the nationalist movements grew in the 1930s, showcasing the role of health in the state building and reform project (Longuenesse 1995; Hanna 1996). In liberal Egypt, physicians were actively involved in developing a theoretical framework for public health that aimed explicitly and unprecedentedly at social reform. Even though this took place only through a few pilot projects, it was an important forerunner of what would be the model for public health medicine after independence (Chiffoleau 1997).

The Welfare State and Public Health: Between Socialism and "Patrimonialism"

Arab states emerging from independence wars and struggles in the 1950s and 1960s faced deplorable health conditions: infant mortality rates (IMR) were 145/1000 in Morocco, 155–160/1000 in Tunisia, Algeria, and the Arabian Peninsula and 179/1000 in Egypt. Such rates had not been seen in Western Europe since the late nineteenth century. The situation was better in Lebanon (61/1000) and Kuwait (80/1000). Life expectancy at birth was less than 50 years almost everywhere, except in Lebanon (around 62 years) and in the smaller Gulf States (55–60 years) (Tabutin & Schoumaker 2005). The new states inherited health systems built after the colonial model, oscillating between charity and a colonialist preoccupation with public health. Health facilities and medical centers were ill-equipped and hospitals were concentrated in large cities, where the bulk belonged to religious missions. The medical workforce was meager: Egypt had one physician/ 2700 population in 1952 (Chiffoleau 1997) while Syria had one physician/4000 population in 1955. After many foreign doctors left the Maghreb countries upon their independence, the region needed several years to catch up to an already low rate of specialized medical staff at the end of the colonial period (Camau et al 1990).

Health as a Right for All

The activist elites, who led the national liberation struggles, considered misery, poverty, and injustice as rooted in the colonial domination. Adopting the ideals of the French Revolution, they claimed health as a right for all in a more just society. The strong representation of doctors in the nationalist movements reflected their mobilization in the social struggle, and illustrated the close link between the fight against disease and the fight against injustice.

Having inherited economies and societies profoundly disrupted by colonialism, Arab states had to shoulder missions assigned elsewhere to the private sector. The growing state control of the national

economy meant high expectations from the public. Health and education became the two symbols of social progress and the preferred source of legitimacy of the "new state" (Camau et al 1990). State action to protect the health of the population was not just meant to enhance human productivity. From Syria to Saudi Arabia, health was gradually considered as a right that must be guaranteed by the state. Undoubtedly, the discourse justifying health policies and their implementation varied in different countries, but ultimately, the logic remained the same. The Egyptian constitution of 1952 guarantees free access to health services for all, while the Statute of the Ba'th Party maintains that "the state must create medical institutions capable of meeting the needs of all citizens and guarantee them free health care" (Ba'th 1993). In 1956, President Bourguiba of Tunisia declared: "The world needs to know that the government is determined to make every effort to serve the people, and cannot tolerate that some compatriots are left without care"; he added that he was ready to enroll doctors by force if necessary (Camau et al 1990 p. 180). Similarly, and surprisingly, such states whose political choices seemed radically opposed, drawing their legitimacy from their adherence to traditions rather than from their claim to progress, development, and modernity, also based their health policies on similar concepts. Saudi Arabia proclaims that "the state has the duty to provide free medical care to all citizens, as well as to pilgrims." The Jordanian Royal Medical Systems provides free health care to an increasing proportion of the population (Longuenesse 1992).

Broadly speaking, health was part of a dynamic package that was meant to push the society upward, creating a process of major social mobility through the development of the governmental institutions and public services, including public sector employment, urbanization, and education. However, the development of health services, embodying this vision, was only one factor in the process of improving population health.

Rapid improvements

Throughout the region, there were remarkable improvements in population health between 1950 and 1980. In 20 years between the early 1960s and early 1980s, Morocco under the reign of the Alawite dynasty emulated the achievements of socialist Algeria: In Morocco life expectancy at birth rose from 48 to

59 years while infant mortality rate (IMR) decreased from 145 to 90 per 1000 live births. In Algeria, life expectancy increased from 48 to 61 years, while the IMR decreased from 159 to 84. For the same period, improvements of health indicators in Egypt were slower; life expectancy rose by only 9 years (47 to 56 years) and IMR decreased from 179 to 108/1000. Comparison between socialist-oriented Syria and oil-rich Saudi Arabia shows more impressive improvement in the latter. The causes of such changes are complex, and can be as much related to availability of resources and other indirect factors such as urbanization and development of media and communication as to sanitation measures and health policies.

State Responsibility Toward the People

The idea of the responsibility of the nation state for the development of the health sector and health services accessible to all is closely linked to the importance of medicine in the reform and modernization projects. This was true before, during, and after the colonial era. It was reflected in Egyptian hospitals as early as 1925 with the establishment of free outpatient consultations. In Iraq, all medical students benefitted from scholarships and were offered employment in the public service after graduation. However, it was the revolutions that led to the implementation of proactive policies of health coverage for the whole population in Egypt, Syria, and Iraq.

The development of a national health system and the extension of free health care to all led to a conflict between social health insurance schemes, financed by fees from labor income, and free medical care previously reserved for the poor, and which was eventually withdrawn in Algeria, Egypt, and Syria. The same policies were enacted in Tunisia and later in Algeria. In some countries, medical insurance tied to employment was meant to strengthen the workforce for development goals. In Algeria, financing of all health services by a social security system inherited from colonial times led in the 1980s to a phenomenal budget deficit (Kaddar 1995).

The state's ambitious policies of expanding public health services to all regions and all segments of the population led physicians to find themselves subject to measures that undermined their independent practice of medicine, putting them at odds with the public sector. Physicians were forced to provide a few years of service in rural areas after graduation in Syria and

Egypt (Chiffoleau 1997; Boukhaima 2005), or to work full-time as employees of the public sector in Tunisia. Professionals resisted these constraints; for example in Tunisia during the 1980s, there was a decline in the number of registered doctors to such an extent that the government had to put an end to the requirement of full-time employment in the public sector (Camau et al 1990 p. 184). Except for Algeria, no country fully banned private medical practice; nevertheless the private practice in Tunisia, Syria, or Egypt, remained limited to solo practice, sometimes coupled with a job in the public sector. The only exception was Lebanon, where an extremely profitable private hospital sector developed early in the major cities, in parallel with the public system, aimed at serving rural districts and indigent population.

Oil revenues enabled oil-producing countries to offer free health care services to all their citizens, as early as the 1950s in Kuwait, and the 1960s or 1970s elsewhere. Progress was particularly rapid after the oil embargo of the 1973 war, owing to rising oil revenues and partial or total nationalization of oil companies. The generosity of the state also extended to housing, through heavy home subsidies, and other public services. The social logic behind these social policies was patrimonial: the governed are personally allegiant to the governor. This logic is quite different than the socialistic modernization model illustrated by the Tunisia of Bourguiba, the Algeria of Boumediene, the Egypt of Nasser, or the Ba'thist Syria. Jordan offers a mixed health care model partially comparable to that of countries in the Arabian Peninsula. The "rentier" character of its economy, thanks to British and later American subsidies, allowed the financing of health coverage for the great majority of the population through two institutions: First, through the Royal Medical Services (RMS), which was established in 1963 and was initially reserved for military and security officials and intelligence services and their dependants. In the 1980s, about one third of Jordanians were eligible for RMS coverage through symbolic annual fees; Second, through the medical insurance body covering state servants, allowing them to get free health care in governmental hospitals. In Egypt and Syria too, military hospitals and health services endowed with sophisticated equipment were reserved for military personnel and their dependants. However, the net political impact of such policies, aiming at improving living conditions and at developing public services, may have been the suffocation of political liberties and hindrance of independent political expression, by transforming the relationship of citizens to the state to a pure allegiance to political leaders (Heydemann 2004).

In summary, despite apparently contradictory political rhetoric and ideological references, the combination of authoritarianism and patrimonialism is common to most social schemes in the Arab countries and is translated into broadly comparable health policies.

Neo-liberal Shifts and Public Health Issues

In the years after independence, urbanization, education, and improvement of living conditions have contributed to increased life expectancy, lower infant mortality, and decline of pandemics and epidemics once common in many Arab areas. But from the years 1970 to 1980, continued improvement in living standards and new government policies led to increasing social inequities and a profound transformation of the practices, expectations, and thus demands for health care. Withdrawal of socialist policies and return to economic liberalism gradually happened starting in the 1970s, accompanied by the entry of new local and global actors. Changes occurred over two periods: in the 1970s with the increase of oil prices and the acceleration of migration and in the 1990s with the worsening of external debt, implementation of structural adjustment reforms, explosion of social inequities, and the toll of war and forced exile, in such countries as Sudan, Palestine, and Iraq. During these periods, health policies and on-the-ground developments led to concomitant and opposing trends: governmental efforts to promote community health and the development of lucrative private medical services for the well-off. While in the 1970s Arab states still had resources to invest in social services and health, since the 1990s they were increasingly restricted by budget cuts and pressure from international financial institutions. Reform of social protection systems and health insurance was on the agenda in most Arab countries, as in the rest of the world. Indeed, neo-liberal reforms enforced by the World Bank have been salient in many Arab countries, bringing a wider role for the private sector and changing the meaning and responsibilities of the state in health service provision.

The Increase in Demand and the Deepening of Inequalities

The exponential income growth generated by the oil boom after 1973 disrupted the economic and social equilibrium of the Arab region. The emerging markets in the Arab Peninsula, Iraq, and Libya attracted hundreds of thousands of workers from Egypt, Lebanon, Syria, Jordan, Yemen, and Tunisia. Home remittances sharply increased family income but caused serious discrepancies in the labor market. This led to widening social gaps and promoted new patterns of consumption. While oil revenues benefited the states, directly or indirectly, allowing new social investment programs and delaying the crisis resulting from the multiple failures begotten by bureaucratized economies, they concurrently promoted conspicuous consumption and created new health demands.

Increasing governmental investments and expenditures in the health sector went hand in hand with the growth of private services, including for-profit hospitals targeting well-off clients. Meanwhile, economic liberalization was under way in many countries. International agencies and organizations (World Bank, World Health Organization [WHO], or international NGOs) and local actors including the private sector and NGOs started to have a greater impact on health policies.

By the end of the 1970s, while being pressured by a growing demand for services, the public sector suffered universally from limited resources, neglect, and apathy by disenchanted health professionals who experienced a relative decline in wages due to inflation caused by the influx of migration income. Camau et al (1990) observed a paradox in Tunisia in the 1980s: improved access to health services due to the development of the public sector, whose services were free or at minimal costs, stimulated further demand for private services inversely proportional to the deterioration of the public sector. There was widespread perception that free public health care was medicine for the poor; consequently, the new urban middle class shifted to consuming private medical care assumed to be of better quality. The free nature of services became illusory with public physicians, and there was a common practice of redirecting patients to private offices and soliciting bribes to queue-jump for surgery or to ensure a better treatment (Camau et al 1990; Boukhaima 2005).

In Tunisia, a 1980s survey showed a growing distortion between health care supply and demand and increased inequality in access to health services leading Camau to argue that the earlier improvement in living standards was followed by unequal development, worsening social inequalities, and cultural discontinuities (Camau et al 1990). Faced with growing and heterogeneous demands, the state disengaged, established a new division of labor between the public and the private sectors, privatized some public services and attempted to compensate through assistance programs for the poor. The 1980s witnessed a clear differentiation of the medical profession, with a larger base of generalists and "front-line health care" provided by a new generation of young physicians employed in the rural, poor urban, and community facilities and settings while established and Western trained physicians dominated more lucrative posts.

As is often the case, Egypt demonstrates a particularly striking contrast between the impressive quantitative improvements of the 1950s and 1960s and the appalling deterioration of the health system later on. The influx of students in the provincially based, under-equipped medical schools was associated with a dramatic decline in quality of education. The entry into the labor market of young physicians with little hands-on training and experience affected adversely the quality of health care (Chiffoleau 1997 p. 254–256) The hepatitis C contamination scandal uncovered in the 1990s is a terrible illustration of the dead-end health policies that were pursued. It was a dramatic and unforeseen result of the campaign against schistosomiasis launched in the 1960s and 1970s. Due to lack of resources and ignorance and neglect of underpaid and poorly trained health professionals, contaminated syringes were reused for vaccination causing a rapid spread of hepatitis C, whose prevalence in Egypt still remains unmatched worldwide (Radi 2007; Chiffoleau 2005 p. 221).

The increasing demand for, and consumption of, medical care would eventually contribute to the difficulties ahead resulting from the economic downturn in the 1980s, that resulted from falling oil prices after 1982.

Health Sector Reforms: Between Community Health and Medicine for the Rich

Most Arab countries were signatories to the 1978 Alma Ata declaration and the manifesto of "Health for All. " This led to shy health care reform efforts to promote primary health care, public health, and community medicine. In Egypt, this was attempted in 1982. But the professional elite resisted such reform and hospital physicians hampered the development of public health training, considered of little value. Conversely, the attempt to introduce a cap on numbers of medical students conflicted with the sacrosanct principle of the right for all to access higher education (Chiffoleau 2005).

In the 1980s, international aid agencies played an important and increasing role in promoting specific and vertical public health programs, sometimes referred to as selective primary health care, thought to be of highest "value" such as vaccination and campaigns against respiratory infections and diarrheal diseases (Chiffoleau 2005 p. 221–222). But the success of this first phase of post-Alma Ata reforms was mixed at best. The WHO was not the only international agency promoting community care. The World Bank, USAID, and other international assistance agencies had started to play a prominent role. However, as elsewhere, the new policies had to overcome the lack of trained staff in the public sector and the resistance of university and private hospitals.

A new package of reforms was launched in the 1990s, under the patronage of the World Bank, allied with other aid agencies (particularly USAID) and local actors. These reforms aimed at further liberalization of the health sector. Meanwhile, a non-profit private sector started to develop, in some countries like Egypt, represented by religious charitable institutions around clinics and hospitals attached to mosques and by NGOs. This development was favored by the increasing difficulty for young professionals from modest backgrounds to settle, and by the rise in the cost of health services in the private sector (MOHP & El-Zanaty 2003; Adly 2007).

Syria underwent similar changes to Tunisia's but almost a decade later. In the 1980s, while public sector conditions were deteriorating, small lucrative hospitals proliferated. The medical profession underwent both differentiation and polarization. The growth of medical manpower and the difficulty for newcomers to enter the labor market impelled the government to promulgate a decree in 1991 guaranteeing employment for newly graduated physicians (including an increasing number of women)

(Longuenesse 1993) in the public sector. At the same time, a paradoxical enthusiasm of young doctors to locate their practice in the countryside took place (Longuenesse 1995; Boukhaima 2005). To circumvent rising health care costs, the government started to rely on international assistance but also on local NGOs, sometimes members of international aid networks. A huge "health sector modernization program" was launched, for example in Syria, in cooperation with the European Union in 2004 (European Commission 2004). This way, older health-promoting civic organizations, specialized in the struggle against specific diseases, have reemerged in the country (Boukhaima 2005).

In some Arab countries, health care has become a particularly lucrative industry. In Jordan and Lebanon "investment hospitals" with sophisticated equipment have flourished, attracting wealthy clients from across the region. Medical tourism is also developing in Morocco and Tunisia where Europeans take advantage of less costly medical services. Cosmetic surgery, which benefits particularly from this cost differential, has grown rapidly. During the sanction years in Iraq, it was reported that many rich Arabs and Westerners would travel to Iraq to buy kidneys and have renal implantation.

For other countries, health care remains synonymous with emergency medicine. In refugee camps, in war zones, and in the poor neighborhoods of large cities, the voices of those advocating the universal right to health often seem unrealistic. New health scourges are emerging owing to poverty, poor environmental conditions, and the failure of public services.

Conclusion

In this chapter, we have tried to highlight the importance of public health in the construction of the modern state. In the nineteenth century, the Ottoman and Egyptian modernizing projects did include public health programs. The colonization went on with these programs, but used the medicalization project as a tool for the control of the populations, and for the sake of their own economic and security interests. On the contrary, during the first decades of independence, health became a right that was guaranteed by the state and important progress was realized. But the crisis of the development model in the 1980s and the reduction of public expenditures resulted in the emergence of new international as well as local, but mainly private, actors, and in a context of increasing inequalities, international agencies and NGOs, including charitable and religious ones, played an increasing role.

Today, the goals of social justice and the right to health for all seem far off after the failure of national development policies and the subsequent withdrawal of the state from social programs. The new challenge facing health professionals is to create new social and political dynamics that could make these goals realistic again.

Endnote

* Figures de la santé en Égypte: Passé, présent, avenir, available from http://ema.revues.org/index697.html

References

Adly E (2007) À la polyclinique de l'imam al-Shâfi'î, Egypte/Monde Arabe, No 3 (p. 147–177). Cairo, Egypt: Cedej [In French]

Arnold D (1993) Colonizing the body: State medicine and epidemic disease in nineteenth-century India. Berkeley, CA: University of California Press

Augé M, Herzlich C (1983) Le sens du mal, Anthropologie, histoire, sociologie de la maladie. Paris-Montreux, France: Archives Contemporaines [In French]

Ba'th M (1993) A propos de la 'question de santé'. In: B. Curmi & S. Chiffoleau (eds.) Médecins et protection sociale dans le monde arabe (p. 155–172). Cahiers du Cermoc [In French]

Becker HS, Hughes EC, Strauss AL (1961) Boys in white. Chicago, IL: University of Chicago Press

Boltanski L (1971) Les usages sociaux du corps. Annales, 26: 205–233 [In French]

Boukhaima S (2005) Le système de santé syrien, des réformes nécessaires dans un environnement contraignant. In: S. Chiffoleau (ed.). Politiques de santé sous influence inernationale. Afrique, Moyen-Orient. Paris, France, Maisonneuve et Larose [In French]

Bourmaud P (2008) Ya doktor, Devenir médecin et exercer son art en Terre Sainte, Une expérience du pluralisme médical dans l'empire ottoman finissant, PhD thesis at Université de Provence, Aix en Provence, France [In French]

Camau M, Zaiem H, Bahri H (1990) Etat de santé, besoin médical et *enjeux politiques en Tunisie.* Paris, France: CNRS Editions [In French]

Chiffoleau S (1997) *Médecines et médecins en Egypte, Construction d'une identité professionnelle et projet médical.* Lyon-Paris, France: Maison de l'Orient Méditerranéen-L'Harmattan [In French]

Chiffoleau S (2005) La réforme du système de santé égyptien: un nouveau type de processus politique entre logique internationale et enjeux nationaux. *In:* S. Chiffoleau (Ed.) *Politiques de santé sous influence internationale: Afrique, Moyen-Orient* (p. 213–236). Paris-Lyon: Maisonneuve & Larose [In French]

Chiffoleau S (2007) *Entre initiation au jeu international, pouvoir colonial et mémoire nationale: le Conseil Sanitaire d'Alexandrie, 1865–1938. Egypte Monde Arabe, n°4.* (p. 55–74). Cairo, Egypt: Cedej [In French]

Chiffoleau S (forthcoming) *De la peste d'Orient à l'OMS. Une histoire de la santé publique internationale.* Paris, France: CNRS [In French]

Chiffoleau S, Curmi B (eds.) (1993) *Médecins et protection sociale.* Beyrouth-Paris, France, Cermoc-IRD, Cahiers du Cermoc [In French]

Dewachi O (2008) *The professionalization of the Iraqi medical doctor in Britain: Medicine, citizenship, sovereignty and empire.* PhD Dissertation at Harvard University, Cambridge.

Dodge B (1958) *The American University of Beirut, a brief history.* Beirut, Lebanon: Khayat

Elshakry M (2010) Darwinian conversions: science and translation in late Ottoman Egypt and Greater Syria in Perilous Modernity. *In:* Anne-Marie Moulin and Yesim Isil Ulman (Eds.) *History of medicine in the Ottoman Empire and the Middle East from the 19th century onwards.* (p. 85–95). Istanbul, Turkey: The Isis Press

European Commission (2004) *European delegation to Syria.* Available from http://www.delsyr. ec.europa.eu/en/eu_and_syria_ new/european_union_syrian_ cooperation_projects_lah.htm [Accessed 14 January 2011]

Foucault M (2003) *The birth of the clinic: An archaeology of medical perception.* London, UK: Routledge classics, Edition Reprint, Routledge, 2003, ISBN 9780415307727, (first published in French in 1963, La naissance de la Clinique)

Freidson E (1970) *Profession of medicine.* New York, NY: Harper and Row

Gallagher N (1983) *Medicine and Power in Tunisia, 1780–1900.* Cambridge UK: Cambridge University Press.

Gaudin JP (1987) Savoirs, savoir-faire et mouvement de professionnalisation dans l'urbanisme au début du siècle, *Sociologie du Travail,* 39(2):177–197 [In French].

Hanna A (1996) *Al-Muthaqqafûn fî Sûriya: al-Atibbâ'.* Damascus, Syria: Dar Dimashq [In Arabic]

Heydemann S (2004) Toward a new social contract in the Middle East and North Africa. *Arab Reform Bulletin,* January 20, 2004

Jagailloux S (1986) *La médicalisation de l'Egypte au 19e siècle.* Paris, France: Edition recherches sur les Civilisations [In French]

Kaddar M (1995) Financement et dynamique des systèmes de santé au Maghreb: données et problèmes actuels [in French]. *In:* E. Longuenesse (ed.) *Santé médecine et société dans le monde arabe* (p. 185–198), Lyon-Paris, France: Maison de l'Orient Méditerranéen-L'Harmattan

Khouri R (2010) Histoire de la Medecine au Liban *Journal Medical Libanais,* 58(1): 28–44 [In French]

Kronfol N, Mroueh A (1985) *Health care in Lebanon.* Alexandria, Egypt: WHO

Longuenesse E (1992) Systèmes de protection sociale dans le monde arabe, *Maghreb-Machrek,* 138: 111–128 [In French]

Longuenesse E (1993) Femmes médecins en pays arabes, l'exemple de la Syrie, Islam et santé. *Sociologie santé,* 9: 133–152 [In French]

Longuenesse E (1995) Les médecins syriens, des médiateurs dans une société en crise. *In:* E. Longuenesse (Ed.) *Santé, médecine et société dans le monde arabe* (p. 219–250). Lyon-Paris, France: Maison de l'Orient Méditerranéen-L'Harmattan [In French]

Ministry of Health and Population in Egypt (MOHP-Egypt) (2003) El-Zanaty and Associates, and ORC. *Macro Egypt Service Provision Assessment 2002.* Cairo, Egypt: Calverton MD: ORC Macro

Mitchell T (2002) *Rule of experts: Egypt, techno-politics, modernity.* Berkeley, CA: University of California Press.

Moulin AM (1995) Les instituts Pasteur de la Méditerranée arabe: une religion scientifique en pays d'islam. *In:* E. Longuenesse (Ed.) *Santé médecine et société dans le monde arabe.* Lyon-Paris, France: Maison de l'Orient Méditerranéen-L'Harmattan [In French]

Panzac D (1982) *Endémies, épidémies et population en Égypte au XIXe siècle, GREPO, L'Égypte au XIXe siècle.* Paris, France: Éditions du CNRS [In French]

Panzac D (1985) *La peste dans l'Empire ottoman, 1700–1850.* Louvain, Belgium: Peeters [In French]

Radi S (2007) L'hépathite C et les défaillances du système égyptien de santé publique, Itinéraires thérapeutiques et solutions palliative. *Egypte Monde Arabe,* [In French]

Rivet D (1995) Hygiénisme colonial et médicalisation de la société marocaine au temps du protectorat français: 1912–1956. *In:* E. Longuenesse (ed.) *Santé médecine et société dans le monde arabe* (p. 105–128). Lyon-Paris, France: Maison de l'Orient Méditerranéen-L'Harmattan [In French]

Rivet D (2002) *Le Maghreb à l'épreuve de la colonization*. Paris, France: Hachette [In French]

Suchman EA (1963) *Sociology and the field of public health*. New York, NY: Russel/Sage Foundation

Tabutin D, Schoumaker B (2005) The demography of the Arab world and the Middle East from the 1950s to the 2000s. *Population*, 60, 5–6, 505–591+593–615

Turin Y (1971) *Affrontements culturels dans l'Algérie coloniale: écoles, médecines, religion, 1830–1880*. Alger, Algeria: Entreprise Nationale du Livre [In French]

Watts S (1999) *Epidemics and history: Disease, power and imperialism*. New Haven, CT: Yale University Press.

Watts S (2003) *Disease and medicine in world history*. London, UK: Routledge

Chapter

2

The Political, Economic, and Social Context

Samer Jabbour, Rouham Yamout, Jamil Hilal, and Adib Nehmeh

The Arab uprisings and revolutions of Winter 2010–2011 have refocused attention on the underlying conditions that foster discontent and national indignation among the masses against the tyrannical regimes: lack of freedoms; oppression and abuses of power and rights; social, economic, and political exclusion; high unemployment, especially among the youth; corruption; and poverty. These are the same conditions that underline the challenges of public health, i.e., the social determinants or the "causes of causes" of health and ill-health (CSDH 2008). This chapter describes and analyzes some of the key challenges in the political, social, and economic domains. Because these challenges operate across all areas of public health, we aim to provide background data and analyses that can inform the discussions in other chapters of this volume. The chapter describes a set of political, economic, and social processes that have characterized the development paths in the Arab countries; for example in economic development and social policy, and then examine the social consequences of these processes that are most relevant to public health, such as poverty and unemployment.

At the outset, we stress the need to put development challenges in a historical perspective that incorporates political economy and social theory. The literature of many United Nations (UN) and international agencies (see for example, World Bank 2004; UNDP 2009a) as well as pundits focus on obstacles to development, seeing many to be internal while paying less attention to the history, the wider regional and international context, and the political economy of development and de-development. Much of this literature appears in technical discourse, while in fact it is highly ideological and political as it restricts questions that need to be asked and the ways in which issues are framed. Through the Arab Human Development Report project (five reports have been

released between 2002 and 2009 and are accessible at UNDP [2010a,b]), the UNDP has incorporated more political analysis in approaching problems of development. However, the UNDP's diagnoses for the failure of development have elicited controversy over the relegation of priorities and giving less weight to the impact of external factors (Amin 1999, see also Chapter 36). There is extensive literature that stresses the importance of understanding history as an entry to analyzing the contemporary Arab state, society, economy, and development (for useful readings, see Amin 1978; Amin 1999; Owen 2004; Barakat 2008; Richards & Waterbury 2008). The next section provides a brief historical review as an entry to discussing the problems of development.

A Historical Background

Throughout the modern era, the roles of colonial powers, following the four-century long Ottoman rule, was decisive (this is extensively analyzed in Amin 1999; Hourani et al 2004; Owen 2004). The English helped abort the 1916–1918 "Great Arab Revolution," led by Sharif Hussein that aimed at unifying Arab countries. Western powers divided the region along the famous "Sykes Picot" accord of 1916. The legacies of European "mandates" and Zionist settler colonialism in the Levant and the brutal European colonialism of North Africa have had a decisive impact that persists to this day. The rise of the significance of oil in the global economy was a key factor in the geopolitical importance of the region. European and North American influence has not faded; only its forms and instrument have changed. This takes direct forms such as the Israeli settler-colonialism, the US-led occupation of Iraq, and the substantial US military presence in the Gulf. Less obvious forms include the shaping of the political and the development agendas through bilateral relations and instruments of globalization (see for example, the extensive case studies in Harrigan & El-Said 2009a, 2009b). Calls for resisting foreign domination have overshadowed, in some Arab countries, the need for comprehensive socio-economic development plans. In a few countries, fundamentalist movements built on popular frustrations to pursue their own agendas.

The largely "fragile" Arab states that were created by Western powers in the twentieth century (Owen 2004) inherited widespread illiteracy and poverty, feeble economic infrastructures, hardly any experience in democratic governance, and weak standing in the international political order. Arab states such as Algeria, Egypt, Iraq, Sudan, and Syria, came to be controlled by military regimes and found themselves handicapped in their declared aims of shedding off foreign influence and in seeking Arab unification, socio-economic development, and social equality and justice. The presence of oil necessitated the creation of regimes friendly to international centers of power. Oil wealth produced its own problems to the Gulf States, as they had to increasingly depend on immigrant labor with limited civil and social rights, and no political rights. Recurrent major wars, fear of external threats, and internal strife facilitated the allocation of relatively large resources to the military and to security apparatuses. The regimes effectively used the Arab-Israeli conflict as a pretext to suppress the masses and delay democratization.

Many proposals have been made since the formation of the League of Arab States in 1945 to further pan-Arab economic and political cooperation without much progress owing to the very nature of the fragmented Arab regime created by the Western powers in cooperation with local elites. Rivalries and divergent political systems and ideologies among Arab countries, fueled by international rivalries, hindered cooperation and in some cases led to open hostilities. What could have been considered a regional order (Sayigh 1991) collapsed in the period leading up to and following the 1991 Gulf War. The social impact of this collapse is clear if we examine the repercussions, for example, of the decision of some of the Gulf States to expel hundreds of thousands of workers from Arab countries that did not take a clear position against the Kuwait invasion by Iraq's Saddam.

Since Napoleon's Egypt campaign in 1879, the relentless interests of global powers have defined the "development" options and paths that could be followed (Amin 1999). Between the end of the Second World War and the end of the Cold War, the region was an important stage for competing political and economic interests of the Eastern and Western blocs. After the collapse of the Soviet Union, which exposed the region to US domination, accelerated globalization forces have integrated the region more and more into the global economic capitalist (based on a consumption rather than a productive model along with liberalization of trade and privatization of the economy) and the international political system, especially since the oil boom following the 1973 war (see the extensive examples in Guazzone & Pioppi 2009; and Henry & Springborg 2010). Bilateral relations and aid flows fostered this form of integration. Harrigan & El-Said (2009a) show that the international financial institutions such as the World Bank and IMF pursue policies of most interest to donors rather than guided by poverty reduction or genuine development considerations. This is done according to geopolitical considerations whereby "favored" countries such as Egypt and Jordan receive more aid and loans than needier countries. Between 2000 and 2005, the poorest countries received only 15% of total aid to the region (UN & LAS 2007). Except for Sudan, "development" aid to each of these countries was lower in 2005 than in 1990.

The complex interactions of the dominating global political and economic centers (with their double standards: declaring support for democracy while supporting reactionary and despotic regimes; declaring support for freedom and human rights while supporting Israeli occupation), corrupt, unaccountable, and oppressive regimes, have limited the input of democratic and progressive forces into the building of modern societies and states based on rights, rule of law, and social equality. In this context, opportunities for socio-economic equitable development were undermined (Jabbour 2003). This has shaped the realities of everyday life and posed a set of political, economic, and social challenges that are of direct interest to public health.

General Characteristics

The 22 country members of the League of Arab States share linguistic, cultural, and demographic characteristics but show remarkable diversity of dialects, ethnicities, religious and social composition, economic resources and structures, and political outlooks (Shami 2001). While we focus here on a region-wide analysis, we also attempt to highlight the diversity across sub-regions and states. We do not focus on within-country differences, although important and significant, as this level of analysis requires a dedicated analysis beyond the limited space.

Classification

Because of its complexity and diversity, there are many classifications of the Arab world depending on the framework of analysis and on the area of interest of different actors (see Introduction). Having an idea of the various classifications is important, since they regularly appear in public health and development literature. Researchers might use these classifications, or modifications of (see for example, Rauch & Kostyshak 2009), according to analytical and descriptive need.

The World Bank and UNDP classify the Arab countries according to income and human development index. Because of the increasing importance of the dual dynamics of resource-labor in generating such phenomena as economic migration, recent development documents (for example. UNDP 2009b) might classify countries as resource-rich/labor-abundant (e.g., Syria), resource-rich/labor-poor (GCC countries), or resource-poor/labor-abundant (e.g., Lebanon). Because of the profound impact of conflict, countries can be defined according to their security situation (see also chapters in Section 5). Because of shared histories and socio-economic commonalities, Arab countries can be grouped according to sub-regions: GCC countries (Bahrain, Kuwait, Oman, Qatar, Saudi Arabia, UAE), Mashreq countries (Egypt, Jordan, Iraq, Lebanon, OPT, Syria), Maghreb countries (Algeria, Libya, Morocco, and Tunisia), or by severity of poverty, thus grouping the poorest countries together (Comoros, Djibouti, Mauritania, Somalia, Sudan, Yemen). The latter group is also commonly referred to in the development literature as the "least developed Arab countries." We might also choose to classify countries along less conventional descriptors, for example by human poverty, social inequality, degree of internal political polarization, food security, economic dependency, type of political system, or even health system development.

The Arab State and State–Society Interactions

Historical, geopolitical, and socio-economic factors have produced regimes with all-powerful executive and security apparatuses in both republics dominated by single parties as well as monarchies. The political, economic, and social policies adopted have been basically re-oriented from the ambitious plans of "nation-building" and social and economic development after independence (see also Chapter 1) to serve the primary goal of regime survival. This has produced governance patterns that have stamped the region with authoritarianism and the repression of basic human and civil rights. Thus systems of repression and violations of human rights are widespread (UNDP 2009a). Most Arab states have consistently and severely restricted political participation. In 2008, six countries (Algeria, Egypt, Iraq, OPT, Syria, Sudan) were under a state of emergency (UNDP 2009a). Syria has been under "emergency" since the Ba'ath party came to power in 1963! Beyond political exclusion, emergency laws have been important instruments in economic and social exclusion.

Governance, among the most important elements in health system development as discussed in Chapter 28, has been characterized by a low level of accountability and inclusiveness (UNDP 2009b). Using the Index of Governance Quality, the region has the worst gap compared with other developing regions (World Bank 2003). Voice and accountability is the governance area showing the least improvement between 1996 and 2007 in all Arab countries. Public administration is not clearly subject to accountability: the oil-rich countries perform the best on quality of administration but the worst on public accountability (World Bank 2003). Poor governance, among other factors, has undermined foreign investments (Jafari Samimi & Ariani 2010). The poor quality of institutions has limited the region's integration into the global economy and undermined job creation (Méon & Sekkat 2004). Not surprisingly, corruption is a major challenge (Chêne & Hodess 2007). Guetat (2006) has shown that the impact of corruption and poor institutions is highest in this region compared with other world regions. The cost of corruption is estimated at $1 trillion between 1950 and 2000, or a third of the total income earned by Arab countries (AACO 2010). The health sector is not spared. In a multi-country study, 80% of population respondents in Morocco perceived high corruption in health (Lewis 2006). Public officials, business executives, and the public ranked health among the top four most corrupt sectors.

With corruption and accountability, the benefits of economic growth witnessed in both oil-rich and non-oil economies were not distributed fairly, favoring regime and regime-friendly interests, resulting in widening social inequalities, with profound public health consequences (see the Egypt case study in Chapter 37). The liberalization policies of the preceding three decades further contributed to this process. As public and private interactions were not regularly subjected to the rule of law, the phenomenon of abuse of public power for private gains became widespread. In some countries, such as Egypt, that had nationalized many industries and sectors, re-privatization, both active and passive, including selling public assets at dirt-cheap prices, and privileged the ruling elites and their allies (see Chapter 37).

Under these circumstances, many have argued that the Arab state has obstructed development (Salem 2010). Civic engagement in the public sphere, an important force in modern public health, has been limited except in settings where the state has been weak or absent such as Lebanon and the 1967 Occupied Palestinian Territory. Up until the current revolutions, it appears that the various authoritarian Arab states have found ways to live with and control limited civic action. The recent growth of NGOs has taken place under the close scrutiny of states, and sometimes some NGOs are run by regime loyalists, making these "governmental NGOs" used as means of controlled liberalization (Ben Neffisa et al 2005). The governments have attempted to control even trade unions, so important to securing economic, social, and health rights of workers, but with variable success as shows the case of the Tunisian labor union, which has been a key component of the Tunisian revolution.

Henry and Springborg (2010) have alluded to the capacity of Arab regimes to maintain control despite remarkable international and regional developments, including in the aftermath of 9/11. But this is not to say that Arab regimes have not been changing. Even prior to the onset of the revolutions and protests, change has been under way but in a controlled fashion and with the purpose of serving regime persistence as the case studies about Egypt, Syria, Morocco, and Palestine in Fürtig (2007) show.

Because of lack of public space for social mobilization that can allow the articulation of a vision and strategies for the future, large segments of the population are driven to seek refuge from various forms of marginalization and insecurity to the private sphere and to pre-state forms of social organization such as religious/sectarian, ethnic, or clan formations.

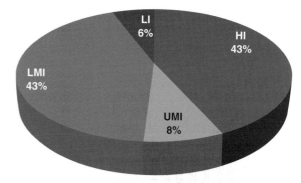

Distribution of regional GDP

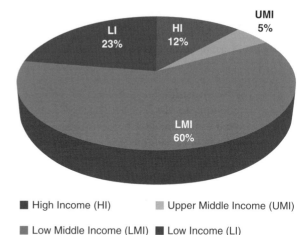

Distribution of regional population

■ High Income (HI) ■ Upper Middle Income (UMI)
■ Low Middle Income (LMI) ■ Low Income (LI)

Figure 1. Distribution of GDP vs. population by country group 2007. Source: UNDP 2009a.

Such developments have fueled ethnic, sectarian, and socio-political polarization that the Arab world has witnessed in recent years (Al Hajj Saleh 2010a). The revolutions have created new spaces for public mobilization, the full effects of which will take years to fully unfold.

The Regional Economy

The Arab world has abundant resources, especially natural ones such as oil, gas, and human resources, but coupled with marked inequalities in wealth distribution and opportunities. The poorest countries house over 23% of the population but enjoy no more than 6% of the region's gross domestic product (GDP) (Figure 1). Inequalities between and within states have profound significance if considered from the viewpoint of regional solidarity in health and the need for a

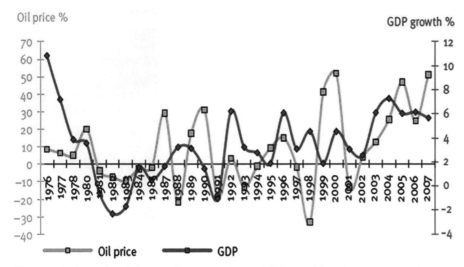

Figure 2. GDP growth volatility in Arab countries. Regional GDP growth based on constant 1990 prices, and growth in nominal oil prices 1976–2007. Source: UNDP 2009a.

common action in health. Such inequalities reflect the failure of attempts to develop a regional economic order, an Arab economic community of sorts, which can benefit all national economies. For instance, intra-regional trade accounts for only 10% of total trade in the region, a figure much lower than in other regions (UNDP 2009a).

Although economies have undergone marked changes over the past two decades, many of the descriptions proposed by Samir Amin (1948) in his 1984 classic, *The Arab Economy Today*, remain true today (Barakat 2008). These economies are diverse in terms of patterns and modes of production and resource ownership with co-existing features of feudalism, primitive capitalism, and even pastoral economy in rural and Bedouin areas. The broad characteristic is that of capitalist "commercial–agricultural" economies. Family and small businesses, not large corporations, remain the center of economic activity. These economies suffer from a high degree of dependency related to its integration in the global capitalist system under the aforementioned historical conditions.

Although different post-colonial states have followed different politico-economic models, reliance on "rent," especially oil, has dominated economic growth especially since the 1970s, with profound political, social, and cultural consequences. The "rentier" economies also include non-oil producing countries, which have also benefitted substantially from remittances of workers employed in oil-producing countries, intraregional investments generated by oil wealth, direct aid from oil

countries, and other sources such as tourism and services also related to oil investments (UNDP 2009b).

For all its resources, the region's economic performance has been disappointing, explaining failures at creating jobs to meet population growth. The UNDP (2009a) reported only a 6.4% increase in *real* GDP per capita between 1980 and 2004. Volatile economic growth (Figure 2) has affected the prospects of economic and job securities in the whole region. Fluctuating oil prices alone do not explain this volatility. With poor performance in other economic branches such as agriculture, industrial production, and manufacturing, Arab countries do not have a strong economic base that can buffer them against oil price volatility. Excluding oil, the region has the lowest export to GDP ratio of all developing regions except sub-Saharan Africa (Méon & Sekkat 2004). The structure of GDP (see UNDP 2009a, Figure 5-4) shows that oil and services dominate the economic sectors while consumption dwarfs both investments and exports.

Investments in industry and agriculture have not increased significantly since the mid-1970s (UNDP 2009a). Arab economies today are less industrialized (contributing less than 10% of GDP) than they were in 1970. Agriculture, historically the backbone of the economies in the Fertile Crescent and Nile valley, has witnessed a dramatic decline due to a decrease in profitability of agriculture due to irresponsible governance of crop trade, coupled with lack of adequate investments, poor land and water management, and climate change. This is particularly worrisome because of the chronic problems of food insecurity (see also Chapter 10). The ambitious but uncoordinated plans set in the 1950s to the early 1970s by post-colonial countries to industrialize and achieve agricultural self-sufficiency did not bear fruit. Consequently, the share of services of the overall Arab economy have increased to account for over 50% of GDP in non-oil producing countries (over 65% in Bahrain, Djibouti, Jordan, Lebanon, and Morocco) and over 50% of employment in most countries. The types and qualities of services do not position the Arab economies well in the global economy (UNDP 2009a).

Social Policy: Focus on Social Protection

A recent review (UNESCWA 2009b) provides a historical perspective on the evolution of socio-economic policies, especially social protection and the changing role of the state in Arab countries in relation to available resources and global pressures. The oil boom of the 1970s provided Arab governments with resources to develop the infrastructure of social protection established in the post-independence era of the 1950s–1960s. Government expenditures increased to 42% with major investments in education, health, and subsidies. Many of these investments were rolled back with falling oil prices in the 1980s and institution of structural adjustment reforms through the 1990s. To ensure minimal levels of social stability, governments maintained reasonable investments in social protection (estimated as percentage of GDP to be 5.7% in Lebanon, 11.2% in Yemen, 12.9% in Egypt, and 17.9% in Jordan) (UNESCWA 2009b).

Trends in the 2000s are mixed as the rise of oil prices have increased social spending by some countries, especially in the Gulf, while the perusal of liberalization policies, the growth of informal employment and decline of public employment, and the increasing needs due to population growth, reduced governmental spending on social protection in others, such as in Egypt, Jordan, and Syria. Nevertheless, Arab countries continue to spend a considerable share of national income on social protection estimated at around 20–25% in Egypt and Jordan (Loewe 2009).

Long-term social investments, coupled with persistent relatively high levels of public sector employment, has helped countries improve social and health indicators despite cycles of economic stagnation and external shocks related to factors such as wars, internal strife, and fluctuating oil prices. This is reflected in the 2010 Human Development Report (UNDP 2010 a,b), whereby 5 of the 10 countries with the largest development gains since 1970 were Arab (Oman, Saudi Arabia, Tunisia, Algeria, and Morocco). The gains are largely in the areas of health and education, the non-income dimensions of UNDP's Human Development Index. Since 1970, life expectancy increased from 51 years to almost 70 years, the largest gain among world regions while infant mortality rates decreased from 98 per 1000 live births to 38, below the world average of 44. Educational gains, discussed below, are also substantial but less so than health gains. The main question is whether ongoing liberalization policies in the region will allow decent levels of social protection in the future and how the revolutions will impact future directions.

Social protection is a broad umbrella that includes wage protection, state provision of assistance, general price subsidies, for example, for food or energy, social security and pensions, social and health insurance and health protection programs, among others. All of these aspects are important and are in use to varying degrees in the region. However, most social protection measures leave significant gaps. The gaps in public health financing, high rates of out-of-pocket expenditures on health, and risks of catastrophic health expenditures are well covered in Chapter 29 and will not be discussed here. The example of pensions demonstrates the inequitable nature of social protection gaps.

While most countries have pension plans, total coverage is low (less than 40% of the working population) (Loewe 2009). Only five countries (Libya, Tunisia, Algeria, Egypt, and Jordan) have coverage rates in the 55–80% commensurate with rates in other world regions. Coverage excludes migrant workers as in the Gulf States where only 5–30% of the working population is covered (Loewe 2009). Pension schemes might benefit the middle- and high-income groups more than the lower income groups. Governments use general tax revenues, to which the poor contribute disproportionately, to support pension schemes, but only parts of the working population can access these schemes. Coverage is influenced by the political orientation of the country, rather than the rights of citizens and their equality under the law. Loewe (2009) notes that coverage rate is double in republics (44%) vs. monarchies (22%), the latter including GCC countries, Jordan and Morocco. He opines that the "stability of the republican regimes depends much more on social achievements than in the case of monarchies."

A significant, although undetermined, proportion of social protection in the region comes from informal, as opposed to formal or state supported, sources. This includes for example remittances from work abroad. Between 1970 and 1995, official remittances to seven labor-exporting countries increased from $0.4 billion to $6.35 billion (Handoussa & Tzannatos 2004, Table 5.3). Remittances are especially important for poor rural areas not well covered by formal protection schemes. In rural Egypt when remittances are included in total income, poverty rate drops by 10%. Other sources of protection include extended family support, and programs of the voluntary non-state sector including religious charities, and social programs of political movements such as Muslim Brotherhood in Egypt and Hezbollah in Lebanon (see case studies in Harrigan & El-Said 2009b). NGOs also commonly provide protection programs funded by foreign or local donors. These sources are likely to become increasingly important with the mounting problems and gaps in the formal protection schemes, the gradual withdrawal of state welfare schemes in many countries, and the growth of informal employment.

In addition to social protection, social policy includes many other domains of direct relevance to public health including employment, education, environmental sustainability, urban planning, and rural development. Because these domains are inter-related and states have to balance investments among them, social policy needs to be developed and implemented in an integrated fashion ensuring that all segments of society are engaged in this process. Arab states have a long way to go to realize this (UNESCWA 2009b).

Society and Social Change

In an overview building on prior work, Barakat (2008) argues that it is possible to describe a "contemporary Arab society," as a unit of analysis that consists of multiple sub-societies and groups in different countries. The reason is the broad commonalities and the inter-connectedness of political, economic, and social developments across the region. The spread of protests in winter 2010–2011 to several Arab countries in a very short period confirms the links between the common struggles of people across Arab countries against systems commonly characterized by oppression and exclusion. Barakat sees the society

as being very diverse in its social structures, which have different origins: "patriarchal" with authoritarian tendencies on multiple levels, and "transitional" in nature and polarized by forces of "modernization" and "traditionalism." These features are at the heart of the struggle of public health for social change (see Chapter 38).

Al Hajj Saleh (2010b) has argued for dispelling the myth that nothing changes in the Arab world. Rather, profound changes have taken place in the era of communication, economic liberalization, and globalization but these changes are externally determined and most take place without the needed political and social control from within the region and therefore remain alien to people. However, the revolutions in Tunisia and Egypt show the potentialities of under-the-surface changes beyond what analysts might predict and that people can take control when the time is right.

Some Development Features

Table 1 presents commonly used development indicators. Other resources (for example, UNDP 2009a, 2009b; UN & LAS 2010) cover an expanded set of indicators. In what follows, we visit a selected set of such features of special interest to public health.

Poverty

The World Bank has shown progress in the reduction of incidence of poverty (using the international poverty line of $2/person/day) in a subset of Arab countries (Middle East and North Africa [MENA] countries) from approximately 32% in 1981 to around 20% in 2005 (Chen & Ravallion 2007). This compares favorably with Asia and Africa. These data did not include assessments of poverty in countries in conflict. Taking the whole region yields higher estimates (UN & LAS 2010). Additionally, the $2/day cutoff may underestimate poverty in some countries that have higher national poverty lines: $2.7/day in Egypt, Jordan, Morocco, and Tunisia and $2.43 in Djibouti, Mauritania, and Yemen. Given the dependence of the Palestinian economy on the Israeli economy, the poverty line is $3.1/day (PCBS 2009). The AHDR 2009 estimates that as many as 65 million people live in poverty. Other sources (UN & LAS 2007) put this figure at 35.4 million. Based on surveys of nine countries, the AHDR 2009 also estimates that 18.3% the poor live in extreme poverty (daily income below the

Table 1a. Selected Development Indicators

	Independence	Population (Mln) 2008	Economic classification #	Economic classification ##	Human Development rank[3] 2010	Gender-inequality rank[3] 2010	GNI per capita*[4] 2007–09	Population below national poverty line (%) (1999–2006)[2] Urban	Rural	National 2008	Net ODA received (% of GNI)[4] 2008	Water access (%)[4] 2008	Sanitation access (%)[4] 2008	Mobile subscribers (%)[4] 2008	Internet users (%)[4] 2008
Algeria	1962	34.37	LARR	MOE	84	70	8,110	10.3	14.7	12.1	0.19	83	95	93	12
Bahrain	1971	0.78	LIRR	OE	39	55	33,690	–	–	–	–	95	36	186	52
Comoros	1975	0.64	Poor	PEE	140	–	1,300	–	–	–	7.01	92	56	15	4
Djibouti	1977	0.85	Poor	PEE	147	–	2,480	–	–	–	11.3	99	94	13	2
Egypt	1922	81.53	LARP	DE	101	108	5,680	10.1	26.8	19.6	0.82	79	73	51	17
Iraq	1932	30.71	Conflict		–	–	3,330	–	–	–	11.9	96	98	57	1
Jordan	1946	5.81	LE	DE	82	76	5,730	12.9	18.7	14.2	3.35	99	100	91	27
KSA	1932	24.81	LIRR	OE	55	128	24,150	–	–	–	–	–	–	145	31
Kuwait	1961	2.73	LIRR	OE	47	43	53,890	–	–	–	–	100	–	107	37
Lebanon	1943	4.19	LE	DE	–	–	13,400	–	–	7.97	3.61	–	97	34	23
Libya	1951	6.29	LARR	MOE	53	52	16,400	–	–	–	0.06	–	–	77	5
Mauritania	1960	3.22	Poor	PEE	136	118	1,960	–	–	46	8.70	49	26	65	2
Morocco	1956	31.61	LE	DE	114	104	4,400	12	27.2	19	1.39	81	69	72	33
Oman	1908	2.79	LIRR	OE	–	–	24,530	–	–	–	0.05	88	89	116	20
OPT	–	3.94	Conflict		–	–	–	–	–	–	–	91	100	29	9
Qatar	1971	1.28	LIRR	OE	38	94	–	–	–	–	–	100	100	131	34
Somalia	1960	8.93	Conflict		–	–	–	–	–	–	–	30	23	7	1
Sudan	1956	41.35	Poor	PEE	154	106	1,990	–	–	–	4.55	57	34	29	10
Syria	1943	20.58	LE	DE	111	103	4,620	8.7	14.2	11.4	0.26	89	96	34	17
Tunisia	1956	10.33	LE	DE	81	56	7,810	1.7	8.3	4.1	1.24	94	85	83	27
UAE	1971	4.49	LIRR	OE	32	45	–	–	–	–	–	100	97	209	65
Yemen	1967	22.92	Poor	PEE	133	138	2,330	20.7	40.1	34.8	1.23	62	52	16	2

Notes: *Current international US$, GNI = Gross national income; PPP; KSA = Kingdom of Saudi Arabia; UAE = United Arab Emirates; OPT = Occupied Palestinian Territory; ODA = official development assistance; the gender inequality index is the rank in Human Development Index after adjustment for gender inequality; Economic Classification: #LARR = Labor abundant, resource rich; LARP = labor abundant, resource poor; LIRR = labor importing, resource rich; LE = labor exporting (Chaaban 2010); ##MOE = mixed oil economies; DE = diversified economies; OE = oil economies; PEE = primary export economies (UNDP 2009b).

Sources: [1]Chaaban 2010; [2]UNDP 2009b; [3]UNDP 2010; [4]World Development Indicators 2010.

Table 1b. Selected Development Indicators

	Corruption Perceptions Index[a,5]	Democracy Index[a,6]	Literacy (% of 15+)	School enrollment (% net)	Unemployment (%)[7]		Life expectancy (years)[8]	U5MR (per 1,000)[8]	Malnutrition (% of children <5) (2000–2008)[8]		MMR (per 100,000 live births)[8]	Skilled birth attendance (%)	Immunization, measles (% 12-23 months)[8]
	2008	2008	2008	2008	Total	15–24	2008	2009	#	##	2008	2000–2008	2009
Algeria	2.9	3.44	–	95	10	45.6	72.4	32.3	6.6	23.3	120	95.2	88
Bahrain	4.9	3.49	91	98	5	20.7	75.9	12.1	–	–	19	99	99
Comoros	2.1	3.07	74	–	–	–	65.3	104.0	25	46.9	340	61.8	79
Djibouti	3.2	2.2	–	41	41	37.8	55.4	93.5	25.4	26.5	300	92.9	73
Egypt	3.1	3.07	78	–	8	25.8	70.1	21.0	6.8	30.7	82	78.9	95
Iraq	1.5	4.00	–	–	30	45.3	67.9	43.5	7.1	27.5	75	79.7	69
Jordan	4.7	3.74	–	89	11	38.9	72.7	25.3	3.6	12	59	99.1	95
KSA	4.7	1.84	69	85	5	25.9	73.1	21.0	5.3	9.3	24	96	98
Kuwait	4.5	3.88	–	88	3	23.3	78	9.9	–	–	9	100	97
Lebanon	2.5	5.82	88	88	12	21.3	72.1	12.4	4.2	16.5	26	98	53
Libya	2.2	1.94	57	–	7	27.3	74.3	18.5	5.6	21	64	–	98
Mauritania	2.3	3.86	56	77	16	44.3	56.7	117.1	23.2	28.9	550	60.9	59
Morocco	3.4	3.79	87	89	10	15.7	71.3	37.5	9.9	23.1	110	62.6	98
Oman	5.3	2.86	94	68	7	19.6	75.9	12.0	–	–	20	98.6	97
OPT	–	5.44	–	75	25	33.1	73.5	29.5	2.2	11.8	–	98.9	–
Qatar	7.7	3.09	86	–	1	17	75.9	10.8	–	–	8	100	99
Somalia	1.1	–	84	–	33	43.4	49.8	180.0	32.8	42.1	1200	33	24
Sudan	1.6	2.42	78	–	21	41.2	58.1	108.2	31.7	37.9	750	49.2	82
Syria	2.5	2.31	–	–	21	19.8	74.2	16.2	10	28.6	46	93	81
Tunisia	4.3	2.79	61	98	14	26.5	74.3	20.7	3.3	9	60	94.6	98
UAE	6.3	2.52	98	–	2	6.3	77.8	–	–	–	10	100	92
Yemen	2.2	2.64	80	73	–	–	62.9	66.4	43.1	57.7	210	35.7	58

Notes: [a]Scale (10 best, 0 worst); U5MR: Under-5 mortality rate; MMR: Maternal mortality ratio; [#]Weight for age; [##]Height for age.
Sources: [5]Transparency International 2010; [6]Economist Intelligence Unit 2010; [7]Chaaban 2010; [8]World Development Indicators 2010.

Table 2. Incidence of Human Poverty (2006)

Income group (# of countries)	Value of Human Poverty Index (%)	Probability of not surviving to age 40	Adult (15 and older) illiteracy rate (%)	Population without access to safe water (%)	Children under-weight for age (%)
Low (4)	35.0	22.8	40.5	31.7	42.1
Lower middle (7)	20.4	7.2	28.9	8.3	6.8
Upper middle (3)	12.0	5.0	11.0	18.0	8.0
High (4)	11.7	5.1	14.7	8.2	13.7
Total (18)	22.3	10.4	29.1	13.9	15.4

Source: UNDP 2009a.

lower national poverty lines, which roughly correspond to $2/day), up from 17.6% based on surveys from the 1990s.

There are important inter-country and within-country differences. Poverty rates range from 28.6% in Lebanon to 59.95% in Yemen (UNDP 2009a). Low-income countries have more extreme poverty than middle-income countries (36.2% vs. 15.9%, respectively). Poverty is more prevalent in rural populations (UNDP 2009b): in a survey of seven countries that house 53% of the population not in conflict countries, 74% of the poor live in rural areas. Since the early 1990s, the rural–urban divide has widened in these countries. In Egypt and Morocco, 1 in 4 people is poor in rural areas in contrast to 1 in 10 in urban areas. Poverty is higher among children than among other age groups (see Chapter 17).

There is also a gender dimension to income poverty. While household surveys in the region do not suggest an *overall* major difference in poverty between female- and male-headed households, sub-group analysis shows important differences (UNDP 2009b). These differences demonstrate interactions between gender, urban/rural status, marital status, and number of children. For example, in Egypt, Lebanon, and Syria, households headed by widows with more than three children have more poverty. In Jordan, separated women are more vulnerable to poverty than all other household groups.

Expanding the focus beyond income, the UNDP has proposed other measures to assess capabilities and opportunities, building on Amartya Sen's work. The composite Human Poverty Index (HPI) is supposed to capture the dimensions of health, education, and standard of living. HPI includes the proportion of the population not expected to reach 40 years of age;

the adult (more than 15 years of age) illiteracy rate; and the composite of the proportion of the population without access to safe water and the proportion of children under 5 years who are under-weight. Table 2 shows the performance on HPI of 18 countries. Interestingly, both middle- and high-income countries also have important gaps, for example unacceptable levels of adult illiteracy and child under-nutrition in high-income countries. This "puts in question the effectiveness of the state in providing, and ensuring access to the basic necessities of life" (UNDP 2009a). While the region's human poverty rate has reportedly dropped by about a third between 1996 and 2005, progress has been unequal, with high- and upper middle-income countries having the most improvement. Considering the levels of GDP and human development, Arab countries, except for Jordan, Lebanon, and Syria, have higher rates of human poverty than countries in other developing regions due mainly to higher rates of adult illiteracy and child under-nutrition in the Arab region.

Inequalities

The Arab region is commonly said to have less inequalities than other regions. However, in their comprehensive review of literature and evidence, Bibi & Nabli (2010) show "moderately high levels" of inequality, based on household expenditures, compared to other regions. Inequalities in earnings are actually higher in this region. The World Bank (2004) estimates that the MENA region has the highest wage inequality of all developing regions; this grim statistic improves if oil-producing countries are excluded. That income data expose more inequality than expenditure data is well known. The Arab countries

Table 3. Inequality in Various Income Groups

	High inequality	Medium inequality	Low inequality
Poorest countries	Comoros	Mauritania	Yemen Egypt
Medium living standards	Morocco Tunisia	Algeria Jordan	Lebanon Syria
Richest countries		Oman United Arab Emirates	Kuwait

Note: *Inequality is assessed based on Gini coefficient.
Source: Bibi & Nabli (2010).

show more inequalities in the distribution of other non-income variables such as health, land ownership and education. There is variation between countries even within each national income bracket (Table 3).

Trends in income inequality are difficult to discern. Bibi & Nabli argue that regional inequality has been relatively stable, or not significantly changed, over the past two to three decades reflecting two opposite trends: increasing inequality in countries that started with low levels of inequality (e.g., Syria and Yemen since the late 1990s due to liberalization reforms) and decreasing inequality in those that started with initial high inequality (e.g., Morocco and Tunisia). Benar (2007), on the other hand, shows increasing income inequalities in seven studied countries (Algeria, Egypt, Jordan, Kuwait, Morocco, Syria, Tunisia). Like Benar, Ali (2009) showed increasing inequalities, based also on consumption data, between 1995 and 2004. Ali argued for a political economy perspective and that inequalities might have contributed to civil unrest in the first decades after independence in some Arab countries. Inequalities are undoubtedly an important factor in today's revolutions.

Bibi & Nabli note that when excluding GCC countries, inequality in the region appears driven mainly by inequalities *within* countries rather than *between* countries. When rich GCC countries are included in the analysis, inter-country inequality appears to contribute significantly to overall inequality. This reflects the wealth difference between GCC and other Arab countries. That most inequality is national in non-GCC countries relates to factors such as access to various sources of income, land ownership, education, and gender. In Egypt inequality between governorates

accounted for 87% of the national inequality in 1995/1996 and 82% in 1999/2000. These inequalities are reflected in health outcomes, which are examined in details in many chapters throughout the volume.

Employment

Poor governance and economic performance of Arab countries have limited job creation; coupled with continued population growth, this has led to high unemployment especially among youth and those with higher education. This is at the heart of the recent protests.

Chaaban (2010) estimates the Arab world's labor force at over 100 million, half of it in Egypt and the other labor-exporting countries of Jordan, Lebanon, Morocco, Syria, and Tunisia. About 60% of workers are in agriculture and social and personal services. Agriculture and fishing employ 50% of workers in poor countries, which might explain the profound impact on the livelihoods and health of these people under the current projections of environmental change. Labor force participation is low at one third of the working age population, mainly because of low participation among women, who have the lowest rates (around 30%) in the "developing" world (UNDP 2009a). This is despite major increases in female education. About 29% of employment is still in the public sector, which remains attractive to job seekers despite low wages compared with the private sector because of job security and other privileges.

Based on studies from five countries conducted between 1994 and 2003, UNDP (2009a) estimates that informal employment (defined as % of non-agricultural employment) is 40–50% in Algeria, Egypt, Morocco, and Tunisia and over 20% in Syria. This has tremendous implications as informal workers are not covered by protection programs, as defined by ILO standards, and may not be able to lift themselves and their families from poverty and low education.

Unemployment around the region is about 13% and disproportionately affects women willing to participate in the labor market, youth, and individuals with higher education. About a quarter of the youth (15–24 years old), who constitute a third of the population, are unemployed (international average is 14%) (Chaaban 2010). In the poor and conflict-ridden areas where about 80 million people live, the unemployment rate is more than double the Arab world's average (Chaaban 2010). Not unexpectedly, youth unemployment is very high in conflict countries and in the poorest countries (Table 1). In economic terms, Chaaban (2008) estimated the cost of youth exclusion in Egypt and Jordan as percentage of GDP to be almost 17.4% and 7.3%, respectively.

Chaaban (2010, Figure 11) eloquently showed that structural adjustment, as measured in share of government expenditures in GDP and average applied import tariff rates, along the Washington Consensus did not reduce unemployment rates. Poor countries showed doubling of unemployment rates between 1997 and 2005 under such policies.

The future outlook for employment does not seem bright. For five countries with diversified economies (Egypt, Jordan, Morocco, Syria, Tunisia) and Algeria with a mixed oil economy, UNDP (2009b) estimates that creating employment to match population growth requires an average GDP growth rate of 7.62% (range 5.08% for Jordan and 10% for Tunisia), as compared with the actual rate of 4.91%. Looking at the past records does not provide inspiration either. Many countries that have followed neoliberal reforms have not been able to reduce unemployment, challenging the orthodox economic wisdom of the Washington Consensus (Chaaban 2010). Creating employment opportunities is undoubtedly one of the greatest challenges facing the Arab world today.

Education and Literacy

We have alluded to the mixed progress on education. UNESCO (2010) estimates that 29% of the adult population (approximately 58 million) lack basic literacy and numeracy skills. Egypt is among the top 10 countries in the world in number of illiterates (17 millions). Women account for 65% of illiterate adults. Obviously, illiteracy starts much earlier in life. The regional net enrollment rate in primary education increased from 70% around 1990 to 80.5% in 2004/2005 (UN & LAS 2007). The disappointing rate (78.2%) in GCC countries raises questions about the impact of social investments from oil wealth.

There are important inequalities in education. Primary education enrollment rate in the poorest countries is only 54.6%. Almost one in two children was out of school in 2005. There are also inequalities within countries. In Egypt, as compared with better-off children, the percentage of poor children is lower for all levels of education (UNDP 2009a). Conflict worsens education for children. Enrollment in 1967

OPT dropped by 16% since 1999 but was back to over 98% in 2010 (information from the Palestinian Ministry of Higher Education). Patterns of completion rates of primary education are similar to those of net enrollment in primary education. For example, the poorest countries have a completion rate of only 48.3% (UN & LAS 2007). In Morocco, around 25% of children aged 10 to 15 years have not completed elementary school because of poverty (UNDP 2009a). Building on enrollment and completion rates, youth (15–24 years) literacy rate was 83.4% in 2006 (UN & LAS 2007). In the poorest countries, almost a third of young people are illiterate. Gender gap in education is decreasing. In 2004/2005, the ratio of girls to boys reached 0.9, 0.91, and 1.0 at the primary, secondary, and tertiary levels, respectively. Again, the gender gap is higher in the poorest countries where the ratio is only 0.81 at the primary level.

This brief discussion does not address the issue of quality of education. There is a common view of the mismatch between what students are taught and the skills needed by the job market. This adds another challenge to the issue of ensuring employment and sustaining economic and social development.

Millennium Development Goals (MDGs)

The United Nations and the League of Arab States have launched three MDG progress reports, the last in December 2010 (UN & LAS 2007). The second report (UN & LAS 2007) provides a "youth lens." Many countries have made important improvements in MDGs. From an equity perspective, large gaps between the poorest and other countries remain striking. For example, maternal mortality, per 100,000 live births, ranges from below 10 in some GCC countries to around 1600 in Somalia. Civil society researchers rightly critique a narrow focus on development through the MDGs, lens but still see MDGs as presenting an opportunity to hold Arab governments accountable to their own commitments (Mahjoub et al 2010). They have lamented the poor progress in many areas and document that MDGs are neither mainstreamed nor properly addressed in national policymaking processes. Governments have not carried out serious and inclusive consultations about how to make progress. Gender dimensions of MDGs and bridging the gaps between the poorest countries and others are not seriously addressed either. In terms of addressing the gaps between the poorest countries and the rest,

Mahjoub et al discussed that, between 2000 and 2006, Arab countries contributed only 4.7% of official development assistance to the region (OECD contributed 77.6%), which indicates lack of commitment to regional solidarity in development. With street protests underway, an Arab Economic, Social and Development Summit in Egypt in January 2011 (the first one held in Kuwait in January 2009) issued promises to make more investments in social and economic development. But the Arab street seems to think that the problem is in the regimes themselves and not just in their investments.

need to situate the discussions of health and well-being, and of public health education, research, and practice, in relation to these determinants and challenges. The problems are many and concern the use of the vast natural resources, tapping into people's capacities, economic performance, governance and accountability, poverty and inequalities, and policies relating to education, employment, and social protection. But even as these challenges appear monumental today, so do the possibilities for change that are unfolding under the wave of revolutions sweeping the Arab world today.

Conclusions

This brief review has attempted to outline some of the determinants and challenges of development facing the Arab world today. We have done so because there is a

Acknowledgment

The views expressed herein are those of the authors and do not necessarily reflect the views of the United Nations.

References

AACO (Arab Anti-Corruption Organization) (2010) *Corruption cost Arabs $1 trillion.* Beirut, Lebanon: AACO

Al Hajj Saleh Y (2010a) *[Regarding escalating divisions and the void of the public space in our modern societies]* Al Hewar Al Mutamadden. Available from http://www.ahewar.org/m.asp?i=3 [Accessed 26 May 2010] (In Arabic)

Al Hajj Saleh Y (2010b) *[Are our situations really static without change?]* Al Hewar Al Mutamadden. Available from http://www.ahewar.org/m.asp?i=3 [Accessed 26 May 2010] (In Arabic)

Ali AAG (2009) *The political economy of inequality in the Arab region and relevant development policies.* Working Paper No. 502. Cairo, Egypt: Economic Research Forum

Amin G (1999) *[Globalization and Arab development].* Beirut, Lebanon: Center for Arab Unity Studies (In Arabic)

Amin S (1978) *The Arab nation: Nationalism and class struggles.* London, UK: Zed Books

Amin S (1984) *The Arab economy today.* London, UK: Zed Books

Barakat H (2008) *[Contemporary Arab society: A study of transformation in*

circumstances and relations]. Beirut, Lebanon: Center for Arab Unity Studies (In Arabic)

Ben Neffisa S, Abd Al Fattah N, Hanafi S, Milani C (2005) *NGOs and governance in the Arab World.* Cairo, Egypt: American University in Cairo Press

Benar H (2007) Has globalization increased income inequality in the MENA Region? *International Journal of Economic Perspectives,* 1(4): 193–206

Bibi S, Nabli MK (2010) *Equity and inequality in the Arab region.* ERF Policy Research Report No. 33. Cairo, Egypt: The Economic Research Forum

Chaaban J (2008) *The costs of youth exclusion in the Middle East. The Middle East Youth Initiative Working Paper* (No. 7, May 2008). Dubai, UAE: Wolfensohn Center for Development, Dubai School of Government

Chaaban J (2010) *Job creation in the Arab economies: Navigating through difficult waters. Arab Human Development Report Paper Series, No 03.* New York, NY: UNDP Regional Bureau for Arab States

Chen S, Ravallion M (2007) *Absolute poverty measures for the developing world, 1981–2004.* Policy Research Working Paper,

No. 4211. Washington, DC: the World Bank

Chêne M (Author), Hodess R (Reviewer) (2007) *Overview of corruption in MENA Countries.* Bergen, Norway: Anti-Corruption Research Centre

CSDH (Commission on the Social Determinants of Health) (2008) *Closing the gap in a generation: health equity through action on the social determinants of health, Final Report of the Commission on Social Determinants of Health.* Geneva, Switzerland: World Health Organization

Economist Intelligence Unit (2010) Democracy index 2010. Available from http://graphics.eiu.com/PDF/Democracy_Index_2010_web.pdf [Accessed 8 March 2011]

Fürtig H (Ed.) (2007) *The Arab authoritarian regime between reform and persistence.* Newcastle, UK: Cambridge Scholars Publishing

Guazzone L, Pioppi D (2009) *The Arab state and neo-liberal globalization: the restructuring of state power in the Middle East.* Reading, UK: Ithaca Press

Guetat I (2006) The effects of corruption on growth performance of the MENA countries. *Journal of Economics and Finance,* 30(2): 208–221

Handoussa H, Tzannatos Z (2004) *Employment creation and social protection in the Middle East and North Africa, The Third Mediterranean Development Forum.* Cairo: American University in Cairo Press

Harrigan J, El-Said H (2009a) *Aid and power in the Arab world: IMF and World Bank policy-based lending in the Middle East and North Africa.* UK: Palgrave Macmillan

Harrigan J, El-Said H (2009b) *Economic liberalisation, social capital and Islamic welfare provision.* UK: Palgrave Macmillan

Henry CM, Springborg R (2010) *Globalization and the politics of development in the Middle East.* Cambridge, UK: Cambridge University Press

Hourani A, Ruthven M (2003) *A history of the Arab Peoples* (2nd edition). Cambridge, MA: Belknap Press of Harvard University Press

Hourani AH, Khoury P, Wilson M (Eds.) (2004) *The modern Middle East: Revised edition.* New York, NY: I. B. Tauris

Jabbour S (2003) Health and development in the Arab world: which way forward? *British Medical Journal*, 326(7399): 1141–1143

Jafari Samimi A, Ariani F (2010) Governance and FDI in MENA region. *Australian Journal of Basic and Applied Sciences*, 4(10): 4880–4882

Lewis M (2006) *Governance and corruption in public health care systems.* Working paper No. 78. Washington, DC: Center for Global Development

Loewe M (2009) *Pension schemes and pension reforms in the Middle East and North Africa.* New York, NY: UNRISD (United Nations Research Institute for Social Development)

Mahjoub A, Abdel Halim MM, al Khouri R (2010) *Assessing the millenium development goals process in the Arab region: A survey of key issues.* Beirut, Lebanon: Arab NGO Network for Development

Makhoul J, El-Barbir F (2006) Obstacles to health in the Arab world. *British Medical Journal*, 333(7573): 859

Maziak W (2009) The crisis of health in a crisis ridden region. *International Journal of Public Health*, 54(5): 349–355

Méon PG, Sekkat K (2004) Does the quality of institutions limit the MENA's integration in the world economy? *The World Economy*, 27: 1475–1498

Owen R (2004) *State, power and politics in the making of the modern Middle East* (3rd edition). New York, NY: Routledge

PCBS (Palestinian Central Bureau of Statistics) (2009) *On the eve of International Population Day 11/7/2009.* Ramallah, Occupied Palestinian Territory

Rauch JE, Kostyshak S (2009) The three Arab worlds. *Journal of Economic Perspectives*, 23(3): 165–188

Richards A, Waterbury J (2008) *A political economy of the Middle East* (3rd edition). Boulder, CO: Westview Press

Salem P (2010) *The Arab state: Assisting or obstructing development?* Carnegie Papers Number 21. Beirut, Lebanon: Carnegie Middle East Center

Sayigh Y (1991) The Gulf crisis: Why the Arab Regional Order failed. *International Affairs*, 67(3): 487–507

Shami S (2001) Middle East and North Africa: Sociocultural aspects. *In*: NJ Smelser, PB Baltes (Eds.) *International encyclopedia of the social & behavioral sciences* (p. 9792–9796). Amsterdam: Elsevier

Transparency International (2010) Corruption Perceptions Index 2010. Available from http://www.transparency.org/policy_research/surveys_indices/cpi/2010/results [Accessed 8 March 2011]

UN & LAS (United Nations and League of Arab States) (2007) *The millennium development goals in the Arab region 2007: A youth lens.* New York, NY: United Nations and Cairo: League of Arab States

UNDP (United Nations Development Programme) (2009a) *Arab Human Development Report 2009: Challenges to human security in the Arab Countries.* New York: UNDP Regional Bureau for Arab States

UNDP (2009b) *Development challenges for the Arab region: A human development approach (vol. 1).* New York, NY: UNDP Regional Bureau for Arab States

UNDP (2010a) Human Development Report 2010. *The real wealth of Nations: Pathways to human development.* New York, NY: UNDP

UNDP (2010b) Human Development Report: Indices and Data, available from http://hdr.undp.org/en/statistics/

UNESCO (United Nations Educational Sceintific and Cultural Organization) (2010) *Education for all global monitoring report: Reaching the marginalized.* Paris, France: UNESCO & Oxford: Oxford University Press

UNESCWA (United Nations Economic and Social Commission for Western Asia) (2009a) *Social policy and the state in comparative perspective: Tracking change in Arab countries.* Beirut, Lebanon: UNESCWA

UNESCWA (2009b) *Integrated social policy: visions and strategies in Arab countries.* Beirut, Lebanon: UNESCWA

World Bank (2003) *Better governance for development in the Middle East and North Africa. Enhancing inclusiveness and accountability.* Washington, DC: World Bank

World Bank (2004) *Unlocking the employment potential in the Middle East and North Africa: Toward a new social contract.* MENA Development Report 28815

Chapter

3

The Demographic Transitions: Characteristics and Public Health Implications

Dominique Tabutin and Bruno Schoumaker

Demography has a central place at the intersection of several key domains in the Arab world. These include development strategies and employment potentials (see also Chapter 2), environmental sustainability in an arid region (see Chapter 4), and international migration patterns. Demography is also important to politics as the size of population groups is at the center of discussions of refugees and minorities in the region, impacts the competition between social groups in countries such as Lebanon, and is a key factor in the Arab–Israeli conflict (Fargues 1993; Fargues 2000).

The demographic transitions in the Arab world also have profound impact on all aspects of life including health. Several chapters in this volume refer to this impact: the "youth bulge" (Chapter 18), population ageing (Chapter 20), and health system challenges (see chapters in Section 6). This chapter aims to provide a broad overview of the main demographic trends to facilitate the discussion of various public health issues, directly or indirectly linked to demography.

Approach

This chapter engages the demographic transition through three axes: through describing the main characteristics of the demographic changes over almost half a century (1960–2005), based on analyzing population growth rates and age structures; through describing the correlates of four key demographic features: fertility, mortality, international migration, and refugees; and last, through a focused discussion of the public health implications of the demographic transitions. Although our approach is primarily descriptive, we synthesize the data to identify trends, characteristics, and future challenges. Regional and sub-regional trends are expressed in average indicators. Additionally, we briefly discuss disparities

across and within countries, noting that other chapters will explore the health aspects of inequalities in more details.

Our main sources are the databases of the various United Nations agencies (Population Division, UNDP, WHO), which provide comparable records of the major changes since 1950 and key specific indicators, and various national demographic and health surveys over the past 20 years. These surveys are generally of good quality and provide the most reliable and recent information on demography and child and maternal health (see Tabutin & Schoumaker 2005). All indicators (for the whole region, sub-regions, and countries) and their definitions are presented in Web Appendix Tables.

Figure 1 depicts the chapter's conceptual framework (Demographic terms used in this chapter are defined in Tabutin & Schoumaker 2005). Population growth of a country depends on three phenomena: fertility (births), mortality (deaths), and migration (immigration and emigration). In this chapter, we also consider the issue of political refugees and stateless people because of its importance in the Arab world. The demographic transition model (Caldwell 2009) describes the passage from the traditional situation with high death rates and high birth rates, to a situation of low death rates and low birth rates, leading to low natural growth rates. The duration of transition depends on the rhythm of changes in the two main contributors: fertility and mortality declines. This rhythm may vary considerably across countries and regions depending on numerous economic (urbanization, standard of living), social (education and health), cultural (family structures, gender, religion), and political factors (population policies), which vary across regions and countries and over time. These transitions have short- and long-term consequences that are important to public health.

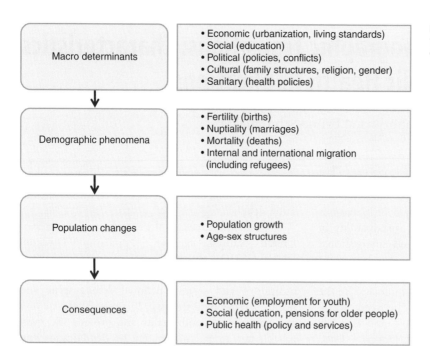

Figure 1. A conceptual framework of the demographic and population change.

Characteristics of the Demographic Transitions

We describe the characteristics of the demographic transitions in relation to past and projected population growth rates and changing population age–sex structures.

Fast Growth Rates and Varied Demographic Transitions Since 1950

Generally speaking, the entire region (Figure 2, diagram 5) began its demographic transition in the 1960s and followed the standard pattern. Mortality, initially very high (crude death rate close to 25 per 1000 population, life expectancy ~40 years), fell sharply with social, economic, and sanitary improvement. The birth rate, among the highest in the world with 50 births per thousand, corresponding to 7.5 children per woman, remained more or less constant until the early 1980s and then started to fall more quickly, with the rise in age at marriage, cultural changes, economic conditions, and national family planning policies. Earlier mortality declines leveled off, taking the region into a slower population growth. Around 2005, with a birth rate of 28‰ and a death rate of 7‰, the Arab world still experiences a fast population growth of 2.1% per year (Web Appendix Table A1).

Four models of demographic transition can be distinguished (Figure 2, diagrams 1–4): *quasi-pre-transitional model* (Occupied Palestinian Territory [OPT], Somalia, Yemen, and Comoros) with high birth rates (close to 40‰) and very rapid growth (>3% in OPT); *early but hesitant transition* (Egypt and Iraq) with birth rates ~30‰ and growth rate >2%; *classic model of ongoing transition* (Morocco, Saudi Arabia, Algeria, Libya, Oman, Syria, and Jordan) with a steady and irreversible decline of birth rates (currently ~25‰); and *advanced transition* (Lebanon, Tunisia, Bahrain, United Arab Emirates [UAE], Kuwait, and Qatar), with birth rates <20‰ and growth rates still >1%. As a result of varied demographic histories, disparities in population growth rates across the region are much larger today than in the past. Future transition in each country will be determined by economic, educational, and cultural development and various social policies.

Very Strong Demographic Pressures up to 2040

Although growth rates are indeed declining, absolute population growth and hence demographic pressure on essential goods and services (such as education, housing, food, employment, and health) is still very strong. The Arab world's population has more than

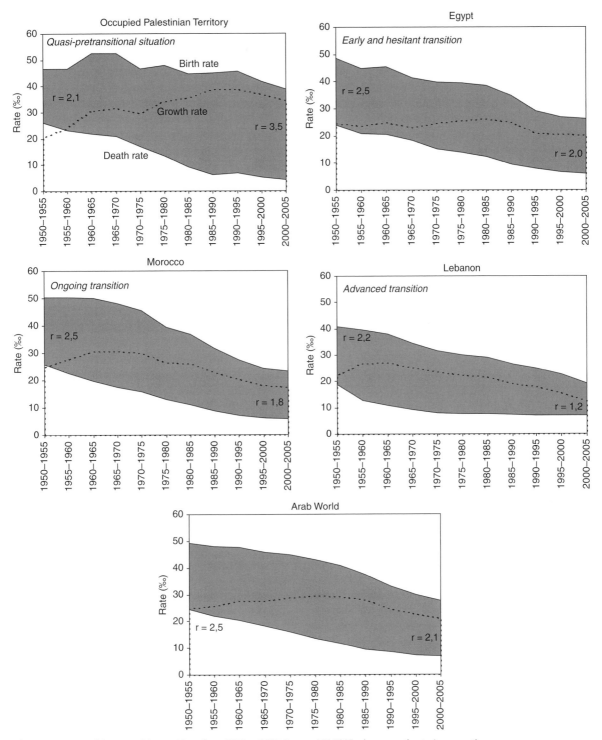

Figure 2. Types of demographic transitions from 1950 to 2005. Source: UN 2007a. (r = growth rate in percent).

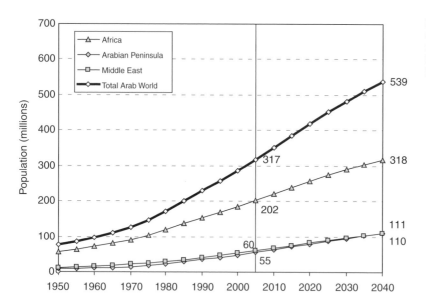

Figure 3. Population change since 1950 and projections up to 2040 for the whole region and the three sub-regions. Source: UN 2007a, medium variant for projections.

tripled since 1960 (Web Appendix Table A1). As a consequence of fertility history but also, in some cases of international migration (refugees, workers), the population of some countries, such as Saudi Arabia, Jordan, Libya, Iraq, OPT, and Yemen, has more than quadrupled in 50 years.

Although fertility and growth rates are expected to slow down (see Web Appendix Table A1 for projected rates of natural increase in 2040, around 1%), rapid population growth will continue over the next 30 years (Figure 3), from 317 million in 2005 to 539 million by 2040, and will double to 700–750 million by 2100.

While future population growth will be undoubtedly large, the situation will vary among countries (UN 2007a). Growth rates will be very rapid in some countries (Yemen, Saudi Arabia, Somalia, Iraq, Mauritania, and especially OPT), leading to a doubling of population size in 35 years. Growth rates will be more modest in others (Morocco, Lebanon, Algeria, and Bahrain). By 2040, Egypt alone will have more than 110 million inhabitants; Sudan, Algeria, Morocco, Iraq, Saudi Arabia, and Yemen will each have 40 to 65 million.

Changes in Population Age–Sex Structures

The region has a fairly young population with a median age of 22, one-third under the age of 15 and almost 60% below the age of 25. Only 6% of

the population is 60 and older. By comparison, the world's median age is 28, the developing world's 26, and East Asia's 34. There is heterogeneity within the region. Some countries have populations among the youngest in the world (notably OPT, Somalia, Yemen with median ages around 17 years), while others are well engaged in the ageing process (Tunisia, Lebanon, UAE, Kuwait, Bahrain with median ages around 28 years) (UNESCWA 2009; UN 2009). Saxena (2008) suggests three ageing patterns with profound future impact on population age–sex structures. The fast ageing countries include the United Arab Emirates, Tunisia, Kuwait, Bahrain, Qatar, Lebanon, Algeria, Libya, and Morocco. The medium ageing countries include Syria, Jordan, Saudi Arabia, Egypt, and Oman. The remaining eight countries were classified as slow ageing countries. Ageing is observed also in rural areas where it is related to rural-to-urban migration of younger people (UNESCWA 2007).

Allowing for the caution needed when using projections, in 2040 people aged 60 and over will probably account for 13–17% of the population, compared with 6–8% today, of many countries, corresponding to nearly 90 million older people vs. 20 million at present. The population percentage of people 65 years and older, currently 4%, is expected to grow to 5.7%, or 26.3 million people, by 2025 before it begins to rise more rapidly (UNESCWA 2009). The current rapid increase in the number of people aged 25–64 years in

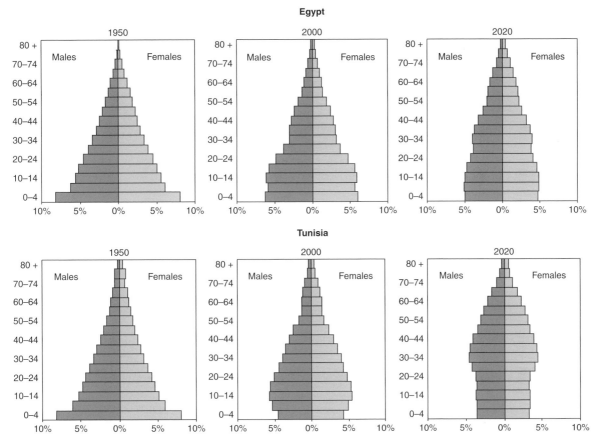

Figure 4. Population pyramids in 1950, 2000, and 2020 in Egypt and Tunisia. Source: UN (2005). Population pyramids represent the proportions (%) of each age–sex group in the total population.

the Arab countries may result in a much accelerated population ageing in the near future.

While population ageing is still at an early stage, the increase in absolute numbers of older people will present challenges to health systems, pension schemes, and rural and economic developments. Compared to the world average, the Arab region currently has one of the lowest old age dependency ratios (estimated at 5%). This ratio is expected to rise to 8% in 2025 and 13% by 2050 and will affect the total dependency rate (young and old) in the region, where the responsibility of the workforce would increasingly shift from the support of children to the simultaneous support of children and older persons.

Egypt and Tunisia illustrate past trends and future prospects of demographic transitions (Figure 4). In 1950, both countries had similar age–sex structures typical of young populations not having

undergone a fertility transition. By 2000, faster and more consistent fertility decline in Tunisia led to an older aged structure than in Egypt. These trends are expected to continue between 2000 and 2020 leading to a population with more adults and older people and less young people in Tunisia than in Egypt.

Understanding the Demographic Transitions

The determinants of population change are very complex and can be pursued in the political, economic, social, cultural spheres at the local, national, regional, and international levels. We attempt here a focused discussion of some of the correlates of three key features underlying the demographic transitions in the Arab region, which are of special interest to public health.

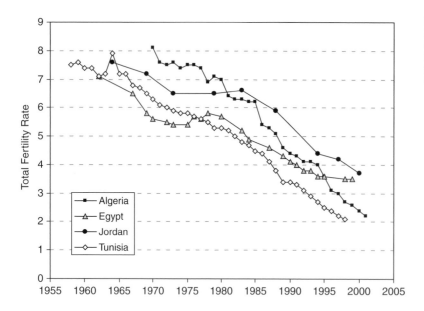

Figure 5. Total fertility rate from 1960 to 2000 in four countries (average number of children per woman). Source: Tabutin & Schoumaker (2005). Definition of the total fertility rate is provided in note 1, Web Appendix Table A2.

The Fertility Transitions: Spectacular Decline in Fertility Rates

The region as a whole has experienced a spectacular fertility decline over the past 50 years (see examples of countries in Figure 5), and especially since 1985 (number of children per woman, to which we will refer here as fertility rate was >7 in 1965, 6 in 1980, 3.7 in 2005) (Web Appendix Table A2). This decline has come fairly late compared with other developing regions. As elsewhere, there is marked diversity in the pace of change between countries and according to social stratifiers and an increase in heterogeneity over time (Web Appendix Table A2 presents regional comparisons of fertility rates in 1960–64 and 2000–04). For example, in the 1960s, fertility rate in Yemen, Somalia, Sudan, and Mauritania was 7–8; by the year 2000, the rate still hovered around 5–6. In contrast, rates in GCC countries dropped from about 7 to 2–4. Lebanon actually has a rate below the replacement level of 2.

There are multiple inter-related drivers of fertility declines which reflect change in a complex set of inter-related social, economic, and cultural realities (Darrat & Yousef 2004) in addition to the impact of policies and services. In any one country, different drivers may be at play at different periods (Khawaja 2009) but common regional drivers and patterns can be described. In every Arab country, while the demand for children remains strong and family image

highly valued, the number of desired children has been declining for the past 15–20 years among married women, notably among the youngest cohorts and among those who already have three children (Tabutin & Schoumaker 2005). Couples of higher social groups have fewer children. New social realities, such as urban living coupled with limited availability of childcare services, increasing costs of child-rearing, increasing numbers of working women, and increasing access to education, especially among women, and health services, including contraception, are important drivers of fertility decline.

Two factors, i.e., changes in timing of marriage (Fargues 2005; Eltigani 2009) and in age patterns of contraceptive use (Courbage 1999), are the two major proximate determinants of fertility decline. Changes in timing of marriage and births reflect profound and ongoing changes in the traditional family models in the region, with a shift from the large family to the smaller nuclear unit. This is undoubtedly due partly to the difficult living conditions (employment, housing, cost of living) in many countries but also because of urbanization, cultural changes, and declines in child mortality (more surviving children mean less need for more births).

Traditional marriage regimes in Arab countries, such as early marriage for women, large age differences between spouses, polygyny, endogamy, and repudiation, have changed greatly over the past decades. Indeed, some countries have undergone what we can call a marriage revolution (Ajbilou 1999; Eltigani 2000; Rashad & Osman 2001; Tabutin & Schoumaker 2005). The mean age at first marriage for women increased from 19 years some 30 years ago to the current level of 24.3 years. In 2007, this figure was 30 years in Algeria, Tunisia, Libya, and Lebanon, perhaps the highest in the developing world. Ages at marriage among men have also risen, although more slowly, now standing at around 28 or 29 in a majority of countries. Differential increases in the age at marriage between men and women have reduced the age differences between spouses: from 5 to 7 years, depending on the country, to around 4 years in a majority of countries. Only Egypt, Sudan, and Mauritania still have rather "traditional" age gaps between spouses.

Marriage at later ages, leading to an increasing mean age at child-bearing (now around 30 years in countries with the most advanced fertility transition), represents a major change in women's social responsibilities, with a shift away from complete dedication to marriage and child-bearing beginning during or just after adolescence. Women now commonly experience an extended period of single life, particularly in Lebanon and North African countries: in Algeria, the proportions of never-married women are currently 58% at ages 25–29, 34% at 30–34, and 17% at 35–39. Later marriage is likely related to the longer time spent in education, cultural factors, unemployment among young people, and housing shortages. The extended single life is still frequently lived within the family sphere, in contexts often characterized by low female economic activity and by a strong social and family control over the personal choices and sexuality of young people, especially young women (Obermeyer 2000).

The importance of the aforementioned changes is reflected in the observation that in a majority of Arab countries, fertility has decreased at all ages with the sharpest declines in women below age 25 and above age 40. Given that infant mortality is higher among offspring of younger and older women, the noted change in timing of births contributed to declining infant mortality. In turn, lower child mortality may have contributed to lower fertility, as couples perceive that fewer "replacement" births are needed. This showcases the complexity of factors contributing to the demographic transitions.

There are additional contributors to fertility decline. Polygyny has been practiced in all Islamic societies and remains authorized by all Arab states (except Tunisia since 1956). Compared with sub-Saharan Africa, it has never been a dominant marriage system in the region and is showing clear signs of decline in a majority of countries, notably in North Africa. Abortion, legal only in Tunisia since 1965, is a taboo subject that receives little attention in official surveys, although clinicians acknowledge its daily occurrence. Limited data from Morocco and Egypt suggest possibly the growing importance of this issue (Johnston & Hill 1996). Other factors include postpartum abstinence and insusceptibility (which depends on the duration of breastfeeding, Web Appendix Table A2), fecundability, sterility, and fetal mortality (Ben-Salem & Locoh 2001; Eltigani 2000).

The Mortality Transitions: Falling Death Rates and Rising Life Expectancies

The Arab world has experienced remarkable reduction in death rates and prolongation of life expectancy over the past few decades. This mortality transition began slightly later than in other developing regions but was very rapid thereafter. Crude deaths rates dropped from approximately 24 per 1000 around 1950 to approximately 7 around 2000 (Saxena 2008). Correspondingly, life expectancy rose from a very low level of 46.5 years in the 1960s (Web Appendix Table A3) to almost 67 years now, matching Southeast Asia's (67.2 years), but trailing Latin America's (71.3 years) and East Asia's (72.6 years). Large sub-regional inequalities persist today. Life expectancies range from below 57 years in the poorest countries (Sudan, Somalia, Djibouti) to 70 years or more in countries of North Africa, Mashreq, or GCC. Life expectancies in Kuwait and UAE (around 78 years) are close to those in Western countries.

All population groups have seen mortality declines but to different degrees. Mortality and morbidity patterns of different population groups are discussed in chapters of Section 4. There are many determinants of, and contributors to, the patterns of mortality transitions in the Arab world, some of which are already discussed under the fertility transitions. Very diverse social, economic, environmental, and public health factors highlight the importance of enlightened policies. Some of these factors will be examined later and in other chapters.

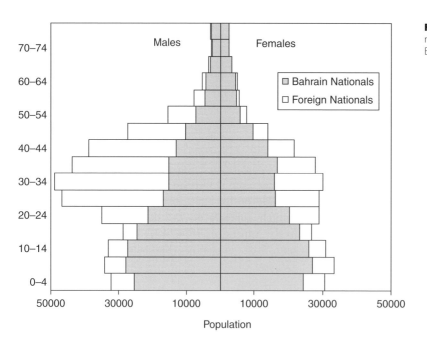

Figure 6. Age and sex structure by nationality of the resident population of Bahrain in 2001. Source: 2001 Census Data.

International Migration: Intense and Sharply Polarized Migration Flows

Despite its acknowledged importance in the Arab region, international migration as a demographic phenomenon with profound public health implications is under-studied. In 2005, international migrants (those born outside their current country of residence) made up over 10% of the population in 10 of the 22 Arab countries and more than a third of the population in the six GCC countries (69% in Kuwait, 70% in UAE, and almost 87% in Qatar) (ILO 2009). A growing share of workers in the GCC countries is from South and Southeast Asia as compared with earlier trends of having predominantly workers from other Arab countries (Kapiszewski 2004). Some countries, such as Morocco and Algeria, also have considerable emigration (Humphrey 1993; Fargues 2004; LAS 2004). Other countries, such as Lebanon, are both a source of migrant workers, for example to Gulf states and other destinations with better job opportunities, and a destination for migrant workers, for example for domestic workers and other unskilled workers from East Asia and Africa.

Migratory movements can exert strong influences on population structures in some countries (Figure 6). For the Bahrain nationals, the population pyramid has a fairly classic shape with a slight narrowing of

the base indicating a fall in fertility. However, the structure of the total population is very different, with a distinct "bulge" at the working ages (20–55 years), associated with the presence of foreign workers, with men being heavily over-represented (160 men for 100 women). There is limited literature on migrant populations, especially manual laborers who often live and work in difficult conditions and face health problems linked to long working days, accidents, and stress (see also Chapters 16, 21 and 22).

Emigration from the Arab world, especially to the Western hemisphere, has also been intense for several decades. In 2000, there were more than two million North African emigrants in six European countries (France with over half, Germany, Belgium, Netherlands, Italy, and Sweden). Approximately 1 million migrants from the Mashreq (mainly Lebanese, Iraqis, and Syrians) were recorded in these countries and in the US, Canada, and Australia (60% of them in the latter three). In contrast, emigrants from the Arab Peninsula are very few in Western countries. In addition to home remittances, emigrants participate in the flows of information and values contributing to changing social ideals and consequently demographic behaviors.

Finally, for African migrants heading to Europe, North African countries are transit countries, in which they sometimes settle for long durations. These migrant populations are not well known – as they are often in irregular situations – but are widely thought to be increasing.

Political/Security Refugees and Stateless People

The Arab world has large numbers of political refugees and stateless people who present important demographic and public health challenges. Most refugees are from the Arab world itself, with Palestinians being the oldest group and the largest stateless population group in the world. After the creation of Israel in 1948, around 750,000 Palestinians fled or were expelled to neighboring countries, mainly to Jordan, Syria, and Lebanon (Morris 1987). A large number relocated to the GCC countries, most notably after the 1967 war (Russell 1992), many of whom (up to 400,000 in some estimates) had to move again after the 1991 Gulf war due to policies in response to the position of the Palestinian leadership in support of Saddam Hussein. Most of the population of Palestinian origin (5–5.5 million out of 9) now lives outside historic Palestine (Courbage 2005) with the majority in neighboring Arab countries (3.5 million in Jordan, Syria, and Lebanon) and Israel (around 1.2 million). At the end of 2002, nearly half the Palestinian population had refugee status. Almost one-third of UNRWA refugees live in 59 camps in OPT, Jordan, Syria, and Lebanon, where living conditions are often deplorable (FAFO 2005; Rabah et al 2005).

The region has other stateless groups. The Bidoons (an Arabic term meaning literally "those without" citizenship) in the Arab Peninsula might number up to 500,000 but there has been recent progress in addressing their situation (Blitz & Lynch 2009). For several decades, Syria has had stateless Kurds, now numbering 300,000, whose political, cultural, and social demands, including health ones, remain to be addressed (Lynch & Ali 2006).

The region also has large numbers of "stateful" refugees. Iraq has millions of internally (within Iraq) displaced people (IDPs) and hundreds of thousands of refugees in neighboring Arab countries and elsewhere (see Chapter 25). Chronic conflicts in Sudan and Somalia have produced large numbers of IDPs and refugees, including Somali refugees to poor neighboring countries such as Yemen, which can barely cope with the demands of their own populations.

Public Health Implications

Because public health is implicated in every, and all, demographic issues thus far discussed, it is only practical to focus this discussion on a limited set of issues. The first concerns the speed and context of demographic transition. In Western populations, transition took a long time. The transition in the Arab world is happening over a shorter period and in the context of rather limited resources. The second concerns the nature of the health transition associated with the demographic transition and the emergence of the double burden of disease due to continued burden of infectious diseases, especially in lower socioeconomic strata, and the rise of non-communicable and chronic diseases. These issues are discussed in more details in chapters of Section 3.

The third concerns the contribution of public health policies to observed demographic transitions. While research has not fully addressed this issue, increased availability of, access to and utilization of health services (see also Chapter 28) must have played important roles. These services include contraception, prenatal care and skilled birth attendance, measures to reduce child mortality such as mass vaccination (Tabutin & Schoumaker 2005), and use of oral rehydration therapy for diarrhea (Miller & Hirschhorn 1995). Many examples are presented throughout this volume. We examine here one example most relevant to demographic change.

The use of modern contraception, an important contributor to fertility decline, has considerably increased since the early 1980s from a low prevalence among married women (4%–10% in most countries except Tunisia and Egypt), to about 36% across the region today, and, impressively, above 50% in several countries (Algeria, Egypt, Morocco, Tunisia, Jordan, and Lebanon). Low levels of use (<6%) in the African Arab countries persist (Web reference Table A2). Knowledge is no longer a major obstacle as more than 90% of married women in most countries report knowing at least one modern contraceptive method (Tabutin & Schoumaker 2005). Nevertheless, there are still unmet needs for family planning, for example estimated at 16% in a national survey in Jordan (Mawajdeh 2007), in less educated as well as younger and older women.

Differences in country use of contraception reflect not only different demands for contraception due to social, cultural, and economic factors, but also family planning policies and services. In Morocco, Steele et al (1999) examined how provision improves use. In Egypt, Hong et al (2006) correlated increased use of contraception with client perception of better quality services. The relative contribution of contraceptive use vs. social, cultural, and economic factors is highlighted in the case of Lebanon, which has the same rates of contraceptive use as in Jordan, OPT, and Syria but has lower fertility rates, probably due to higher age at first marriage and the increasing numbers of never married women and men. Despite the disparities, and consistent with what is observed in other regions, there is a strong inverse relationship between contraceptive use and total fertility in the Arab countries. Today, contraception progress remains a key factor for fertility changes.

The fourth concerns whether population and public health policies can respond to the challenges of the current and projected demographic situations. Population growth will lead to more pressures on key social and environmental determinants of health, such as land and water, housing and employment, as well as more demands for public health and social services, such as reproductive health for young people and health and living arrangements for the growing older populations (UNESCWA 2009). We see limited literature that shows planning of public health and health services based on population projections. Additionally, there is limited literature that examines population policies (see UN 2007b) from a public health perspective. We consider this to be a priority area for future research and public health planning.

Finally, understanding the magnitude, direction, and drivers of demographic changes and developing ways in a public health scope requires better integration of demography and social sciences into core public health research and actions. There is limited research that demonstrates such integration.

Conclusions

Demographic transitions in the Arab world, still under way in many countries, have been similar to those of other regions although changes have come later in this region. The three major demographic challenges that require health and social policy responses are: the short-term challenge of large numbers of youth, the medium-term challenge of population ageing, and the challenge of migrant, refugee, and stateless populations.

The speed of demographic change varies from one country or sub-region to another, reflecting differences in histories, political regimes and crises, in economic systems, and in demographic and social policies. Observing the diversity of transitions, we can draw the conclusion that Islam has not in itself constituted, or at least no longer constitutes, an effective barrier to socio-demographic change (Obermeyer 1992; Tabutin & Schoumaker 2005).

Compared to other developing regions, the Arab world's demographic history exhibits paradoxes that challenge the robustness of demographic transitions. For example, how can we explain the late fertility decline in the OPT, knowing that the country has high child school attendance and low child mortality (Courbage 2006)? Or the relative slowing-down of demographic transition in Egypt? Or the rapid changes in Morocco where access to education and social development were far behind neighboring Algeria and Tunisia during the 1980s and 1990s? Or the considerable changes that have occurred in a large number of Arab societies, where women's economic activity is relatively low, where their education is far from universal, and where their emancipation is far from complete? We hope that future research will address some of these questions.

References

Ajbilou A (1999) Crise et montée du célibat en Afrique du Nord (in French). In: D Tabutin, C Gourbin, G Masuy-Stroobant, B Schoumaker (Eds.) Théories, paradigmes et courants explicatifs en démographie (p. 641–660). Louvain-la-Neuve/Paris: Academia/L'Harmattan

Ben-Salem L, Locoh T (2001) Les transformations du mariage et de la famille (in French). In: J Vallin, E Locoh (Eds.) Population et développement en Tunisie, La métamorphose (p. 143–169). Tunis, Tunisia: Editions Céres

Blitz BK, Lynch M (2009) Statelessness and the benefits of citizenship: A comparative study. Geneva, Switzerland: Geneva Academy of International Humanitarian Law and Human Rights

Caldwell JC (2009) Demographic transition theory. Dordrecht, Netherlands: Springer

Courbage Y (1999) Issues in fertility transition in the Middle East and North Africa. Cairo, Egypt: Economic Research Forum for the Arab Countries, Iran and Turkey

Courbage Y (2005) L'enjeu démographique en Palestine à l'aube du 21ème siècle (in French). *In:* B Khader (Ed.) *Palestine: mémoire et perspectives.* Alternatives Sud, Paris, France: Editions Syllepse

Courbage Y (2006) Les enjeux démographiques en Palestine après le retrait de Gaza (in French). *Critique internationale,* 31(2): 23–38

Darrat AF, Yousef DA (2004) *Fertility, human capital and macroeconomic performance: Long-term interactions and short-run dynamics.* Cairo, Egypt: Economic Research Forum for the Arab Countries, Iran and Turkey

Eltigani E (2000) Changes in family building patterns in Egypt and Morocco: A comparative analysis. *International Family Planning Perspectives,* 26(2): 73–78

Eltigani E (2009) Towards replacement fertility in Egypt and Tunisia. *Studies in Family Planning,* 40(3): 215–226

FAFO (2005) *Palestinian refugees: Information for policy.* Borgata: FAFO

Fargues P (1993) Demography and politics in the Arab world. *Population: An English Selection,* 5: 1–20

Fargues P (2000) Protracted national conflict and fertility change among Palestinians and Israelis. *Population and Development Review,* 26(3): 441–482

Fargues P (2004) Arab migration to Europe: trends and policies. *International Migration Review,* 38(4): 1348–1371

Fargues P (2005) Women in Arab countries – challenging the patriarchal system. *Reproductive Health Matters,* 13(25): 43–48

Hong R, Montana L, Mishra V (2006) Family planning services quality as a determinant of use of IUD in Egypt. *BMC Health Services Research,* 6: 79

Humphrey M (1993) Migrants workers and refugees. The political economy of population movements in the Middle East. *Middle East Report,* 181: 2–7

ILO (International Labour Organization) (2009) *International labor migration and employment in the Arab region: Origins, consequences and the way forward.* Switzerland: International Labour Organization

Johnston HB, Hill K (1996) Induced abortion in the developing world: indirect estimates. *International Family Planning Perspectives,* 22(3): 108–114

Kapiszewski A (2004) Arab labor migration to the GCC states. *In:* IOM/League of Arab States (Ed.) *Arab migration in a globalized world* (p. 115–133). Geneva, Switzerland: International Organization for Migration

Khawaja M, Assaf S, Jarallah Y (2009) The transition to lower fertility in the West Bank and Gaza Strip: Evidence from recent surveys. *Journal of Population Research,* 26: 153–174

LAS (League of Arab States) (2004) *International migration in the Arab region and suggestions for key actions. Third Coordination Meeting on International Migration.* New York: United Nations, Population Division

Lynch M, Ali P (2006) *Buried alive: Stateless Kurds in Syria.* Washington, DC: Refugees International

Mawajdeh S (2007) Demographic profile and predictors of unmet need for family planning among Jordanian women. *Journal of Family Planning and Reproductive Health Care,* 33(1): 53–56

Miller P, Hirschhorn N (1995) The effect of a national control of diarrheal diseases program on mortality: The case of Egypt. *Social Science and Medicine,* 40: S1–S30

Morris B (1987) *The birth of the Palestinian refugee problem, 1947–1949.* New York, NY: Cambridge University Press

Obermeyer CM (1992) Islam, women and politics: The demography of Arab countries. *Population and Development Review,* 18(1): 33–60

Obermeyer CM (2000) Sexuality in Morocco: Changing context and contested domain. *Culture, Health and Sexuality,* 2(3): 239–254

Rabah J, Lapeyre F, Husseini J, Daneels I, Brunner M, Bocco R (2005) *Palestinian public perception of their living conditions. The role of international and local aid during the second Intifada.* Ramallah, OPT: IUED/UNDP

Rashad H, Osman M (2001) Nuptiality in the Arab countries: Changes and implications. *In:* NS Hopkins (Ed.) *The new Arab family* (p. 20–50). Cairo Paper in Social Science, Cairo, Egypt: The American University in Cairo Press

Russell S (1992) International migration and political turmoil in the Middle East. *Population and Development Review,* 18(4): 719–727

Saxena P (2008) Ageing and age-structural transition in the Arab countries: Regional variations, socioeconomic consequences and social security. *Genus,* LXIV (12): 37–74

Steele F, Curtis SL, Choe M (1999) The impact of family planning service provision on contraceptive-use dynamics in Morocco. *Studies in Family Planning,* 30(1): 28–42

Tabutin D, Schoumaker B (2005) The demography of the Arab world and the Middle East from the 1950s to the 2000s. A survey of changes and a statistical assessment. *Population (English Edition),* 60(5–6): 505–616

UN (United Nations) (2005) *World population prospects. The 2004 revision.* New York: Department of Economic and Social Affairs, Population Division

UN (United Nations) (2007a) *World population prospects. The 2006 revision.* New York: Department of Economic and Social Affairs, Population Division

UN (United Nations) (2007b) *World population policies*. New York: Department of Economic and Social Affairs, Population Division

UN (United Nations) (2009) *World population ageing 1950–2050*.

New York: Department of Economic and Social Affairs, Population Division

UNESCWA (UN Economic and Social Commission for West Asia) (2007) *The demographic profile of Arab countries: Ageing of*

rural populations. New York, NY: United Nations

UNESCWA (UN Economic and Social Commission for West Asia) (2009) *The demographic profile of Arab countries*. New York, NY: United Nations

Chapter

4

Environmental Degradation: The Challenge of Sustaining Life

Mey Jurdi, Rim Fayad, and Abbas El-Zein

No region in the world is safe from environmental challenges, but the ones facing the Arab region are especially severe. While the region is rich in some natural resources such as oil and gas, it faces critical shortages in others such as water and cropland needed to support growing demands. When considered in the context of projected demographic transitions and population growth (see Chapter 3), past and ongoing environmental degradation, as well as the impact of globalization and climate change, these deficits raise a serious question: can environmental resources support life for future generations in the Arab world? This question is commonly posed at the global level in relation to widespread environmental degradation, resource depletion, species extinction, and climate change. However, owing to its unique environmental profile, the Arab region may be among the first regions of the world to confront the question directly. The challenge is not just about achieving sustainable development, a concept which first received global attention with the Bruntland (1987) Commission and later in the Earth Summit in Rio de Janeiro in 1992 (UNCED 1992) and more recently made part of the Millennium Development Goals (MDGs). It is about the survival, prosperity, and quality of life of a large proportion of the region's population.

Approach

There are multiple ways of framing and approaching environmental issues. Environmental degradation can be seen as a "development" failure and thus discussed from that perspective. Increasingly, environmental challenges are framed as security issues (Brown & Crawford 2009). This is especially the case for water scarcity, which can lead to conflicts and wars in a region already blighted by political violence. Because security and development perspectives are discussed in other chapters (see Chapters 2 & 36), we focus here on environmental problems, determinants, consequences, responses, and implications for public health. We use the DPSIR (Drivers-Pressures-State-Impact-Response) framework (Smeets & Weterings 1999) loosely, realizing critiques and alternatives (Niemeijer & de Groot 2008).

Our analysis is informed by the regional realities. The Arab world has a unique environmental profile that reflects its natural resources and characteristics and sets it apart from other regions of the world. At the same time, the region boasts significant ecological diversity (e.g., seasonal snow in the mountains of Lebanon and Morocco and water scarcity in the Gulf countries and the North African Sahara). A region-wide ecosystem review affords the reader a broader perspective. Nevertheless, we attempt to expose different environmental endowments in different countries and sub-regions, as well as the variety of environmental challenges that reflect the different political, economic, and social drivers at play.

Before proceeding further, two points need clarification. First, although we focus here on the environment–public health connections we recognize that a broader perspective on the environment should go beyond an anthropocentric approach and recognize that preserving the environment is itself a vital and moral goal that requires no justification. Second, we devote more attention to the "natural" environment rather than to the "built" environment. The latter, such as housing, exposure to pollutants, and access to sanitation, has tremendous relevance for public health and typically receives more attention in public health research and practice in the region but requires a dedicated review.

Drivers of Environmental Change and Degradation

Evaluating environmental conditions in the region and their implications for public health research and action requires a good understanding of the drivers of environmental degradation, as well as those that create opportunities for positive environmental and public health action. Various drivers across the region reflect different political and socio-economic profiles in different countries and sub-regions. Nevertheless, some key drivers are at play, and have impacts, across the region.

In the past century, and especially in the past 50 years, the region has experienced profound economic, cultural, political, and social changes (see also Chapter 2), all reflected in increased environmental pressures. The rise of the oil economy, especially since the boom of the 1970s, has profoundly affected the whole region. The increased availability of resources and investments happened at a time when most Arab countries were in need of such resources in the post-independence era for development purposes (see also Chapter 1). In oil-rich countries, resource revenues were used to fund massive development projects. For non-oil producing countries, home remittances from laborers working in oil-rich countries, as well as aid and investments from these countries, also supported development projects. In addition, international aid and the politics of the Cold War played a role, for example, in the Soviet support of the massive High Dam project in Egypt and Furat Dam in Syria.

The consequent rapid development has not been particularly environmentally friendly. For example, while the region today has a weak manufacturing sector, it carries the burden of many energy-intensive industries, especially those related to petrochemicals. Both oil and gas dependence and the related industries are not considered environmentally sustainable in the long run. Similarly, while countries have invested heavily in agriculture, investment options that were pursued have not been environmentally sustainable and have not managed to bring food security to the Arab world (see Chapter10).

Increased wealth and more availability of resources for social and health programs have resulted in improved life expectancy, exponential population growth (see Chapter 3), and a shift toward consumption-intensive lifestyles. All these changes, coupled with a weak public culture of environmental protection, have major environmental impacts. As in the rest of the world, cities became the engines of economic growth, giving rise to increased urban–rural differentials in opportunities and unprecedented (and largely unmanaged) urbanization (El Batran 2008). This has stressed natural resources and environmental amenities (water, sanitation, solid waste management) (El Araby 2002) and has led to the emergence of the slums, a phenomenon previously unknown in the Arab world, with significant public health implications. For example, roughly 1.1 million people in Cairo live in "unsafe areas" (Khalifa 2010).

Conflicts (wars, occupations, and civil strife) in the region have had tremendous environmental and public health impacts. War can destroy ecosystems. For example, Israeli bombardments of a petrochemical storage facility in the July 2006 war in Lebanon led to a significant oil spill in the Eastern Mediterranean. The use of cluster bombs made many forests and rangelands in south Lebanon unsafe and often inaccessible. The deliberate drying of the southern marshes of Iraq by the regime of Saddam Hussein in its pursuit of rebels after the first Gulf War (see Chapter 25) wreaked havoc with a valuable and fragile ecosystem. The use of depleted uranium by US forces in the same war led to persistent radioactive pollution. More generally, civil wars in Iraq and Lebanon degraded and deeply changed urban environments in many affected cities, partly because of priorities given to security over other considerations. What is perhaps more pernicious is the way conflicts disrupt the ability of countries to set priorities and plan strategically. Resources are consumed in response to health, economic, and social emergencies while environmental degradation progresses, adding to the overall socio-economic burden (see also Chapter 23).

While regional dynamics have dictated specific patterns of environmental degradation, global drivers can be just as important. International patterns of trade, manufacturing, energy demand and supply, and long-range pollution such as global warming are significant determinants of environmental dynamics in the region. Global warming has especially dire consequences in this arid and dry part of the world. On the other hand, a rising global conscience concerned about threats to environmental sustainability and the pressure of international agencies for attention to these threats are now slowly being reflected in regional discussions (Tolba 2008).

Much of what happens to the environment comes down to who has the power to influence environmental policies and impact on-the-ground practices, especially in the era of dominance of the neoliberal economic framework. Policies can facilitate or mitigate the impact of various environmental drivers and processes. However, the environment has not been high on the political, and thus policy, agenda. The regional budgetary allocations for environmental safeguard do not exceed the 1% of GDP in best cases. Moreover, the existing environmental agencies lack legislative mandates, and have limited effectiveness (Nielsen & Adriansen 2005; Tolba & Saab 2009). It is safe to say that focus on economic growth and the power of special interests have delayed environmental awakening of Arab governments. There are signs that the situation may possibly be changing.

The complex inter-play of the different drivers discussed above makes it very difficult or impossible to isolate and model the impact of any one driver or set of drivers on the environmental situation. This is an important area for future environmental health research. Nevertheless, whatever drivers are at play, we can distinguish three key processes through which those drivers have impacted, and will continue to impact, the environment. These include the following: (1) resource depletion and scarcity usually due to over-exploitation of natural resources, reminiscent of patterns in middle- and low-income countries, and worsened by the impacts of global climate change; (2) rising consumerism, reminiscent of patterns in high-income countries, with over "development" and increasing energy and resource use and consequent environmental degradation; and (3) direct environmental destruction and degradation related to conflict, corruption, or irresponsible use. These processes are interrelated and play out across the region, albeit to different degrees in different sub-regions and countries. For example, rising consumerism is especially prominent in Gulf countries, which already have scarce natural resources other than oil and gas. In Lebanon, on the other hand, rising consumerism adds to the challenges of accelerated over-utilization of abundant natural resources and the environmental impacts of multiple wars and recurrent civil strife (Partow 2009).

Environmental Conditions and Challenges for Sustainability and Public Health

We present here a limited review of environmental conditions; the reader is referred to recent extensive reports (Tolba & Saab 2008; Tolba & Saab 2009; UNEP 2010) on which this review draws heavily.

Water Scarcity and Access to Water and Sanitation

Water scarcity is a defining environmental feature of the region (UNEP 2010). Various factors have led to a reduction in the annual per capita renewable fresh water availability from 3500 m^3 in 1960 to the current 1000 m^3 (compared with the global average of 7240 m^3), a level considered to represent water poverty. This will fall further to 740 m^3 by 2015 and to 550 m^3 by 2050. Only five countries, namely Sudan, Syria, Iraq, Morocco, and Lebanon, have sufficient freshwater resources to expand agriculture. The rest of the region suffers from water scarcity (Mubarak 1998). Some countries, especially Egypt and Syria, have done well in reusing wastewater. For example, in 1999, Egypt used 5228 million m^3 while Syria used 1200 million m^3 (Al Salem 2005). The GCC countries rely on desalination plants to secure 79% of their fresh water needs (UNEP 2010), up from 65% in 2000 (Al-Mumtaz 2000). This percentage is rising with the increased need, triggering growing energy, environmental, and economic concerns. It is easy to understand the security implications of water scarcity considering that 81% of regional supply comes from surface sources and that 66% of such resources are rivers that originate outside the region and are not governed by permanent treaties for fair resource sharing. This situation makes the Arab region among the least water-secure in the world (AWC 2009). Food production presents a special challenge for both water and land management: agriculture consumes 88% of water but with a limited productivity that does not allow the region to reach food security. Access to safe water and sanitation is still a challenge (Figure 1). About 83 million people lack access to safe water. Access rates showed improvement between 1990 and 2002, but this is variable (86.7% of urban and 72% of rural population). About 96 million lack adequate sanitation. Most of these people are either

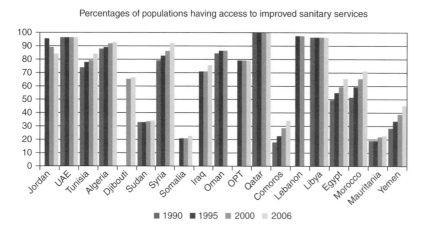

Percentages of populations having access to improved sanitary services

■ 1990   ■ 1995   ■ 2000   ■ 2006

Figure 1. Access to sanitation in Arab countries 1990–2006. Source: UNEP (2010).

in low-income countries or among the marginalized in richer ones. If these problems are not addressed, access rates will continue to decline in the future with profound impacts on public health and well-being, equity, and economic performance (UNEP 2010).

Land Resources

About 90% of the land in the Arab region is arid with annual rainfall of less than 250 mm (range, 50–500 mm). Various factors, including population growth, economic policies, and changing consumption habits, have put tremendous stress on land in the past 25 years, which, coupled with the effects of global warming (El Bagouri 2007), led to degradation of 68.4% of total land (UNEP 2010). About 98% of degradation is attributed to human activities. Food productive land now accounts for 14.1% of total land, which includes 5.1% (global average 11.5%) agriculture-ready land. This represents a drop of about 72% compared with 1980. Land degradation is equally alarming in the fragile rangelands, which represent 33% of the total land surface in the Arab world. Various factors, including cultivation and overgrazing, have affected these ecosystems, leading to soil deterioration and desertification. Between 1980 and 2005, per capita share of rangeland dropped by 33%. The Arab region has limited forests, now only 6.4% of total land (global average 30.3%), three quarters of which are in Sudan. Loss of forests is no less significant with a 34% loss over the last 25 years (Abahussain et al 2002). Land degradation takes many forms, including soil salinity, soil erosion, desertification, and loss of habitat and biodiversity. Desertification embodies well the seriousness of the region's

environmental problems, having affected 68% of the total land and threatening another 20% in the future (JCEDAR 2007).

Biodiversity and Livelihoods

The region's biodiversity is challenged by progressive destruction and degeneration of both land and marine habitats. Protected areas currently constitute less than 5% of the total land area, well below the world average (13%). Extinction threatens 1084 species (24% of fish, 22% of birds, and 20% of mammals) in the region (UNEP 2010). This unprecedented situation has profound implications for livelihoods, sustainability, and public health. Many of the region's ecosystems are already adapted to scarcity and aridity. Local crops and lands are often resistant to disease and stress. However, habitats and species in such environments often live close to their environmental tipping points (temperature, water availability, soil nutrients, etc.). North Africa is one of the top 25 global biodiversity hotspots with traditions of medicinal plant use among the oldest and richest in the world. Biodiversity loss can further worsen food insecurity and weaken the ecological basis of public health. Considering the growing importance of biodiversity in the global economy, where 40% of economic activities depend on biological products and processes, many opportunities for sustainable development will be missed in this region if the current risks of extinction persist (Diaz et al 2006).

Air Quality and Greenhouse Gases

Air quality deterioration in the cities of the Arab world is well documented and becoming a major challenge. With high private car ownership (El Raey 2006; Shaaban 2008), transportation is a leading source of emissions, contributing 90% of overall carbon monoxide. Fossil fuel energy production and consumption is a major emitter of carbon dioxide whose emissions increased by 15% between 1990 and 2003 mainly due to increased industrial and development activities. Various industrial activities produce many other greenhouse gases (GHG) and pollutants. Overall, Arab countries contribute 4.7% of world emissions of GHG. Seasonal sands and dust storm are crucial in transporting and dispersing various air pollutants within and across countries, further stressing the need for region-wide approaches (El Raey 2006).

Solid Waste

Since 1970, municipal solid waste has increased by 900% (from 4.5 M tons/year to a current 81.3 M tons/year) and is expected to increase by over 2200% (to 200 M tons/year) in 2020. This is a major problem considering the inability of current waste management systems to meet demand. Only 20% of generated waste is properly treated and less than 5% is recycled. In some countries, more than 50% of such waste combined with industrial and medical waste is managed by primitive methods of open dumping and open burning (LAS 2009). Managing hazardous waste (1.6 to 3.2% of municipal solid waste) is even more problematic given the higher risks involved. Some countries are progressing in the development of legal frameworks for proper waste management (Abou-Elseoud 2008). However, this remains the exception rather than the rule.

Environmental Conditions Through a Sub-regional Lens: The Example of the Gulf Countries

It is not possible in this limited space to take account of the remarkable differences in the environmental conditions and challenges among the different sub-regions, countries, and localities. However, understanding these differences has profound implications for regional action, as we will show later, and for locality- or country-specific solutions. For example, rapid population growth in the rich economies of the Gulf countries, mostly due to migrant workers and accelerated economic development has given rise to a whole set of environmental challenges. These include marine and coastal ecosystem destruction, large-scale construction- and demolition-related solid waste production, and high emissions of GHG amounting to 50% of the region's problems (El Raey 2006; Shaaban 2008; El-Sayyed 2008). These challenges have added to chronic problems such as land degradation, food insecurity, and critical water deficits, leading to reliance on technology to generate water through desalination. These countries often attempt to water down international agreements on reducing greenhouse gas emissions, further increasing their ecological footprints. On the other hand, some of these countries have recently enacted environmental policies and projects such as the Masdar City, projected to become the "greenest" city in the world, near Abu Dhabi and green building codes in Dubai, United Arab Emirates (Reiche 2010).

The Toll of Environmental Degradation and Scarcity on Livelihood and Public Health

While the future appears to be dire if current environmental problems are not addressed, the effects of these problems are already with us. In economic terms, the cost of environmental degradation, estimated as a percentage of GDP, is at 2–5% (Algeria 3.6%, Egypt 4.8%, Lebanon 3.4%, Morocco 3.7%, Syria 3.5%, and Tunisia 2.1%). These figures are estimated to be 1.5–2 times higher than those in industrialized countries (Tolba & Saab 2008; UNEP 2010). Tunisia's lower burden may reflect a generally better environmental performance as illustrated by international indices, to be discussed later.

The cost of the damage to the global environment is about 0.5–1.6% of GDP (Hussein 2008). These figures may underestimate true costs as they are based on studies conducted in only six countries in the late 1990s and early 2000s. Another potential source of underestimation is the methodology and the data sources. Costs are usually estimated for three types of losses: (1) loss of healthy life, estimated to contribute 60–65% of overall costs; (2) economic losses from reduced value of natural resources and drop in international tourism; and (3) loss of environmental opportunities and costs of rehabilitation to reverse or correct environmental degradation. Lack of regular monitoring and deficiencies in data reporting systems in these areas, including burden of disease and

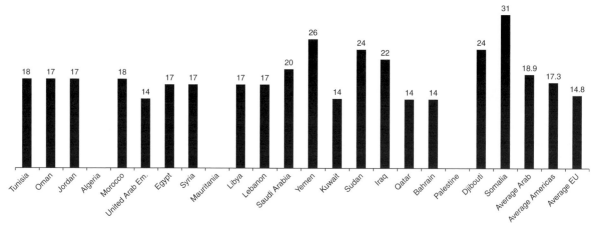

Figure 2. Environmental burden of disease (% of total disease burden) in Arab countries. Source: WHO (2007).

ill-health, may also significantly underestimate the losses and associated costs.

Environment–health connections are complex with multiple cause and effect pathways that can be explored within different frameworks (WHO & UNEP 2008). These frameworks include, for example, the narrower lens of disease burden of specific environmental exposures, or the broader scope of an ecosystem approach to health and environment (sometimes referred to as eco-health). The latter examines, in addition to negative effects, the positive health impacts of favorable environments and sees multiple pathways rather than single risk factors and disease outcomes. There are more data and research in the Arab region within the first framework rather than the latter. However, a systematic review of various exposures and disease outcomes has not been carried out. Globally, it is estimated that about 25% of disease burden results from environmental exposures. Environmental degradation-associated disease burden, as a percentage of the total burden, varies across the region (Figure 2), with the poorest countries having the highest burden.

From an equity perspective, poorer countries and vulnerable populations within all countries (approximately 60% of people live under the poverty line [UNDP 2009] and experience more environmentally related disease burden. Waterborne diseases, attributed to unsafe potable water quality and poor sanitation and unhygienic practices, are major contributors to disease burden and death, especially in the poorest countries of Comoros, Djibouti, Mauritania, Somalia, and Yemen where diarrheal diseases alone cause an estimated 16–19% of deaths among children

(Abouzaid 2008). Approximately 36% of malaria burden is attributable to environmental deterioration (deficient policies and practices regarding land use, deforestation, water resource management, and settlement location). This burden again is concentrated in the poorest countries of Mauritania, Somalia, Sudan, and Yemen (which account for 98% of reported cases). These countries have high rates of childhood deaths due to malaria (Prüss-Üstün & Corvalán 2006).

Climate change presents a new set of health challenges for the region, which are more pronounced in poorer countries (Nuwayhid et al 2009). Evidence points to the risk of spread of vector-borne diseases, such as malaria and schistosomiasis in Egypt, Morocco, and Sudan; more allergies and pulmonary disease in Lebanon, Saudi Arabia, and UAE; and worsening health impacts of heat waves in countries with hot climates.

Policy Framework for Environmental Action

Since 1986, Arab countries have signed several declarations on environment and development and adopted a regional action program on sustainable development in 1992 following the Rio summit. In 2002, under the League of Arab States banner, countries committed to a "Sustainable Development Initiative in the Arab region" aiming to develop strategies to meet the MDG 7 on environmental sustainability (UNDP 2009). Most countries today have national sustainable development strategies. However, the integration and operationalization of this concept in decision making, governance and day-to-day practice, and thus the impact on the ground, differs among countries. They are especially poor in countries with a high level of political and security instability.

Because environmental action occurs at many levels, understanding the different challenges in different sub-regions, countries, and even localities must form the basis for action especially within a framework of regional coordination, cooperation, solidarity, or integration. For example, variable rates of land degradation across the region (35.6% in Mashreq countries vs. 89.6% in the Arabian Peninsula) raise the importance of land preservation in land-rich countries such as Egypt, Sudan, Syria, and Tunisia to improve the chances for food security for the whole region. Reliance on export-oriented but soil-degrading and water-intensive crops such as cotton by some of these countries such as Egypt and Syria to generate foreign currency has contributed to land degradation. This degradation has region-wide implications that should be addressed through region-wide action to secure resources for environmental protection.

For all the work that has gone into developing regional frameworks and national strategies for sustainable development, it is widely recognized that the overall environment, policy framework, technical capacity, and state institutions for environmental work are still weak (Khordagui 2004; Tolba & Saab 2009; UNEP 2010). In most countries, the health, environment, and development/economy functions are addressed separately by different ministries and institutions rather than in integrated fashions to ensure sustainability. National environmental institutions and ministries of environment are recent, underfunded, much weaker than social and economic ministries, and have limited mandates and powers to make the needed change. Institutional capacity building activities for environmental sustainability have been ongoing since the 1992 Rio Summit with modest results. Many joint projects between international agencies and ministries employ contracted personnel who will quit the governmental units upon project completion. This undermines the sustainability of such projects. Capacities for carrying out environmental impact assessment (EIA) are variable among countries. UN-ESCWA's efforts to harmonize EIA for member countries have not been successful.

The legal framework for environmental protection, let alone sustainability, is still weak. Environmental legislation is not well developed and is usually reactive to environmental damages rather than proactive and forward looking. Laws are not well enforced. The lack of regular monitoring and reporting and the powers of political and economic actors further undermine law enforcement. Many environmental cases are settled by civil and commercial courts that do not comprehend the seriousness of environmental degradation.

The environmental priority setting process is not necessarily strategic even if national sustainable development strategies exist. Interests of political groups and investors, availability of project funding and loans, globally defined UN projects, direct short-term outputs, and aggressive competition among the different development sectors influence the priority setting. Many selected projects may have limited impact on the high cost of environmental deterioration, the attributed burden of disease, and the progress toward sustainable development.

Traditional and New Environmental Actors

While the state remains the main actor responsible for environmental sustainability, other actors have emerged to advocate for stricter laws and policies and better enforcement, to challenge the state, and to hold it accountable. At the global level, UN agencies have pushed governments to respond to environmental problems. Civil society contributes locally innovative approaches to handling environmental problems (see example below). Many international and local NGOs throughout the region devote resources to enhancing environmental awareness, advocating environmental change, and carrying out demonstrative projects in environmental sustainability. Some of these NGOs, especially local ones, are limited by financial and human resources. Lack of governmental accountability and responsiveness undermines their impact. Criticizing government environmental policies can be risky if NGOs cross the line and threaten powerful interests. Within the current political environment of the Arab world, it is not surprising that environmental political action is still weak. Exceptionally, Lebanon is now home to three environmental political parties. Regardless of their motives and current impact, which is still small, the mere establishment of such parties holds promise for future environmental action.

Do different actors work together? Our experiences indicate this is not usually the case. This and other questions related to opportunities and frameworks for common action are clearly important research questions. Whatever the answers, the seriousness of environmental challenges indicate that different actors, including public health, must re-examine their roles. We will consider this issue later.

Support for Environmental Programs

Since the early 1990s, Arab countries have implemented, or have been in the process of implementing, various projects that aim to protect and sustain the environment. Many of these projects receive aid from international organizations, including the Global Environment Facility (GEF) an inter-country institution established in 1991 to support environmental efforts on global environmental issues. An Arab Environment Facility was established in 2007 for the same purpose. The GEF lists 169 national projects in 15 Arab countries with a total cost of almost $2 billion, of which GEF contributes 19% (see GEF project database; Global Environment Facility 2011). Egypt alone accounts for 51.3% and Morocco, Jordan, and Mauritania account for another 35.8% of these costs. NGOs and academia also raise funds from national resources and receive support for participating in regional and global environment projects. Several countries provide small grant programs to support environmental projects and research. This means that environmental efforts have received logistic and financial support and that such support remains available today through various mechanisms. The more difficult question relates to the impact and sustainability of these projects. Although some of the aforementioned projects have received favorable evaluation, long-term follow-up is not usually done. Whether the various environmental projects have been able to offset the drivers of environmental degradation and stress is unknown. We are not aware of longitudinal or modeling studies that have studied this question. An indirect way to answer this question is to look at the performance of Arab countries on indices of environmental sustainability over the years that these countries have engaged in environmental sustainability projects. We visit this issue later on.

Examples of Environmental Programs and Activities

Environmental challenges are usually addressed through work on environmental stressors (e.g., water scarcity), risk exposures (e.g., urban air pollution), health outcomes (e.g., vector-borne diseases), or ecosystems (e.g., shared marine ecosystem). These approaches are not mutually exclusive. Because of limited space, we present only a few examples.

The Challenge of Addressing Water Scarcity and Quality

From nation-defining projects such as the High Dam in Egypt to regional cooperation on water sharing to local programs on increasing water productivity, water has received tremendous attention as a top environmental issue with important security implications. Integrated water resources management (IWRM) is now considered an essential approach to water scarcity in the region (UNEP 2010). Countries are at different stages of implementing national IWRM strategies but obstacles are many (Jurdi et al 2003). These include regional geopolitics and conflict, the needs of food security vs. sufficiency, and water productivity. However, opportunities are many as well, including regional cooperative strategies, substituting water consuming crops with dry land crops, and engaging the public in addressing water stress.

A recently reported case study from Jordan (WHO & UNEP 2008, p. 50–57) illustrates how improved domestic and agricultural water management, by reducing domestic water leakage and using drip irrigation techniques, can simultaneously benefit the economy (water savings), the environment (reduced aquifer depletion and reduced energy demand for water pumping), and health (reduced rates of diarrhea). The aggregate benefit/cost was estimated to be more than 2.4:1. Inspiringly, public health professionals played a key part in this example.

Success in Reducing Consumption of Ozone Depleting Substances

Measures and projects are currently being implemented, or planned, in different areas to mitigate the impact of climate change (CAMRE 2007). Arab countries have invested considerable efforts in implementing the Montreal Protocol to reduce ozone depleting substances (ODS). Legislation and programs to reduce, control, and monitor ODS consumption, especially chlorofluorocarbons, have been enacted. Since 2000, all countries started reporting drops in total ODS consumption, the most significant

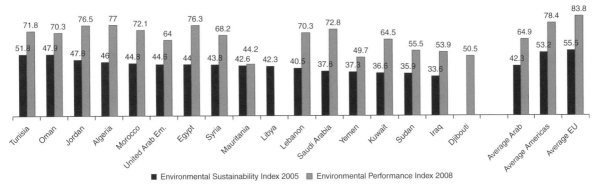

Figure 3. Computed sustainability indices for the Arab countries. Source: YCELP & CIESIN (2005 & 2008).

of which is that reported for the Mashreq countries (40% reduction rates) (UNDP 2009). The major challenge is to sustain programs and achieve set targets. There are still untapped resources that can reduce fossil energy dependence. The Arab region has high potentials for renewable energy resources such as solar resources, hydropower, wind power, and biomass (CAMRE 2007). The development of these alternatives is still limited and heavy reliance on fossil fuel remains the norm.

Civil Society–State Conflict Over Solid Waste Management

The 60,000 Zabbaleen (Arabic for garbage collectors) of Cairo have been collecting and reusing or recycling both organic and inorganic garbage for at least five decades (UN 2005). Reuse/recycle rates are quite high, up to 85% according to some reports. In 2005, conflict arose when the Cairo governorate decided to contract out the garbage collection services to three foreign companies, reportedly to "rehabilitate" Cairo's image as a modern city (Fahmi & Sutton 2006). Another conflict erupted over government-mandated large-scale slaughtering of pigs, to which Zabbaleen fed the organic garbage, during the H1N1 pandemic, a measure which was seen as over-reactive and politically motivated.

Measuring Environmental Performance of Arab Countries

The most recent comprehensive report on the environment (UNEP 2010) draws a grim picture of current conditions and trends since the early 1970s. In the face of this situation, it is useful to know how well Arab countries are responding. Many global indices

measure country environmental performance (for a review, see Böhringer & Jochem 2007). While such indices might be useful as advocacy tools, these must be approached critically and used cautiously. In addition to technical critiques of how different indices are developed, some authors (for example, Morse & Fraser 2005) have warned that some of these indices favor Northern countries and do not take stock of their true contribution to global environmental degradation.

An Arab world perspective can be illuminating in this respect. For example, if the countries that participated in the US-led invasion and occupation of Iraq were held accountable for the environmental damage they caused in Iraq, their performance on global environmental indices would drop considerably. It is no coincidence that Iraq and Occupied Palestinian Territory have made the least progress toward achieving MDG 7, similar to poorer Arab countries. Another problem with country-based global indicators is that they do not consider regional cooperation in environmental action as an indicator of success. Despite these reservations, indices can allow comparison among Arab countries and between the Arab region and other regions. For example, the overlap between middle- and high-income countries on two commonly used indicators, Environmental Performance Index and Environmental Sustainability Index (Figure 3), indicate the need to examine factors beyond national wealth.

The Role of Public Health

What can public health hope to achieve in light of the formidable environmental challenges and the obstacles to action? There are indeed many opportunities for research and practice that have been discussed at the global (Griffiths 2006; UNEP & WHO 2008) and regional levels (Nuwayhid et al 2009). There is still a paucity of research from the Arab world on a variety of critical topics. For example, the health–environment links are especially important considering that the Arab region is projected to suffer the most severe consequences of climate change. The capacities and preparedness of community and local health systems to respond to environmental threats and extreme weather events can form the basis for future interventions. Understanding the positions, capacities, and practices of public health institutions and practitioners toward environmental sustainability and threats are important research questions. Research results can be powerful tools in the hands of environmental actors to advocate for priorities in different localities, countries, and sub-regions.

Demonstrative projects that show the effectiveness of ecosystem-based approaches can prove useful in encouraging, and pressuring if needed, governments for their adoption on larger, even national scale. The global importance of such projects is underscored by the finding that health and environmental sustainability research, for example in the area of climate change, commonly focuses on health impact and proposed policies and strategies with very little emphasis on examples and implementation of actual strategies (Nichols et al 2009). Through community partnerships and participatory research (see Chapter 35), public health can learn from and support indigenous efforts by the communities to solve environmental problems at the local level and encourage innovation in different settings.

Curative care-oriented health systems in the Arab world (see chapters in Section 6) are ill-prepared to respond to environmental sustainability challenges. This provides another imperative for health system change based on a population health perspective. For example, many of the climate change-related effects on health can be mitigated through public health and health system action such as vaccines, vector control, disaster preparedness, and surveillance. Because environmental degradation affects the poor and vulnerable more, these populations may experience more inequitable health outcomes providing another imperative for social justice-oriented work for public health in this area. Public health's credibility, strengthened through earth-friendly and sustainable practices within our health institutions, can be useful in increasing public awareness of the urgency of environmental issues, the costs of inaction, and the potential benefits of prevention.

It is hard to foresee how public health, as a collective force, can make a stronger contribution beyond provision of limited technical capacity without becoming itself an important environmental actor working alongside others. This process implies a transformative process for public health, a process that necessitates introspection by public health researchers, academics, and practitioners about the place of the environment on their own agendas vis-à-vis the many other issues competing for their attention and the institutional set-ups needed to respond to environmental challenges. For example, public health academic institutions might consider integrating environmental sustainability across all activities rather than assign it to a department of environmental health. A more difficult question concerns resolving the inherent tensions between improving population health, which might consume resources, and ensuring environmental sustainability (Rainham & McDowell 2005), within our regional context. Such introspection might lead to identifying what it takes to develop an institutional framework for action on various environmental issues, nurture a critical mass of researchers and practitioners to carry out the work, and build partnerships with other actors.

Conclusions

The environmental situation in the Arab world is alarming, with formidable threats to sustainability that raise the question of the future survival of the region's inhabitants. In this chapter, we have examined the various drivers that impact environmental degradation, identifying three key drivers: rapid development linked especially to availability of oil and post-independence investments, population growth and increasing consumption, and conflict. We have identified three major processes through which drivers operate: resource depletion and scarcity, rising consumerism, and conflict-related destruction. In reviewing the environmental conditions in the region, we report on important challenges in the areas of water scarcity and access to water and sanitation, land resources, biodiversity and livelihoods, air quality and greenhouse gases, and solid waste management. Environmental degradation and scarcity have an important toll on livelihoods and public health. This is demonstrated through percentage of GDP, which is

1.5–2 times higher than in industrialized countries, and through the burden of disease, which varies from 14% (Kuwait and Bahrain) to 33% (Mauritania), raising important equity concerns.

Environmental action is slowly gaining strength in the region. The policy framework is becoming increasingly supportive of stronger action but is hampered by limited funding, inadequate intersectoral collaboration, limited regional cooperation, outdated legal framework, and poor strategies of priority setting. In addition to the state, new environmental actors, such as NGOs, are emerging. However, political environmental action remains weak. Only a few countries have green parties. The global support for environmental action holds promise in this regard. We have reviewed examples of environmental programs in the areas of water scarcity and quality, reduction of ozone depleting substances, solid waste management, and innovative ecosystem approaches. However, measures of environmental performance of Arab countries indicate the need for improvement.

This chapter has highlighted several roles for public health in addressing environmental degradation. This includes research on environment–health links, capacities of communities and health systems to respond to environmental threats, and the positions of various actors; demonstrative projects of ecosystem-based approaches; and health system changes to respond to environmental challenges. It is hard, however, to foresee a strong impact of public health without becoming itself an important environmental actor. This is our challenge today.

References

Abahussain AA, Abdu ASh Al-Zubari W, El Deen NA, Abdul-Raheem M (2002) Desertification in the Arab Region: analysis of current status and trends. *Journal of Arid Environment*, 51(4): 521–545

Abou-Elseoud N (2008) Waste management. *In*: MK Tolba, N Saab (Eds.) *Arab environment: Future challenges* (p. 111–126) Report of the Arab Forum for Environment and Development (AFED). Beirut, Lebanon: AFED

Abouzaid H (2008) Health and the environment with focus on the Eastern Mediterranean region. *Eastern Mediterranean Health Journal*, 14(Suppl.): 32–142

Al-Mumtaz M (2000), Water desalination in the Arabian Gulf region. *In*: MFA Goosen, WH Shayya (Eds.), *Water management, purification & conservation in arid climates, Volume 2: Water purification* (p. 245–265). Pennsylvania: Technomic Publishing Company, Inc

Al Salem S (2005) *Overview of the water and wastewater reuse crises in the Arab world.* Available from http://www2.mre.gov.br/aspa/semiarido/data/saqer_al_salem.htm [Accessed 15 January 2011]

AWC (Arab Water Council) (2009) Arab countries regional Report, Bridging the Water Divide between the Arab States and Their Neighboring Countries. Available from http://portal.worldwaterforum5.org/wwf5/en-us/worldregions/MENA%20Arab%20region/Consultation%20Library/MENA-Arab%20Regional%20Report.pdf [Accessed 15 January 2011]

Böhringer C, Jochem P (2007) Measuring the immeasurable: A survey of sustainability indices. *Ecological Economics*, 63: 1–8

Brown O, Crawford A (2009) *Rising temperatures, rising tensions: Climate change and the risk of violent conflict in the Middle East.* Manitoba, Canada: International Institute for Sustainable Development

Bruntland G (Ed.) (1987) *Our common future: The World Commission on Environment and Development.* Oxford: Oxford University Press

CAMRE (Council of Arab Ministers Responsible for the Environment) (2007) *Arab Ministerial declaration on climate change.* Available from http://www.docstoc.com/docs/19648772/The-Arab-Ministerial-Declaration-on-Climate-Change [Accessed 15 January 2011]

Diaz S, Fargione J, Chapin FS, Tilman T (2006) Biodiversity loss threatens human wellbeing. *PLoS Biology*, 4(8): 1300–1305

El Araby M (2002) Urban growth and environmental degradation: The case of Cairo, Egypt. *Cities*, 19(6): 389–400

El Bagouri IHM (2007) Interaction of climate change and land degradation: The experience in the Arab Region. *United Nations Chronicle*, 44(2): 50–53

El Batran M (2008) Urbanization. *In*: MK Tolba, N Saab N (Eds.) *Arab Environment: Future challenges* (p. 31–45). Report of the Arab Forum for Environment and Development (AFED). Beirut, Lebanon: AFED

El Raey M (2006) *Air quality and atmospheric pollution in the Arab Region.* Report of the Joint Arab Secretariat of the Arab States and The United Nations Economic and Social Commission for West Asia and the United Nations Environmental Program for West Asia

El-Sayyed MK (2008) Marine environment. *In*: MK Tolba, N Saab (Eds.) *Arab environment: Future challenges* (p. 75–85). Report of the Arab Forum for Environment and Development (AFED). Beirut, Lebanon: AFED

Fahmi WS, Sutton K (2006) Cairo's Zabaleen garbage recyclers: Multinationals' takeover and state relocation plans. *Habitat International*, 30: 809–837

Global Environmental Facility (GEF) Available from http://www.gefonline.org [Accessed 15 January 2011]

Griffiths J (2006) Mini-symposium: Health and environmental sustainability: The convergence of public health and sustainable development. *Public Health*, 120(7): 581–584

Hussein MA (2008) Cost of environmental deterioration: An analysis in the Middle East and North Africa. *Management of Environmental Quality*, 19(3): 305–317

JCEDAR (The Joint Committee on Environment and Development in the Arab Region) (2007) *Sustainable development of land resources, agriculture and rural areas of the Arab Region (Draft Report) Presented at the Ninth Session of JCEDAR. 4–6 November 2007.* Cairo: JCEDAR

Jurdi M, Abed Al-Razzzak M, Basma S (2003) The introduction of water resources management in Western Asia region. *Water Policy*, 5(3): 253–268

Khalifa MA (2010) Redefining slums in Egypt: Unplanned versus unsafe areas. *Habitat International*, 35(1): 40–49

Khordagui H (2004) *Sustainable development in the Arab region: From concepts to implementation. Proceedings of the Regional Workshop on National Sustainable Development Strategies and Indicators for Sustainable Development in the Arab Region.* 12–14 December 2004. Cairo, Egypt

LAS (League of Arab States) (2009) *Report of the Council of Arab Ministers responsible for Environment.* Available from http://www.preventionweb.net/files/10868_AbdulAzizAlSaud1.pdf [Accessed 15 January 2010]

Morse S, Fraser EDG (2005) Making 'dirty' nations look clean. The nation state and the problem of selecting and weighting indices as tools for measuring progress towards sustainability. *Geoforum*, 36: 625–640.

Mubarak JA (1998) Middle East and North Africa: Development policy in view of a narrow agricultural natural resource. *World Development*, 26(5): 877–895

Nichols A, Maynard V, Goodman B, Richardson J (2009) Health, climate change and sustainability: A systematic review and thematic analysis of the literature. *Environmental Health Insights*, 3: 63–88

Nielsen TT, Adriansen HK (2005) Government policies and land degradation in the Middle East. *Land Degradation and Development*, 16: 151–161

Niemeijer D, de Groot RS (2008) A conceptual framework for selecting environmental indicator sets. *Ecologic Indicators*, 8: 14–25

Nuwayhid I, Youssef R, Habib RR (2009) Human health. *In*: MK Tolba, N Saab (Eds.) *Arab environment. Climate change: Impact of climate change on Arab countries* (p. 88–98). Report of the Arab Forum for Environment and Development (AFED). Beirut, Lebanon: AFED

Partow H (2009) Environmental impact of wars and conflicts. *In*: MK Tolba, N Saab (Eds.) *Arab environment: Future challenges* (p. 159–171). Report of the Arab Forum for Environment and Development (AFED). Beirut, Lebanon: AFED

Prüss-Üstün A, Corvalán C (2006) *Preventing disease through healthy environment: Towards an estimate of the environmental burden of disease.* WHO. Available from http://www.who.int/quantifying_ehimpacts/publications/preventingdiseasebegin.pdf [Accessed 15 January 2011]

Rainham DGC, McDowell I (2005) The sustainability of population health. *Population and Environment*, 26(4): 303–324

Reiche D (2010) Energy policies of Gulf Cooperation Council (GCC) countries – possibilities and limitations of ecological modernization in rentier states. *Energy Policy*, 38(5): 2395–2403

Shaaban F (2008) Air quality. *In*: MK Tolba, N Saab (Eds.) *Arab environment: Future challenges* (p. 45–60). Report of the Arab Forum for Environment and Development (AFED). Beirut, Lebanon: AFED

Smeets E, Weterings R (1999) *Environmental indicators: Typology & overview. Technical report No 25.* Copenhagen, Denmark: European Environment Agency

Tolba MK, Saab N (Eds.) (2008) *Arab environment: Future challenges.* Report of the Arab Forum for Environment and Development (AFED). Beirut, Lebanon: AFED

Tolba MK, Saab N (Eds.) (2009) *Arab environment: Climate change. Impact of climate change on Arab countries.* Report of the Arab Forum for Environment and Development (AFED). Beirut, Lebanon: AFED

Tolba MK (2008) Integrating environment in development planning. *In*: MK Tolba, N Saab (Eds.) *Arab environment: Future challenges* (p. 13–30). Report of the Arab Forum for Environment and Development (AFED). Beirut, Lebanon: AFED

UN (United Nations) (2005) *Changing unsustainable patterns of consumption and production. Human settlement and water.* New York, NY: UN Division for Sustainable Development

UNDP (United Nations Development Programme) (2009) *Development challenges for the Arab Region: A human development approach.* New York: UNDP

UNEP (United Nations Environment Programme) (2010) *Environment outlook for the Arab Region: Environment for development and human well-being.* Nairobi, Kenya: UNEP

UNCED (United Nations Conference on Environment and Development) (1992) The Earth Summit in Rio de Janeiro, 3–14 June 1992. Available from http://www.un.org/geninfo/bp/enviro.html [Accessed 15 January 2011]

WHO (World Health Organization) (2007) Environmental burden of disease: Country profiles. Available from http://www.who.int/quantifying_ehimpacts/countryprofiles/en/ [Accessed 15 February 2010]

WHO & UNEP (World Health Organization and United Nations Environment Programme) (2008) *Health and environment: Managing the linkages for sustainable development,*

Synthesis Report of the WHO/UNEP Health and Environment Linkages Initiative (HELI). Geneva, Switzerland: WHO & UNEP

YCELP & CIESIN (Yale Center for Environmental Law and Policy & the Center for International Earth Science Information Network) (2005, 2008) 2005 and 2008 reports. Available from http://sedac.ciesin.columbia.edu/es/esi/ [Accessed 15 January 2010]

Chapter

5

Health Inequities: Social Determinants and Policy Implications

Zeinab Khadr, Hoda Rashad, Susan Watts, and Mohamed E. Salem

This chapter presents evidence for health inequities, seen within a social-determinants-of-health (SDH) framework, and attempts to investigate the structural root causes of such inequities. It also attempts to assess whether declared health policies include an equity lens and to present the progress of a recent initiative attempting to support the adoption of inter-sectoral policies and SDH-based action for health equity in some Arab countries. Our driving question is whether the Arab countries are in need for policy reform to prioritize health equity not just in health policy but in all social and economic policies.

The chapter is divided into five sections. The first includes a brief overview of the concept of health inequity within the SDH framework and its measurements. The second provides examples of cross- and within-country inequities and briefly discusses their underlying determinants. The third focuses on examining the place of health inequities in health policies. The fourth describes a regional initiative to promote intersectoral action to address health inequities and their social determinants. The final section provides a brief synthesis of the findings and their implications.

The Concept of Health Inequities

Definitions and Framework

Health is known to be linked to the biological background, behavioral choices, or the psychological status of individuals, which are shaped by the social conditions in which people are born, are raised, live, and age. When different populations, or different social groups within a particular population, which have different levels of socio-economic or political advantage exhibit different rates of health indicators, disparities in health acquire the characteristic of being systematic and patterned. While health inequalities are defined as the differences in health between social groups of population regardless of any assessment of their structural pattern (Solar & Irwin 2007), sources, or fairness, health inequities refer to a subset of these health inequalities that are deemed systematic, socially produced, and unfair (Whitehead & Dahlgren 2006). The unfairness qualification of health inequities entails a value judgment that strongly relates to health as a basic human right and ideas of distributive justice as applied to health.

The social justice perspective entails that health inequities do not relate only to inequities in health outcomes but also to inequities in health opportunities. Such framing traces the origin of health inequities and links them to the performance of the political, social, and economic institutions and their success in securing equitable opportunities for health for all. This approach in interpreting health inequities broadens the scope of the efforts and policies for tackling them beyond the biomedical sphere. Health in all policies is one reflection of the social justice model.

The links between health inequities and social determinants are well articulated in the final report of the Commission on Social Determinants of Health (CSDH 2008), where social position is central to understanding distribution of health and well-being. But the framework moves beyond the proximate determinants defined by daily living conditions and their manifestations in material conditions, psycho-social support, and behavioral options, into the structural root causes of inequities such as socio-economic context, politics and governance, policy, and cultural and societal norms and values. Root causes may operate on the global and the national levels. Social institutions, such as the healthcare system, play a role in modifying or producing health inequities.

Public Health in the Arab World, ed. Samer Jabbour et al. Published by Cambridge University Press. © Samer Jabbour et al., 2012.

Measurements and Analysis

Health inequities are commonly assessed by comparing social categories through linking a measure of health with a "stratifier," a characteristic that reflects degrees of social advantage/disadvantage. Because of availability of data, we focus in this chapter on a limited set of stratifiers such as wealth and education. Several measures are commonly used to capture and display inequities and we use herein two measures. *Absolute differences* assess the range of the gap in rates of a health indicator between two or more social groups. This measure is influenced greatly by the prevalence of the indicator assessed, and cannot be used in comparisons between populations exhibiting different prevalence rates of the studied outcome. *The relative risk* calculates the risk of acquiring a health outcome given a negative exposure, and is independent of the prevalence of the studied outcome. Measures of health and of social disparity can be shown by the *gradient* between the different social categories or the gap between the "most" and the "least" disadvantaged. We use both measures when data are available.

Quantitative methods do not always capture the complete relationships between health indicators and social and areal stratifiers and often reduce mechanisms that produce health inequities to mere statistical artifacts. Such methods often treat determinants as sole "causes" when more than one determinant operate in complex multi-level and multi-factor processes. Therefore, an in-depth understanding of the interplay of several layers of social determinants in influencing health inequities, within a particular context, is imperative. This requires complex and inequity-informed quantitative analysis and targeted qualitative research. Such research is only slowly emerging in the Arab region.

In terms of available data, the Arab region lacks national databases which can be mined to identify health inequities and their social determinants. However, many countries have population surveys based on cluster sampling techniques that can provide representative data in certain areas of health equity. Most countries have one or more Demographic and Health Surveys (DHS) carried out since the mid-1980s. Those surveys were originally designed by USAID to monitor their child and maternal health interventions. DHS data – the sole source for World Health Statistics on health inequity – has limited, but important, use for health equity analysis as it collects data

only on married women of reproductive age and their young children, excluding large portions of the population. These surveys are rarely able to include clinical examinations and rely on reported health status.

The PanArab Project for Family Health (PAPFAM) surveys from 1995 onward organized by the League of Arab States, with the support of several international agencies, have been implemented cyclically in Arab countries. Compared to DHS, these surveys have a wider general health perspective and apply special modules for population segments neglected in the DHS such as youth and older population. Data on health inequities also can be retrieved from other national sample surveys in the region such as the PAPCHILD surveys conducted in five Arab countries during the first half of the 1990s and Multiple Indicator Cluster Surveys, which is a global project of UNICEF conducted in about 10 countries. None of these surveys were originally designed to identify health inequities. Thus, they use standardized components that are likely to omit relevant questions.

Health-focused surveys might also provide useful equity data but are not commonly national. Nationally representative health surveys have been carried out in various Arab countries, for example the Palestinian Family Health Survey and the Sudan Household Health Survey. However, health surveys do not use the same methodologies and instruments, rendering cross-country comparisons difficult, unlike the case with DHS and PAPFAM.

This chapter is not designed to present a review of existing literature on health inequities in the region. There is limited but growing peer-reviewed research on health inequities, some of which is reviewed below, with many researchers relying on analyzing datasets from the above surveys. The WHO has carried out a useful review of health inequities and their social determinants in several countries in the region (WHO 2008a; 2008b).

The key challenge of the aforementioned surveys is their limited focus on few aspects of maternal and child health and inability to represent a wider set of stratifiers. They further lack the capacity to capture context of the rapid changes in the Arab world, where many countries are challenged by conflict, water and food insecurity, and economic crises. We analyze data from available surveys while understanding their limitations with the hope that future surveys will allow us to better capture health inequities and their social determinants.

Health Inequities and Their Determinants

This section aims to demonstrate that, regardless of the level of economic development and health achievements, Arab countries do reflect a large degree of patterned inequalities, and to bring out the unfairness of these inequalities through the application of a social model approach sensitive to structural root causes. Several chapters in this volume (for example, see Chapter 7 and chapters in Section 4) provide and analyze various examples of health inequities. To achieve our aim and supplement the examples from other chapters, we carry out analyses using PAPFAM and DHS data of some Arab countries. We supplement our analyses with data from published and unpublished regional literature. The evidence reviewed here is shaped by the available datasets, which are constrained by lack of precise information on structural root causes.

If we group Arab countries according to national income (Table 1), we can readily observe that the variations in national health status indicators correspond reasonably well with the variations in income. However, if we look at health variations, measured for example by the gap in under-5 mortality, within countries according to different social stratifiers, for example between the two extreme categories of wealth or educational attainment or urban/rural residence, we see that improved national health indicators (i.e., averages) do not necessarily mean a smaller gap between the more and the less advantaged within a particular country (see Web Appendix). It is expected that these gaps tend to increase with the neo-liberal policies adopted by many Arab governments recently (Ali 2009).

Inequalities According to Classical Social Stratifiers

There is increasing research on health inequities according to well known social stratifiers. For example, wealth has been correlated with under-5 mortality rates in Morocco (Garenne & Hohmann-Garenne 2003), with healthcare utilization in Lebanon and Egypt (Elgazzar 2009), and with health expenditures (Salti et al 2010). To illustrate the degree of within-country health inequities, we analyze different measures of child, adult, and women's health (see Web Appendix) as well as healthcare utilization

according to key social stratifiers such as wealth, education, residence, and gender. With very few exceptions, these stratifiers are systematically linked to the health outcome examined. The exceptions concern child health in Lebanon and adult and women's health in Algeria and Morocco, where disadvantaged social groups exhibit better health status. These exceptions are probably due to inadequate sample sizes or to policies of positive discrimination whereby disadvantaged social groups receive more targeted health services.

Wealth (Figure 1): Health differentials by wealth (measured based on possession of consumer durable goods and household amenities) are substantial. This is particularly true for child health, where the relative risk (RR) exceeds 1.5 for under-5 mortality and for the proportion of stunted children less than 5 years of age for almost all studied countries. The situation is worse in the case of under-5 mortality with RR exceeding 2 in Algeria, Egypt, Morocco, Tunisia, and Yemen. As for adults, chronic disease RR between the poorest and richest wealth quintiles ranges between 1.02 (Tunisia) to 1.65 (Yemen). The RR for the proportion of anemic women of reproductive age ranges between 1.03 (Lebanon), and 2.42 (Djibouti).

Education (Figure 2): Health differentials by educational attainment are also substantial with the RR comparing the uneducated vs. those with secondary or higher exceeding 2 in one or two health indicators in the majority of the studied countries.

Place of residence (Figure 3): Rural residents are more likely to experience heavier burden of ill health than their urban counterparts. The differences are small in magnitude; in the majority of cases, RR for the health indicators in all countries ranges between 1.02 and 1.4. However, for four health indicators, i.e., the prevalence of anemic women in Djibouti, under-5 mortality in Morocco and Tunisia, and proportion of stunted children under 5 in Morocco, RR exceeded 1.8. Health differentials related to urban vs. rural residence are smaller than those related to wealth and education differentials. It is possible that these smaller differences are attributed to the composite nature of this stratifier reflecting both the distribution and interaction of different separate determinants such as education and income.

Health inequalities along the three previous stratifiers are not only apparent in indicators of health status but also in indicators of health care utilization.

Table 1. A Profile of Some Health Indicators in the Arab Countries by Their Income Categories

Income status	GDP/capita (2005)	LEB (years)	HALE (years)	MM/100,000 LB	IMR/1000 IB	U5MR/1000 LB
Low-income countries[1]	<2,000	52–64	45–54	430–1400	55–88	73–142
Middle-income countries[2]	4,000–9,000	63–72	54–64	62–300	15–36	17–45
High-income countries[3]	>15,000	71–78	62–69	4–64	7–20	8–25

Notes: GDP/capita = gross national product per capita category; LEB = life expectancy at birth; HALE: healthy life expectancy; MM = maternal mortality; LB = live birth; IMR = infant mortality rate; U5MR = under-5 mortality rate.
[1]Djibouti, Somalia, Sudan, Yemen.
[2]Algeria, Egypt, Iraq, Jordan, Lebanon, Libyan Arab Jamahiriya, Morocco, Syrian Arab Republic, Tunisia.
[3]Bahrain, Kuwait, Oman, Qatar, Saudi Arabia, United Arab Emirates.
Source: WHO (2008).

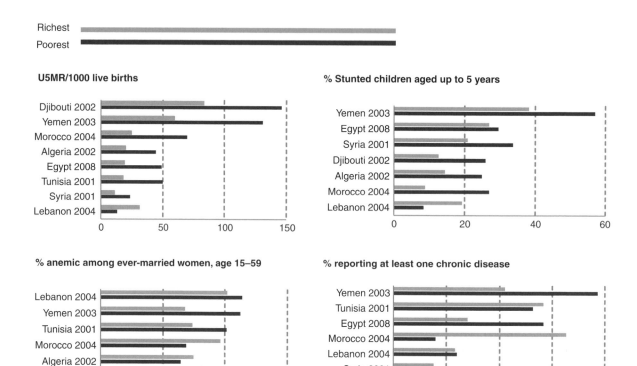

Source: calculated from special tabulations of DHS and PAPFAM data

Figure 1. Disparities in selected health indicators by extreme categories of wealth quintiles.

This is well demonstrated in Table 2 which reports on two indicators well known to be associated with health outcomes. Inequalities in births attended by skilled personnel are particularly pronounced.

Gender: Gender differentials in under-5 mortality and stunting confirm the biological advantage of female children over their male counterparts in all countries except for Lebanon and Djibouti, where girls

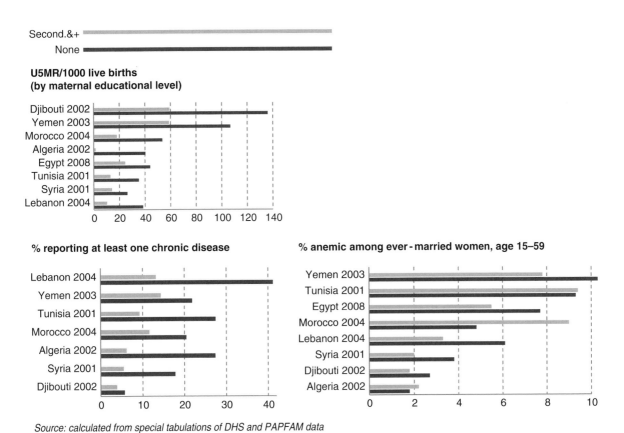

Source: calculated from special tabulations of DHS and PAPFAM data

Figure 2. Disparities in selected health indicators by extreme categories of educational attainment.

experience higher levels of mortality and Yemen, where mortality rates are equal between girls and boys (RR 1.77, 1.07 and 0.99, respectively). As for adults, the biological advantage of females seems to fade: women report higher levels of morbidity with the relative risk for having at least one chronic disease ranging between 1.32 (Tunisia) and 1.52 (Morocco). Similar findings are seen from health surveys in the Gulf countries (Table 3), which show the biological advantage of female infants (except in Saudi Arabia) and the loss of this advantage for adult females. The magnitude of the differences in adult morbidity in both analyses is too large to be attributed to biological factors and clearly reflect the impact of gender dynamics in these countries. Chapters 7 and 17 explore gender dynamics in health in more details.

Less Visible Inequalities and Unfairness of Their Root Causes

There is a large degree of interaction between various stratifiers. Actual inequalities are expected to be larger

than portrayed in the previous section given the tendency of stratifiers such as wealth, education, and place of residence to cluster in social groups. For example, postnatal mortality rate (per 1000 live births) is 6.8 for urban areas but increases to 11.5, 13.8, and 17.5, in Upper Egypt, among the uneducated in Upper Egypt, and among the poor and uneducated in Upper Egypt, respectively (source: Egyptian Demographic & Health Survey 2008).

Gender is particularly important in this regard as gender dynamics operate differently across social groups and reflect themselves differently across the other stratifiers. Females who are in the lowest wealth status, who are uneducated, and who reside in disadvantaged regions experience a much higher degree of gender biases and much higher health disadvantage by sex. A study on urban inequity in Cairo governorate shows the impact of gender dynamics on self-rated health (SRH) by social status (Figure 4). In the more privileged groups, the difference between men's and women's reports of poor SRH is small (5%) to the advantage of women. This pattern is reversed in the

Table 2. Births Attended by Skilled Health Personnel, and Measles Immunization Coverage by Residence, Wealth, and Maternal Education

Country	Year	Births attended by skilled health personnel (%)						Measles immunization coverage among 1-year-olds (%)					
		Place of residence		Wealth quintiles		Maternal education		Place of residence		Wealth quintiles		Maternal education	
		Rural	Urban	Lowest	Highest	Lowest	Highest	Rural	Urban	Lowest	Highest	Lowest	Highest
Yemen	1997	14.3	46.9	6.8	49.7	16.4	62.5	–	–	–	–	–	–
Sudan	1990	59.3	85.9	–	–	52.6	95.5	56.3	69.9	–	–	50.3	84.8
Comoros	1996	43.1	78.9	26.2	84.8	40.8	82.9	63.5	63.0	51.1	86.0	58.7	75.5
Mauritania	2000–2001	28.9	85.8	14.7	92.8	40.4	91.6	53.0	74.3	42.0	86.2	44.2	55.4
Egypt	2005	65.8	88.7	50.5	95.7	54.3	89.1	96.5	96.8	95.1	97.2	96.0	97.6
Morocco	2003–2004	39.5	85.3	29.5	95.4	65.9	48.8	85.9	94.2	83.1	97.6	87.6	96.3
Jordan	2002	96.8	98.8	–	–	90.7	98.7	94.2	95.4	–	–	80.8	95.9

Source: World Health Organization. World Health Statistics 2008.

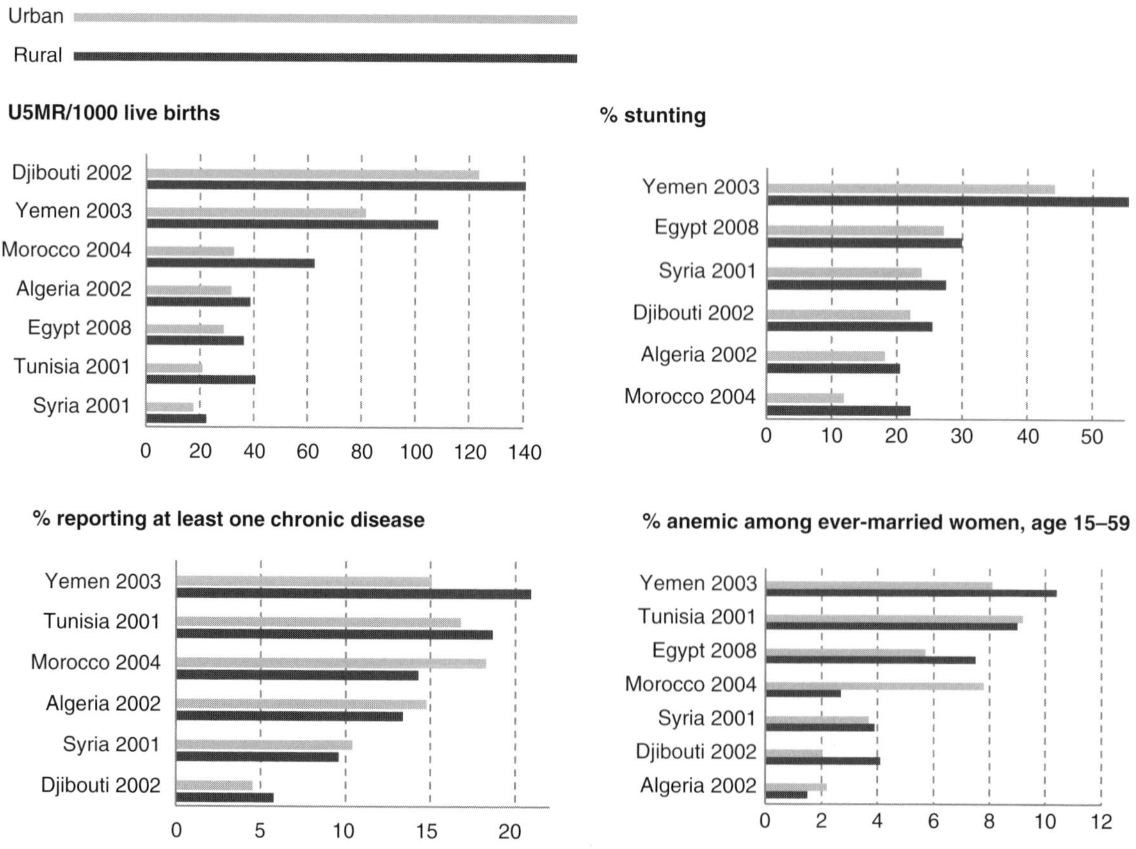

Urban

Rural

U5MR/1000 live births

Djibouti 2002
Yemen 2003
Morocco 2004
Algeria 2002
Egypt 2008
Tunisia 2001
Syria 2001

0 20 40 60 80 100 120 140

% stunting

Yemen 2003
Egypt 2008
Syria 2001
Djibouti 2002
Algeria 2002
Morocco 2004

0 10 20 30 40 50

% reporting at least one chronic disease

Yemen 2003
Tunisia 2001
Morocco 2004
Algeria 2002
Syria 2001
Djibouti 2002

0 5 10 15 20

% anemic among ever-married women, age 15–59

Yemen 2003
Tunisia 2001
Egypt 2008
Morocco 2004
Syria 2001
Djibouti 2002
Algeria 2002

0 2 4 6 8 10 12

Source: calculated from special tabulations of DHS and PAPFAM data

Figure 3. Disparities in selected health indicators by residence (rural/urban).

Table 3. Infant Mortality Rates[a] and Burden of Ill Health[b] by Sex for Some Gulf Countries

Country	Infant mortality rate			Longstanding illness		
	Male	Female	RR	Male	Female	RR
Bahrain 1995	15.1	13.2	0.87	18.1	26.2	1.45
Kuwait 1996	11.9	10.6	0.89	20.1	27.1	1.35
Oman 1995	21.4	19.2	0.9	13.1	21.4	1.63
Qatar 1998	10.2	8.2	0.8	20.2	27	1.34
KSA 1996	21.1	21.8	1.03	18.6	25.4	1.37
UAE 1995	14.5	10.5	0.72	16.3	22.5	1.38

Sources: Family Health Survey Reports.
[a]For the 10-year period preceding the survey.
[b]Among persons 15 years and over.

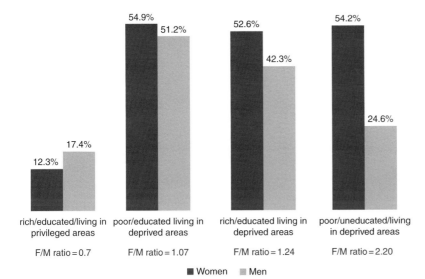

Figure 4. Percents reporting poor self-rated health by gender within different social groups, and female/male ratio calculated for each group. Source: Special Tabulation from Khadr (2008).

least privileged group where women reported poorer SRH than men and the difference is as large as 30%.

The inequalities related to the four stratifiers considered herein are quite visible and recognized in the public health domain. There are, however, many other inequalities that are less visible and tend to be ignored. Two recent studies point to such inequalities. Using a new categorization of Cairo governorate neighborhoods to high, medium, or low physical deprivation, based on land use and availability of social services (Khadr et al 2010), Khadr (2008) showed that for all age groups the percentage of sick household members was higher in the highly deprived

neighborhoods compared to the two other categories and the differences became more pronounced in the older age groups (Figure 5). El Sheneity (2008) showed a positive relationship between women's financial autonomy and a composite index that includes physical and psychological health. Report of poor health increased along a clear gradient from 20.2% among women with the highest financial autonomy to 28.1% among those with the lowest financial autonomy.

Variations in health outcomes could be explained by the variations in intermediate determinants such as behavioral forces. For example, under-5 mortality

Table 4. Intermediate Determinants of Child Mortality in Egypt by Wealth Quintiles (2000)

Intermediate determinants of child mortality	Wealth quintiles					Low/high	Low/high
	First	Second	Third	Fourth	Fifth	*Ratio*	*Difference*
Fertility related							
Total fertility rate	4	3.4	3.3	3.2	2.9	1.38	1.1
Teenage fertility rate	57	71	55	44	16	3.56	41
Antenatal and delivery care							
Antenatal visit to medically trained personnel	31.1	41.3	52.4	68.1	84.4	0.37	53.3
Delivery by medically trained personnel	31.4	45.5	61.1	76.2	94.2	0.33	62.8
Treatment of childhood diseases							
Medical treatment ARI	52.5	63.7	66.8	81.2	74	0.71	21.5

Source: Gwatkin et al (2007).

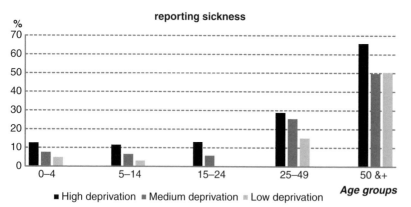

Figure 5. The proportion of the household population reporting being sick and that their sickness had affected their activities of daily living; by age group and the neighborhood classification on the deprivation scale. Source: Khadr (2008).

is shaped by many behaviorally mediated factors: maternal factors (age at first birth, number and spacing of birth, mother's health), health care factors (antenatal care and care during delivery), child care (immunization; treatment of illness), exposure to risks (hygienic practices), and nutritional factors (food quantity and composition). Such determinants are always less favorable and create more risks among socially disadvantaged groups. Table 4 (extracted from Gwatkin et al 2007) demonstrates the differences of behavioral determinants of child mortality among different wealth quintiles. Gwatkin et al report similar findings for Jordan, Morocco, and Yemen.

Why are behaviors less favorable in the disadvantaged groups? Are these behaviors governed by preferences and/or uninformed choices? Traditional health interventions and programs appear to favor such explanations and tend to engage heavily in awareness campaigns and information dissemination. Such framing does not pay adequate attention to the contextual and structural forces that shape the choices and preferences and hence do not make "healthy choices easy choices." For example, uneducated poor girls with no skills for productive careers who live in a context of biased gender relations would understandably opt for the security of early marriage and give in to the pressure of the family for a large number of children that would secure old age. Similarly, poor families without access to affordable and/or good quality health facilities would not have an adequate opportunity to use antenatal and delivery care for mothers or medical treatment of childhood diseases.

Health interventions based on understanding these determinants would have a different focus. For example, rather than preach to families against early marriage, they might support female education and employment opportunities for the disadvantaged groups.

From an equity perspective, the alternate question that needs to be asked is not just why the disadvantaged social groups behave in less favorable ways, much of which can be explained by the disadvantaged status itself, but why these groups are disadvantaged in the first place. Unequal opportunities commonly underpin the disadvantaged status. Unfair resource allocation provides an illustration of the structural roots of poor health. This is demonstrated in a study of health inequities among the five main regions in Egypt (Zaky 2009) which showed that Upper Egypt has persistently the highest infant mortality rate (Table 5). Being the most disadvantaged region, Upper Egypt is subjected to multiple inequities which add to its disadvantaged social status. For example, Upper Egypt exhibits the lowest income level and the highest prevalence of poverty, ultra-poverty, and unemployment. It suffers from significant shortages in infrastructure and the quality of the educational system is much lower than in the other regions. Health system inequities further disadvantage Upper Egypt, with this region having the lowest averages for health system inputs, which in turn are reflected in Upper Egypt's lower levels of access to health services. In brief, the structural determinants of social and economic policies manifest themselves in inequitable distribution of resources and opportunities, resulting in the clustering of deprivation in Upper Egypt, which largely explains ill-performance on health measures.

The story of Upper Egypt is not uncommon and underlies the patterned geographic health inequalities in the majority of the Arab countries. Limited systematic and comprehensive data and research from around the region about health inequities and their determinants greatly impedes the discussion of such inequities.

The Place of Health Equity in Health Policies

The framework proposed earlier in this chapter strongly suggests that governments have the main role in improving social and health equity (Blas et al 2008). Policies are the means by which governments show their political will to promote equity. In this section, which is based on Salem (2009), we examine whether Arab countries have articulated policies relating to health inequities and whether these policies are confined to the health sector alone or include social policies and/or intersectoral actions for health equity. This is carried out through exploring the existence of an equity lens in health policies in the Arab countries.

The term *policy* is defined here in terms of any official statement of health goals and the plans set to achieve these goals. Existence of health policy is assessed through studying health policy documents, such as policy papers, short- and medium-term strategic plans, goals, and objectives, published on the Web sites of the ministries of health. The limitation of the Web search is acknowledged. As noted by Ritsetakis (1987), policy is not always presented in forms of documents or text and might be expressed in administrative decisions or ministerial directives. Hence, not having a written policy on equity does not necessarily mean that equity is away from the policymaker's agenda. It is possible to have an equity oriented strategic direction without naming it as such. Furthermore, a ministry may not have a Web site or may not post or update policies on a Web site. The absence of such information may in itself reflect a weak commitment to equitable sharing of information and to equitable access to a ministry's vision and future directions. Despite these limitations, a Web analysis is a step toward a much needed and more expansive policy analysis.

Published studies on health policy analysis in general and equitable health policies in particular, in low- and middle-income countries (LMICs) are still limited. Gilson & Raphaely (2008) reviewed the published English literature on health policies in LMICs between 1994 till 2007 and identified only 164 studies. To our knowledge, an analysis of health policies in the Arab world from an equity perspective has not been previously conducted.

An Internet search in November 2010 showed that all the 22 Arab countries have official Web sites for the ministry of health. Thirteen of these had their health policies, documents on their Web sites. Only the policy documents on Comoros ministry of health had no clear statements regarding fair distribution of health in their population or equitable health access. The documents from the remaining 12 countries exhibited varying level of emphasis on health equity as one of their health policy or strategy objectives.

Table 5. Comparison of the Various Structural Determinants of Health by Region in Egypt

	Urban governorates	Lower Egypt	Upper Egypt	Frontier governorate	National indicators
Health indicator[a]					
IMR 2000	37.4	45.3	**71.2**	37.3	54.7
IMR 2005	26.0	32.7	**51.6**	33.3	23.0
IMR 2008	29.7	21.3	**36.3**	24.1	28.6
Low birth weight/100 livebirth	12.4	9.1	**12.5**	7.7	11.1
Less than average child size (%)	13.4	9.7	**16.1**	13	12.9
Health system inputs[b]					
No. of physicians per 10,000 people (MOH) (2006)	7.2	6.8	**2.1**	11.5	6.5
No. of nurses per 10,000 people (MOH) (2006)	9.4	17.1	**4.1**	36	13.8
No. of hospital beds per 10,000 people	39.6	17.9	**16.6**	32.9	21.9
No. of health units per 100,000 people (MOH) (2005)	5.5	3.4	**3.3**	6.8	3.8
Access to health services[b]					
Contraceptive prevalence	65.2	64.3	**52.7**	52.3	60.3
Receiving regular antenatal care	85.1	67.7	**56.4**	64.7	66
Delivery at health care facility	89.4	78.1	**57.5**	72.9	71.7
Delivery assisted by medical provider	92.3	85.3	**66.4**	79.1	78.9
Had postnatal care for the child within 2 working days (%)	83	69.4	**50.9**	65.7	64.6
Women reporting distance to health facilities as an obstacle to access to health care	13.7	16.5	**19**	37.3	17.1
Housing environment[a]					
Household with access to sanitation (%)	90.8	48.5	**30.5**	49.5	50.5
Educational conditions[a]					
Adult literacy rate	80.5	69.1	**63.6**	76.2	69.5
Primary pupil/teacher ratio	23.5	23.5	**30.3**	13.8	28
Primary class density	44.1	40.6	**42.9**	25.6	42.8
% of unfit school buildings	14.4	19.8	**25.5**	8.6	19.8
Economic conditions[a]					
Real GDP per capita (PPP$) (2006)	*5641.9*	*6399.1*	***5431.9***	*5903.3*	*5899.7*
% poor people of total population	*5.7*	*14.5*	***32.5***	*14.5*	*19.6*
% ultra poor of total population	*0.7*	*0.5*	***8.3***	*4.8*	*3.9*
Unemployment rate (2006)	*10.8*	*9.3*	***19.4***	*6.3*	*9.3*

Sources: [a]UNDP 2008; [b]El-Zanaty & Way 2009.

Eight of these countries, namely Lebanon, UAE, Djibouti, KSA, Iraq, Bahrain, Puntland State of Somalia, and Qatar, reported health equity as a part of their mission statements or health goals but there was no mention of clear strategies or action plans to achieve this goal. Except for Qatar, all these countries limited their understanding of health equity to the narrow perspective of equal health services provision not to the wider social determinants of health approach. Qatar, unlike the other seven countries, has recently stepped forward after establishing the supreme council of health in 2009. The council was given the responsibility to guide health reform in Qatar, to create a clear vision for the nation's health direction, set goals, and formulate policies and programs to achieve the vision. This council is headed by the crown prince. The establishment of this council reflects the significant positive steps toward adopting an intersectoral action in tackling health inequity. The remaining four countries (Oman, Sudan, Jordan, and Morocco) were more implicit in adopting equity-oriented policies in their strategic health plans. We examine these statements below.

Morocco's health strategic plan for 2008–2012 mentioned plans to adopt a multisectoral approach in the health strategy in which the health sector, other governmental departments, civil society, and the private sector actively engage in setting this strategy. The plan identified the "Difficulty in accessing health services among the marginalized population groups and rural population as well as inequitable distribution of health services across the country" are the first shortcomings in the health system. Consequently, two of the plan's main objectives were (1) to secure equity in health with particular emphasis on differentials between urban and rural areas, and (2) to increase access to health services among marginalized population groups and the rural population.

In Jordan, a higher health council was established in 1965, headed by the prime minister with the representation of several mainline ministries such as health, planning, finance, social development, labor, and others to ensure a comprehensive multisectoral engagement in setting health policies. The high level commitment to health is reflected in the statements used in the 2006–2010 health strategic plan. Terms such as *health for all* and *equity* were used in the ministry of health's mission. "Enhancing intersectoral action" was one of the main principles underlying the functioning of the ministry of health. Inequity was

reported as one of the major challenges facing the health system in Jordan.

The Federal Ministry of Health in Sudan has the longest forward-looking strategic plan in the region, spanning over 25 years. The plan, to be executed by peripheral authorities, aims to fulfill the Millennium Development Goals and improve equity across and within states, and among vulnerable groups. The plan clearly emphasizes equity in its vision for health, specifically "provision of *equitable and quality health services*" and advocates removal of barriers to access through the adoption of pro-poor policies, fostering equity, and recognizing health as a basic human right. Equitable access to health services and pro-poor policies were mentioned in 6 of the 18 strategic objectives. Nevertheless, the health strategy adopts a narrow focus on the health sector and lacks the multisectoral approach in its development and implementation.

Oman is a special case having comprehensive documents that specify health policy goals, directions, objectives, and indicators. The seventh five-year strategic plan for health development, 2006–2010, is exemplary and is based on three main pillars. The National Strategic Plan is concerned with the general goals and objectives and specifies targets using evidence-based management philosophy. The Regional Operational Plans, addressed to directorates at regional or central levels, include targets, operational activities, and the needed resources to execute and achieve desired outcomes. The Local Supportive Plans are short-term plans for one year built by each "Wilaya" (governorate system in Oman) based on local needs and developed with community participation. Oman's health development strategies have working plans and expected actions in 30 different health domains. However, there is no mention of social interventions with the objective of tackling the wider determinants of health. For instance, in tackling AIDS, eight actions are suggested to improve health and psychological conditions of people living with HIV but none address the critical issues of gender and stigma. The strategy shows, theoretically, a commitment to provide equal services for Omani and non-Omani expatriates but this is not reflected in the monitoring indicators since there is no disaggregation by the nationality status.

In conclusion, based on a simple review of Web-published health strategies and plans, it is clear that although health equity is acknowledged by almost all Arab countries and is emerging as a major concern among policy makers, it has not been sufficiently translated into comprehensive strategies tackling inequities or their social determinants. Policy documents have adopted the rhetoric of "equitable health status for all population" and "equity" but none have detailed the processes based on which these policies came to recognize the existence of health inequities and their levels and magnitudes. Although many countries such as Sudan, Bahrain, Jordan, and Oman indicated the need for strengthening the research component in their health system, there was no mention of health equity research. Our review of the processes by which countries in other global regions launched equity-oriented health policies shows a different approach. In the latter countries, policies were built on thorough documentation of health inequities, and called upon all stakeholders to contribute in identifying priority intervention areas before setting out health strategic plans (Starfield 2001).

A Regional Initiative to Address Health Inequities

The WHO's Eastern Mediterranean Regional Office has launched an initiative to address health inequities and their social determinants that is inspired by the recommendations of the WHO's Commission on Social Determinants of Health (CSDH). To address the determinants of health inequities, many of which lie outside the health sector, the initiative calls for using intersectoral action (ISA) as a key strategy. This poses a challenge in the region as the work of ministries of health and WHO offices have rarely reached beyond the health sector.

The initiative builds on reviews of SDH and health inequities in seven countries, five of which are Arab (Egypt, Jordan, Morocco, Occupied Palestinian Territory, and Oman) (WHO EMRO, 2008a) and a separate review of SDH in countries in conflict (WHO EMRO 2008b). The initiative, which has been taken up in Egypt, Jordan, Morocco, and Yemen, follows a step-by-step model to facilitate the achievement of sustainable and effective ISA.

The first recommended activity is a national stakeholders meeting to prioritize SDH and health inequities, debate next steps and identify opportunities and challenges for country action. This involves assessing national commitments and capacities to address SDH and health equity, identifying a national organization that can act as an umbrella organization for ISA, and

a Technical Working Group to translate ISA concepts into action. The first country stakeholders meeting, held in Jordan in July 2009, became a model for later meetings held in 2009 in Morocco and Egypt. In Jordan, participants came from the High Health Council, ministries of health and five other line ministries, municipal and water authorities, UNICEF, universities, and civil society. The meeting's recommendations identified the High Health Council as the most appropriate umbrella organization for the various sectors and agencies involved, and set up a Technical Working Group which later identified lifestyles, specifically female obesity, as a target for action. A variant of this approach was followed in Morocco, when the Ministry of Health Commission on Primary Health Care, at its first meeting in November 2009, identified the need to prioritize one health inequity issue, maternal mortality.

Some countries already have effective institutional structures for ISA, as in Oman with the Inter-Ministerial Health Committee at the national level and Wilayat Health Committees at the local levels. Others may have suitable structures that can undertake these responsibilities, if terms of reference are suitably revised, as in Jordan. All countries in the region are in the process of identifying SDH focal points in WHO country offices and in-country agencies, usually in ministries of health or social welfare, who will be provided with information and networking facilities to enable them to advance the ISA agenda.

At the operational level, a plan is needed to facilitate ISA, with national and field monitoring activities planned for all partners, and a corresponding communication strategy. At the local level, community structures need to be identified, perhaps modeled on local activities under the rubric of the WHO Community Based Initiative/Basic Development Needs projects (Assai et al 2006). Training and operational research activities are important contributors to these efforts. Documentation of ISA activities is already taking place, as in the case of the recent national report from Yemen.

This model is being developed in the region in an iterative manner: learning by doing and by sharing experiences. ISA activities have so far focused on countries that have some experience of activities they wish to share, or to develop further. There remains a number of countries in which ministries of health are reluctant to move beyond what they regard as their only, and unique, responsibility, the prevention, diagnosis, and treatment of disease. The reasons for this reluctance are those that hinder intersectoral cooperation and action everywhere: ISA may appear to endanger the already small funds received from central governments, to extend already overstretched capacity, and to upset established presumptions and practices. In time, it is hoped that the power of example will persuade all parties of the advantages of ISA that it is not about competition but rather cooperation for mutual advantage and toward achieving shared aims.

Summary and Implications

Until the recent past, health inequalities have been investigated and accepted as part and parcel of the inequalities in the social fabric in any society including those of the Arab countries. It is only recently and with the concerns for the widening health gaps among and within countries that the concept of social justice was introduced in the discussion of health inequalities. This concept emphasizes the need to deepen our understanding of the real causes of health inequalities and to go beyond the usual proximate determinants of health and to trace the root and structural causes of these inequalities. Social justice was clearly articulated in the conceptual framework proposed by WHO's Commission on Social Determinants of Health.

This chapter presents an overview of health inequities among and within Arab countries. A reasonably patterned association between the countries' income levels and their health status indicators appears but improved national health indicators is not necessarily associated with reduced inequities. Within countries health inequalities are investigated using illustrative examples of selected health indicators classified by simple and single stratifiers (wealth, education, place of residence, and gender) and demonstrate the persistence of health inequalities along all stratifiers. These inequalities, while variant by type of stratifiers and by country, reach significant magnitude. For example, under-5 mortality and child stunting is strongly associated with all stratifiers, particularly wealth, where RR exceeded 2 in many countries. Clustering of less favorable categories of

stratifiers translates into larger degree of health inequities. The chapter also draws attention to less recognized dimensions of health and social stratifiers.

A major contribution of this chapter is to draw attention to structural root causes and to demonstrate the unfairness of health differentials. The structural root causes discussed are not confined to health system inputs but covered social and economic determinants shaped by social policies and allocation of resources as demonstrated by the empirical case study of Egypt. Inequitable distribution of resources and opportunities plays a significant role in explaining health inequalities and in determining their unfairness.

A novel assessment of Web-posted health policy documents that, while health policies and strategies in many countries specify health equity and fair distribution of health as one of their objectives, only few countries, Oman, Sudan, Jordan, and Morocco, are making health equity a priority, and implementing strategic plans for placing health in "all policies."

The WHO EMRO has pursued an initiative to promote the inclusion of "Health in All Policies" through promoting a model of intersectoral action. This model aims to challenge the health system monopoly of actions to tackle health inequities and allow other national stakeholders to understand and actively engage in these actions. Activities to promote the ISA agenda in the area of health inequity are under way in some countries, Jordan, Morocco, and Egypt. There is clearly room for a serious policy reform supported by a research program and a process of engagement of other social sectors and members of the society.

Acknowledgment

Special thanks to Dr. Ahmed Abdel Monem, PAP-FAM manager, for providing the health indicators requested by the authors from the recent PAPFAM datasets. Susan Watts is a staff member of the World Health Organization. The author alone is responsible for the views expressed in this publication and they do not necessarily represent the decisions or policies of the World Health Organization.

References

Ali AAG (2009) *The political economy of inequality in the Arab region and relevant development policies. Arab Planning Institute working paper Series 0904.* Kuwait: Arab Planning Institute

Assai M, Siddiqi S, Watts S (2006) Tackling social determinants of health through community based initiatives. *British Medical Journal,* 333: 854–855

Blas E, Gilson L, Kelly MP, et al (2008) Addressing social determinants of

health inequities: What can the state and civil society do? *The Lancet,* 372: 1684–1689

CSDH(2008) *Closing the gap in a generation: Health equity through action on the social determinants of health. Final Report of the*

Commission on Social Determinants of Health. Geneva, Switzerland: World Health Organization

Elgazzar H (2009) Income and the use of health care: An empirical study of Egypt and Lebanon. *Health Economy, Policy and law*, 4(Pt 4): 445–478

El-Sheneity S (2009) *Diagnosis of women's needs and challenges. Unpublished Technical report submitted to UNIFEM*. The Social Research Center, America University in Cairo

El-Zanaty F, Way A (2009) *Egypt Demographic and Health Survey 2008*. Cairo, Egypt: Ministry of Health, El Zanaty Associates and Macro International

Garenne M, Hohmann-Garenne S (2003) A wealth index to screen high risk families. *Journal of Health and Population Nutrition*. 21(3): 235–242

Gilson L, Raphaely N (2008) The terrain of health policy analysis in low and middle income countries: A review of published literature 1994–2007. *Health Policy and Planning*, 23(5): 294–307

Gwatkin DS, Rutsteun K, Johnson E, Suliman A, Wagstaff B, Amouzou A (2007) *Socio-economic differences in health, nutrition and population: Egypt. Country Reports on HNP and Poverty*. The World Bank. (Similar studies by the same authors are available for Jordan, Morocco, and Yemen)

Khadr Z (2008) Comparative study of living conditions among Cairo neighborhoods. *In: Unpublished final report for the Urban inequity study*. Cairo, Egypt: the Social Research Center, The American University in Cairo

Khadr Z, Nour-el-Dein M, Hamed R (2010) Using GIS in constructing area-based physical deprivation index in Cairo Governorate, Egypt. *Habitat International*, 34: 264–272

Ritsetakis A (1987) *Frame for the analysis of country* (HFA) policies. WHO/EUR/HFA

Salem M (2009) *Health for all: Inequity in health policies in the Arab countries. Paper presented at the IUSSP international seminar "Social and health policies for equity: Approaches and strategies."* London, UK: 2–4 November 2009

Salti N, Chaaban J, Raad F (2010) Health equity in Lebanon: A micro-economic analysis. *International Journal for Equity in Health*, 9: 11

Solar O, Irwin A (2007) *A conceptual framework for action on the social determinants of health. Discussion paper for the Commission on Social Determinants of Health*. Geneva, Switzerland: World Health Organization

Starfield B (2001) Improving equity in health: A research agenda. *International Journal of Health Services*, 31(3): 545–566

UNDP (United Nations Development Program) (2008) *Egypt human development report: Egypt social contract: The role of civil society*. Cairo, Egypt: Institute of National Planning

Whitehead M, Dahlgren G (2006) *Leveling up (part 1). A discussion paper on concepts and principles for tackling social inequities in health, Studies on Social and Economic Determinants of Population Health No 2*. Copenhagen, Denmark: WHO Regional Office for Europe

WHO (World Health Organization) (2008) *Introduction and overview in 2008 World Health Report. Primary health care: Now more than ever*. Geneva, Switzerland: World Health Organization

WHO EMRO (Eastern Mediterranean Regional Office) (2008a) *Building the knowledge base on the social determinants of health. Review of seven countries in the Eastern Mediterranean Region*. Cairo, Egypt: WHO EMRO

WHO EMRO (2008b) *Social determinants of health in countries in conflict: A perspective from the Eastern Mediterranean Region*. Cairo, Egypt: WHO EMRO

Zaky H (2009) *Health system indicators with an equity lens: A case study of Egypt. Paper presented at the IUSSP international seminar "Social and health policies for equity: Approaches and strategies."* London, UK: 2–4 November 2009

Chapter

Assets and Health: Toward a New Framework

Marwan Khawaja, Mona Mowafi, and Natalia Linos

Research over the past three decades has documented the importance of social factors in determining health status, health behavior, and health care delivery. Genetics and biomedical factors alone have proved insufficient to explain variations in disease distribution and survival chances within and across countries. The sub-discipline of social epidemiology has stemmed from a research agenda, which has expanded beyond the traditional boundaries of epidemiology to include a wider array of health determinants such as the social environment (Berkman & Kawachi 2000). Engagement with social science disciplines such as anthropology, sociology, and political science has promoted a more integrated approach to health program and policy development. Socioeconomic factors, including poverty, social capital, and assets, are now considered important determinants in the global health agenda (CSDH 2008).

This chapter introduces a framework on the role of assets in the production of health and disease distribution, reviews evidence of links between assets and health status among various populations in the Arab region, and identifies research gaps and areas of possible interventions. It also elucidates some policy implications for improving health and health equity in the Arab world through strengthening assets, especially in disadvantaged communities.

An Assets Framework

Within the social determinants of a health framework (CSDH 2008), assets play a central role in understanding disease distribution. Prior literature linking poverty and health has traditionally emphasized income as the key asset. In this chapter, we propose expanding the traditional emphasis on a single asset such as income with a broader framework that incorporates economic, social, and cultural assets.

In doing so, we draw on the asset accumulation framework proposed by Moser (2007), addressing problems of poverty and household vulnerability, and Bourdieu's (1984; 1986) work on social reproduction. We believe that these frameworks are complementary. An in-depth understanding of the impact of various assets on health is required to develop a nuanced approach that can inform a new public health action agenda which traditionally focuses on deficits (Morgan & Ziglio 2007). We therefore devote a considerable portion of this chapter to discussing the conceptual basis of an assets framework.

Moser's framework elucidates the temporal dynamics of poverty, particularly the process of coping with and cycling in and out of poverty at the household level. Drawing on Amarya Sen's (1981) work on famine and entitlements and other research (e.g., Ford Foundation 2004), Moser defines assets as various stocks – including financial, human, physical, and social resources – which can be acquired and developed across generations. Assets are not viewed merely as resources to be disposed of, but also as sources of capability for people (Bibbington 1999). Unlike traditional analyses that rely solely on income, this framework analyzes how the poor mobilize their assets and entitlements to cope or "resist" economic and political shocks as "the more assets people have, the less vulnerability and insecurity they experience in the face of risk, insecurity and violence" (Moser 1998). Moser's analysis suggests that households in disadvantaged communities rarely rely on a single asset, such as income, to advance their livelihood or cope with crisis; households act strategically in managing their asset portfolios and balance the "trade-offs" between different investments. She suggests that in a context where the state's ability to provide welfare is weak, asset accumulation is more challenging than initial asset building.

Public Health in the Arab World, ed. Samer Jabbour et al. Published by Cambridge University Press. © Samer Jabbour et al., 2012.

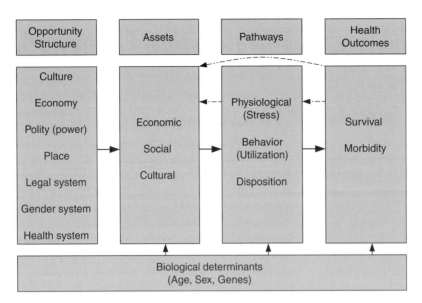

Figure 1. Conceptual framework linking assets with health outcomes.

Likewise, Bourdieu acknowledges the importance of both material and non-material assets but also emphasizes cultural and symbolic resources. His concept of capital as "the set of actually usable resources and powers" (Bourdieu 1984 p. 114) was developed within a broader study of social reproduction in French society, based on researching education and stratification. Bourdieu demonstrated that "economic obstacles are not sufficient to explain" differences in the educational success of children from various social classes (Bourdieu & Passeron 1979 p. 8), and highlighted the importance of "cultural habits and dispositions" of children. His concept of culture departed from the traditional anthropological view of it as shared norms and values, arguing that much like economic capital, cultural "habits" are assets that can be both *profitable* and *transmitted* across generations. Cultural practices constitute "status groups" or collectivities made by drawing symbolic boundaries between individuals occupying different positions in the class structure. "Social space" is structured by the *volume* and *composition* of different kinds of capital. Although Bourdieu repeatedly talks about an array of "species of capital," which cannot be subsumed under a single category, he singles out three forms in his studies: economic, cultural, and social capitals (Bourdieu 1986; Bourdieu & Wacquant 1992).

Informed by Moser and Bourdieu's work, we define assets in terms of economic, social, and cultural capital to describe varying mediating pathways through which the structures of unequal opportunity influence health and health inequities in the Arab world. A simplified schematic diagram of these links is shown in Figure 1. The proposed framework includes three different "levels" of determinants. The formation and accumulation of assets at the individual and household levels are clearly determined by broad structural arrangements in society, particularly forces that shape "life chances," as well as genetic/biological factors. The "distal" level consists of the society's opportunity structure and includes diverse institutional, political, socio-economic, and cultural factors. Biological characteristics such as age, sex, and genes are positioned at the lower level because they can affect health through intermediate factors at the individual and household levels. Both sets of determinants can influence proximal determinants and directly impact individual health; they are more relevant, however, in terms of increasing or decreasing an individual's predisposition toward ill health through their effects on assets and where the person is placed within the society's hierarchy. At the intermediate level of the framework, three broad categories of mediating risk factors with a direct impact on health outcomes are identified: behavioral, psychosocial, and individual dispositions. Figure 1 also shows that health outcomes can modify the links between the various components of the framework, including formation and accumulation of assets (Deaton 2002; Palloni et al 2009).

Economic Capital

This form of capital refers to the variety of material resources that help individuals and households manage their financial needs, including those related to health. Economic assets are not limited to disposable income, but include wealth from physical goods, durable goods that enable livelihood (such as cars and stoves), financial remittances, inheritance, land, and home ownership. Although conceptually straightforward, measuring economic capital is rather difficult, especially in low- and middle-income countries (LMICs). Studies focusing on socio-economic inequalities and health have largely focused on financial assets, although occupational class is also considered an important indicator of economic capital as well as status and power. In LMICs, monetary assets are often assessed using expenditure data and data on use of basic necessities such as food, clothing, and shelter since individuals are often more willing to report spending habits than income to data collectors. Several surveys, including the Demographic and Health Survey (DHS), collect information on household characteristics, including on the materials and quality of houses, and detailed information on household possessions, such as the presence of a radio, automobile, refrigerator, and the like. This information is often used to construct a single index, which reflects the economic capital of the household and is a reliable proxy for consumption and expenditure data (Gwatkin et al 2007).

Regional characteristics need to be considered for measuring economic capital in the Arab world. For example, household ownership or other traditional measures of wealth may be inappropriate in certain communities such as Palestinian refugees or expatriate workers where legal barriers may prevent land ownership. Similarly, in this region housing characteristics may reflect political conditions and recent conflict (i.e., damage due to war) rather than simply economic capital. Some may argue that status group (i.e., regional, family, or ethnic background) could be more important than income or social class in stratifying people in the Arab world, and that there may be important interactions between economic capital and these characteristics.

Social Capital

This concept has roots in the social sciences going back to Durkheim and Marx in the nineteenth century and generally refers to the quantity and quality of social relations (and sometimes norms) embedded in social structures which enable individuals and communities to solve problems of common concern (Portes 1998; Putnam 1993). Sociologists Bourdieu (1986) and Coleman (1988) popularized the term during the 1980s, with the former focusing on social connections and resource flows in networks, and the latter highlighting the role of social norms as social control, and the accumulation of this capital for social mobility, which ultimately yields health benefits (Edmonson 2003). In the 1990s, Putnam conceived it in structural terms – as a characteristic of communities rather than individuals, and underscored the notions of belonging, trust, and engagement (1993).

Drawing on social science, recent public health research has made useful distinctions between different forms of social capital, for example between structural and cognitive social capital (Harpham et al 2002). *Structural social capital* refers to observable social relations, and includes size and patterns of social networks, levels of civic engagement, social support, and reciprocal exchange. *Cognitive social capital* refers to "soft" unobservable elements, including norms, values, and attitudes. Szreter and Woolcock (2004) distinguished between bonding (connections within small, social homogeneous groups such as family or occupational groups) and bridging/linking (relations across social categories such as ethnic, class, or occupational groups) social capital.

A lack of consensus remains regarding the definitions of social capital as a concept as well as its measurement. Furthermore, there is considerable disagreement regarding applicability and measurement of the concept across varied cultural settings (Baum & Ziersch 2003). At the same time, until recently much of the social capital literature discounted the importance of structural inequalities (e.g., due to race, gender, and class) on the inequitable distributions of resources in society (Lynch et al 2000; Muntaner & Lynch 1999; Navarro 2002), suggesting that if individuals could only increase their social capital, that would fix their problems without resort to major social change (Harris 2001). This notion was criticized as neo-liberal discourse that advocated for individual level changes over intervention on structural inequalities (Szreter & Woolcock, 2004). Other studies in the social epidemiologic literature over the past decade have addressed issues such as discrimination, political orientation, and gender inequalities, and they have considered how these factors influence an individual's ability to gain from social assets. Box 1

Box 1. Social Capital Instruments

Nour Kibbi

Harvard Kennedy School of Government's Social Capital Benchmark Survey

- Assesses social capital in the United States (Hudson and Chapman 2002).
- Includes items to evaluate individuals' sense of belonging to a community as well as structural and cognitive displays of group membership.
- Asks about participation in formal and informal networks.

UK Department of Health

- Developed a condensed survey similar to the Social Capital Benchmark Survey for the assessment of social capital in 21 British communities.
- Includes both area level and individual level measures pertaining to levels of social participation and support, perceived levels of reciprocity and trust, civic participation, and views of the local area.

The World Bank's Social Capital Assessment Tool

- Aimed at creating an integrative instrument to assess social capital in the developing world (Healy 2002).
- The components of SCAT are tri-partite: qualitative observations made at the community and organization levels, and quantitative data collected through individual-level surveys.
- Observations of community-level concerted action, solidarity, community assets and public services, conflict resolution, institutional networks, and organizational density are included.
- Community-level perspectives offer the bigger picture of the strength of the linking capital ties.
- By conducting group interviews and making field observations of the "community at work," researchers arrive at a definition of the community and an idea of the degree of social cohesiveness.
- At the organizational-level, the channels of support and participation in formal and informal networks of an organization are identified.
- At the household level, the components of structural and cognitive capital are assessed.
- To evaluate the cognitive aspects, respondents are asked about trust, solidarity, norms, and attitudes.
- Respondents are also asked to describe structural features, including the horizontal organizational

structure, i.e. evaluate the quality of relationship they have with their coworkers or colleagues.
- (To the best of our knowledge, only two surveys on social capital are available in the Arab world.)

The Palestine Social Capital Survey

- Pioneering study in that it provides an instrument to measure social capital under condition of conflict and prolonged foreign occupation.
- Also measures bridging and bonding capital.
- Departs from OECD definition of social capital, and includes a lengthy questionnaire with 81 items covering four pre-defined domains of (1) trust in individuals and institutions (e.g., governmental, religious, political, news media, and judicial); (2) civic engagement and political participation (e.g., membership in networks and social, professional, civic, and political institutions; participation in electoral process; number of institutions in the locality and the number of its members; etc.); (3) informal social networking and social support (e.g., communicating with family and friends inside and outside Palestine, visiting neighbors, reliance on others in emergencies); (4) norm and values (e.g., volunteer work, charity work and donations, views about the future).

American University in Beirut's Urban Health Study

- Includes detailed modules on three forms of capital: economic, social, and cultural.
- Social capital indicators were intended to capture culture-specific determinants of group connectedness, inclusion, social cohesion, and degree of trust.
- Social capital concepts and indicators were organized in two clusters: community-based and individual-based (Table 1), although they capture various forms of capital including cognitive and structural components as well as bonding, bridging, and linking ties.

describes a few social capital instruments, including those used in two studies from the Arab world.

Cultural Capital

This concept has not been used extensively in public health research, but is an important component of our framework. Bourdieu (1986) introduced the term and distinguished three forms of cultural capital.

First, an "embodied" form refers to the "long lasting dispositions of the mind and body" (1986 p. 243) and includes the tastes, skills, or judgmental competences inherited or gained through extensive learning during one's upbringing. Second, objects such as book collections or musical instruments function as a form of cultural capital; their "consumption" reflects an amount of embodied cultural capital. Finally, cultural capital exists in an institutionalized state, namely educational degrees and competencies.

In *Distinction*, where Bourdieu elaborated and applied the concept most fully, cultural capital is defined broadly as a form of knowledge, a cognitive acquisition of artistic competence and talent which equip its bearer with empathy toward, and aesthetic appreciation of, cultural artifacts (1985). Such competencies often result in increased power and advantage. Although there is disagreement on how best to capture the concept in empirical studies, most social analysts define it in terms of aesthetic pursuits, consumption, and attitudes. In one of the earlier empirical studies, DiMaggio (1982; DiMaggio & Mohr 1985) conceptualized the term as multilayered, consisting of three related dimensions: (1) attitudes toward art, music, and literature; (2) activities, including the creation of artifacts, attending art events, and reading; and (3) information, including knowledge about music, literature, and art. In addition, material objects of artistic or intellectual nature may be included as a distinct form of cultural capital.

Unlike the concept of "culture," cultural capital refers to concrete practices and assets that are acquired or otherwise home-cultivated, enabling people "to generate relations of distinction which are instituted as social or status hierarchies" (Fyfe 2004). This capital plays a pivotal role in stratifying people by creating a "market of symbolic goods" (Bourdieu 1985). Taste, language, music, and other forms of cultural embodiments are conceived of as commodities that may be used by their bearers for personal gain, much like other forms of economic and social capital. Cultural capital is also similar to economic capital in that it may be unequally distributed, and hence may create opportunities for "exclusive advantage."

Since cultural capital has comparable qualities to other forms of assets, its accumulation also influences health outcomes and may be important independently or in combination with other forms of capital. While cultural assets have been largely ignored in the social epidemiologic research, there have been a few attempts to extend work in this field by exploring the link between cultural capital, social hierarchies, and health outcomes (see for example Abel 2008; Haines et al 2009). Specific characteristics of the Arab world may impact how "cultural capital" is defined and operationalized in public health research in this region. For example, in older generations, a woman's lack of a higher education degree may not reflect low "cultural capital" but simply reflect social norms at the time around female education. At the same time, given the varying artistic opportunities available in different countries of the region, an individual's lack of attendance at art/music events may simply reflect the scarcity of these events in their country or city, reflecting a structural inequality rather than lack of investment in cultural capital at the individual level.

Pathways of Influence of Assets on Health

Most of the research associating assets (economic, social, and cultural) with various health outcomes is based on observational studies, making it difficult to assess causality. Literature on socio-economic inequalities in health, however, suggests that availability and accumulation of assets may impact health outcomes through various mechanisms in complex, multilayered, and often indirect ways. Two main mediating pathways are widely cited: material and psychosocial (Marmot 1999; Lynch 2000). In other words, the debate is framed into whether health inequality is caused by absolute deprivation (material) or relative deprivation (psychosocial). This debate may be relevant to cultural and social capital as well.

Proponents of the "material deprivation" argument assert that material assets are related to health outcomes through nutrition, good quality housing, hygiene, and other aspects of living or working conditions, all of which are linked directly to socio-economic status. A related mechanism is access to and utilization of services, especially health care. While deprivation mostly affects the poorest, it can also affect health across socio-economic strata at the community or neighborhood levels. Satisfying basic needs, rather than tackling issues of inequality per se, is the main goal of proponents of this approach.

Proponents of psychosocial mediators argue that relative position in the social hierarchy impacts health outcomes through increased stress and other adverse physiological effects (Wilkinson 1996). Involvement in social or cultural activities may lead to changes in critical hormone levels or other psychosomatic responses. Inequality in assets can also influence health through emotions and affective states (Gallo & Matthews 1999). For cultural participation especially, a growing body of research demonstrates the healing potential of creative, arousing, emotionally or intellectually stimulating activities (see for example, Bojner-Horwitz et al 2003). People at the lower end of the socio-economic spectrum can suffer from hopelessness, anger, anxiety, and depression, and these may be associated with higher risks of mortality and disease. Wilkinson (1997) argues that socio-economic equality is associated with better health at the macrolevel because the former leads to improvement in social cohesion, security, and high self-esteem.

In addition to material and psychosocial pathways, social and cultural capital can affect health in other indirect ways. At the individual and family levels, "bonding" social capital may lead to instrumental and emotional support. Social capital may enhance participation in local governance at the neighborhood or community level and may provide opportunities for empowering marginalized and underserved groups to share information and coordinate their efforts for challenging inequity and injustice. Well connected and cohesive communities can also change policy and practices either directly or through influencing prevailing norms and values concerning the health and well-being of vulnerable groups. A related pathway is vertical, *linking social capital* where social movement organizations can play a role in advocacy and in mobilizing people for demanding access to resources and infrastructure (Korten 1990). Although such organizations may not explicitly be focused on improving health, their actions can have spill-over effects by intervening on critical social determinants of health.

Two notes are important to consider. First, reverse causality between social capital and health may make it difficult to interpret research findings. For example, healthy individuals and families may be in a better position to cope with stressful situations and to participate in economic and community activities. Second, while social capital is usually perceived in positive terms, it may have deleterious effects on health. Publication bias may play a role in this perception. While having dense social networks and multiple social resources may lead to positive health outcomes, they may also increase burdens on individuals who are often the caretakers in relationships. In "traditional" societies in which social structure is often organized around the collective rather than the individual, this factor may be significant. In such an environment, having more individuals in one's network could mean an increase in daily responsibility and stress, resulting in poor health outcomes. We need to test such hypotheses to better understand the complex associations between social capital and health status.

With regard to cultural capital, cultural participation may impact family health by making women more self-confident, improved problem solvers, and better care providers (Khawaja et al 2007). In largely patriarchal contexts such as those found in the Arab world, watching entertainment programs on television and going to movies and art exhibitions may provide women with opportunities for exposure to more autonomous female role models as well as alternative perspectives on living. People who accumulate cultural assets are capable of generating "relations of distinction which are instituted as social or status hierarchies" (Fyfe 2004). They are also more likely to have better social skills, including more effective negotiation and communication skills which enable them to transform this cultural capital into tangible health benefits for them and their families. Maternal education is one example of this link between cultural capital and health.

Assets and Health in the Arab World

While evidence linking assets and health is still limited in the Arab world, published studies suggest that economic, social, and cultural resources play a varied role in health and survival chances. Before reviewing this evidence, we must stress the importance of a sound conceptualization to understanding and measuring assets in the region. Our approach would utilize the proposed framework while adopting it to regional realities and specificities. For example, with regard to measuring economic capital, we must bear in mind that this region has one of the lowest female labor force participation in the world. In such a case, wage data or occupational class may not be very useful in research that explores links between women's health and economic assets. High youth unemployment may make a corresponding measure inappropriate for this group. As mentioned earlier, household ownership may be a problematic measure in communities such as Palestinian refugees where legal barriers may prevent land ownership. Some argue that status group (i.e., family, or ethnic background), which incorporates social and cultural assets, could be more important than income or social class in stratifying people. Similarly, when measuring social capital in certain countries in the region it may be necessary to take into account political aspects, including how social networks may be influenced by historic or current civil conflict.

Understanding the macro-level cultural, social, and economic features that directly impact asset accumulation and its consequences in the Arab world also requires assessments of legal and regulatory frameworks governing markets and state–society relations, type of political regime, inter-organizational relations, strength of civil society groups, political stability and conflict, overall economic conditions, as well as cultural norms or values. These dimensions are interrelated, and the capacity of people and communities to access and accumulate assets often depends on these macro-level conditions.

In the remainder of this section, we review the current literature on assets and health in the Arab region following the proposed framework. Synthesis of this evidence (currently limited in quantity and scope) is important to identifying gaps that can be addressed in future research.

Economic Capital and Health

The link between economic wealth and health has been well established in the literature. Many studies show health inequities associated with inequitable distribution of economic resources (Kawachi 2000; Subramanian & Kawachi 2007). In the Arab context, household income may not be the most crucial source of economic buoyancy, and may have a relatively weak association with health outcomes compared to Western nations. The income–health links vary between Arab countries, depending on their sources of economic wealth and level of development. Oil-rich nations differ dramatically from poorer countries such as Yemen and Sudan. While Kuwait protects against poverty by distributing an annual stipend to its citizens, the equivalent of a "dividend" from national profits, poorer Arab countries do not have this type of economic security. On the contrary, the latter have high poverty and unemployment rates, making access to liquid assets a major challenge.

In poorer Arab contexts, land ownership, heredity of durable goods (which may be sold), and social networks may help protect against limited financial resources and provide access to cash when needed (e.g., to access health services). In the current health system, financing arrangements with high rates of out-of-pocket health expenditures in the region (see Chapter 29) is a reality for many families. The situation may be less problematic in more socialized health care systems such as in Syria, where access to financial assets may matter less. However, these safety nets may be eroding as such countries propose liberalization policies. In countries with strong social welfare programs (often an artifact of pan-Arab socialist policies of the 1960s), economic assets may not contribute to health disparities in the way that is observed in other countries and regions. For example, a study of the possible association between multiple dimensions of socio-economic status (SES) and obesity in Cairo found that obesity was generally evenly distributed across SES groups in this population (Mowafi et al 2008). One explanation may be that individuals at the lower end of the SES spectrum gain access to excess calories through the national food subsidy program, whereas the wealthy gain access to greater quantity and variety of foods through their personal wealth.

In situations of conflict, access to economic resources (regardless of type) may matter less than access to services. In the Occupied Palestinian Territory, the greatest determinant of malnutrition among children was closures and roadblocks preventing ease of movement from one area to another (Abdeen et al 2003; FAO 2003). In Iraq, childhood mortality increased after the Gulf War and under UN sanctions directly or indirectly from blockades of goods and a dearth of services available to the population in the south/center regions, despite high literacy and significant oil wealth (Ali & Shah 2000).

Social Capital and Health

Over the past three decades a growing literature has linked social capital and health (Islam et al 2004), but only in the past few years has this work percolated into the Arab world. To those who live and interact in the region, "Arab hospitality" is well-known, and the benefits of closeness among friends and neighbors may have real health benefits. But the dynamics of social capital in the Arab context may also be complicated, especially for more vulnerable groups such as women given the dominant patriarchal structures in addition to political instability and conflicts endemic to many parts of the region. The nature and effect of social capital may vary intra-regionally as do cultural norms and customs.

The international literature largely points to a positive association between social capital – exemplified by large social networks, interpersonal trust, civic engagement, and social participation – and health. There are few published studies in the Arab world on social capital and health, with preliminary evidence suggesting variation in this association across populations. For example, a study of the association between civic engagement and health of Palestinian refugees in refugee camps in Jordan found that men who were not members of clubs or associations reported poorer health. However, this relationship was absent among women (Khawaja et al 2006). Another study exploring the relationship between social capital and health among adolescents in three impoverished communities on the outskirts of Beirut, Lebanon, found that, although social capital was associated with better health outcomes, Palestinian adolescents living in a refugee camp had poorer self-reported health (controlling for age, sex, and household income) even though they displayed high levels of social capital (Khawaja et al 2006).

Cross-national research suggests that social capital does not uniformly benefit individuals in the same community and that there may be cross-level interactions between individual and contextual factors (Poortinga 2006; Mansyur et al 2008; Subramanian et al 2002). In the Arab region, legal and economic exclusion as well as discrimination based on gender and ethnicity may attenuate the process of transforming social capital into individual health benefits. A recent study of the association between individual social capital and self-rated health in Israel found difference among Jews and Arabs. Arabs displayed overall lower levels of social capital compared to Jews in the study, and the association between social capital and health was much stronger among Jews (Baron-Epel et al 2008). This finding, the authors suggest, could be due to a stronger effect of social capital on health in wealthier communities or in contexts that have a higher level of aggregate social capital. The social, legal, and economic exclusions facing Arabs likely influences the association between social capital and health, similar to what was seen among Palestinian communities

experiencing discrimination in Lebanon described above (Khawaja et al 2006).

Another explanation for the different results on the relationship between social capital and health may be that the quality and type of social capital are not adequately captured in survey instruments in the region. The populations showing a smaller association between social capital and health described above, namely women and Palestinian refugees, also tend to be less mobile, more socially excluded, and largely discriminated against. Given that socially excluded groups may have a harder time in building broad networks outside their communities, *bridging capital*, which captures the cross-group relationships and may be more important for improving health outcomes (Harpham et al 2002), but may be limited in these communities. If surveys still rank these groups as having high social capital because they have strong *bonding capital* with their peers who are equally socially excluded, the "null" results with regard to health outcomes may simply signal that we need a more nuanced operationalization of this concept in this region.

Data from the fourth wave of the World Values Survey (undertaken in the 2000s) provide insights into comparative levels of common measures of social capital, such as trust, perceived fairness, and civic engagement in selected Arab countries: Algeria, Egypt, Iraq, Jordan, Morocco, and Saudi Arabia. Levels of trust varied from a high of 51% in Saudi Arabia to a low of 11% in Algeria (Figure 2). There was no clear pattern in the levels observed, and contrary to expectations, level of trust did not correspond with level of economic development, population health, or democracy. With regard to general perceptions of "fairness" in how individuals deal with one another in society, nearly one half of Iraqis and Egyptians believed that most "people try to be fair" compared to about one quarter of those in Algeria and Morocco. Interestingly, Algeria and Morocco ranked among the lowest levels of perceived fairness among all countries, just before Uganda, at 21%. Jordan and Saudi Arabia had relatively higher levels of perceived fairness, with 37% and 45%, respectively. Algerians and Moroccans were additionally asked about their participation in civic groups, but both countries ranked low, with only 14% in Algeria and 3% in Morocco involved in any group. Of those who participated, involvement in sporting groups ranked as the most popular social activity.

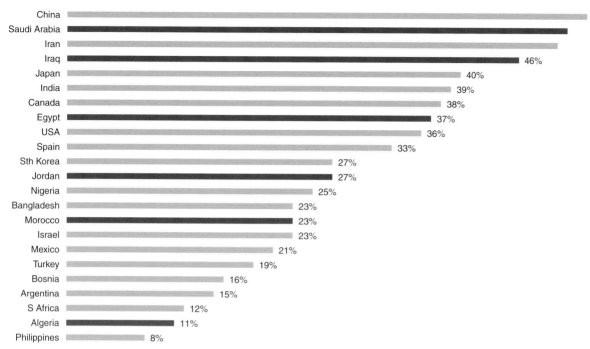

Figure 2. Proportions of population with generalized trust by selected countries, World Values Survey, fourth wave (1999–2004). Source: The World Values Survey, microdata.

Two large scale studies in the region have examined various dimensions of social capital, including trust. The Urban Health Study, which covered three low-income neighborhoods in greater Beirut, Lebanon, provides a thorough assessment of social capital across ethnically closed communities. Figure 3 shows selected measures of social capital for the components of the study looking at adolescent and women's health. The majority of adolescents and women in these communities have close relatives and friends living nearby, yet levels of social ties, group membership, exchange relations, and trust are relatively low. It is unclear whether these features of social fragmentation are unique to these poor urban communities or transcend them to Lebanon as a whole. The sectarian makeup of Lebanon as well as the national experience of prolonged civil war may account for interpersonal distrust and low levels of social cooperation and connectedness. Low trust despite a high level of social relationships is demonstrated in another example from Palestine (Box 2). The issue of trust and its implications for health needs to be further explored in future studies.

Cultural Capital and Health

Cultural assets may also play a unique role in attenuating negative health outcomes, independent of the effect of social and economic capital, or as a modifying variable that interacts with these other forms of capital (Abel 2008). Only three studies in the Arab world have looked at the association between cultural capital and health status. All three studies are from the Beirut Urban Health Study. They focus on the association of cultural engagement (production versus consumption) and women's health. Cultural engagement was measured by asking about whether participants were actively engaged in the arts, for example, or passively engaged by watching cultural television programs, reading, etc.

In one study, low cultural capital was associated with poor general health and poor mental health, after controlling for social capital, SES, demographic, community, and other health risk factors (Khawaja & Mowafi 2006). A similar study found that with the exception of art production, lower cultural capital (measured in terms of not watching cultural TV

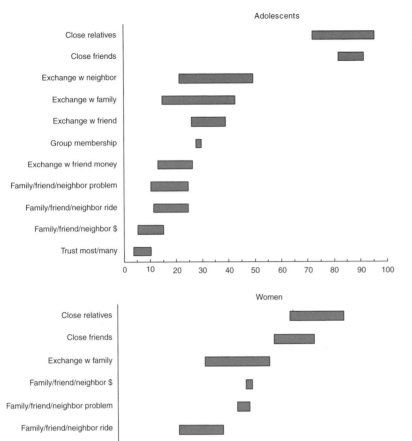

Figure 3. Community differences in social capital (%), Urban Health Study, 2003. Source: The Urban Health Study, Center for Research on Population and Health, micro data.

programs or not consuming art or literature) increased the odds of poor health among women, adjusting for socio-demographic factors and social capital (Khawaja & Mowafi 2007). The third study found a significant positive association between two indicators of maternal cultural participation (watching entertainment TV programs and going to the movies/exhibitions) and child health status, as reported by the mother, after controlling for other risk factors, including household income (Khawaja et al 2007).

Conclusions and Implications

In this chapter, we underscore the importance of exploring various kinds of assets in seeking to understand the social determinants of health. We suggest a simple assets framework consisting of three forms of capital: economic, social, and cultural. The field of social epidemiology has traditionally focused on income, and more recently on social capital, as they relate to health outcomes. Our proposed framework incorporates social capital and economic resources, but also includes cultural capital as an additional, potentially powerful, stratifying factor. Although the three forms of capital can be interrelated and future studies could explore interactions, we suggest that each has its unique, or otherwise additive, contribution to health status.

There are several research and policy implications of our discussion. First, we know very little

Box 2. The Palestine Social Capital Survey

Awad Mataria

To conceptualize, describe, and explain social capital in the Occupied Palestinian Territory (OPT), a special questionnaire was designed to cover four pre-defined domains: trust, participation, networking, and values (Naser and Hilal 2007). Results reveal low generalized trust, with less than one fifth of the study sample reporting trusting others, but relatively high membership rates in civic (58.5%), political (21.1%), religious (27.6%), social (18.8%), and professional (15.4%) associations among Palestinian adults. Networking seems high; over half communicate (through visits, telephone, or email) with relatives inside or outside OPT. More than half report having a family *"diwan"* (meeting place) or *"hamola"* (clan), and around 40% declare having participated in its activities during the last year. Around 40% report taking part in voluntary work and around 60% declared donating for charity activities.

Factor analysis *revealed a six-factor solution to be the most appropriate*, including trust in political institutions; social, professional, civic and political participation; behavioral values; trust in local and international institutions; informal social networks and social support; and social values. Subjects ranked trust as the most important dimension, followed by participation, values, and finally networks. Men had higher overall social capital scores than women.

about levels and quality of social and cultural assets in the Arab world. Traditionally, Arab society is known to have strong primordial loyalties, cohesive families, extensive inter-familial ties and support (Khawaja & Blome Jacobsen 2003), hospitality, interpersonal trust, and strong attachments to places of origin (Barakat 1993). Whether these features still persist is unknown. Given the wide diversity of economic and socio-cultural conditions across the region, we need baseline data on social and cultural capital in various settings. We also need to develop and validate culturally appropriate instruments to capture social and cultural capital in the region. There are only a few studies on the association between asset accumulation and distribution of health-related outcomes or mortality. We know of no study exploring various aspects of social capital such as bonding or bridging and their relationships to health in the region. Nor do we have any study

conceptualizing and testing the impact of "negative social capital" on health. Little is known about changes in asset accumulations across the life course, particularly shifts in assets formations by age and cohort and the possible impact of generational differences on health status. Such causal links are best captured by carefully designed longitudinal studies on assets and population health, which are currently lacking in the region. Also needed are in-depth qualitative studies to better understand the various constructs described here as well as the possible pathways linking social and cultural assets to health within and across countries.

Although the evidence base on social and cultural capital, especially in the Arab countries, is largely based on observational studies and limited in scope, we argue that strengthening the assets base of marginalized groups needs to be built into health and social sector programs that address social determinants of health. If it is true that social connections and participation in cultural and recreational activities are important to health, then "signs" of social fragmentation and inactivity need to be identified and efforts made to address them. We have argued here that the accumulation of assets is probably context dependent; so strengthening individual and group assets requires thorough assessments of the enabling environments, including the existing legal and policy frameworks as well as social sector programming.

While there is a growing consensus on the importance of social determinants of health among health policy makers and practitioners, incorporating structural factors into health policy programs, is not an easy task. Health policy making is often dominated by biomedical science and economics, two disciplines oriented toward analysis of individual behavior, leading to individual-level interventions. Even among many public health professionals, concerns for individuals can take precedence over contextual, macro-level determinants of population health. Structural factors that transcend the individual, such as social and cultural capital, are often viewed as elusive (i.e., less scientific), and therefore difficult to include. Incorporating structural factors into health development plans will probably necessitate an expanded public health workforce that includes professionals and others such as community health workers sensitized to community concerns. Ultimately, building and strengthening economic,

Table 1. Social Capital: Concepts and Measures, AUB Urban Health Study, 2003

Concepts and measures

A. Community-related

1. Community Attachment (3 main items)
Respondents were asked if they enjoy living in the neighborhood, length of residence in years, and rating of several services, including health, schools, electricity and water supply, on a Likert-type scale (good to bad).

2. Safety/Victimization (2 main items)
If the respondent feels safe walking in the neighborhood at night (yes, no), and whether or not s/he was victimized during the past 6 weeks. Theft, physical and verbal assaults were included in the victimization questions.

3. Civic engagement (5 items)
The number of formal and informal groups the respondent belongs to, and the type of group (sport, cultural etc) in case s/he is involved in any group. Three cognitive questions are also asked, including the feeling of efficacy in influencing decisions affecting local areas (yes, no), activities undertaken to influence decision (protest, writing to newspapers etc), and whether or not the respondent feels well informed about community issues.

4. Trust (3 items)
If the respondent trusts (most-none) people in neighborhood, trust (most-none) shopkeepers/traders, and whether s/he agrees (or not) that one must be careful in dealing with people in the neighborhood.

5. Reciprocity (7 items)
If the respondent thinks that people in the neighborhood try to be helpful to others or look out for themselves. In addition, the respondent is asked about exchange of favors and money during the last month from family, friends, and neighbors.

B. Individual-related

6. Social networks (6 items)
The number of relatives and close friends living nearby and if the respondent knows (most-none) people in the neighborhood s/he lives in. Also, if the respondent is satisfied or not with the number of relatives and close friends living nearby. In addition, there are items about contacts, including frequency of visiting relatives, friends, and neighbors.

7. Social support (18 items)
Items pertaining to both hypothetical and actual support received and given during the past month are included. For hypothetical support, the respondent is asked to identify the source of in kind support (household chore, shopping, during sickness) if needed. The respondent was also asked if s/he can raise $100 in case of need and the source of support. There are several items pertaining to actual exchange of in-kind and financial help (given and received) with family, friends, and neighbors by kind of help (e.g., transportation).

social, and cultural capital requires assessing institutional capacity at the local level, mobilizing resources, and creating demand for inter-sectoral collaborations and advocacy for change at the grass-roots level.

Acknowledgment

The views expressed herein are those of the authors and do not necessarily reflect the views of the United Nations.

References

Abdeen Z, Qasrawi R, Greenough G, Dandeis B (2003) *Nutritional assessment of the West Bank and Gaza Strip.* Emergency Medical Assistance Project (CARE/USAID)

Abel T (2008) Cultural capital and social inequality in health. *Journal of Epidemiology and Community Health,* 62: e13

Ali M, Shah I (2000) Sanctions and childhood mortality in Iraq. *The Lancet,* 355(9218): 1851–1857

Barakat H (1993) *The Arab world: Society, culture and state.* Los Angeles, CA: University of California Press

Baron-Epel O, Weinstein R, Haviv-Mesikab, Garty-Sandalonb N, Green MS (2008) Individual-level analysis of social capital and health: A comparison of Arab and

Jewish Israelis. *Social Science and Medicine*, 66: 900–910

Baum FE, Ziersch AM (2003) A glossary of social capital. *Journal of Epidemiology and Community Health*, 57: 320–323

Berkman LF, Kawachi I (Eds.) (2000) *Social epidemiology* (p. 76–94). Oxford, UK: Oxford University Press

Bibbington A (1999) Capitals and capabilities: A framework for analyzing peasant viability, rural livelihood and poverty. *World Development*, 27: 2021–2044

Bojner-Horwitz E, Theorell T, Anderberg UM (2003) Dance/movement therapy and changes in stress-related hormones: A study of fibromyalgia patients with video-interpretation. *Arts Psychotherapy*, 30: 255–264

Bourdieu P (1984) *Distinction: A social critique of the judgment of taste.* Cambridge, MA: Harvard University Press

Bourdieu P (1985) The market of symbolic goods. *Poetics*, 14: 13–44

Bourdieu P (1986) The forms of capital. *In: J Richardson (Ed.) Handbook of theory and research for the sociology of education.* Westport, CT: Greenwood Press

Bourdieu P, Passeron JC (1979) *Reproduction in education, society and culture.* London, UK: Sage

Bourdieu P, Wacquant LJD (1992) *An invitation to reflexive sociology.* Chicago, IL: University of Chicago Press

Coleman J (1988) Social capital in the creation of human capital. Washington: *American Journal of Sociology*, 94: S95–S120

CSDH (Commission on Social Determinants of Health) (2008) *Closing the gap in a generation: Health equity through action on social determinants of health.* Geneva, Switzerland: World Health Organization

Deaton A (2002) Policy implications of the gradient of health and wealth. *Health Affairs (Millwood)*, 21(2): 13–31

DiMaggio P (1982) Cultural capital and school success. *American Sociological Review*, 47: 189–201

DiMaggio P, Mohr J (1985) Cultural capital, educational attainment and marital selection. *American Journal of Sociology*, 90: 1231–1261

Edmonson R (2003) Social capital: A strategy for enhancing health? *Social Science and Medicine*, 57: 1723–1733

FAO (Food and Agriculture Organization) (2003) *Food security assessment West Bank and Gaza Strip. Food and Agriculture Organization of the United Nations in collaboration with World Food Programme*, Rome. Available from ftp://ftp.fao.org/docrep/fao/006/j1575e/j1575e01.pdf, July, 2003 [Accessed 15 January 2011]

Ford Foundation (2004) *Building assets to reduce poverty and injustice.* New York, NY: Ford Foundation

Fyfe G (2004) Reproductions, cultural capital and museums: aspects of the culture of copies. *Museum Society*, 2: 47–67

Gallo LC, Matthews KA (1999) Do negative emotions mediate the association between socio-economic status and health? *Annals of the New York Academy of Sciences*, 896: 226–245

Gwatkin DR, Rutstein S, Johnson K, Suliman E, Wagstaff A, Amouzou A (2007) *Socio-economic differences in health, nutrition, and population within developing countries: An Overview.* World Bank

Haines RJ, Poland BD, Johnson JL (2009) Becoming a 'real' smoker: cultural capital in young women's accounts of smoking and other substance use. *Sociology of Health & Illness*, 31(1): 66–80

Harpham T, Grant E, Thomas E (2002) Measuring social capital within health surveys: key issues. *Health Policy and Planning*, 17: 106–111

Harris J (2001) *Depoliticizing development: The World Bank and social capita.* Delhi, India: Leftworld

Healy T (2002) *The measurement of social capital at the international level. National Economic and Social Forum, Ireland. Presented at the International Conference on the Measurement of Social Capital*, London, UK: September 2002

Hudson L, Chapman C (2002) *The measurement of social capital in the United States, Presented at the International Conference on the Measurement of Social Capital.* London, UK: September 2002

Islam MK, Merlo J, Kawachi I, Lindstrom M, Gerdthan UG (2006) Social capital and health: Does egalitarianism matter? A literature review. *International Journal for Equity in Health*, 5: 3

Kawachi I (2000) Income inequality and health. *In: L Berkman & I Kawachi I (Eds.) Social epidemiology.* New York, NY: Oxford University Press

Khawaja M, Abdulrahim S, Afifi RA, Karam D (2006) Distrust, social fragmentation and adolescents' health in the outer city: Beirut and beyond. *Social Science Medicine*, 63: 1304–1315

Khawaja M, Barazi R, Linos N (2007) Maternal cultural participation and child health status in a Middle Eastern context: evidence from an urban health study. *Child: Care, Health and Development*, 33: 117–125

Khawaja M, Blome Jacobsen L (2003) Familial relations and labor market outcomes: The Palestinian refugees in Lebanon, *Social Science Research*, 32: 579–602

Khawaja M, Mowafi M (2006) Cultural capital and self-rated health in low income women: Evidence from the Urban Health Study, Beirut, Lebanon. *Journal of Urban Health*, 83: 444–458

Khawaja M, Mowafi M (2007) Types of cultural capital and self-rated health among disadvantaged women in outer Beirut, Lebanon. *Scandinavian Journal of Public Health*, 35: 475–480

Korten D (1990) *Getting to the 21st century-voluntary action and the global agenda*. West Hartford, CT: Kumarian Press

Lynch JW (2000) Income inequality and health: Expanding the debate. *Social Science and Medicine*, 51: 1001–1005

Lynch J, Davey Smith G, Kaplan G, House J (2000) Income inequality and mortality: Importance of health of individual income, psychosocial environment, or material conditions. *British Medical Journal*, 320: 1200–1204

Mansyur C, Amick BC, Harrist RB, Franzini L (2008) Social capital, income inequality, and self-rated health in 45 countries. *Social Science and Medicine*, 66: 43–56.

Marmot MG (1999) Epidemiology of socio-economic status and health: Are determinants within countries the same as between countries? *Annals of the New York Academy of Sciences*, 896: 16–29

Morgan A, Ziglio E (2007) Revitalizing the evidence base for public health: an assets model. *Promotion and Education*, (Suppl. 2): 17–22

Moser C (1998) The asset vulnerability framework: Reassessing urban poverty reduction strategies. *World Development*, 26: 1–19

Moser C (2007) *Reducing global poverty. The case of asset accumulation*. Washington DC: The Brookings Institution

Mowafi M, Khadr Z, Subramanian SV, Kawachi I, Bennett G (2008) *Socioeconomic status and obesity among adults in Cairo: A heavy burden for all?* unpublished draft

Muntaner C, Lynch J (1999) Income inequality, social cohesion, and class relations: A critique of Wilkinson's Neo-Durkheimian research program. *International Journal of Health Services*, 29: 59–81

Naser M, Hilal J (2007) *Raas al-Mal al-Ijtimai' fi al-Mujtama' al-Falastini* [*Social Capital in Palestinian Society*]. Ramallah, OPT: MAS (in Arabic)

Navarro VA (2002) Critique of social capital. *International Journal of Health Services*, 32: 423–432

Palloni A, Milesi C, White RG, Turner A (2009) Early childhood health, reproduction of economic inequalities and the persistence of health and mortality differentials. *Social Science and Medicine*, 68(9): 1574–1582

Poortinga W (2006) Social capital: An individual or collective resource for health? *Social Science and Medicine*, 62: 292–302

Portes A (1998) Social capital: Its origins and applications in modern sociology. *Annual Review of Sociology*, 22: 1–24

Putnam R (1993) *Making democracy work: Civic tradition in modern Italy*. Princeton, NJ: Princeton University Press

Sen A (1981) *Poverty and famine: An essay on entitlement and deprivation*. Oxford, UK: Clarendon Press

Subramanian SV, Kawachi I (2007) Income inequality and health: What have we learned so far? *Journal of Epidemiology and Community Health*, 61: 802–809

Subramanian SV, Kim DJ, Kawachi I (2002) Social trust and self-rated health in US communities: A multilevel analysis. *Journal of Urban Health*, 79: 21–34

Szreter S, Woolcock M (2004) Health by association? Social capital, social theory, and the political economy of public health. *International Journal of Epidemiology*, 28: 650–667

Wilkinson RG (1996) *Unhealthy societies: The afflictions of inequality*. London, UK: Routledge

Wilkinson RG (1997) Health inequalities: Relative or absolute standards? *British Medical Journal*, 314: 591–595

Chapter

7

Gender Disparities in Health

Kathryn M. Yount

Few issues have solicited as much attention in scholarship on the Arab world as gender has. Our purpose here is to focus on the gender–health links, seeing these within the profound diversity and ongoing changes across the region. From the perspective of the social determinants of health, *gender*, a multi-dimensional social construct of the socially, culturally, and historically prescribed and experienced aspects of femaleness or maleness (Johnson et al 2009), is key (see Chapter 5). Differential social roles between the sexes create different behaviors, interests, expectations, and divisions of labor (Johnson et al 2009), all of which affect health and cause some of the observed differentials between men and women. Also, because gender categories are socio-political, whereby "maleness" is typically favored with greater power and access to more resources and opportunities, gender inequalities are of a structural nature, and produce inequities in health. Micro-level rules and practices and macro-institutions reinforce gender roles by affecting a person's *gender identity* (self-perception on the continua of female or male) and *gender relations* (interactions with others based on one's ascribed gender) (Johnson et al 2009). Gender norms and hierarchies intersect with other hierarchies in variable ways to provide complex inequities in health.

In the Arab world, understanding the gender situation, and consequently its relation to health, requires a broad outlook on the prevailing political, economic, and social processes, and the structures these processes have produced, that shape the life conditions of women and men (see Chapter 2). The gender situation, in terms of roles and powers, is as diverse as those processes and structures. Gender characteristics vary within and across countries, even communities, rendering generalizations about gender across the region difficult. Nevertheless, there are shared characteristics.

Gender inequality favoring men is the norm in this region (Moghadam 2004, 2009; World Bank 2004), as in most others. This inequality is observed for example in patriarchal kinship structures (see for example Charrad 2001; Joseph 1993) and in family laws that "typically place women in the position of minors and dependents" (Moghadam 2009, p 10). In some parts, *classic patriarchy*, as defined by Kandiyoti (1988), is still observed and may foster sharp distinctions in gender roles and power, contributing to gender *inequities* in health. However, women may perceive benefits, including to health of gender role distribution and even patriarchal kinship (Charrad 2001; Kandiyoti, 1988), such as protection and economic support. Endogamy, often along patrilineal lines, occurs in one-to-two thirds of couples (Tabutin & Shoumaker 2005), and married daughters typically live patrilocally (see for example, Yount 1999). This practice increases the woman's value to, and leverage with, her natal kin, which can prove crucial in instances of marital conflict and may be associated with lower risks of women experiencing intimate partner violence (IPV) (Yount 2005).

Perhaps the most common feature of gender across the region is the profound *and ongoing* changes in definitions of roles and powers as a result of globalization and economic liberalization, urbanization, legal reforms, and most importantly the expansion of girls' schooling (Charrad 2001; Fargues 2005; Moghadam 2004; Tabutin & Schoumaker 2005). Kandiyoti (1988) has attributed *crises of patriarchy* to these factors and especially economic changes that disrupt the gendered division of labor. Over time gender changes have contributed to changes of profound public health impact such as increases, especially among women, in the mean age at marriage and the proportion never married.

Despite increasing nuclearization, the family remains a key factor in determining rules about gender.

Women's domestic roles are still strong (Moghadam 2004; Yount 2004b), and their participation in the documented formal workforce lags behind the world average (33% versus 55%) (Fargues 2005). Yet, declines in men's real wages in urban areas force wives to work outside (Fargues 2005 p. 47), without exempting them from domestic work, thus shouldering a double burden.

Gender and Health

There are many ways to explore the links between gender and health. For example, we can examine gender differentials in the social determinants of health (see Chapter 2), in access to and utilization of health services (see also Chapter 31), or in outcomes of medical and public health interventions. Because of limited space, I examine evidence for gender inequities in three domains of health. The reader is also referred to the many examples of these inequities presented throughout the volume, e.g., in relation to health inequities (see Chapter 5), health of population groups (Section 4), or specific diseases and conditions (Section 3), as well as other reviews (e.g., WHO 2007; World Bank 2004).

Differential Risks of Under-5 Mortality and Their Causes

Boys are biologically more vulnerable to mortality from endogenous causes that dominate in infancy. Such causes are diminished by early childhood (ages 1–4 years), when parents are most able to influence child health and survival. Studies in the 1980s and 1990s documented "excess" mortality among girls aged 1–4 years (see for example, Arnold, 1992; Coale & Banister 1994; Hill & Upchurch 1995; Waldron 1987), especially in South Asia (see Das Gupta 2005). The "Middle Eastern Crescent" had unusually high excesses for prevailing levels of under-5 mortality in the 1990s (Hill & Upchurch 1995; Yount 2001). I review estimates from regional surveys of female: male ratios in the neonatal (0–28 days), post-neonatal (1–11 months), and early child (1–4 years) periods (Table 1) and then discuss some of the hypothesized causes of historical excesses in girls' 1–4 mortality.

Female-to-male ratios of neonatal mortality show a consistent male disadvantage (e.g., ratio less than 1.0) for all countries and years for which data are available. In the post-neonatal period, there is an excess in girls' mortality in some settings. This excess

persists only in Egypt, where it peaks in the late 1980s and early 1990s because of faster declines in post-neonatal mortality among boys. By 2000, girls' excess post-neonatal mortality in Egypt remains apparent but is lower than in prior years, most likely because of faster declines in post-neonatal mortality among girls than boys between the 1990s and 2000s.

Across the years for which data are available, Egypt, Morocco, and Yemen exhibit persistent excess 1–4 mortality among girls, with the percentage of excess ranging from small (1%) to large (47%) (Table 1). Girls' excess 1–4 mortality in Egypt was highest in the 1980s (47%) but had declined to 8% by the late 1990s and early 2000s. A similar pattern of decline was apparent in Morocco and Yemen until the mid-to-late 1990s, when girls' 1–4 mortality exceeded that of boys by about 20% (Table 1). This general pattern of decline in girls' excess 1–4 mortality corroborates research for the 1970s and 1980s (e.g., Tabutin 1992; Yount 2001). Yet, comparing regional 1–4 mortality rate ratios to those for historical northwest Europe at the same level of under-5 mortality reveals persistent excesses in girls' 1–4 mortality in the region. (The differences in girls' and boys' 1–4 mortality, which are shown in the Web Appendix, become smaller with overall declines in mortality.) Thus, the Arab Middle East during the second half of the twentieth century experienced marked declines in the risk of under-5 mortality, a persistent, and probably biological, male excess risk of neonatal mortality, a decline in girls' excess risks of post-neonatal and 1–4 mortality, but high excess 1–4 mortality of girls when compared to other regions at the same level of under-5 mortality.

Biases in the Allocation of Food and Health Care to Sons and Daughters

Girls' excess 1–4 mortality generally is attributed to conscious or unconscious discrimination by parents, especially in allocating food and health care. Breastfeeding is one possible marker of this discrimination. Table 1 shows female/male (F/M) ratios of estimates of the median duration of any and exclusive breastfeeding for boys and girls less than 6 months. The median durations of exclusive breastfeeding are below the recommended duration, ranging from 0.4 to about 3 months regardless of the child's gender (see Web Appendix). Yet, median durations of *any* breastfeeding are much longer, ranging from 11.4 to 20.8 months for girls and from 12.6 to 21.8 months

Table 1. Female/Male Ratios for Selected Child Health Indicators in Selected Arab Countries

Year	Dates of estimate	Child mortality			Child care				Child nutrition		
		NN	PNN	1–4	Imm	Diar.	No treat	BF	Stunted	Wasted	U/W
Comoros											
	1980–1996	0.78	0.84	0.94	1.06	1.16	1.23	1.00	0.89	0.74	0.87
Egypt											
1992	1982–1992	0.75	1.09	1.47	0.95	0.93	0.97	1.06	1.00	1.03	1.02
1995	1985–1995	0.74	1.40	1.29	1.01	0.84	2.00	1.11	–	–	–
1997	1987–1997	0.69	1.39	1.13	–	–	–	–	–	–	–
1998	1988–1998	0.94	0.99	1.00	–	–	–	–	–	–	–
2000	1990–2000	0.77	1.31	1.10	1.00	0.97	0.88	0.94	–	–	–
2005	1995–2005	0.71	1.08	1.08	1.00	0.97	1.08	1.06	0.87	0.95	0.81
Jordan											
1990	1980–1990	0.94	1.16	0.93	1.00	1.00	–	1.00	0.96	0.63	0.93
1997	1987–1997	0.69	0.67	1.78	1.02	0.93	1.11	1.00	–	–	–
2002	1992–2002	0.94	1.00	1.00	1.05	0.96	0.82	1.71	1.18	0.78	1.15
2007	1997–2007	0.81	1.75	1.50	1.03	0.97	1.19	1.00	–	–	–
Morocco											
1987	1962–1966	0.70	1.18	1.04	–	–	–	–	–	–	–
1987	1967–1971	0.67	0.98	1.26	–	–	–	–	–	–	–
1987	1972–1976	0.80	0.72	1.12	–	–	–	–	–	–	–
1987	1977–1981	0.99	1.06	1.14	–	–	–	–	–	–	–
1987	1982–1986/7	0.89	0.98	1.01	0.97	0.87	0.78	1.25	–	–	–
1992	1982–1992	0.75	0.94	1.14	1.01	1.07	0.98	0.96	0.98	0.77	0.88
1995	1985–1995	0.84	1.00	0.89	0.95	0.91	1.19	1.00	–	–	–
2003/4	1993–2003	0.70	0.78	1.22	1.05	0.98	0.85	1.25	0.90	0.98	0.96
Mauritania											
2003	1993–2003	0.73	1.06	0.96							
2001	1997	–	–	0.88	1.11	0.87	1.02	–	1.01	0.72	0.96
Sudan											
1990	1980–1990	0.72	1.03	1.01	0.95	1.00	0.95	–	–	–	–
Tunisia											
1988	1963–1967	0.62	0.79	0.82	–	–	–	–	0.61	1.05	0.97
1988	1968–1972	0.81	0.86	1.61	–	–	–	–	–	–	–
1988	1973–1977	0.50	1.03	1.42	–	–	–	–	–	–	–
1988	1978–1982	0.85	1.45	1.36	–	–	–	–	–	–	–
1988	1983–87/8	0.75	0.89	0.77	0.90	0.78	0.99	1.00	–	–	–

Table 1. *(cont.)*

Year	Dates of estimate	Child mortality			Child care				Child nutrition		
		NN	PNN	1–4	Imm	Diar.	No treat	BF	Stunted	Wasted	U/W
Yemen											
1991/2	1972–1976	*0.81*	1.04	1.13	–	–	–	–	–	–	–
1997	1973–1977	*0.70*	0.99	0.99	–	–	–	–	–	–	–
1991/2	1977–1981	*0.76*	0.91	0.94	–	–	–	–	–	–	–
1997	1978–1982	*0.80*	0.93	1.15	–	–	–	–	–	–	–
1991/2	1982–1986	*0.71*	0.89	1.07	–	–	–	–	–	–	–
1997	1983–1987	*0.78*	0.95	1.02	–	–	–	–	–	–	–
1991/2	1987–1991	*0.86*	0.94	–	0.95	0.86	1.03	1.00	–	–	–
1997	1993–1997	*0.79*	0.73	1.18	0.93	0.96	0.78	0.83	0.98	0.88	0.96

Notes: NN = Neonatal mortality; PNN = Post-neonatal mortality; 1–4 = mortality from 1 to 4 years; Imm = Fully immunized, or having received at the age of 12–23 months, 3 polio DPT, 1 BCG, and measles/MMR vaccination; Diar = sought provider for treating diarrhea; No Treat = reports an episode of diarrhea that has not been treated; BF = Median duration of exclusive breastfeeding; Stunted = Height-for-age >2 standard deviations below the reference median Wasted = Weight-for-height >2 standard deviations below the reference median; UW = Weight-for-age >2 standard deviations below the reference median.

Sources: Mondoha et al (1997); El-Zanaty et al (1993); El-Zanaty & Way (2006); Zou'bi et al (1992); DOS-Jordan & ORC (2003); ONS & ORC Macro (2001); Azelmat et al (1993); Ministère de la Santé [Maroc], ORC Macro, et Ligue des États Arabes (2005); Aloui et al (1988); CSO & MI (1998); Demographic and health surveys in the cited Arab countries.

for boys. Compared to girls in four of seven settings (Egypt, Jordan, Mauritania, and Morocco), the median duration of any breastfeeding is longer for boys, and this gap is fairly consistent over time. These findings support evidence from Jordan that birth weights are higher for prenatally known males than females (Al-Qutob et al 2004). Thus, in some settings, it seems girls receive fewer benefits of any breastfeeding and maternal prenatal care. Intra-regional variation in the extent of these biases may reflect intra-regional variation in maternal preferences for sons (Akin et al 1986; Al-Qutob et al 2004). Qualitative research is needed to clarify the nature and reasons for these preferences.

The timely introduction of complementary foods is another key measure of nutritional intake and psychosocial care in early life. The DHS surveys in Egypt (2008) and Jordan (2007) collected data on complementary feeding of children 6–23 months old (El-Zanaty & Way 2009; DOS-Jordan & MI 2008). Only one-third to two-fifths of children this age receive the recommended intake of milk products and food groups, as well as the recommended frequency of eating solid or semi-solid foods (Web Appendix). Feeding practices are similar for boys and girls in Egypt as well as for non-breastfed boys and girls in Jordan; however, fewer breastfed girls than boys in Jordan are fed three or more food groups daily (76% versus 81%) and the minimum recommended number of times per day (57% versus 67%). These differences may result from real or perceived sex differences in energy requirements; yet, the evidence for fetal care, lactation, and complementary feeding reveals a consistent preference for sons in the context of Jordan.

Greater parental investment in sons' preventive and curative care is thought to be the main proximate determinant of girls' historical excess mortality (Yount 2001). Table 1 presents female/male ratios of vaccination and curative care for appropriate age groups of children in selected countries. Historical gaps in preventive care corroborate those for 1–4 mortality, yet are smaller than those observed in South Asia (see for example, Pande 1999). In the late 1980s and early 1990s, full coverage of basic vaccinations among children 12–23 months was lower for girls than boys in Egypt, Morocco, Sudan, Tunisia, and Yemen (see Yount 2001, for a review of other studies.). By the late 1990s, such gaps had largely disappeared in all countries with data, except for Yemen. Thus, as full coverage of basic vaccinations rose for all children

12–23 months, most gender gaps in coverage diminished or disappeared.

Gender gaps in curative care have also been documented in parts of the region. In Minya, Egypt, in the mid-1990s, boys were more likely to receive any health care and private care from a trained provider, an earlier first treatment, more treatments, and greater expenditures on care per episode of illness (Yount 2001, 2003a, 2003b, 2004a). Girls with diarrhea less often have received private care (Egypt and Yemen), oral rehydration (Egypt, Jordan, Turkey, and Yemen), and treatment at a medical facility or health provider (Egypt, Morocco, and Tunisia) (Yount 2001). Girls also less often have received any treatment for diarrhea and fever (Yemen), antibiotics for respiratory problems (Sudan), and any treatment or antibiotics for respiratory problems (Egypt) (Yount 2001). Table 1 shows the F/M ratios of children aged less than 5 years who saw any provider or received no treatment during an episode of diarrhea in the 2 weeks before interview. In the 1980s, girls less often saw any provider and more often received no treatment for diarrhea. Yet, inequities in care for episodes of diarrhea diminished into the 1990s and early 2000s, which parallels the regional decline in girls' excess 1–4 mortality.

Thus, overall, Egypt and Jordan are two settings where gender biases in children's care are still observed. Compared to Egypt, however, Jordan exhibits higher *overall* levels of curative care and lower *overall* risks of under-5 mortality (see Web Appendix). If parental inequalities in care do not contribute to large absolute gender gaps in 1–4 mortality, such inequalities still may affect gaps in child development. Research in this direction is needed.

Nutrition Across the Life Course

Nutritional status in fetal and early life is crucial for health and future development. Gender may influence nutrition in various ways across the life course (Sweeting 2008). In early childhood (e.g., ages 1–4), children are naturally able to regulate their food intake, yet parents can override this ability by controlling access to food. In parts of South Asia and the Arab Middle East, son preference has contributed to greater investments in sons in early life (e.g., Pande 1999; Yount 2001, 2003a, 2004a). Such biases may lead to disproportionate under-nutrition in girls where under-nutrition remains a prevalent problem (see for example, DeRose et al 2000). In the school

years, when *direct* parental control over food intake and activity subsides, gendered socialization may encourage different dietary practices and physical activities, contributing to gender *inequities* in overweight and obesity (e.g., Sweeting 2008). As argued elsewhere (see for example, Nelson & Olesen 1977), norms of *gender complementarity* are common in many Arab populations and define men as economic providers and women as mothers and homemakers. Although gender *practices* vary widely across Arab populations (World Bank 2004), women less often are economically active than men, and when women are active, they more often occupy more sedentary service and public-sector positions (see for example, ESCWA 2002; World Bank 2004). Also, working women often leave the labor force around the time of marriage or child-bearing (World Bank 2004), and a high percentage of women in some settings report restrictions to their public movement (see for example, El-Zanaty et al 1996). There also is greater physical inactivity in women than men, especially in Gulf countries (see for example, Guthold et al 2008; Mabry et al 2009). Thus, more sedentary social roles for women than men may foster behavioral differences into adulthood (see for example, Batnitzky 2008; James et al 2001), leading to more frequent overweight and obesity in women.

Sex contributes to susceptibility to overweight and obesity in women and men (see for example, James et al 2001). Noting the simultaneous influences of gender and sex on nutrition, we examine below the evidence regarding differences in nutrition in childhood and adulthood.

Under-nutrition in Early Childhood

In the 1980s in some settings and at some ages, girls have been more malnourished than have boys. In Cairo and squatter settlements in Amman, Jordan, girls were underweight more often (Ahmed et al 1981; Tekce & Shorter 1984; Doan & Bisharat, 1990; Tekce 1990). In Egypt, girls 24–29 months had higher odds of being underweight and less than 85% of the Harvard standard height-for-age at higher birth orders and in Lower Egypt (Makinson 1985); yet, after age 30 months, girls were better off than were boys in WAZ, HAZ, and WHZ scores.

By the late 1990s, the prevalence of stunting had declined in several Arab countries (De Onis et al 2000, Table 1), and F/M ratios in wasting and underweight often were smaller than those for stunting. Table 1 shows the F/M ratios for stunting (height-for-age), wasting (weight-for-height), and under-weight (weight-for-age), for selected countries between 1988 and 2005 (absolute differences and z-scores for deviations from the reference population's median levels are provided in the Web Appendix). Gaps in under-nutrition between girls and boys are small, and if anything, with a slight female advantage. Differences in wasting and under-weight are similarly small, and for selected countries, no clear pattern in the gap over time is apparent. These results corroborate those from older studies in the Gaza Strip and Basrah, Iraq (Mahmood & Feachem 1987; Schoenbaum et al 1995). Thus, *gender* gaps in under-nutrition from *unequal* parental investments generally have been small in Arab and Middle Eastern countries, even when under-nutrition was common. Sex/gender gaps moreover have remained small as child under-nutrition has declined. Thus, throughout the 1990s and early 2000s, disparities in under-nutrition *across* Arab and Middle Eastern countries were more salient than were sex differences or gender disparities *within* countries.

Over-nutrition in Youth and Adulthood

Overweight and obesity are already major public health problems in the Arab world (see Chapters 10, 12, and 13). Estimates are compiled of mean BMI and sample distributions of bodyweight categories on both youth and adults from studies published since the late 1990s identified in a PubMed search and originating from diverse countries (see Web Appendix). While comparisons across studies are limited by use of different criteria for establishing cutoffs for weight categories, broad patterns in overweight and obesity are noteworthy and I discuss these in two age groups. Summary indicators are presented in Table 2.

The rising incidence of obesity in childhood and adolescence is an emerging public health issue for many low and middle-income countries (LMICs), including in the Arab world. While there are no clear global sex/gender differences in obesity in children less than 19 years (Sweeting 2008), there are notable differences in this region. The combined prevalence of overweight and obesity varies widely, from 5% to 48%. In a majority of studies, girls are more often overweight or obese, most notably in later adolescence and in Gulf countries. This pattern corroborates a review that included selected studies in Arab

populations (Sweeting 2008) and suggests that sex/gender interact to produce gender inequalities in overweight/obesity, especially in the Gulf. Possible contributors include low woman's labor force participation (Fargues 2005) and less physical activity among women, especial in Gulf countries (Guthold et al 2008; Mabry et al 2010). Thus, despite small sex/gender gaps in early-life under-nutrition, adolescent girls in selected countries are at higher risk of overweight and obesity than same-aged boys, perhaps partly because of more sedentary social roles and consequently lower levels of physical activity.

The Arab world has some of highest rates of adult overweight and obesity in the world (James et al 2001). This review of PubMed studies since the late 1990s (see Web Appendix) suggests several noteworthy patterns. In most cases, the combined prevalence of overweight and obesity is especially high, exceeding 40% for men and women in a majority of settings. Also, the prevalence of overweight and obesity is higher among women in a majority of settings (9 of 17 with estimates and 16 of 19 with estimates, respectively).

Gender may explain part of the variability within the region in male–female differentials in overweight and obesity. This conjecture departs from the classic nutrition transition theory, which identifies shifts toward urbanization and industrialization as the underlying causes of changes in diet and physical activity (see for example, King et al 2001; Popkin 1999) and which gives passing attention to shifts in women's roles and the disproportionate burden of over-nutrition in women (see for example, Batnitzky 2008). According to Batnitzky (2008, p. 447), "macro-level processes may have differential effects on the diet and physical activity patterns of men and women... [and] [t]he differential effects of such macro-level processes have yet to be incorporated into a framework of social, epidemiological, demographic, and economic change." Batnitzky's work was in Morocco, but her assertions that gendered social roles predict women's obesity is possibly relevant elsewhere in the region.

Violence Against Women and Men

Various forms of violence are associated with physical and mental health; these relationships, along with the high prevalence of violence regionally, motivate attention to the gendered bases of violence. *Gender-based*

Table 2. Gender Differential in Overweight/Obesity Among Different Age Groups in Arab Countries

	Authors	Date	Location	Setting	Age	N	% Overweight		% Obese	
							Males	Females	Males	Females
Children	Al-Isa & Moussa	1998	Kuwait	Community	'0–5	7,419	–	–	8	9
	Al-Isa & Moussa	2000	Kuwait	Elementary school	6–10	8,957	–	–	16	14
	Al-Isa	2004	Kuwait	Children	10–14	14,659	30	32	15	13
	Musaiger & Gregory	2000	Bahrain	13 Schools	6–18	1,586	–	–	–	–
	Al-Sendi et al	2003	Bahrain	School	11–18	506	–	–	21	35
	Ghannem et al	2000	Tunisia	Urban school	6–18	1,569	11	16	6	10
	El-Hazmi & Warsy	2002	KSA	School children	1–18	12,701	11	13	6	7
	Sibai et al	2003	Lebanon	School children	3+	2,104	23	8	16	3
	Jabre	2005	Lebanon	Children	6–8	234	26	25	7	6
	Lafta & Kadhim	2005	Iraq	6 Schools	7–13	8,300	18–21	18–22	21–26	21–27
	Raja'a & Mohanna	2005	Yemen	Urban schools	7–18	1,253	5.6	10.5	–	–
	Qotba & Al-Isa	2007	Qatar	Elementary school	6–7	271	3	9	2	5
	Mali & Bakir	2007	UAE	Preschool	5–7	789	10	14	11	10
				Elementary school	8–10	1,190	25	24	13	10
				Intermediate school	11–13	1,816	23	25	16	12
				Secondary school	14–17	586	19	17	13	18
Adolescents	Salazar- et al	2006	Egypt	Public schools	10–19	1,502	7	13/25	6/7	8/9
	Bener	2006	Qatar	Urban schools	12–17	3,923	29	19	8	5
	Chakar & Salameh	2007	Lebanon	Private schools	10–18	12,299	29	19	10	4
	Aounallah	2008	Tunisia	Adolescents national	15–19	2,872	17	21	4	4
Adults	Al-Nuaim et al	1996	KSA	Community	16–50	13,177	29	27	16	24
	Al-Nuaim et al	1997	KSA	Community	20–50	10,651	33	29	18	27
	Al-Nuaim et al	1997	KSA	Community	20–50	10,651	33	29	18	27
	Warsy & el-Hazmi	1999	KSA	Community 92–96	15+	–	27	25	13	20
	Al Turki	2007	KSA	Medical setting	18+	3,205	40	24	37	58
	Al-Othaimeen et al	2007	KSA	From HHS	18+	19,598	31	28	14	24
	Musaiger	2001	Bahrain	Natives	30–79	514	35	31	21	49
	Abdul-Rahim et al	2001	Palestine	Rural	30–65	497	–	–	17	36
				Urban	30–65	492	–	–	30	49
	Moktar et al	2001	Tunisia	20+ from HHS	20–60	2,760	23	28	7	23
				Young adults	19	–	5	10	–	–
	Moktar et al	2001	Morocco	Community	18+	17,320	28	33	6	18

Table 2. (cont.)

Authors	Date	Location	Setting	Age	N	% Overweight		% Obese	
						Males	Females	Males	Females
Benjelloun	2002	Morocco	Adults (1984)	18+	–	19	32	–	–
			Adults (1998)	18+	–	25	45	–	–
Tazi et al.	2003	Morocco	Community	20+	–			–	–
Rguibi & Belahsen	2007	Morocco	National (1984)	20+	41,526	17	26	2	6
			National (1998)	20+	14,028	21	29	4	16
Lahmam et al.	2008	Morocco	Adult Amazigh	20+	436	22	33	2	13
Al-Lawati & Jousilahti	2008	Oman	Community	20+	1,421	–	–	41	42
Yahia et al.	2008	Lebanon	University students	18–22	220	38	14	13	3
Zindah et al.	2008	Jordan	Medical setting	18+	710	–	–	21	42

Notes: Overweight = BMI >85th; obesity = BMI >95th percentiles, of the National Center for Health Statistics (NCHS) reference data. References can be found in the Web Appendix.

violence is defined as "any act...that results in, or is likely to result in, physical, sexual or psychological harm or suffering to women, including threats of such acts, coercion or arbitrary deprivation of liberty, whether occurring in public or in private life" (UN General Assembly 1993). Such acts include but are not limited to physical, sexual, or psychological assault or aggression occurring in the family or general community or perpetrated or condoned by the State. As Linos (2009) has noted, this definition equates gender-based violence with violence against women. Here, I adopt a broader definition of gender-based violence to include any form of sexual, psychological, or physical assault or aggression against individuals or groups because of their ascribed gender, or perceived failure to conform to their ascribed gender. This definition acknowledges that both men and women may experience gender-based violence, although the forms, magnitudes, and effects of such violence may differ. Social scientists see the roots of gender-based violence in social norms and structural inequalities in resources and power. Wide variability in various forms of gender-based violence suggests that such violence is not inevitable (see Yount 2005; Yount and Li 2009). While various forms of gender-based violence exist in the region (e.g., Yount 2002, 2004b; Yount & Carrera 2006; Yount & Balk 2004), limitations of space lead me to focus on two forms: intimate partner violence (IPV) and violence in conflict and post-conflict settings.

Intimate Partner Violence

Intimate partner violence refers to "assaultive and coercive behaviors that adults use against their intimate partners" (Holden 2003 p. 155). In North America and Europe, studies of often non-representative samples show that men and women commit physical and psychological IPV at similar rates (Straus 2004; Swan et al 2008); yet, men's physical violence is thought to be more injurious, and men more often stalk, sexually assault, and use coercive tactics of control (Swan et al 2008). Women in poorer, more gender-stratified settings experience physical IPV more often (ORC Macro n.d.). In surveys in LMICs including some Arab settings, 12%–71% of women report a prior experience of physical IPV (Douki et al 2003; Garcia-Moreno et al 2006; Hindin et al 2008; Watts & Zimmerman 2002). According to reports by women or men, women have initiated such violence less often (Kishor & Johnson 2004; ORC Macro n.d.). Thus, IPV occurs asymmetrically in ways that disproportionately burdens women.

Despite high levels of IPV against women in other regions, research on such violence in the Arab world is sparser (Boy & Kulczycki 2008). Table 3 summarizes English-language articles on domestic violence against women in selected Arab settings. Some of these studies have been cited elsewhere (Boy & Kulczycki 2008), and

Table 3. Prevalence of Intimate Partner Violence as Reported by Women Participating in Studies in Middle Eastern and North African Populations

Author(s)	Date	Country	Location	Characteristics	Sample size	Physical		Psychological		Sexual		While pregnant
						L/T	p/yr	L/T	p/yr	L/T	p/yr	
El-Zanaty et al	1996	Egypt	National	Representative (15–49)	7,121	34.4	12.5					
Ramiro et al	2004	Egypt	Ismailia	Urban EMW (15–49)	590	–		10.5	10.8			
Hassan et al	2004	Egypt	Ismailia	Urban mothers (15–49)	631	11.1	10.5					
Bakr & Ismail	2005	Egypt	Cairo	Women at OP clinic	509	34.2				17.1		
Yount	2005	Egypt	Minya	EMW (15–54)	2,522	26.8	9.1					
El-Zanaty & Way	2006	Egypt	National	Representative (15–49)	5,613	33.2	20.4	17.5	10.7	6.6	3.8	6.2
El Nashar et al	2007	Egypt	Dakahlia	Married (16–49)	936					11.5		
Fahmy & Abd El-Rahman	2008	Egypt	Zagazig	18–50 years	500	22.4		74.0		19.6		
Khawaja & Barazi	2005	Jordan	Camps	Currently married	262	42.5	19.2					16.6
Dept. of Stats (Jordan)	2008	Jordan	National	EMW (15–49)	3,444	20.6	12.2	20.0	14.0	7.6	5.6	5.4
Clark et al	2009	Jordan	–	Literate, EMW	390							15.4
Khawaja & Tewtel-Salem	2004	Lebanon	Beirut	Married refugees	417	22.0	9.1					6.9
Hammoury & Khawaja	2007	Lebanon	Sayda	Pregnant in PN clinic	349	59.0	19.1				26.2	11.5
Usta et al	2007	Lebanon	Beirut	Women in PHC	1,382	23.0						
Khawaja & Hammoury	2008	Lebanon	Sayda	Pregnant In PN clinic	349						26.2	
Hammoury et al	2009	Lebanon	Sayda	Refugees (15–42)	351	59.0	19.1					11.4
Haj-Yahia	1999	OPT	National	Representative	2,410		52		90.9		386	
Rachana et al	2002	KSA	National	Married pregnant	7,105							21
Ahmed & Elmardi	2005	Sudan	Omdurman	Literate, married/MC	394	41.1						6.9
Maziak & Asfar	2003	Syria	Aleppo	≥13 years in PCCs	411	23.1						
Maziak & Asfar	2003	Syria	Aleppo	Married ≥13 years	362	26.2						

Notes: EMW = ever-married women; L/T = Lifetime prevalence; p/yr = during the prior year; OP = outpatient clinic; PN = prenatal centers; PHC = primary health care center; MC = medical center; Age range of study participants is reported between brackets in 'characteristics' when available. References can be found in the Web Appendix.

others were identified in a PubMed search. Several cautionary notes are warranted. First, the definitions of IPV and its various types differed across studies, limiting comparisons of prevalence across studies. Second, a majority of studies focused only on physical IPV, and so less is known about psychological and sexual forms of such violence. Third, most studies are based on small, clinic-based samples, precluding inferences to national populations. Finally, 8 of the 21 identified studies were conducted in Egypt, and so other Arab settings are under-represented.

Table 3 offer useful insights. Estimates vary widely, suggesting that IPV against women is neither universal nor inevitable in the region. Levels of lifetime *physical* IPV range from 11% of ever-married women in Ismailia, Egypt, to 59% of pregnant clinic attendees in Saidon, Lebanon. Estimates of lifetime *psychological* IPV vary more widely, from 10% to 74% in parts of Egypt. Levels of lifetime *sexual* IPV are not negligible, ranging 7%–20% in parts of Egypt. In the three national surveys, rates of physical, psychological, and sexual IPV in the prior year were 12%–52%, 11%–91%, and 4%–37%, respectively. These rates fall within the range of those reported for other world regions and are unacceptable in this region as they are elsewhere.

Feminist scholars have argued that women's experiences of IPV are rooted in systems of gender stratification (Kalmuss & Straus 1982). One link between women's structural subordination and experiences of violence is ideological. Namely, men's preponderance in economic, social, legal, and political institutions legitimizes and sustains policies and practices that naturalize their dominance. A discussion of laws, institutions, and related gender norms in Egypt is illustrative. A woman who seeks to marry, travel, or open a business, for example, must by law obtain permission to do so from a male relative (Joseph 2000). Women, moreover, still receive less schooling than do men, less often participate in formal work after marriage, and are less well-represented in public positions of power (El-Zanaty & Way 2006; Hoodfar 1997; UNDP & INP 2005). Finally, norms of *gender complementarity*, which partly are rooted in Islamic prescripts, uphold "separate but balanced" family roles for men and women, in which the husband/father is the economic provider and the wife/mother is the obedient housekeeper and childrearer (Nelson & Olesen 1977).

With regard to the laws, institutions, and norms pertaining to violence, Egyptian women who experience IPV have little recourse. Family violence falls under the provisions of general law covering all cases of abuse, and so spousal violence is not explicitly forbidden (Ammar 2006). Accordingly, only 65 of the total 2896 legal complaints to police during 2002–2004 pertained to allegations of violence against women, and more than two fifths of reported cases of IPV were soon-after withdrawn (Ammar 2006). In 2000, women earned the right to divorce on grounds of *incompatibility*, but in such cases must relinquish their financial and custodial claims as wives (Ammar 2006). Divorce, moreover, is often seen as a disobedience to God and is stigmatizing for women, who in most cases remain unmarried (Ammar 2006). Few organizations offer direct services to women who experience IPV. The few shelters typically have rigid rules for admittance, and like law-enforcement, prioritize spousal reconciliation (Ammar 2006). As a result, few Egyptian women of reproductive age are divorced (2%) and, even fewer (< 1%) who have experienced recent physical or sexual IPV seek formal recourse (El-Zanaty & Way 2006). Thus, patriarchal values and a view of violence against wives as discipline lead to "passive acquiescence in its inevitability" (Ammar 2006 p. 249) and a minority (35%) of wives seeking any recourse in cases of IPV (El-Zanaty & Way 2006). Still, women at least in some Middle Eastern settings draw on their natal kin ties for protection, although natal kin may also recommend tolerance (Yount 2010).

While IPV against women may be rooted in gender systems, inequalities in the family and experiences of violence in childhood also have predicted a woman's risk of IPV. In Egypt, atypical wives who have much less or more schooling than their husbands are at higher risk of experiencing physical and psychological IPV (Yount 2005; Yount & Li 2010). For a less-schooled wife, severe dependence may limit her alternatives to an abusive marriage. For a more-schooled wife, her transgression of status expectations may provoke violence as "compensatory masculinity." Finally, a woman who has been exposed to normalized violence in childhood, including physical IPV by a parent and female genital cutting, has higher odds of experiencing psychological and physical violence (Yount & Li 2010). Such associations suggest that prior experiences of violence teach women to view IPV as normal (Yount & Li 2009).

Indeed, a high percentage of women in Arab countries view IPV against women as justified. Table 4 summarizes studies on this subject. A recent partial review (Boy & Kulczycki 2008) complemented by a PubMed search reveals only a few surveys of women's attitudes about IPV against women. Available data have limitations of comparability and country and population coverage (only four of nine studies are nationally representative and are on Egypt and Jordan), and only one study asked men about their attitudes regarding IPV against women (Khawaja 2004). Still, these data offer tentative insights. In all samples a majority of women, 50% in Egypt (2005) to 90% in Jordan (2008), agree that wife-beating is justified for at least one reason. Attitudinal change may be occurring in Egypt as the rate changed from 86% in 1995 to 50% of women in 2005 (although changes to the question may partly account for such trends). In Jordan, women's attitudes seem more stable, with around 90% of women in 2002 and 2008 agreeing that domestic violence was justified for some reason.

Also notable in Table 4 are the circumstances for which women most and least often justify wife-beating. Where the question was asked, the highest percentage of women reported that a husband was justified in beating his wife for neglecting her responsibilities and disobedience, including refusing sex to her husband. In most cases, women least often agreed that wife-beating was justified if she burned the food or did not prepare it properly. Accordingly, certain ascribed roles for women may be more salient than others, in part because they are tied to personal and family reputation. If women are vested in maintaining gender structures and perceive benefits of conforming to gender scripts (see Kandiyoti 1988), then they may also see violent responses to a wife's gender transgressions as legitimate forms of disciplinary action (Yount and Li 2009).

Conflict-Related Violence and Trauma

This form of gender-based violence has received increased attention in research and humanitarian aid (WHO 2008). Until recently, the focus was on violence perpetrated against women (e.g., WHO 2008) which is a major concern before, during, and after conflict (Hynes et al 2004). Linos (2009), however, has questioned the assumption that women are the only recipients of gender-based violence during conflict, suggesting that male civilians also experience such violence and this may be less visible, however, if men disproportionately under-report it.

Data on exposure to conflict-related violence and trauma are surprisingly limited for Arab populations, and gender disaggregated data on such exposures are even more sparse. Studies in selected settings suggest high exposure among adults in certain circumstances. Among male Iraqi refugees arriving in the United Kingdom during 1990–1993, 10%–62% reported various forms of physical torture, including sexual assault (14%) (Gorst-Unsworth & Goldenberg 1998). Between 23% and 67% of these refugees also reported various forms of psychological torture, such as sensory (67%) and sleep (51%) deprivation (Gorst-Unsworth & Goldenberg 1998). Among 106 mostly young Lebanese men who were released from the Israeli Khiam prison in 1990–1996, 85% reported at least one experience of torture, 75% a lack of food or water, 68% solitary confinement, 64% loss or kidnapping, 18% heavy fighting, 17% murder of a family member or friend, 16% serious injury, and 5% rape or sexual assault (Saab et al 2003). Among adults 20 years or older in two towns in Southern Lebanon, most (87%) had experienced at least one of 25 traumatic events, including confinement to the home because of danger (66%), forced hiding (37%), murder of a family member or friend (28%), and bodily beating (8%) (Farhood et al 2006). Among adults 18 years or older in Juba, Southern Sudan, one half or more were exposed to a lack of food or water, the unnatural death or murder of a family member or friend, or a combat situation (Roberts et al 2009). Around one fifth also reported physical torture or beating or forced isolation, and about 7% reported rape or sexual assault (Roberts et al 2009).

Such exposures also have at times been high among youth. Among 309 preschool children in part of the Gaza strip, 92% reportedly witnessed mutilated bodies and wounded people on television, 51% witnessed the airborne bombardment of other people's houses, and 3% witnessed the beating or killing of a close relative (Thabet et al 2006). High levels of exposure to traumatic events also have been reported among parents and children aged 9–18 years in the north and east of Gaza (Thabet et al 2008). Among high school students from the Ramallah District of the West Bank, more than 60% reportedly were

Table 4. "Causes" of Intimate Partner Violence as Reported by Women From Some Selected Countries

Author(s)	Year	Country	Sample[a]	(n)	Goes out w/out telling him[c]	Burns food[d]	Neglects children	Argues with him[e]	Insults him	Disobeys him	Refuses him sex	Commits infidelity[f]	Behaves in way he dislikes	Doesn't do chores properly	Violates his religion	Doesn't respect his family	≥one reason
El-Zanaty et al.[f]	1996	Egypt	EMW 15–49	(7,121)		27.2	50.9	69.1			69.9						86.4
El-Zanaty & Way[f]	2005	Egypt	EMW 15–49	(19,474)	40.4	19.0	39.8	37.4			33.5						50.0
Yount	2005	Egypt	EMW 15–54	(2,522)													72.9
Amowitz et al.	2004	Iraq	Women 18–95	(814)						54							
Haj Yahia	1998	Israel	Arab MW 16–65	(425)				42		35	25	69					
Haj Yahia	2000	Israel	Arab women 19–77	(291)			55	61				73					
Khawaja	2004	Jordan	Palestinian MW Palestinian MM	(162)	39.5 36.5	19.6 16.8	32.5 28.9	35.2 37.6		48.6 50.4			36.8 37.2	22.0 18.4		43.4 39.0	61.8 60.1
Govt of Jordan & ORC Macro[f]	2002	Jordan	EMW 15–49	(6,006)	24.1	59.5	36.6	4.2	10.4	52.3	83.4				0.2	0.2	87.0
Dept. of Stats Jordan & Macro Int[g]	2008	Jordan	EMW 15–49	(10,876)	34.9	7.7	41.8	16.3	65.9	55.3	87.5						90.0

Notes: MW = married women; MM = married men; EMW = ever-married women.
[a]Where no ages are listed, the age range of study participants was not reported.
[b]In some surveys, the phrasing read "hitting or beating."
[c]In some surveys, the phrasing read "goes out in public unaccompanied."
[d]In some surveys, the phrasing read "doesn't have meals prepared properly or one time."
[e]In some surveys, the phrasing read "talks back," "answers back," "insults," or "argues with the husband or "speaks in a hostile manner."
[f]In Jordan, the phrasing read "betrays the husband."
[g]Nationally representative estimates.
References can be found in the Web Appendix.

exposed to tear gas, sound bombs, the arrest of a stranger, and the humiliation of a stranger (Giacaman et al 2007b). Among other exposures, 11% also had seen a friend or neighbor killed, and 7% had seen a family member killed (Giacaman et al 2007a).

Exposure to certain forms of conflict-related violence and trauma appear to be higher among men. Among adults 16–60 years old in Gaza, men were exposed to more traumatic events over their lifetimes (4.7 versus 1.1), and proportionately more men (86%) than women (44%) have ever experienced at least one traumatic event (Punamäki et al 2005). Compared to women in Juba, Southern Sudan, men more often reported exposure to 8 or more of 16 trauma events (28% versus 18%), lifetime serious injury (32% versus 20%), torture or beating (26% versus 15%), and imprisonment (17% versus 10%) (Roberts et al 2009); yet, surprisingly, men and women reported comparable rates of rape or sexual abuse (5% versus 8%).

Similarly gendered patterns of exposure to conflict-related violence or trauma are observed among older adults and youth. During the civil war in Lebanon, middle-aged and older adult men more often experienced any traumatic event (68% versus 63%) (Sibai et al 2001). Men also experienced personal traumas (13% versus 4%), property losses (40% versus 30%), and displacement (29% versus 25%) more often; whereas, women more often witnessed or heard about the traumas (31% versus 27%) and property losses (11% versus 7%) of other family members (Sibai et al 2001). Among 10th and 11th graders in the Ramallah District of the West Bank, boys were exposed more often to tear gas (72% versus 50%) and sound bombs (71% versus 56%) and have more often seen the arrest (74% versus 50%) and humiliation (72% versus 62%) of a stranger (Giacaman et al 2007b). Boys also have more often been beaten by the Israeli army (30% versus 2%), used as a human shield (10% versus 3%), bodily searched (54% versus 9%), shot at or hit (38% versus 13%), detained or arrested (29% versus 6%), and interrogated (22% versus 5%), among other exposures (Giacaman et al 2007b). Thus, boys in Ramallah have experienced more often than girls both individual and collective forms of conflict-related violence and trauma (Giacaman et al 2007a, 2007b).

Exposure to conflict-related violence or trauma has been associated with various psychological and physical health outcomes. In Gaza, exposure in children was associated with symptoms of post-traumatic stress disorder and anxiety (Thabet et al 2006). In Ramallah,

both individual and collective forms of violence were independent predictors of depressive symptoms among high school students (Giacaman et al 2007b). Among Kuwaiti preadolescents during the Gulf War of 1990, war-related trauma was associated with higher odds of a reported diagnosis of heart disease, hypertension, diabetes, or high cholesterol, and the magnitude of the odds was comparable with those reported in studies of childhood abuse and neglect in US adults (Llabre & Hadi 2009).

Although girls' and women's lower exposure to certain forms of conflict-related violence and trauma, such exposures may also impact them but the patterns of impact among men and women may not be consistent. In adult Palestinians in Gaza, exposures are associated with PTSD in both genders but with anxiety, mood, and somatoform disorders only in women (Punamäki et al 2005). Among Somali, Afghan, and Iranian refugees and asylum-seekers to the Netherlands, women have higher odds of more than one chronic condition, symptoms of PTSD, and symptoms of depression/anxiety (Gerritsen et al 2006). Among 6–16 year-old schoolchildren in Gaza, aggression was reported more often for boys than girls, but exposure to military violence was associated similarly with aggression among boys and girls (Qouta et al 2008). The health impacts of conflict-related violence and trauma may, therefore, depend not only on gender, but also on the particular trauma, age at exposure, and concurrent environmental conditions.

There is limited evidence from the region on the links between political and IPV. Clark et al (2010) showed that women in the OPT whose husbands were *directly* exposed to political violence had increased odds (1.89) of physical as well as sexual (2.23) violence. Corresponding odds for women whose husbands were *indirectly* exposed were 1.61 and 1.97, respectively. Usta et al (2007) linked political and IPV in the context of the 2006 war in Lebanon and reported that women experienced domestic violence during (27%) and after (13%) the conflict.

In summary, women suffer disproportionately from various forms of IPV, whereas men more often suffer from certain types of conflict-related violence and trauma. Women's minority status in the marital home may enhance their risks of IPV, while gender norms and structures that limit women's mobility and public roles may lessen their risks of certain forms of conflict-related violence. These conclusions do not imply that men and women share equally the benefits and harms of dominant gender role distribution. Rather, men and women suffer unique forms of violence, which are rooted in these local forms of gender roles.

Conclusion

This chapter has explored the evidence for gender differentials in three prominent domains of health in the Arab world. Substantial but often variable differences are apparent and do not lend themselves to easy summary statements. A historical excess in girls' post-neonatal and 1–4 mortality diminished as under-5 mortality declined, making boys' endogenous excess neonatal mortality the most apparent differential in under-5 mortality. Gaps in under-nutrition in early life have been smaller in the Arab world than in South Asia, but boys in selected settings have received preferential treatment in breastfeeding and health care. Girls' greater overweight and obesity than boys' in later adolescence is both a common and a distinguishing feature of the region compared to elsewhere. Women's greater overweight and obesity than men's especially in the Gulf point to women's more sedentary roles in these countries. Levels of domestic violence against women vary considerably but fall within the rates observed in other regions. Men's greater exposure to certain forms of conflict-related violence in some settings suggests that local gender roles have unique adverse effects on women and men. In short, gender roles, norms and structures, and associated differences in power and opportunity have distinct health impacts for women and men in the region. These impacts must be continuously monitored, especially in light of the ongoing changes in gender roles and relations.

References

Ahmed W, Beheiri F, El-Drini H, Manala OD, Bulbul A (1981) Female infant in Egypt: Mortality and childcare. *Population Sciences*, 2: 25–39

Akin J, Bilsborrow R, Guilkey D, Popkin B (1986) Breastfeeding patterns and determinants in the Near East: An analysis for four countries. *Population Studies*, 40: 247–262

Al-Qutob R, Mawajdeh S, Allosh R, Mehayer H, Majali S (2004). The effect of prenatal knowledge of fetal sex on birth weight: A study from Jordan. *Health Care for Women International*, 25(3): 281–291

Ammar NH (2006) Beyond the shadows: Domestic violence in a "democratizing" Egypt. *Trauma, Violence and Abuse*, 7(4): 244–259

Arnold F (1992) Sex preference and its demographic and health implications. *International Family Planning Perspectives*, 18(3): 93–101

Batnitzky A (2008) Obesity and household roles: Gender and social class in Morocco. *Sociology of Health & Illness*, 30(3): 445–462

Boy A, Kulczycki A (2008) What we know about intimate partner violence in the Middle East and North Africa. *Violence Against Women*, 14(1): 53–70

Charrad MM (2001) *States and women's rights: The making of post-colonial Tunisia, Algeria, and Morocco*. Berkeley, CA: University of California Press

Clark CJ, Everson-Rose SA, Suglia SF, Btoush R, Alonso A, Haj-Yahia MM (2010) Association between exposure to political violence and intimate-partner violence in the occupied Palestinian territory: a cross-sectional study. *The Lancet*, 375(9711): 310–316

Coale AJ, Banister J (1994) Five decades of missing females in China. *Demography*, 31(3): 459–479

Das Gupta M (2005) Explaining Asia's "missing women": A new look at the data. *Population and Development Review*, 31(3): 529–535

De Onis M, Frongillo EA, Blössner M (2000) Is malnutrition declining? An analysis of changes in levels of child malnutrition since 1980. *Bulletin of the World Health Organization*, 78(10): 1222–1233

Doan RM & Bisharat L (1990) Female autonomy and child nutritional status: The extended-family residential unit in Amman, Jordan. *Social Science and Medicine*, 31(7): 783–789

DOS-Jordan (Department of Statistics-Jordan) & Macro International Incorporation (MI) (2008) *Jordan population and family health survey 2007*. Calverton, MD: Department of Statistics and Macro International Inc

DeRose LF, Das M, Millman SF (2000) Does female disadvantage mean lower access to food? *Population and Development Review*, 26(3): 517–547

Douki S, Nacef F, Belhadj A, Bouasker A, Ghachem R (2003) Violence against women in Arab and Islamic countries. *Archives of Women's Mental Health*, 6: 165–171

El-Zanaty F, Hussein EM, Shawkey GA, Way A, Kishor S (1996) *Egypt demographic and health survey 1995*. National Population Council, Cairo. Calverton, MD: Macro International

El-Zanaty F, Way A (2006) *Egypt demographic and health survey 2005*. Ministry of Health and Population. National Population Council. El-Zanaty and Associates. Cairo, Egypt: ORC Macro

El-Zanaty F, Way A (2009) *Egypt Demographic and Health Survey 2008*, Ministry of Health, El-Zanaty and Associates and Macro International, Cairo. Egypt. ORC Macro

ESCWA (United Nations Economic and Social Commissions for Western Asia) (2002) Women and men in the Arab countries: Employment, March, 2002. ESCWA/STAT/ 2002/1

Fargues P (2005) Women in Arab countries: Challenging the patriarchal system? *Reproductive Health Matters*, 13(25): 43–48

Farhood L, Dimassi H, Lehtinen T (2006) Exposure to war-related traumatic events, prevalence of PTSD, and general psychiatric morbidity in a civilian population from Southern Lebanon. *Journal of Transcultural Nursing*, 17(4): 333–340

Garcia-Moreno C, Jansen HA, Ellsberg M, Heise L, Watts CH (2006) Prevalence of intimate partner violence: Findings from the WHO multi-country study on women's health and domestic violence. *The Lancet*, 368: 1260–1269

Gerritsen AA, Bramsen I, Devillé W, van Willigen LH, Hovens JE, van der Ploeg HM (2006) Use of health care services by Afghan, Iranian, and Somali refugees and asylum seekers living in the Netherlands. *European Journal of Public Health*, 16(4): 394–399

Giacaman R, Abu-Rmeileh NM, Husseini A, Saab H, Boyce W (2007a) Humiliation: The invisible trauma of war for Palestinian youth. *Public Health*, 121: 563–571

Giacaman R, Shannon HS, Saab H, Arya N, Boyce W (2007b) Individual and collective exposure to political violence: Palestinian adolescents coping with conflict. *European Journal of Public Health*, 17(4): 361–368

Gorst-Unsworth C, Goldenberg E (1998) Psychological sequelae of torture and organized violence suffered by refugees from Iraq. *British Journal of Psychiatry*, 172: 90–94

Guthold R, Ono T, Strong KL, Chatterji S, Morabia A (2008) Worldwide variability in physical inactivity: A 51-country survey. *American Journal of Preventative Medicine*, 34(6): 486–494

Hill K, Upchurch DM (1995) Gender differences in child health: Evidence from the demographic and health surveys. *Population and Development Review*, 21(1): 127–151

Hindin MJ, Kishor S, Ansara DL (2008) *Intimate partner violence among couples in 10 DHS countries: Predictors and health outcomes.* DHS Analytical Studies No. 18. Calverton, MD: Macro International Inc

Holden GW (2003) Children exposed to domestic violence and child abuse: Terminology and taxonomy. *Clinical Child and Family Psychology Review*, 6: 151–160

Hoodfar H (1997) *Between marriage and the market: Intimate politics and survival in Cairo.* Berkeley, CA: University of California Press

Hynes M, Robertson K, Ward J, Crouse C (2004) A determination of the prevalence of gender-based violence among conflict-affected populations in East Timor. *Disasters*, 28(3): 294–321

James PT, Leach R, Kalamara E, Shayeghi M (2001) The worldwide obesity epidemic. *Obesity Research*, 9(4): S228–S233

Johnson JL, Greaves L, Repta R (2009) Better science with sex and gender: Facilitating the use of a sex and gender-based analysis in health research. *International Journal for Equity in Health*, 8: 14

Joseph S (1993) Connectivity and patriarchy among urban working-class Arab families in Lebanon. *Ethos*, 21(4): 452–484

Joseph S (2000) *Gender and citizenship in the Middle East.* Syracuse, NY: Syracuse University Press

Kalmuss DS, Straus MA (1982) Wife's marital dependency and wife abuse. *Journal of Marriage & the Family*, 44: 277–286

Kandiyoti D (1988) Bargaining with patriarchy. *Gender and Society*, 2(3): 274–290

Khawaja M (2004) Domestic violence in refugee camps in Jordan. *International Journal of Gynecology and Obstetrics*, 86: 67–69

King GA, Fitzhugh EC, Bassett DR Jr et al (2001) Relationship of leisure-time physical activity and occupational activity to the prevalence of obesity. *International Journal of Obesity*, 25: 606–612

Kishor S, Johnson K (2004) *Profiling domestic violence: A multicountry study.* Calverton, MD: ORC Macro

Linos N (2009) Rethinking gender-based violence during war: Is violence against civilian men a problem worth addressing? *Social Science and Medicine*, 68(8): 1548–1551

Llabre MM, Hadi F (2009) War-related exposure and psychological distress as predictors of health and sleep: A longitudinal study of Kuwaiti children. *Psychosomatic Medicine*, 71: 776–783

Mabry RM, Reeves MM, Eakin EG, Owen N (2010) Evidence of physical activity participation among men and women in the countries of the Gulf Cooperation Council: A review. *Obesity Reviews*, 11(6): 457–464

Mahmood DA, Feachem RG (1987) Feeding and nutritional status among infants in Basrah City, Iraq: A cross-sectional study. *Human Nutrition*, 41C(5): 373–381

Makinson C (1985) *Age and sex differences in treatment of childhood diarrheal episodes in rural Menoufia,* Unpublished manuscript. Cairo, Egypt: American University in Cairo, Social Research Center

Moghadam V (2004) Patriarchy in transition: Women and the changing family in the Middle East. *Journal of Comparative Family Studies*, 35, 137–162

Moghadam V (2009) Feminism, legal reform and women's empowerment in the Middle East and North Africa. *UNESCO*, 9–16

Nelson C, Olesen V (1977) Veil of illusion: A critique of the concept of equality in Western thought. *Catalyst*, 10: 8–36

ORC Macro (n.d.) Surveys with the domestic violence module. Available from http://www.measuredhs.com/topics/dv/dv_surveys.cfm [Accessed 19 April 2009]

Pande R (1999) *Grant a girl elsewhere, here grant a boy: Gender and health outcomes among rural Indian children*. Baltimore, MD: Johns Hopkins University

Popkin BM (1999) Urbanization, lifestyle changes and the nutrition transition. *World Development*, 27: 1905–1916

Punamäki RL, Komproe IH, Qouta S, Elmasri M, De Jong JT (2005) The role of peritraumatic dissociation and gender in the association between trauma and mental health in a Palestinian community sample. *American Journal of Psychiatry*, 162: 545–551

Qouta S, Punamaki RL, Miller T, El-Sarraj E (2008) Does war beget child aggression? Military violence, gender, age and aggressive behavior in two Palestinian samples. *Aggressive Behavior*, 34: 231–244

Roberts B, Damundu EY, Lomoro O, Sondorp E (2009) Post-conflict mental health needs: A cross-sectional survey of trauma, depression and associated factors in Juba, Southern Sudan. *BMC Psychiatry*, 9: 7

Saab BR, Chaaya M, Doumit M, Farhood L (2003) Predictors of psychological distress in Lebanese hostages of war. *Social Science and Medicine*, 57: 1249–1257

Schoenbaum M, Tulchinsky TH, Abed Y (1995) Gender differences in nutritional status and feeding patterns among infants in the Gaza Strip. *American Journal of Public Health*, 85(7): 965–969

Sibai AM, Fletcher A, Armenian HK (2001) Variations in the impact of long-term wartime stressors in mortality among the middle-aged and older population in Beirut, Lebanon, 1983–1993. *American*

Journal of Epidemiology, 154(2): 128–137

Straus MA (2004) Prevalence of violence against dating partners by male and female university students worldwide. *Violence against Women*, 10: 790–811

Swan SC, Gambone LJ, Caldwell JE, Sullivan TP, Snow DL (2008) A review of research on women's use of violence with male intimate partners. *Violence and Victims*, 23: 301–314

Sweeting HN (2008) Gendered dimensions of obesity in childhood and adolescence. *Nutrition Journal*, 7: 1

Tabutin D (1992) Excess female mortality in Northern Africa since 1965: A description. *Population: An English Selection*, 4: 187–207

Tabutin D, Schoumaker B (2005) The demography of the Arab World and the Middle East from the 1950s to the 2000s: A survey of changes and a statistical assessment. *Population (English Edition)*, 60(5/6): 505–615

Tekce B (1990) Households, resources, and child health in a self-help settlement in Cairo, Egypt. *Social Science and Medicine*, 30(8): 929–940

Tekce B, Shorter F (1984) Determinants of child mortality: A study of squatter settlements in Jordan. *Population and Development Review*, 10(1): 257–280

Thabet AA, Karim K, Vostanis P (2006) Trauma exposure in pre-school children in a war zone. *British Journal of Psychiatry*, 188: 154–158

Thabet AA, Tawahina AA, El Sarraj E, Vostanis P (2008) Exposure to war trauma and PTSD among parents and children in the Gaza strip. *European Journal of Child and Adolescent Psychiatry*, 17: 191–199

UNDP (United Nations Development Programme) & INP (the Institute for National Planning) (2005) *Egypt 2005 human development report*. Cairo, Egypt: UNDP

UN (United Nations) General Assembly (1993) *Declaration on the elimination of violence against women*: A/RES/48/104

Usta J, Farver JA, Pashayan N (2007) Domestic violence: the Lebanese experience. *Public Health*, 121(3): 208–219

Waldron I (1987) Patterns and causes of excess female mortality among children in developing countries. *World Health Statistical Quarterly*, 40, 194–210

Watts C, Zimmerman C (2002) Violence against women: Global scope and magnitude. *The Lancet*, 359: 1232–1237

World Bank (2004) *Gender and development in the Middle East and North Africa*. Washington, DC: World Bank

WHO (World Health Organization) (2007) *Cross-cutting gender issues in women's health in the Eastern Mediterranean Region, Cairo, Egypt*. WHO Regional Office for the Eastern Mediterranean

WHO (World Health Organization) (2008) *Preventing violence and reducing its impact: How development agencies can help*. World Health Organization

Yount KM (1999) *Persistent inequalities: Women's status and differentials in the treatment of sick boys and girls*. Case Study of Minia, Egypt. Baltimore, MD: Johns Hopkins Bloomberg School of Public Health

Yount KM (2001) Mortality of girls in the Middle East in the 1970s and 1980s: Patterns, correlates and gaps in research. *Population Studies*, 55(3): 291–308

Yount KM (2002) Like mother, like daughter? Female genital cutting in Minia, Egypt. *Journal of Health and Social Behavior*, 43(3): 336–358

Yount KM (2003a) Gender bias in the allocation of curative care in Minia, Egypt. *Population Research and Policy Review*, 22: 267–295

Yount KM (2003b) Provider bias in the treatment of diarrhea among boys and girls in Minia, Egypt. *Social Science and Medicine*, 56: 753–768

Yount KM (2004a) Maternal resources, proximity of services, and the curative care of boys and girls in Minya, Egypt. *Population Studies*, 58(3): 345–355

Yount KM (2004b). Symbolic gender politics, religious group identity, and the decline in female genital cutting in Minia, Egypt. *Social Forces*, 82(3): 1063–1090

Yount KM (2005) Resources, family organization, and violence against married women in Minya, Egypt. *Journal of Marriage and Family*, 67(3): 579–596

Yount KM (2010) Women's conformity as resistance to intimate partner violence in Egypt. *Sex Roles*, DOI 10.1007/s11199–010–9884–1

Yount KM, Balk D (2004) A demographic paradox: Causes and consequences of female genital cutting in Africa. *In:* V Demos, M Segal M, J Kronenfeld (Eds.) *Advances in gender research volume 8: Gendered perspectives on reproduction to sexuality* (p. 199–249). Oxford, UK: Elsevier JAI

Yount KM, Carrera JS (2006) Domestic violence against married women in Cambodia. *Social Forces*, 85(1): 355–387

Yount KM, Li L (2009) Women's 'justification' of domestic violence in Egypt. *Journal of Marriage and Family*, 71(5): 1125–1140

Yount KM, Li L (2010) Domestic violence against married women in Egypt. *Sex Roles*, 63: 332–347

Knowledge Gaps: The Agenda for Research and Action

Hoda Rashad and Zeinab Khadr

This chapter concludes the section on social determinants of health, in which other chapters have examined key determinants, by attempting to frame a future agenda for research and action in the Arab region. It is clear that the conceptualization of this section, which starts with highlighting health inequities before proceeding to examine other key determinants, makes explicit choices in terms of identifying equity as a clear need with the social domain as the promised arena for action. This section is thus in accord with current international thinking on equity, a previously neglected terrain, and in the renewed calls for broader social policy reforms and for actions on structural social determinants (for example as expressed in the report of the Commission on the Social Determinants of Health; CSDH 2008).

Many Arab scholars, including the authors (see for example Rashad 2005a; 2005b; 2006; Khadr 2008; Khadr et al 2008; Khadr 2009) endorse such framing. Before highlighting the many knowledge gaps and drafting a very much needed research and action agenda, it may be prudent to step back and ask a couple of key questions: Do we have enough consensuses in the Arab region that health equity is a priority? If so, is it recognized that research and actions on social determinants are promising routes to address health inequity? It is our judgment that, excepting a small group of public health professionals, social scientist and a few civil actors, there is no real outcry for health equity and no serious call for social actions to address health inequity. By analyzing health policy documents, Chapter 5 demonstrates that many health authorities do not appear ready to embrace equity and/or social actions for equity as priority concerns within the health domain. The same may be true for policy makers outside health ministries, the society at large and even researchers and civil actors concerned with health and human development.

Many would argue to the contrary: that in the Arab region equity as a value reflected in policies and programs was central to the post-independence development agenda in many countries but that this concern weakened after the adoption of neo-liberal policies of the 1980s and 1990s. The shift to market forces and redefining the state's roles as encouraged by the international financial institutions through structural adjustment programs and sustained by the forces of globalization are seen as underlying such a transition. Ali (2009a) has shown that the Arab region enjoys a medium degree of social inequality, attributing it to the redistributive social contracts that prevailed earlier. He documented a recent trend of increased inequality and linked this to a context of tolerance toward inequality shaped by the argument of "a real tradeoff between policies for economic growth and those for reducing inequality" (Ali 2009a, p. 2).

Evidence supports the argument that social/economic equity, focusing on income distribution and equality of opportunities such as education, health services, women's empowerment, was once a cornerstone of the state agenda. However, this is not clearly the case for health equity. The discussion of the distribution of health outcomes was rarely explicitly linked to social policies and the patterned differences between social groups were never linked to bad politics. Health equity was not discussed as a responsibility of public policies and as such not prioritized as a goal and was confined to the domain of the health care sector and addressed through the fair distribution of health services and resources.

Given this context, the first part of this chapter will propose an agenda for research and action to achieve a major paradigm shift in relation to health equity and its social determinants. This shift entails prioritizing health equity, changing the way social determinants of health are viewed and understood

Public Health in the Arab World, ed. Samer Jabbour et al. Published by Cambridge University Press. © Samer Jabbour et al., 2012.

and more importantly valuing actions on social determinants of health as social policy objectives. Such a shift is imperative to allow the formation of a conscious public and political will to address health equity through the social domain.

The second part discusses the knowledge gaps and the agenda for developing a comprehensive policy reform that frames health equity as a state corporate priority in public policies and intersectoral actions. Such policies and actions should target the root causes of health inequity, which are the inequitable distribution of power, money, and resources that shapes social stratification patterns and impact people's health opportunities (CSDH 2008), and adopt intersectoral actions to achieve health equity.

In the third part, we discuss how to move from research and knowledge into policies and actions. This entails developing the political will, translating that will into initiatives and programs as well as ensuring that development initiatives succeed in achieving their highest impact on health both in terms of improvement in national averages as well as in distributions. We argue for the need to engage with forces of policy change and move beyond elucidating the social determinants of population health into proposing and supporting actions in the social domain that have the potential to address the health gaps and gradients among various social groups.

Toward a Paradigm Shift in Relation to Health Equity and the Potential Contribution of Actions in the Social Domain

A research and action agenda is needed to support the desired paradigm shift of pushing equity to the forefront and questioning the health system monopoly of the solution. Foremost, research needs to unveil the unfairness of existing health inequities and to express the urgency, feasibility, and practicality of health equity actions, as well as the potential significant contribution of actions in the social domain. We can benefit here from the lessons of the revolutionary leap that had occurred on the economic front in tackling poverty.

First and foremost, poverty levels and trends have become central to all discussion of development with poverty alleviation topping the Millennium Development Goals (MDGs) which all Arab countries have

adopted. Second, it is now well accepted that reducing poverty through the trickle-down effect of growth is not enough and there is a need for explicit and comprehensive strategies and public policies. Consequently, it has become accepted that there is a need to mainstream poverty alleviation in all policies and to formulate national integrated strategies addressing poverty's structural drivers. Lastly, a developmental right-based approach in tackling poverty has clearly replaced the charity short-term solution. Targeted developmental programs and intersectoral initiatives are now recognized as necessary to produce significant impact on the most vulnerable groups.

Poverty alleviation efforts have benefitted from major advances on the research and action fronts. One such advance is improving the science and tools for measuring and monitoring poverty and its unequal distribution. For example, World Bank researchers have refined tools of poverty measurement that allow disaggregation and differentiation of groups according to poverty prevalence and severity never previously feasible given the information constraints in low- and middle-income countries (for details see for example Klugman 2002). Another advance comes from the documentation of experiences and lessons from poverty alleviation programs which have demonstrated the much larger impact of interventions couched in a developmental model as compared to the charity-like direct cash transfers that alleviate suffering but do not address the root causes of entrapment.

Achieving a similar paradigm shift on the health front in the Arab world requires a research and action agenda for: 1) improving diagnosis and monitoring of health inequity and 2) improving the knowledge on the potential role of social actions in achieving health equity. Such knowledge can contribute to policy change but does not guarantee such a change. The latter demands additional transformative forces that are social and political in nature. We will visit this point later.

Improving Diagnosis and Monitoring of Health Inequities

Health disparities between social groups are widely recognized and are frequently analyzed by residence, sex, education, age-groups and sometime by income and socio-economic conditions (see for example Al-Kebsi 2008; Halas 2008; Khawaja et al 2008; Osman 2008). Chapter 5 examines evidence from the Arab countries about these disparities and describes them as inequities because of their patterning along social categories, with the disadvantaged commonly displaying worse indicators in both outcome measures and structural determinants, making them unfair. However, the appreciation of the unfairness of these differences is not fully captured by the public as well as policy makers. The reason for the absence of this appreciation draws on two ways of thinking. The first readily attributes these differences to biological/genetic or behavioral risk factors. Hence these factors are seen as either inevitable or shaped by individual choices (whether preferences and/or weak information). The role of the context in governing such choices tends to be ignored. The second way of thinking simply conceptualizes the context as influenced by the normal process of socio-economic development. What is being missed is the unequal opportunities for health and the unfair allocation of the existing resources. Both ways of thinking tend to blur the structural origins of health inequities.

There is weak recognition, among the public as well as many policy makers and researchers, of the ethical and moral imperatives for addressing health inequities. When discussed, these imperatives are commonly misunderstood as ideological impracticalities. Many believe that the health sector can adequately meet its responsibility toward the disadvantaged through its general quest for improvement of public health as well as more equitable health care services and financing, primary care, and community health interventions. The progress in *average* health and health system indicators in Arab countries over the preceding decades seems to contribute to this confusion. Between 1990 and 2006 average life expectancy improved in all countries, regardless of national income (WHO 2008b). Several countries are reported to be on track to achieving health-related target national MDGs; Egypt, for example, was reported to be on the right track to achieve all health-related Millennium Development Goals in particular with regard to child and maternal health and combating major infectious diseases (UNDP 2010). Furthermore, countries like Yemen and Djibouti are reported to be on track for achieving MDGs for infant and child mortality, although achieving other health goals requires more efforts (UNDP 2009).

From the perspective of health equity, there are several problems with this sense of good progress. First, the degree and nature of the trickle down of the documented progress, particularly for the poor and disadvantaged, is not commonly discussed and is frequently unknown. The focus on averages has displaced meaningful discussions of the distribution of health among different social groups. The current information base in the region does not capture the range and the magnitude of health inequities, precluding an assessment of whether health progress has been equitable. Second, if countries perceive that they are doing well then the logical next step is to continue the current path, by fine-tuning programs and interventions of the same biomedical nature, rather than shift direction to address causal pathways of inequities originating in social/political domains. Indeed, discussions of the latter are grossly missing. Third, the diagnosis of public health priorities is distorted if an equity lens is not considered. Risk factors, behaviors, and disease consequences become the most important rather than inequities and their underlying determinants. For example, Mourshed et al (2007) did not identify equity issues when evaluating health system challenges in the Gulf countries. The three priorities were population growth, aging and conditions such as Type 2 diabetes, cardiovascular diseases, and obesity. Fourth, lack of attention to equity derails reform efforts. The health sector reform movement that is sweeping the region – that was originally targeting pro-poor policies – has been quickly redirected toward health sector efficiency including better financing and cost recovery, efficient use of resources as well as health care insurance for those unable to pay (Gwatkin 2001). The public health priorities are defined around specific diseases or broad health dimensions of general groups (women, children) and the way forward does not demand a "new way of doing health".

Pushing equity to the forefront of the political agenda requires a solid program of research to generate data on inequities that advocates can use to push for change. This research effort, however, will have to address the current weaknesses in documenting the nature of health inequities and their underlying causes. Previous research (see Chapter 5) has documented health disparities and differentials by various social stratifiers. However, this research has five main shortcomings:

- Research has mainly focused on a pathology-oriented medical model for a few conditions. Dominated by mortality indicators, it lacks a broader conceptualization of health that includes information on mental, social, and subjective dimensions of ill-health and its burden on individuals and households. This limited focus tends to underestimate the magnitude of inequality and support action on biomedical individual risk factors. Broadening conceptualization of health is likely to document larger inequities and provide a clearer link to social policies. For example, Rashad (2005a) showed that Arab countries with the highest survival rates and life expectancies at birth do not necessarily show large differences by gender. However, investigation of the burden of ill health showed much larger differences. In Bahrain, the life expectancy at birth was 74 years for men and 76 for women but women have higher prevalence of chronic health problems (26% vs. 18%, respectively).

- Research has examined the relationship between health and a limited set of characteristic-oriented stratifiers, such as geographic location (mostly rural/urban), sex (male/female) and very few individual characteristics (mostly education of mother) and sometimes household economic levels (see Chapter 5). Stratifiers that capture social position and social capital and environment, shown to have an important impact on health (see for example Kawachi et al 1999; Kavanagh et al 2006; Yen & Syme 1999) are rarely used. Some chapters in the current volume (see for example Chapter 6) attempt to address this shortcoming and propose using a wider set of stratifiers in analyzing health inequities. A study on urban inequity in Egypt, using an expanded battery of health stratifiers such as social capital and environment, shows significant health inequities (Khadr et al 2008).

- Another drawback of using simple and single stratifiers is the inability to identify vulnerable groups. As Östlin et al note (2009), "When social context is studied as a determinant of health, it tends to be broken into discrete aspects (e.g., poverty, or discrimination by gender or ethnicity, or exposure to occupational hazards) rather than being seen in terms of interacting processes of social stratification, marginalization and exclusion" (p. 4). We need a more sensitive configuration of factors that better identify special groupings and reflect the clustering of risks and their life course cumulative effects. This can encourage integrated actions and the needed focus on structural drivers.

For example, Rashad (2003) showed while post-neonatal mortality for girls is slightly higher than that for boys, the combination of rural residence and mothers' low educational attainment increases the girls' rates to almost two-fold of that for boys (see also Chapter 5).

- Research has not used summary measures needed to rally the general public and policy makers around sticky messages of inequity. In other settings, rising concerns for health inequities have led to the development of numerous tools and measurement approaches for the assessment of health inequity with varying complexity to suit varying audiences (O'Donnell et al 2007). This is rarely done in the Arab countries (See for example Khadr 2009)

- Research has not attempted to track changes in health inequity over time and to introduce the temporal dimension and its link to social policies. Only recently have Arab scholars paid attention to these changes (Khadr 2009). Monitoring of inequity trends, greatly hampered by the existing databases, can be the rallying point to raise the questions around who benefits from inequities and how much. Health policy makers may be more prone to address health inequity issues that show increasing gaps among social groups over time.

These shortcomings are not unique to the Arab region and researchers are developing the conceptual, methodological, and analytical base for addressing them (see for example the WHO Task Force on Research Priorities for Equity in Health Report (2005), updated by Östlin et al (2009). Researchers in the Arab region need to be part of these endeavors.

The aforementioned challenges call for major regional research efforts that revisit the conceptualization of health, its operationalization and the appropriate measurement tools, map and assess the potentials of health information systems in different countries, and recommend practical steps for improving these systems to better contribute to understanding and monitoring health inequities.

Improving Knowledge on the Potential Role of Social Actions in Achieving Health Equity

Recognizing health inequity as a concern is not enough for its prioritization. Appreciating the potential, feasibility, and practicality of social actions in achieving health equity is a cornerstone for pushing health equity to the forefront. This would first require challenging the implicit assumption that health inequities can be adequately addressed through improved health system functioning and would also require demonstrating the success of social policies in this regard. The sense of positive health achievements in the Arab countries has not just ignored the role of societal actions but has also created an implicit assumption that health inequities can be addressed through business as usual coupled with some health sector reforms.

That health improvements are readily attributed to the health system is well known in the international experience. Evans (2008) notes that "The general public is happy to give modern medical care credit for the great benefits, and the providers of care have been willing to accept" is as valid for the Arab region as for the general overview he was presenting. Assigning credit for health improvement to health systems, as opposed to social actions, can heavily influence options for future action in favor of health system interventions (Östlin & Diderichsen 2001). While health care is an undisputed powerful social determinant of health, it has limits in addressing inequities. The key questions are not what the health system can achieve but what are the weights of other social factors in reducing health inequity and what is the knowledge base required to establish the relationships between these social factors and health inequities? Two types of research are needed to answer these questions. The first draws lessons from the international experience and the second revisits the misguided focus of current analytical research on proximate and intermediary determinants of health inequities.

There are enough international experiences to move the discussion of health inequities beyond the entrapment of economics, health expenditures, and health care. Some low- and medium-income countries, such as Cuba, Costa Rica, Thailand, Sri Lanka, the state of Kerala in India, and the state of Porto Allegre in Brazil, have achieved adequate levels of public health indicators despite relatively low national incomes with many showing better health gradient/distribution than economically advanced countries (Bertodano 2003). We need a research repository of international experiences synthesizing principles and lessons for success. The Commission on the Social Determinants of Health has attempted to do this but

more work is still needed. The knowledge base on the experience of the Arab countries is quite limited. Recently, EMRO in collaboration with the Social Research Center of the American University in Cairo undertook an exercise to mainstream an equity lens in the health system observatory for the East Mediterranean region. This exercise attempted to identify health inequity indicators and main health stratifiers with an application on the health system in Egypt. The exercise remains limited in scope as it focused mainly on inequities in the health care services (Zaky & Abdel-Mowla 2009). A comprehensive health repository would dispel popular myths about ill health, demonstrate how ill health is shaped by poor politics, unfair economic arrangements and bad policies, and provide role models for success and illustration of feasible, practical, and affordable social policies that managed to address health inequities.

Another research call is to refocus attention from the usual behavioral proximal causes to the structural root causes. For example, research on education of mothers and influence on child health has commonly emphasized the behavioral mechanisms linking education to child health. As a result, health policies have tended to adopt simplistic ineffective strategies for behavioral changes which do not recognize the contextual constraints facing behavioral change and do not pay needed attention to enabling environments and structural forces. This call fits with the recommendations of a recent WHO initiative to broaden the health research focus and adopt methodologies and strategies to better examine and address health inequities (Östlin et al 2009).

Comprehensive Policy Reforms Framing Health Equity as a Corporate Priority in Public Policies and Intersectoral Actions

We need comprehensive policy reforms if we recognize that ministries of health are not the sole producers of health and agree to reorient the current focus of public health from intermediate determinants to structural drivers many of which lie outside the health sector. The objectives on a public health level are to push the boundaries for defining what constitute public health programs beyond intermediate factors and toward social policies as well as for how public health programs are organized and implemented. On the broader policy level, we need to mainstream health in all policies: public policies whose aim is not health but which influence health need to mainstream health in its strategy.

The proposed reform entails a number of elements. Within the health sector, public health needs to be strengthened and re-oriented away from focusing on changing behaviors, lifestyles, and single risk factors toward assuming new roles of securing intersectoral actions to address health inequity and their underlying contextual forces. This requires redefining the stewardship role of ministries of health to develop effective approaches for intersectoral engagement (Walley et al 2008) and beyond this to ensuring health in all social policies (WHO/Europe 2006).

The CSHD (2008) emphasized the need for comprehensive policy reforms that frame health as a corporate priority in public policies and intersectoral action. This does not mean a line extension to current medical structures or services but a far reaching configuration with integrated change in political, economic, social, environmental, and cultural dimensions. There is a need for health policies and actions that aim for universal coverage with the purpose of addressing the health gradient across the full spectrum of social economic positions. This implies a revamping of current policies and the development of more comprehensive and integrated health policies and strategies.

Redefining stewardship and corporate prioritization are not easy tasks. Inter-sectoral action is challenging and requires the strong endorsement and support of the highest political levels (Saltman & Ferroussier-Davis 2000) to secure the alignment of the various sectors and their genuine commitment toward collaborative actions on health inequity.

The proposed research activities focus on learning from regional and international experiences and role models on how to develop national strategies for health that are both inclusive and participatory and involve relevant policy sectors in the pursuit of health equity. On a regional level, many Arab countries have taken some steps toward building the needed knowledge base to support action on tackling health inequities. These include Bahrain, Egypt, Jordan, Morocco, and Oman. Unfortunately, these efforts have not yet been consolidated as a national strategy for health inequity. On the international front, the Swedish National Health strategy can provide an illustrative example of the feasibility and steps involved in formulating national health strategies. The following is a brief review of the Swedish

National Health strategy formulation process. This review relies heavily and uses a number of extracts from two published texts, Mannheimer et al (2007) and Östlin & Diderichsen (2001).

The National Public Health Strategy for Sweden is considered exemplary as it adopts intersectorality in addressing health inequities. The strategy's main objective was to create a "pro-active multisectoral public health approach at all levels" (Mannheimer et al 2007). It aimed to involve sectors and actors at different levels, such as experts, the civil society, trade unions, and general public, in developing public health policy throughout all phases including initiation, setting the agenda, and implementation. A strong political support to health inequity was demonstrated by appointing a parliamentary commission that consists of politicians and number of experts from academia, trade union authorities, and civil society organizations. The commission formulated the aim and scope of the policy, "health on equal terms."

The formulation of the strategy proposal was based on many working reports prepared by public health experts and advisors that were made available and understandable to the general public. Comments on the proposal were provided by more than 200 stakeholders representing authorities, universities, municipalities, counties, trade unions, and civil society organizations and were incorporated in the final proposal. The main targets in the final proposal focused on reducing exposure to determinants of diseases and injuries making explicit the connections between health targets and responsibilities of different actors and policy areas. Identification of health determinants was based on sound scientific evidence carried out by 14 expert groups on exposure areas such as employment and work conditions, economic factors, and social insurance, and for some diagnostic groups including injuries and mental health. The final strategy included 11 public health targets/health determinants including 3 targets for societal structure and living conditions, 5 for settings and environments and 3 for lifestyle and health behavior (Östlin & Diderichsen 2001).

The implementation of the strategy was assigned to the National Institute of Public Health (NIPH). NIPH was established in 2003 and was chaired by the minister of public health and included several members from the local, regional, and national health authorities, representatives from the education, employment, and integration sectors, the policy authority and representatives from all major ministries. Its mandate was to provide advice on priorities, lead the discussion regarding the policy, coordinate public health policy activities in all sectors, and report on the implementation every four years (Mannheimer et al 2007).

The success of the Swedish National Health strategy can be summarized in the following: Politicians and experts working together; focus on determinants of health and multisectoral implementation; demands for strong scientific evidence; and strong emphasis on the democratic process behind the development of the strategy.

From Research to Policy and Action

The previous two sections emphasize the importance of research and knowledge for action. Knowledge on the need to act and to identify what actions to take does not guarantee the decision and the ability to act. Indeed some writers have linked this apathy on behalf of the policy makers to governance-related factors including corruption, lack of democratic accountability, and the overall weakness of civil society. This divide between research and policy is not limited to the Arab countries. In the World Health Assembly (2005) WHO's Director-General declared the need "to assist in the development of more effective mechanisms to bridge the divide between ways in which knowledge is generated and ways in which it is used, including the transformation of health-research findings into policy and practice."

Prior literature suggests that supportive policy and socio-political context are major factors in bridging the gap between research and policy and enhancing the interaction between the researchers and policy makers (Lavis 2008; Jones & Sumner 2008; Chaskin 2009). The supportive context allows organizational readiness and receptivity of major actors that lead to identification of strategic portals for engagement among actors. This requires clear mapping of relevant actors and building alliances among them. Portals of engagement can take many forms, including continuing, multiple, deliberative and reinforced interactions (Chaskin 2009) among actors. Such interactions in the process of priority-setting, systematic reviews, and policy analysis of current policies and initiatives allow actors to define policy problems, workable policy options, and approaches to policy implementation.

A policy maker-targeted research repository that provides "one-stop-shopping" for optimal high-quality and high-relevance problem reviews can be useful in this regard (Lavis 2008).

The literature on bridging the gap between research and policy has persistently emphasized the importance of systematic reviews and policy analysis of current policies. These activities allow the extraction of valuable lessons from current experiences and their use to advocate and lobby for policy changes. This is done through identifying the factors that hinder or contribute to achieving the full potentials of the policies, along with evaluating the role of various policy actors, including implementers and beneficiaries, in policy changes and implementation. The influence of the rules, laws, norms, and customs over the behavior of the actors and stakeholders and the influence of the global interests and forces over national and local actors are among the most important factors. The end -product of this type of research is to generate the necessary political awareness for evidence-based strategic leadership needed to develop future policies.

In the Arab region, one route to influence policies is to address the clear deficit in the production of evidence for informing the choice of initiatives and actions and for ensuring that the implementation of such actions achieves their highest impact on health as well. Many existing opportunities invite the engagement of researchers to operationalize the social determinants frameworks to ensure the achievement of greater impact on health. These opportunities need to be seized.

One example is the revival of attention to comprehensive primary health care (PHC). With its focus on responding to needs, its concern with the circumstances in which people live, its adoption of intersectoral actions, and its emphasis on community empowerment and participation (WHO 2008a) PHC is potentially an excellent vehicle that ministries of health can use to apply the social determinants of health framework. The Arab region prides itself on the widespread implementation of PHC but a large number of PHC models adopt a biomedical model and simplistic translation of its key elements (Shawky 2008). There is an identified need to move the research focus from documenting the weaknesses into proposing and operationalizing actions for successful implementation of the visionary approach of PHC. The 2008 Doha Declaration on PHC, to which most Arab countries signed, offers a step in the right direction.

Another example comes from the development sector. Ali (2009b) estimates that more than 65 million Arabs live in extreme poverty (under $2 per day) accounting for more than 20% of the total population. Arab countries have committed to achieving the first MDG of eradicating extreme poverty, with many declaring their political commitment and launching ambitious initiatives, many of which adopt new models couched in an empowerment frame. In Tunisia, the anti-poverty strategy adopts a two-dimensional integrated approach: a priority *economic* approach to ensure adequate growth and encourage the integration of vulnerable populations into the production; and an accompanying *social* approach to secure social protection and special support to the hard core of poor. The strategy's main pillars are: (i) financial assistance to guarantee a minimum income for all citizens especially the most underprivileged; (ii) specific development programs to improve general development dynamics and contribute to growth; and (iii) regional action for social promotion and the improvement of socio-economic conditions of the populations living in the deprived areas (UNDP 2004).

In Egypt, the government has prioritized and committed to combating poverty and launched many initiatives. This includes two complementary programs ("Geographic targeting of the poorest 1000 villages" and "Supporting most vulnerable families") that include a form of application of Conditional Cash Transfer model emphasizing empowerment and intergenerational mobility.

These two initiatives (revival of PHC and Poverty alleviation) provide a precious opportunity for evidence-base knowledge and research in their implementation which would contribute not just to the national context, but also to the international literature. Furthermore, both initiatives adopt the empowerment framework that focuses on intersectoral actions and initiatives that target changing the contexts of people's lives. As such, this framework poses great challenges to line ministries unaccustomed to venturing beyond sectoral boundaries. The involvement of researchers in these demonstration models can help in addressing these challenges and should be structurally encouraged and facilitated. The success of these models can support the articulation, planning, and implementation of policies that address the wider set of forces (economics, social policies, and politics) that shape people's health contexts.

The movement from the confinement of the research world into the implementation realms is not an easy process that is welcomed by either the research social or policy circles. The constraints are manifold and include structural as well as conceptual hindrances (Jabbour et al 2009). Researchers may not be ready to embrace such opportunities and to tolerate different rules of engagement imposed by contextual realities and state politics. Another hindrance is the lack of organizational readiness of policy makers to seek the support of the research community in building the knowledge base for particular policy initiatives or interventions (Chaskin 2009).

Summary

The social determinants of health approach and an equity lens incorporate a vision and a strategic approach. Adopting this vision and implementing the corresponding approach is a long process that needs to be supported by an agenda of research and action. This chapter highlights a large number of gaps in the Arab world, advocates a regional research movement to fill those gaps, and proposes a research and action agenda to achieve three important changes that are necessary to address health inequities:

- A paradigm shift to prioritize health equity as concern, change the way social determinants of health are viewed and understood, and more importantly value actions on social determinants of health as priority social policy objectives. The corresponding research and action agenda focuses on improved diagnosis and monitoring of health inequities and improving the knowledge on the potential role of social actions in achieving health equity.

- Comprehensive policy reforms to frame health equity as a corporate priority in public policies and to prioritize inter-sectoral actions to achieve equity. The corresponding research and action agenda focuses on learning from regional and international experiences and role models on how to develop inclusive and participatory national strategies for health equity; how to carry out policy analysis that can extract valuable lessons from current experiences and use them to lobby for policy changes; and redefining the stewardship role of ministries of health and strengthening the role of public health division within the health sector to enable it to undertake its multiple tasks in pursing health equity.

- Moving from research to policy and action on health equity requires the corresponding research and action agenda to focus on identifying portals for engagement among the main actors and engaging these actors in the process of priority setting, developing systematic reviews, a repository of policy maker-targeted research, and analyses of current policies and initiatives to define policy problems, workable policy options

and approaches to policy implementation, and seizing engagement and political opportunities for interactions between research and policies.

The research and action agenda we propose to address on health inequities in the Arab world is indeed formidable but is not insurmountable. We draw hope from the ongoing work of many colleagues, civil society members, and activists, organizations, and even some governmental institutions in this area. Their work inspires us, and many others, to continue to struggle for health equity.

References

Al-Kebsi T (2008) *Child mortality in Yemen and health inequity, Paper presented at the IUSSP International Seminar on Health Inequity: Current knowledge and new measurement approaches.* Cairo, Egypt: February 16–18, 2008

Ali AAG (2009a) *The political economy of inequality in the Arab Region and relevant development policies.* Cairo Egypt: ERF Working paper series No 502

Ali AAG (2009b) *Development challenges for the Arab Region: A human development approach.* Volume 1. *Development and Social Policies Department.* UNDP Regional Bureau for Arab States & League of the Arab States

Bertodano I (2003) Costa Rican Health System: Low cost, high value, *Bulletin of the World Health Organization*, 81(8): 626–627

Chaskin R (2009) *From research to action: Connecting research, policy and practice for children, Paper presented in the Consortium workshop on Diploma on Public Policy Child Rights and Advocacy.* Cairo, Egypt: UNICEF

CSDH (Comission of Social Determinants of Health) (2008) *Closing the gap in a generation: Health equity through action on social determinants of health. Final report of the Commission on Social Determinants of Health.* Geneva,

Switzerland: World Health Organization

Evans RG (2008) Thomas McKeown, meet Fidel Castro: Physicians, population health and the Cuban paradox. *Healthcare Policy*, 3(4): 21–32

Gwatkin D (2001) The need for equity oriented health sector reform. *International Journal of Epidemiology*, 30: 720–723

Halas Y (2008) *Wealth inequity and antenatal care in Yemen. Paper presented at the IUSSP International Seminar on "Health Inequity: Current Knowledge and New Measurement Approaches".* Cairo, Egypt: February 16–18, 2008

Jabbour S, Rashidian A, Shawky S, Zaidi S (2009) *Role of academia in public health and health system development in the Eastern Mediterranean Region.* A background paper for the WHO EMRO meeting 7–10 December 2009 in Beirut, Lebanon

Jones N, Sumner A (2008) *Evidence-informed policy influencing childhood poverty as a lens on knowledge, policy and power.* Paper presented at the EADI (European Association of Development research and training Institutes) Conference, 24–28 June 2008 in Geneva, Switzerland.

Kavanagh A, Turrell G, Subramanian S (2006) Does area-based social capital matter for the health of

Australians? A multilevel analysis of self-rated health in Tasmania. *International Journal of Epidemiology*, 35: 607–613

Kawachi B, Kennedy P, Glass R (1999) Social capital and self-rated health: A contextual analysis. *American Journal of Public Health*, 89: 1187–1193

Khadr Z (2008) *Health inequity: Current knowledge and new measurement approaches. Final Report on the IUSSP International Seminar on Health Inequity. Current knowledge and new measurement approaches.* Cairo, Egypt

Khadr Z, Hamed R, Nour-el-Dein M (2008) *Comparative study of living conditions among Cairo's neighbourhoods.* Unpublished Project Report, The Social Research Center, the American University in Cairo

Khadr Z (2009) Monitoring socioeconomic inequity in maternal health indicators in Egypt, 1995–2005. *International Journal for Equity in Health*, 8: 38

Khawaja M, Dawns J, Meyerson-Knox S, Yamout R (2008) Disparities in child health in the Arab region during the 1990s. *International Journal for Equity in Health*, 7: 24

Klugman J. (Ed.) (2002) *A sourcebook for poverty reduction strategies.* Washington, DC: World Bank

Lavis JN (2008) *Knowledge translation for policymakers. Presented in the*

CIHR IHSPR/ IPPH 7th Annual Summer Institute. Cornwall, Ontario, Canada

Mannheimer L, Letho J, Östlin P (2007) Window of opportunity for intersectoral health policy in Sweden: Open, half open or half shut. *Health Promotion International*, 22(4): 307–315

Mourshed M, Hediger V, Lambert T (2006) *Gulf Cooperation Council Health Care: Challenges and opportunities*. Chapter 2.1. Available from www.weforum.org/pdf/Global_Competitiveness_Reports/Reports/chapters/2_1.pdf [Accessed 12 March 2009]

O'Donnell O, van Doorslaer E, Wagstaff A, Lindelow M (2007) *Analyzing health equity using household survey data analyzing: A guide to techniques and their implementation*. Washington, DC: World Bank

Osman K (2008) *Inequity in nutritional status of children under five in Sudan. Paper presented at the IUSSP International Seminar on Health Inequity: Current Knowledge and New Measurement Approaches*. Cairo, Egypt: February 16–18, 2008

Östlin P, Diderichsen F (2001) *Equity-oriented national strategy for public health in Sweden. Policy learning curve series number 1, European center for health Policy*. WHO/Europe. Available from www.who.dk/Document/E69911.pdf [Accessed 9/4/2009]

Östlin P, Schrecker T, Sadana R, et al (2009) *Priorities for research on equity and health – implications for global and national priority setting and the role of WHO to take the health equity research agenda forward*. Draft (9 September 2009) Available from http://www.globalhealthequity.ca/electronic%20library/Priorities%20for%20research%20on%20equity%20and%20health.pdf

Rashad H (2003) *"Health" in a gender assessment*. Egypt: World Bank and National Council for Women; Cairo, Egypt

Rashad H (2005a) *Health research and social equity in the Arab Region: Issues and Challenges. Paper presented to WHO-EM Regional Consultation to Follow up on Mexico Ministerial Summit on Health Research*. Islamabad, Pakistan: 29–30 November 2005

Rashad H (2005b) *The social determinant of health "opening statement". Keynote address presented to the Global Forum on Health Research Annual Meeting (Forum 9)*. Mumbai, India: 11–13 September 2005

Rashad H (2006) Research priorities for improving health: A social model approach, *In*: AM Glimpse (Ed.) *Health research in the cooperation council states*. Prepared and revised by T Khoja Executive Board of the Health Ministers' Council for Cooperation Council States. October 2006

Saltman R, Ferroussier-Davis O (2000) The concept of stewardship in health policy. *Bulletin of the World Health Organization*, 78: 732–739

Shawky S (2008) *Primary health care in the Eastern Mediterranean: From Alma Atta to Doha*. Personal communication

UNDP (United Nations Development Programme) (2004) *Tunisia National Report on Millennium Development Goals*. Available from http://www.undg.org/archive_docs/3665-Tunisia_MDG_Report_-_English.doc [Accessed 17 September 2009]

UNDP (United Nations Development Programme) (2009) *Tracking the millennium development goals: Country profiles*. Available from http://www.mdgmonitor.org/factsheets.cfm [Accessed 14 April 2009]

UNDP (United Nations Development Programme) (2010) *Egypt's progress towards achieving the millennium development goals: Ministry of State for Economic Development & Egypt Information and decision support Center and UNDP*

Walley J, Elawn J, Tinker A, et al (2008) Primary health care: Making Alma Atta a reality. *The Lancet*, 372: 1001–1007

WHO/Europe (World Health Organization/Europe) (2006) *Stewardship*. Available from www,euro.who.int/healthsystems/Stewardship/20061004_1 [Accessed 14 April 2009]

WHO (2008a) *Primary health care. Now more than ever*. World Health Report Geneva, Switzerland: World Health Organization

WHO (2008b) *World health statistics 2008*. Geneva, Switzerland: World Health Organization

WHO Task Force on Research Priorities for Equity in Health & the WHO Equity Team (2005) Priorities for research to take forward the health equity policy agenda. *Bulletin of the World Health Organization*, 83(12): 948–953

World Health Assembly (2005) Resolution on health research. Available from http://www.who.int/rpc/meetings/58th_wha_resolution.pdf [Accessed 15 January 2011]

Yen IH, Syme S (1999) The social environment and health: A discussion of the epidemiologic literature. *Annual Review of Public Health*, 20: 287–308

Zaky H, Abdel-Mowla S (2009) *Health outcome inequities and the health system: A case study of Egypt*. A paper presented to International Seminar on Social and Health Policies for Equity, Approaches and Strategies. London, UK, 2–4 November 200

Chapter

9

Introduction: Health and Disease in the Regional Context

Cynthia Myntti and Rita Giacaman

This section focuses on selected diseases and conditions that are prevalent in the Arab world. It includes chapters on nutritional problems, infectious diseases, the major non-communicable diseases and their risk factors, mental disorders, and injuries. These conditions are commonly examined in the medical and public health literatures, and mortality and morbidity indicators guide the work of clinicians and policy makers in this region and elsewhere.

We suggest that this standard approach is insufficient for understanding health and disease in the Arab world, or anywhere else. For decades this insufficiency has been pointed out by anthropologists and others based on ethnographic research, which reveals not only what conditions motivate what kind of health-seeking behaviors, but the very meanings attached to specific positive and negative conditions. Researchers such as Giacaman et al (2010) write about these states as actually a continuum between "ease" and "dis-ease," reflecting different states of health at particular moments in time.

The standard approach, and its associated indicators, does not capture non-professional sources of knowledge and insights into health. Lay-persons' points of view do matter. These often reveal what strictly biomedical conceptions do not: connections between body and mind, and individual bodies and families and society at large. They underscore the dynamic and syncretic nature of lay-persons' understanding of health and illness; in an increasingly globalized world, many ideas, medicines, technologies, and images shape people's notions about their health (Ghannam 2010). These "popular" connections may also suggest new hypotheses for research and new ways of conceiving interventions beyond the usual individual-focused prevention or treatment. Fundamentally, they tell us about what defines well-being and the greatest threats to it, and many of these are outside a strictly biomedical purview.

Our chapter is organized into three parts. The first addresses the problematic definition of "health," most commonly conceived of in the negative, by its absence. Health is the absence of pain, for example. This "double negative," in fact, needs to be challenged. The second offers a critical examination of "disease," that is, universally recognized morbidities and other negative outcomes. The third part highlights new approaches to research on health and disease, notably self-rated health and quality of life and well-being studies.

Health as a Positive Concept

The World Health Organization has for many years argued that "health is more than the absence of disease," but little systematic thinking has taken place about what this means theoretically or practically in the Arab world. Very occasionally, however, a glimpse of health as a positive state appears in ethnographic and other qualitative research.

In "Fertile, Plump and Strong: the Social Construction of the Female Body in Low-Income Cairo," Ghannam (1997) argues that women in a poor neighborhood in Cairo define their ideal state as being able to bear many children successfully, maintain an attractive, generously proportioned figure, and endure strenuous domestic labor. She later argues (Ghannam 2008) that women from the same class in Cairo spend substantial amounts of money on skin whitening and other beauty products to improve their bodies. Transforming their bodies is key to their own happiness, marital happiness, and family harmony. Based on field research with men in Lebanon, Myntti et al (2002) also identify the issue of fertility as central to health. Men from all sectarian backgrounds practice withdrawal as a method of family planning because it is easier on the health of their wives than other methods of contraception. They believe that withdrawal protects women's future child-bearing potential. In another Lebanon study, Kaddour et al (2005) find that, in disadvantaged suburban communities of Beirut, good health is not just absence of disease and pain but also having the strength to work. These studies suggest that fertility, beauty, and strength are valued components of health and well-being.

Ghannam's incorporation of attractiveness and beauty into women's construction of the ideal female body raises an important question for future research. Working class Cairo may value plump bodies and pale skin, but in other parts of the region, increasing expenditures on diet remedies and plastic surgery suggest that other notions of health and beauty are important for well-being among other groups. These topics are ripe for research, not only because of their implications for the physical and psychological health of individuals, and consequently for public health action, but for the industries they spawn and financial resources they claim.

Work in Palestine underscores the link between the good health of individuals and improved life conditions for the society at large. Respondents told Giacaman and Odeh (2002) "Freedom gives good health," or "In this situation, no one is healthy except for the occupiers, perhaps they are the only ones who are tranquil – hadi al-bal – and in good health." In other words, health is understood in terms of the broader social, economic, and political contexts in which people live. Morsy (1981) makes a similar point based on fieldwork in rural Egypt; the resolution of conflicts is essential for the attainment of health.

The most provocative writing on health as a positive state comes less from the field of public health and more from psychology and philosophy. Ryff and Singer (1998) identify three principles of positive health: First, positive health is not a medical question but a fundamentally philosophical issue. It requires the articulation of the meaning of the good life, whose features include purpose in life, quality relations with others, self-regard, and mastery. Second, human wellness is about the mind and body and their interconnections. Any comprehensive assessment of positive health must include mental and physical components and the ways in which they influence each other. Third, positive human health is not a discrete end state but a dynamic process. Ryff and Singer (1998) summarize the challenge well: "human well-being is ultimately an issue of engagement in living, involving expression of a broad range of human potentialities: intellectual, social, emotional, and physical."

A small qualitative study conducted among older rural women in the Northeastern USA grounds these ideas further (Butler 1993). Five themes emerge as central to the women's health and well-being: the value of giving and caretaking; the importance of staying busy; the centrality of family as social support; resiliency; and the ability to accept difficult life circumstances. Research is needed in the Arab world to define the themes that are important to the positive definition of health here.

Disease, Illness, and Sickness

In public health and medicine, the codification of disease has been aided by increasingly sophisticated and comprehensive international classifications. In 1994, the World Health Organization issued its latest guidelines, the ICD-10, as the international standard for clinical, epidemiological, and health management purposes (WHO 2010). Although standardized definitions, and corresponding indicators, of morbidity, dysfunction, and disorder are vital in public health and medicine, they are not the whole story. These indicators have been subjected to important critique. For example, measures used in the influential global burden of disease study have been critiqued on several accounts (see for example, Arnesen & Nord 1999; Reidpath et al 2003; Mont 2007). The newer version of the study remains focused on fine-tuning the disability weights and addressing technical critiques rather than incorporating a holistic view of health.

Scholars writing on the social meaning of ill health use three terms to bring a more nuanced analysis of negative states of health: disease, illness, and sickness. Two classic articles from medical anthropology define the differences among them: Eisenberg (1977) was first to differentiate between disease and illness; Young (1982) later elaborated them and added the concept of sickness. For the purposes of clarity, we distinguish the basic differences among these concepts.

Disease is an abnormality in the structure and/or function of body systems as defined by the scientific paradigm of modern medicine. Physicians diagnose and treat diseases. Diseases are pathological states whether or not they are individually or culturally recognized. Hypertension, for example, is a disease that may not be acknowledged individually or culturally recognized in the Arab world as elsewhere. Typically, when someone is *marid*, his/her condition has been identified and labeled according to standard disease classifications.

Illness, on the other hand, refers to a person's perceptions and experiences of negative states including, but not limited to, disease. The person identifies the problem and reports the physical or mental symptoms.

The Arabic language is replete with local idioms to describe such negative states. For example, the Palestinian dialect contains a number of expressions that describe a continuum of ill health: something is wrong with him (*malo ishi*), wilted (*dablan*), not happy (*mish mabsut*), not able (*mish qader*), low energy (*habet*), no energy to complete daily activities (*ma fish mrueh*); down (*kayes*); tired (*ta'baan*); broken or achy (*mkasswar*); and ill (*ayyan*); and finally sick (*marid*). These expressions also highlight the inseparability of physical and mental health (Giacaman et al 2010).

Historically, the medical anthropological literature of the region documented many examples of suffering that would not be labeled as disease, for example: spirit possession or *Zar* (Nelson 1971; Constantinides 1985; Boddy 1988, 1994), problems resulting from the evil eye (*al-ʿain* or *nazra*), envy or *hasad* (Early 1982; Giacaman 1988; Sholkamy 2004). These examples illustrate another important issue of popular beliefs about health: unlike the common practice in medicine and public health to compartmentalize well-being into physical and mental health, lay people commonly see them as intimately related if not integrated.

Recent research in the suburbs of Beirut suggests that it is not just "traditional" illnesses that concern women there. Zurayk et al (2007) found that if women are given the chance to talk about their problems, general bodily pain emerges as a major issue for them, one that eschews an easy disease diagnosis. What's more, women readily make the connection between their pains and living in unheated or damp dwellings, memories of the violence of the civil war, or the everyday stresses of poverty.

Inhorn's research on infertility in Egypt, Lebanon, Iran, and the Gulf (1994, 2002, 2004, 2006) raises an issue that may be classified as both disease and illness, but not addressed in the following chapters in this section of the book: sexual dysfunction and infertility. As she notes, the tragic social consequences of infertility on both men and women in the region, and the readiness of sufferers to spend substantial emotional and financial capital to find a cure, argues for more research in this area. Infertility treatment raises a host of new challenges, not least ethical and financial ones.

Sickness, finally, as defined by Young (1982), is the process where worrisome behavioral or biological signs are given socially recognizable meanings. "Being sick" in recognizable ways often allows a person to avoid his or her normal routines or responsibilities. And sickness, rather than illness, often determines the choice and form of treatment. Myntti (1988), for example, found in a Yemeni village that similar symptoms, from the simple headache to more complicated complaints, had different meanings, diagnoses, and treatments, depending on the age and gender of the sufferer, even within one family. Young educated men used modern scientific explanations and sought prestigious and costly modern medicine for their symptoms, whereas women used traditional explanations for the same complaints and free or cheap herbal and household remedies. Obermeyer (2000) similarly reported medical pluralism with regard to women's practices of birth in Morocco.

These three concepts may or may not overlap. "Professional" views and classic public health indicators typically focus on disease and far less on illness and sickness. But overlap is common in popular beliefs about disease etiology; indeed these categories may be inseparable. For example, long-held beliefs about the link between stress (*ghadhab* [anger] and *zaal* [emotional upset]) and cardiovascular disease have been validated physiologically and epidemiologically from this region (Giacaman 1988; Sibai et al 2001).

Sometimes, however, there are important social reasons why an individual may not want to be labeled as sick, even though he or she may be ill and/or diseased. Stigmatizing diseases such as HIV/AIDS offer one example. Occupational health research in northern Europe (Wickman et al 2005) explored the supposed overlap where a person does not feel well, is diagnosed by a physician, and then, when the problems affect his or her ability to work, is labeled sick. The researchers were particularly interested in absence from work due to sickness. In fact, the researchers found no clear overlap between disease, illness, sickness, and sickness absence. In an economic downturn, they found that sickness absence is low, as people are afraid to lose their job if they stay away from work, even if they are ill. These

119

examples suggest that these different aspects of morbidity must be disentangled and analyzed.

New Approaches in Research

There is increasing recognition in the world today of the inadequacies of the narrowly defined concepts of health and disease and the limitations of classical "objective" biomedical measures derived from them, such as malnutrition, stunting, and disease prevalence rates. This is because such measures focus on disease instead of improving the subjective well-being of individuals. The challenge for public health programs is to measure population health and well-being, and not only disease, in order to improve public health planning and programming. This has prompted researchers from the region to call for a different approach. This approach has two key elements: First, it considers and attempts to understand the local meanings and practices of health and illness and integrates various sources of knowledge including popular beliefs; and second, it expands the focus from disease toward health and well-being, and utilizes in addition to classic indicators complementary subjective measures – people's assessments of their own health status – in evaluating health conditions.

We have already discussed the first element of this approach, i.e., the need for understanding local meanings and practices of health. As for the second element, researchers in the region have used various approaches. In addition to anthropological and ethnographic research, there is growing research on *self-rated health* (SRH) one of various subjective health assessment measures (Quesnel-Vallee 2007; Abdulrahim & Baker 2009). Unlike many of the qualitative anthropological studies on positive health and well-being, SRH is quantifiable. Similar to popular perceptions, it is described in the literature as lying at the crossroads of culture and biology, reflecting the states of the human body and mind (Jylha 2009). SRH has been shown to correlate with fatal and non-fatal outcomes, has demonstrated a constant and universal association with mortality, and has been found to predict functional declines and mortality above and beyond objective health indicators; that is, it can be used as a health predictor (de Oliveira Filho et al 2005; Cheng & Chan 2006; Jylha 2010). Furthermore, self-rated health has been proposed as a useful measure for assessing social inequalities in health (Subramanian & Ertel 2009).

Similarly, in the region *Quality of Life* measures have been tested, elaborated, and applied in the Occupied Palestinian Territory. Researchers there argue that such measures are particularly relevant in conflict-affected zones where violence and insecurity are an important part of daily life. Measures of fatal and non-fatal outcomes alone are not sufficient for guiding policy and resource allocation. One qualitative study (Giacaman et al 2007) found that political freedom, feeling of involvement in political decision-making and participation in democratic processes contributes to people's quality of life. In a more extensive survey, Mataria and colleagues (2009) found suggestive differences between women and men. Women reported a higher quality of life than men, explained by being more home-bound and less exposed to the routine humiliations by the Israeli occupying authorities. The researchers argue that quality of life measures, beyond the standard indicators mortality, morbidity, and injury, have helped them measure the complex social suffering and ill health caused by conflict, and aided their struggle for placing rights and justice at the center of public health.

In conclusion, we argue that future approaches to research on health in the Arab world can benefit from conceptual flexibility by subjecting the questions we normally ask and the categories we use in framing our research and practice to greater scrutiny, and by increasing our appreciation of the potential complementarities of biomedical and lay knowledge and popular perceptions of health and disease. Understanding and appreciating how ordinary people define and deal with health problems are also important for guiding future interventions. Furthermore, understanding health in the Arab world requires qualitative and quantitative methods of inquiry, and combining objective and subjective assessments and measures. This can expand the health discourse from the diagnosis of symptoms and the naming of pathologies to encompassing the broader determinants of health, while at the same time incorporating people's voices in defining their health status, determinants, and needs. Finally, a comprehensive line of inquiry offers us the possibility of distinguishing the clinical response from the population-wide response to ill health as it relates to living conditions, poverty, lack of justice, and human rights, all of which are at the core of the concept of the social determinants of health.

References

Abdulrahim S, Baker W (2009) Differences in self-rated health by immigrant status and language preference among Arab Americans in the Detroit Metropolitan Area. *Social Science and Medicine*, 68(12): 2097–2103

Arnesen T, Nord E (1999) The value of DALY life: Problems with ethics and validity of disability adjusted life years. *British Medical Journal*, 319: 1423–1425

Boddy J (1988) Spirits and selves in Northern Sudan: The cultural therapeutics of possession and trance. *American Ethnologist*, 15(1): 4–27

Boddy J (1994) Spirit possession revisited: Beyond instrumentality. *Annual Review of Anthropology*, 23: 407–434

Butler S (1993) Older rural women: Understanding their conceptions of health and illness. *Topics in Geriatric Rehabilitation*, 9(1): 56–68

Cheng ST, Chan ACM (2006) Social support and self-rated health revisited: Is there a gender difference in later life? *Social Science and Medicine*, 63: 118–122

Constantinides P (1985) Women heal women: Spirit possession and sexual segregation in a Muslim society. *Social Science and Medicine*, 21(6): 685–692

De Oliveira Filho GR, Sturm EJ, Sartorato AE (2005) Compliance with common program requirements in Brazil: Its effects on residents' perceptions about quality of life and the educational environment. *Academy of Medicine*, 80: 98–102

Early E (1982) The logic of well-being: Therapeutic narratives in Cairo. *Social Science and Medicine*, 16(16): 1491–1497

Eisenberg L (1977) Disease and illness: Distinctions between professional and popular ideas of sickness. *Culture, Medicine and Psychiatry*, 1: 9–23

Ghannam F (1997) Fertile, plump and strong: The social construction of the female body in low-income, Cairo, Egypt: Monographs in reproductive health No 3. The Reproductive Health Working Group and the Population Council

Ghannam F (2008) Beauty, whiteness and desire: Media, consumption and embodiment in Egypt. *International Journal of Middle East Studies*, 40(0404): 544–546

Ghannam F (2010) Personal communication

Giacaman R (1988) *Life and health in three Palestinian villages.* London, UK: Ithaca

Giacaman R, Odeh M (2002) Women's perceptions of health and illness in the context of national struggle in the old city of Nablus, Palestine, Monographs in Reproductive Health No. 4, 2002, Reproductive Health Working Group, The Population Council Regional Office for West Asia and North Africa

Giacaman R, Mataria A, Ngyyen-Gillham V, Abu Safieh R, Stefanini A, Chatterji S (2007) Quality of life in the Palestinian context: An inquiry in war-like conditions. *Health Policy*, 81(1): 68–84

Giacaman R, Nguyen-Gillham V, Rabaia Y, Batnijie R, Punamaki RL, Summerfield D (2010) Mental health, social distress and political oppression: The case of the occupied Palestinian territory. *Global Public Health*, 23: 1–13

Inhorn M, Buss K (1994) Ethnography, Epidemiology and infertility in Egypt. *Social Science and Medicine*, 39(5): 671–686

Inhorn M (2002) Sexuality, masculinity and infertility in Egypt: Potent troubles in marital and medical encounters. *The Journal of Men's Studies*, 10(3): 343–359

Inhorn M (2004) Middle Eastern masculinities in the age of new reproductive technologies: Male infertility and stigma in Egypt and Lebanon. *Medical Anthropology Quarterly*, 18(2): 162–182

Inhorn M (2006) "He won't be my son". *Medical Anthropology Quarterly*, 20(1): 94–120

Jylha M (2009) What is self-rated health and why does it predict mortality: Towards a unified conceptual model. *Social Science and Medicine*, 69: 307–316

Jylha M (2010) Self-rated health between psychology and biology. A response to Huisman and Deeg. *Social Science and Medicine*, 70: 655–657

Kaddour A, Hafez R, Zurayk H (2005) Women's perceptions of reproductive health in three communities around Beirut, Lebanon. *Reproductive Health Matters*, 13(25): 34–52

Mataria A, Giacaman R, Stefanini A, Naidoo N, Kowal P, Chatterji S (2009) The quality of life of Palestinians living in chronic conflict: Assessment and determinants. *European Journal of Health Economics*, 10: 93–101

Mont D (2007) Measuring health and disability. *Lancet*, 369: 1658–1663

Morsy SA (1981) Towards a political economy of health: A critical note on the medical anthropology of the Middle East. *Social Science and Medicine*, 15B(2): 159–163

Myntti C (1988) Hegemony and healing in rural North Yemen. *Social Science and Medicine*, 27(5): 515–520

Myntti C, Ballan A, Dewachi O, El-Kak F, Deeb ME (2002) Challenging the stereotypes: Men, withdrawal, and reproductive health in Lebanon. *Contraception*, 65(2): 165–170

Nelson C (1971) Self, spirit possession and world view: An illustration from Egypt. *International Journal of Social Psychiatry*, 17(3): 194–209

Obermeyer CM (2000) Pluralism and pragmatism: Knowledge and practices of birth in Morocco. *Medical Anthropology Quarterly*, 14(2): 180–201

Quesnel-Vallee A (2007) Self-rated health: Caught in the crossfire of the question for 'true' health? *International Journal of Epidemiology*, 36(6): 1161–1164

Reidpath DD, Allotey PA, Kouame A, Cummins RA (2003) Measuring health in a vacuum: Examining the disability weight of the DALY. *Health Policy and Planning*, 18: 351–356

Ryff C, Singer B (1998) The contours of positive human health. *Psychological Inquiry*, 9(1): 1–28

Sholkamy H (2004) The medical cultures of Egypt. *In*: H Sholkamy, F Ghannam (Eds.) *Health and identity in Egypt* (p. 111–128). Cairo, Egypt: The American University in Cairo Press

Sibai AM, Fletcher A, Armenian H (2001) Variations in the impact of long-term wartime stressors on mortality among the middle-aged and older population in Beirut, Lebanon, 1983–1993. *American Journal of Epidemiology*, 154(2): 128–137

Subramanian SV, Ertel K (2009) Self-rated health may be adequate for broad assessments of social inequalities in health. *International Journal of Epidemiology*, 38: 319–324

Wickman A, Marklund S, Alexanderson K (2005) Illness, disease, and sickness absence: An empirical test of the differences between concepts of ill health.

Journal of Epidemiology and Community Health, 59: 450–454

WHO (World Health Organization) (2010) The International Classification of Diseases ICD-10. Available from http://www.who.int/classifications/icd/en/ [Accessed 4 December 2010]

Young A (1982) The anthropologies of illness and sickness. *Annual Review of Anthropology*, 11: 257–285

Zurayk H, Myntti C, Salem M, Kaddour A, El-Kak F, Jabbour S (2007) Beyond reproductive health: Listening to women talk about their health in disadvantaged Beirut neighborhoods. *Health Care for Women International*, 28(7): 613–637

Chapter

10

Nutrition and Food Security: The Arab World in Transition

Abdulrahman O. Musaiger, Hala Ghattas, Abdelmonem S. Hassan, and Omar Obeid

The Arab world faces important challenges in relation to nutrition and food security, which are projected to become more severe over the next decades. The nutritional situation has changed drastically over the past 50 years. A double burden of nutritional disorders exists today with both under- and over-nutrition and their associated public health consequences. Diverse social, economic, political, and demographic changes contribute to the different forms of malnutrition with contributing factors varying across countries, but also within countries. Food insecurity, manifested in rising food supply and trade deficits, has local as well as global determinants and poses major public health threats. The global food crisis has accelerated initiatives to address regional food insecurity; however, programs to prevent and control manifestations of malnutrition are insufficient. This chapter will describe the double nutritional burden and the situation of food security and examine their political, economic, and social determinants, provide a brief review of the most important malnutrition disorders and their public health consequences, and allude to various initiatives to address malnutrition and food insecurity.

The Double Nutritional Burden and Its Determinants

The Arab region is highly diverse in terms of ecological structures, agricultural resources, political stability, and economies with varying consequences for the health and nutritional status of populations (Galal 2003). In the past six decades as a result of social, economic, and political changes, rapid demographic transitions (see Chapter 3) have been paralleled by epidemiologic transitions from prevalent infectious diseases related to malnutrition and poor sanitation, to chronic diseases associated with Westernized

lifestyles and population aging (see other chapters in this section). Different countries are at varying stages of these transitions. The *nutrition transition*, due to changes in the nature of diets in terms of both structure and composition, is a major contributor to these transitions.

Increasing calorie availability and intake, changed lifestyles, and reduced physical activity have led to rampant increases in over-nutrition manifesting as over-weight and obesity and their most commonly associated health outcomes: diabetes and cardiovascular disease. Many countries in the region, such as Arab Gulf countries, have one of the highest rates of obesity in the world (WHO 2010a). At the same time, rates of malnutrition among under-5 children in the poorer countries remain alarmingly high: 57.7% had stunting (low height-for-age) in Yemen in 2004 and 21% had wasting (low weight-for-height) in Sudan in 2007 (WHO 2010b) (see also Chapter 17). This double nutritional burden can largely be explained by social, economic, and political disparities between and within countries. While poverty and conflict strongly predict under-nutrition, urbanization and food market globalization predict over-nutrition and its associated morbidities (UNDP 2009). Nonetheless, globalization also contributes to under-nutrition due to increasing food insecurity.

From the limited available data, poverty and under-nutrition correlate, most notably in the lowest-income countries: Mauritania, Sudan, and Yemen (UNDP 2009). However, poverty and food insecurity do not always manifest as under-nutrition. With globalization and availability of cheap, energy-dense, micronutrient-deficient foods, co-existence of over-weight and micronutrient deficiencies is emerging not only within populations but also within households and in individuals. This may result from two scenarios: (1) energy requirements are met but micronutrient

Public Health in the Arab World, ed. Samer Jabbour et al. Published by Cambridge University Press. © Samer Jabbour et al., 2012.

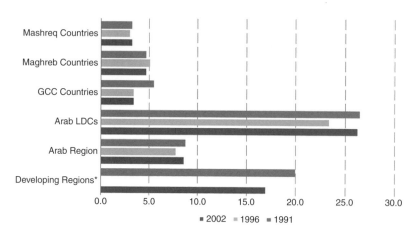

Figure 1. Proportion of population below the minimum level of dietary energy consumption by sub-region, Source: UNESCWA (2007).

deficiencies persist (*hidden hunger*), (2) periods of chronic energy deficiency are followed by periods of abundant energy consumption (*binge-bust eating habits*). In a study that included five Arab countries, stunted preschool children are on average 2–4 times more likely to be over-weight than children with adequate height-for-age (El-Taguri et al 2009).

Food Security

Food security is multidimensional and includes stability of food supplies; availability of food; physical, social, and economic access to safe and nutritious food; and food utilization. We do not have adequate data about all elements of the food security chain. Arab countries are highly reliant on food imports, which account for approximately half of caloric intake, and are the largest net importers of cereal in the world. This reflects low rates of self-sufficiency, or food sovereignty (Abu-Ismail & Mustafa 2009). In 2007, Arab countries faced deficits of 43.9%, 74.8%, and 63.7% in grains, plant oils, and sugar, respectively. Dependence on global markets increases Arab countries' vulnerability to surges in world food prices, as was evident during the 2007–2008 global food crisis. This has increased existing basic food trade deficits, which increased from $11.8 billion in 1990 to $30 billion in 2008 and is projected to increase to $44 billion in 2020 and $71 billion in 2030 (AOAD, 2010). The impact is obviously more evident in low- and middle-income countries.

Despite gains in human development, health, and education in the past two decades, food deprivation rates remain relatively unchanged. Individuals living on less than the minimum level of dietary energy consumption accounted for 8.8% of the Arab population in 1991, and 8.6% in 2002 (Figure 1). Both low-income (Djibouti, Mauritania, Somalia, Sudan, and Yemen) and middle-income (Maghreb and Mashreq) countries made no noticeable progress, with the population proportion living below the food deprivation line remaining unchanged at 26% and 4%, respectively. Only the Arab Gulf countries showed progress, attributed mainly to improvements in the first half of the 1990s. Wide disparities between countries exist in hunger prevalence and progress toward its reduction. In 2002, the proportion of the Somali population below the minimum level of dietary energy consumption intake was 73% (equivalent to 29 times the prevalence in UAE and Morocco) (UNESCWA, 2007). Obviously, conflict has detrimental effects on the nutritional status of populations, especially vulnerable subgroups. We will examine this next.

Conflict, Food Insecurity, and Malnutrition

Populations in countries under violent conflict (Iraq, Morocco/Western Sahara, Occupied Palestinian Territory [OPT], Somalia, and Sudan) face complex humanitarian emergencies, including food insecurities (see chapters in Section 5). Since the beginning of the Al Aqsa Intifada in 2000, the occupation has threatened the livelihoods of Palestinians in OPT (see also Chapter 24). Serial food security assessments since 2003 have documented increasing food insecurity due to limited physical and economic access to markets associated with curfews, closures, high unemployment and poverty rates, strained social support networks, and exhaustion of coping strategies. In the latest surveys (World Food Programme/Food and Agriculture Organization [WFP/FAO] 2009), only 35% of households in the West Bank were food secure, while 25% were food insecure, 11% vulnerable to food insecurity, and 29% marginally food secure. In Gaza, food insecurity or vulnerability to it affected 60.5% and 16.2%, respectively. Abdeen et al (2007) documented associated acute (3–4%) and chronic (9–13%) malnutrition. Among pre-school children, Halileh & Gordon (2006) documented associated anemia (one third) and stunting (9%). Among pregnant women, anemia was present in 31.1% (West Bank) to 44.9% (Gaza) (Halileh et al 2008).

Sanctions imposed after the 1991 Gulf War greatly affected the food security and nutrition situation in Iraq. Political instability under the US-led occupation, especially the large scale population displacement in 2006, has added to this legacy. Surveys in 2003 and 2005 showed alarmingly high rates of food insecurity or vulnerability to it. A recent survey (Central Organization for Statistics & Information Technology [COSIT] et al 2008) showed that 3.1% and 9.4% of households were food insecure or vulnerable to insecurity without rations. Households with highest vulnerability were those of unskilled workers, agricultural workers, and unemployed heads of households. Low income and expenditure, low education levels, rural dwelling, and female headed-households were strong determinants of food insecurity. Stunting in primary school children remains relatively high in Baghdad at 18.7%; 13.5% of children were found to have concurrent stunting and low body mass index for age. Girls were found to be at higher risk of under-nutrition than boys, and risk of stunting increased with age (Al Saffa 2009).

Vulnerability to Food Insecurity

Poverty (see also Chapter 2) is a major predictor of food insecurity as the poor spend the largest share of their budget on food. The rural food-insecure poor tend to be landless laborers who do not benefit from farming subsidies and women-led households (Riely et al 1999). While urbanization is usually associated with improved food security, this is not always the case. In large Arab cities, the poor urban slum dwellers are not better off than their rural counterparts. For example, urban Egyptian children have higher rates of malnutrition, diarrhea, fever, and other illnesses than rural children (Barlow 1999).

Sanitary conditions contribute to food insecurity and under-nutrition. Access to safe water for drinking and food preparation is essential for food and water safety and, consequently, food security. Poor sanitation can lead to recurrent infections, which can initiate a vicious cycle of malnutrition and lead to recurrent infections and mortality. The Egyptian example of food-insecure urban dwellers is likely to be due to lack of universal availability of safe water and sanitation (Galal 2003).

Another example of the multilayered determinants of food insecurity concerns the policy. Enlightened policy can mitigate poverty's impact on food insecurity and under-nutrition. For example, Egypt and Yemen have similar proportions of the population living under $2 a day (40% and 45%, respectively), but Egypt has significantly lower rates of under-nutrition, largely due to availability of aid and food subsidy programs that alleviate the burden of under-nutrition (UNDP 2009).

Combating Food Insecurity

This is a pressing issue that requires funds, resources, and comprehensive policies especially as the region's dependence on food imports is projected to increase by over 60% in the next two decades. Various measures are proposed. Regional and country policies do not operate in a vacuum; global food and trade policies also need reform. Most urgently, there is need for food relief to suffering populations in countries such as OPT, Somalia, and Yemen. In the medium and long term, there is no alternative to enhancing regional food sources. This includes increasing investments, improving land and water resource management, and mitigating the impact of climate change. This will improve agricultural productivity and reducing exposure to market volatility. In parallel, poverty reduction, macroeconomic reforms, and social programs, such as safety nets, family planning, and education, are key to making and sustaining progress. Ensuring food security, specifically for the poor, ultimately comes down to recognizing the right to food, which requires political support within the context of stability.

Malnutrition in the Arab World: Manifestations, Determinants and Interventions

This section focuses on current dietary patterns and nutritional practices in the Arab world, their determinants, the consequences for malnutrition and health, and proposed public health nutrition interventions.

Changing Food Consumption and Lifestyle Patterns

Arab countries have seen remarkable Westernization of lifestyles. In addition to alarming rates of reduced physical activity (see also Chapters 12 & 13), remarkable changes in food habits have occurred. In high-income Arab countries, the traditional diet (dates, milk, vegetables and fruits, whole wheat bread, and fish) has changed to a diet with high energy intake based on excess intake of energy-dense foods rich in fat and free sugars and deficient in complex carbohydrates. Sugar consumption continues to rise, and its contribution to the total energy intake ranges from 10% to 15%. Similar trends are witnessed in middle-income Arab countries and in the upper classes of low-income Arab countries (Musaiger 2002a). There are strong socio-economic and demographic correlates with changing eating habits.

Increases in Energy and Fat Intake

During the period 1970–2005, per capita energy and fat intake rose in most Arab countries (range 10% in Sudan to 40% in Egypt). A high percentage of these calories come from animal foods, particularly in high-income countries, with fat supplies showing impressive increases as a proportion of total caloric intake (FAO 2010). In an urban Lebanese population, for example, fat contributed 39% of total calories (Nasreddine et al 2006).

Reduced Fiber Intake

Studies on fiber intake are few. Since fiber is found only in the carbohydrate portion of the diet, it is widely accepted that the level of fiber in the Arab diet is decreasing due to the decrease in the percentage of dietary intake from carbohydrate and the decrease in the consumption of whole grains. As foods in the region become increasingly processed, grain products lose fiber content. For example, food preparation methods in most Arab countries, such as peeling vegetables and fruits and using wheat flours with low extraction rates in breads, are contributing to a lower intake of fiber (Musaiger 2002a).

Fresh fruits and vegetables are rich sources of dietary fiber in addition to mineral, vitamins, and antioxidants and are associated with less chronic disease. WHO Stepwise surveys in six Arab countries (Egypt, Jordan, Iraq, Kuwait, Saudi Arabia, and Syria) indicate low intake of fresh fruit and vegetables (below five servings/day). In Lebanon, and contrary to its image of boasting a Mediterranean diet, 45% of the urban population consumes less than 400 g of fruits and vegetables daily (Nasreddine et al 2006). Increasing individual fruit and vegetable consumption up to 600g per day (the baseline of choice) could reduce many non-communicable diseases. This is a target for public health policy (see also Chapters 12 & 13).

The intake of fiber-rich foods by children and adolescents in most Arab countries is alarmingly low; their dietary habits, characterized by low intake of fresh fruits, vegetables, and milk and a high intake of carbonated beverages and fast foods, particularly in urban areas, have become similar to those in Western communities. This may in part explain the increase in diet-related chronic diseases in some Arab countries (Arab Center for Nutrition 2003).

Salt Intake

Intake of sodium in this region exceeds the daily requirements of no more than 8–10 mmol of sodium or 500 mg of sodium chloride. This is due to several reasons: high use of table salt, spices, and pickles; and the salinity of water (in some countries) (Musaiger 2002a).

Outcomes of Dietary and Lifestyle Changes
Over-weight and Obesity

These are major public health issues in Arab countries with several among the "Top 20" countries in the world in terms of prevalence of adult over-weight and obesity. Rates vary widely across the region ranging from 30% to 60% among adult men and from 35% to 75% among adult women (Musaiger 2007). A review of studies in the Arab Gulf countries found higher rates of over-weight and obesity particularly among women (75–88% of 30–60 year old women in Kuwait, Qatar, and Saudi Arabia were over-weight or obese), with rapidly increasing rates of obesity (Ng et al 2010). The latest review (Mehio Sibai et al 2010) documents similar findings.

Characteristically, obesity in most Arab countries is more prevalent among women, urban dwellers, married people, non-smokers, and the inactive. The higher prevalence of over-weight and obesity among women has several determinants that show the interaction of structural, social/cultural, biological, and other factors. In Saudi Arabia, mean BMI increased significantly with parity from a mean of 25.1 in nulliparous women to 27.1, 29.8, and 31.7 in women with 1–2, 3–4, and more than 4 parities, respectively (Musaiger 2007). Obesity is more prevalent among women in urban areas. In Jordan, for example, it's 56% in urban areas versus 44% in rural areas. There are similar trends in Egypt, Morocco, Oman, and Tunisia. Lebanon is an exception, as obesity is more prevalent among rural women, probably related to urban cultures. Women's employment affects obesity: Rates among unemployed vs. employed women are 47% vs. 34%, 79% vs. 53%, and 24% vs. 15%, in Kuwait, Saudi Arabia, and Tunisia, respectively (Musaiger 2007). In qualitative surveys, women typically cite various barriers to overcoming over-weight/obesity, including lack of culturally sensitive facilities for physical activity and socio-cultural factors (Ali et al 2010). In contrast to Western countries where the poor carry most of the burden of obesity, there is more obesity in the high socio-economic classes.

The roots of the adult obesity epidemic are growing, with extremely high rates of pediatric and adolescent over-weight (see also Chapters 17 & 18). This is problematic as studies indicate that childhood over-weight predicts adult over-weight and obesity. About 8%–9% of Kuwaiti and Saudi pre-schoolers are obese; Kuwait has one of the highest rates of adolescent over-weight and obesity in the world (40%–46%). This high rate of obesity among adolescents in many Arab countries may be attributed to long periods of watching television or using the Internet, beliefs and attitudes toward obesity and physical inactivity, food advertisements, high intake of fast foods, and an increase of food intake outside the home (Musaiger 2007; Nasreddine et al 2010). Under-nutrition, especially stunting, may be another contributing factor to the high prevalence of over-weight. Stunted children in Djibouti, Libya, Morocco, Syria, and Yemen had higher rates of over-weight compared to their non-stunted counterparts. Metabolic alterations in under-nourished children promote energy conservation. Stunted children have impaired regulation of food intake and have higher susceptibility to the effects of high fat diets, and when energy intake improves, deposition of fat over time may result (El-Taguri et al 2009).

There are no comprehensive programs to prevent and control obesity across the Arab world or in

---

Box 1. Prevention and Control of Obesity in Arab Countries

Summary of the Recommendations of the First Arab Conference on Obesity and Physical Activity, held in Bahrain, 24–26 September, 2002.

1. Government sectors should establish regulations, programs, and activities that can help to reduce obesity and encourage physical activities in the Arab communities.
2. To provide sufficient treatment of obesity, health care providers should have an adequate understanding and training on assessment and management of obesity.
3. Non-governmental organizations and private sector should participate in carrying out training courses, conferences, workshops, and educational programs to prevent and control obesity.
4. The mass media organizations should provide sound and reliable information on the prevention and control of obesity. Regulation of food advertisements, especially those targeting children should be considered. It is important to prepare programs to educate the public on causes, prevention, and management of obesity.
5. Information on causes and management of obesity should be introduced into relevant school and university curricula.
6. It is necessary to establish an Arab Task Force for Obesity and Physical Activity, to increase the awareness of the public in Arab countries on the causes and prevention of obesity, as well as to carry out research and programs on obesity.

Source: Musaiger (2003)

---

individual countries. Some countries have activities to promote physical activity and reduce high energy intake but with limited effect (Arab Center for Nutrition 2003; Musaiger 2007). The 2002 Arab conference on Obesity and Physical Activity in Bahrain proposed recommendations to prevent and control obesity (Musaiger 2003) (Box 1) but these recommendations have not been picked up as policy objectives.

Diet-Related Chronic Non-communicable Diseases

The nutrition transition is associated with the rise of various risk factors, such as hypertension, physical inactivity, and smoking, all of which are closely linked to the epidemiologic transition and the rise of non-communicable diseases (NCDs), including diabetes, heart disease, stroke, and cancer. There are no estimates of the contribution of dietary vs. other factors

Table 1. Life Expectancy and Burden of Nutrition-Related Chronic Diseases in the Arab World (2004–2006)

Health indicators	Low-income countries	Middle-income countries	High-income countries
Life expectancy (years)	47–64	60–74	72–78
Death, heart disease (%)	–	16–30	30–35
Death, cancer (%)	–	3–10	10–16
Adult over-weight and obesity (BMI > 25)			
Male (%)	5–15	14–20	30–50
Female (%)	15–25	25–60	40–70
Adult diabetes (%)	2–7	6–20	12–30

Source: Data available from WHO/EMRO, 2008; UNICEF (2007).

to NCDs in the region. Table 1 provides estimates of the burden of diet-related NCDs. Chapters 12 and 13 focus on NCDs.

Infant Feeding Practices and Child Under-nutrition

Studies on dietary habits linked with prevalence of under-nutrition in the region are scarce. Weight at birth is clearly linked to nutrition; low birth weight (LBW) is one of the most important factors contributing to infant mortality (see Chapter 17). The prevalence of LBW (<2.5 kg) in Arab countries ranges from 6% in Lebanon to 32% in Yemen. Studies on factors associated with LBW in the region are few and limited. LBW can result from malnutrition among mothers, as is the case in Iraq, Djibouti, Somalia, Sudan, and Yemen (UNICEF 2007). Women who were stunted girls are more likely to give birth to LBW infants, creating an intergenerational cycle of under-nutrition. Studies suggest that female sex, low socio-economic status, older mothers, and smaller interval between pregnancies are the main risk factors for LBW. Gestational iron deficiency anemia may also play an important role. Diet and nutrition in utero and in early infancy can affect risk of metabolic disease in later life. Obesity, hypertension, and cardiovascular disease have been associated with birth weight, growth and feeding patterns, and body composition in early childhood.

Breastfeeding initiation rates are relatively high in the region, but there are problems with exclusivity and duration of breastfeeding. Many mothers introduce supplements such as water, sweetened water, and herbal teas as early as the first or second month of infant life. Bottle feeding is also introduced at an early stage, and this may lead to early cessation of breastfeeding and concomitant exposure of the infant to infection and diarrhea. For example, only 47% of infants in the UAE were still breastfed at 6 months of age, and only 10% of Lebanese mothers provided exclusive breastfeeding to 6 months of age (Batal et al 2006; Oweis et al 2009; Sharief et al 2001).

The Baby Friendly Hospital Initiative, launched jointly by UNICEF and WHO in 1991–1992 to support and promote breastfeeding in different countries, has been relatively successful in the region. The proportion breastfed for 6–9 months with complementary feeding increased from 38% in the period 1990–1996 to 45% in the period 1995–2002; about one third are now breastfed for 20–23 months (Djazayery 2004). Obstacles to extended breastfeeding remain and include monitoring for compliance to these initiatives, cultural beliefs, and lack of education regarding the introduction of food at an early stage of infant life.

Under-nutrition, which can be categorized as being under-weight (low weight for age), stunting (low height for age), and wasting (low weight for height), is common among pre-school children (<5 years) in all Arab countries. Stunting is the indicator of chronic food deprivation and is the most common type of under-nutrition, followed by under-weight and wasting. Prevalence of stunting among under-5 children ranges from 8% (Qatar) to 53% (Yemen) (see Chapter 17). Prevalence of under-weight, commonly due to acute health conditions, ranges from 3% to 61%; wasting rates are 3% to 16% (UNICEF 2007).

Chronic diarrhea and recurrent infections is the main contributor to stunting in the poorest segments of population lacking adequate hygienic housing conditions and access to health care. Stunting in richer countries is chiefly the consequence of unhealthy dietary habits and lack of nutritional awareness (UNICEF 2007; UNESCWA, 2007).

Under-weight has also been reported among school children (6–11 years) and adolescents (12–18 years) in many Arab countries. Studies in Egypt, Lebanon, Tunisia, Jordan, Yemen, and Arab Gulf countries report a prevalence of 10% to 35% among school children and 5% to 25% among adolescents. Despite not being nationally representative, these studies raise alarm. Unhealthy dietary habits such as skipping breakfast (Eapen et al 2006), low intake of nutritious foods (such as milk, fruits, and vegetables), high intake of foods with empty calories (such as soft drinks and sweets), and lack of nutritional knowledge are the main contributors (Baba et al 1997).

We must note that child malnutrition and mortality have declined in most Arab countries in the past three decades as a result of socio-economic improvements and progress in health and social services. The oil wealth has done much to lower child mortality, particularly in the Arab Gulf countries. Child malnutrition is sensitive to both health programs and socio-economic conditions such as income, unemployment and illiteracy (El-Ghannam 2003).

Micronutrient Deficiencies

Over a third of the Arab population suffers from micronutrient deficiencies, making this an important public health problem particularly among children and adolescents. Indicators show that daily intakes of iron, calcium, and vitamins D and C in the region are below the recommended dietary allowance (RDA).

Iron Deficiency Anemia

About 50% of cases of anemia are attributable to iron deficiency (IDA), although this varies between population groups and may be overestimated due to misdiagnosis of other etiologies such as sickle cell or thalassemia carrier states. Compared to other middle-income countries, anemia appears to be a moderate public health problem. Prevalence of IDA in Arab Gulf countries is 20–67% among preschoolers, 13–50% among school aged children, and 23–54% in women of childbearing age (Musaiger 2002b; Bagchi 2004).

Low iron intake is the main contributor to IDA and is due to negative iron balance during childhood, adolescence, and pregnancy (Ayoub 1995), low dietary iron intake, and poor iron absorption due to parasitic infections (Musaiger 2002b; Bagchi 2004). IDA is exacerbated by a low intake of foods that enhance iron absorption (e.g., those containing vitamin C) or inhibit iron absorption (e.g., tea, legumes). Consumption of fruits and vegetables is low in all age groups in most Arab countries while tea consumption is relatively high. This may contribute to IDA in poor families who depend on a plant-based diet (Musaiger 2002b). Conditions favoring occurrence of IDA are varied and include economic factors, such as poverty, decreased access to food enhancing

iron absorption, low variety of food; epidemiologic factors such as chronic infectious diseases, such as tuberculosis; parasitic infections, such as ascaris and schistosomiasis; cultural factors, such as the overconsumption of tea; and environmental factors, such as copper deficiency and lead poisoning (Muwakkit et al 2008; WHO 2008). Anemia can have detrimental effects on child development and work capacity of adults therefore affecting the potential productivity of a population.

Vitamin A Deficiency

This deficiency prevails at mild to moderate levels in the region. National surveys conducted between 1990 and 2000 estimated that the prevalence among children 0–72 months decreased from 32.6% in 1990 to 28% in 2000 (Mason et al 2005). According to international studies, this should reduce child morbidity and mortality from infections (Ross 1998). In a prospective study in Sudan, Fawzi et al (1997a; 1997b) found that total dietary vitamin A intake was associated with height and weight attainment among children who were normally nourished at baseline. Vitamin A supplements did not impact height or weight gain (Fawzi et al 1997b). Thus, improving access to vitamin A rich foods rather than giving supplements seems to be of greater effectiveness in improving the nutritional status of malnourished populations in which vitamin A deficiency is an area of concern.

Vitamin D Deficiency

Although Arab countries are sunny, this deficiency, which can result from low sunlight exposure and inadequate dietary intake, is highly prevalent in both adults and children/adolescents (for recent studies, see for example, Meddeb 2005; Allali et al 2009; Bener et al 2009). This is especially the case for women, for whom rates of up to 90% are reported, and is related to parity, low dietary intake, and low sun exposure. In relation to the latter, studies are not always consistent regarding the association with traditional dress in the region. Low dietary intake is common, with more educated women having higher intake (see for example, Gannage-Yared et al 2009).

The burden of the major consequence of vitamin D deficiency, i.e., osteoporosis, is expected to increase with rapid population aging (Maalouf et al 2007). Studies seeking reference ranges for bone mass density (BMD) conducted mainly on female populations in Lebanon (El-Hajj Fuleihan et al 2002), Saudi Arabia

(Ardawi et al 2005), and Kuwait (Dougherty & Al-Mazrouk 2001) found a lower BMD compared to the standard established for Caucasian populations, except in Kuwait, where the BMD reference range was similar to US/European reference data. Risk factors for osteoporosis, such as female sex, age, menopause, and smoking, were similar to those in other populations (Bener et al 2009). Additional risk factors more characteristic of Arab populations include high parity, prolonged lactation, and vitamin D deficiency. These studies suggest that mandatory vitamin D food fortification or supplement use, particularly during the winter time is critical in correcting deficiency and preventing osteoporosis in the longer term. With low sun exposure, some researchers have suggested the need for high doses of vitamin D supplements (Saadi et al 2007).

Iodine Deficiency

Iodine deficiency disorders (IDDs) include a myriad of preventable conditions including goiter, decreased fertility, cretinism, and growth impairment. Based on WHO criteria for iron deficiency, i.e., median urinary iodine (UI) level below 10 µg/dl or goiter prevalence greater than 5% in schoolchildren (WHO 2001), Arab countries have a high burden. Goiter prevalence increased from 23% in 1993 to 37.3% in 2003 (a 63% increase!). In 2003, the proportion of school-age children (6–12 years) and the proportion of the general population with insufficient iodine intake based on urinary iodine levels were 55.4% and 54.1% respectively, placing the region as the second most affected region after Europe (59.9% and 56.9%, respectively) (De Benoist et al 2004). Prevalence of IDDs is considered mild in seven countries (Jordan, Lebanon, Libya, Oman, Syria, UAE, and Yemen) and moderate in four countries (Egypt, Morocco, Saudi Arabia, and Sudan) (Azizi & Mehran 2004). The situation is severe in Iraq due to inadequate intake of dietary iodine, ingestion of goitrogens, and habitation in regions where the soil lacks iodine (Mason et al 2005).

Control programs for IDDs are not usually targeted to specific age or sex groups but rather to whole populations. The region has been very active in this area over the past two decades, with support from international agencies, although not all countries, however, have national control programs. In Tunisia, IDD has been officially declared by WHO to be under control, and in Jordan, Lebanon, Syria, and Yemen, it is said to be almost under control. Seventeen of

Table 2. Prevalence (%) of Micronutrient Deficiencies In the Arab Countries (1995–2006)

Country	Latest survey year	Vitamin A deficiency (children 0–7 years)	Anemia (women) (%)	Total goiter rate (%)
Algeria	2006	29	19–42	8.5
Bahrain	1995	–	40–49	–
Djibouti	2006	–	–	–
Egypt	2005	27	17–79	5.2
Iraq	2006	42	18	24–44
Jordan	2002	19	4–46	32
Kuwait	1996	16	31–42	–
Lebanon	2004	20	27–49	25
Libya	1995	19	23.5	6.3
Mauritania	2000–01	–	42	–
Morocco	2003–04	29	20–40	22
OPT	2006	–	0	–
Oman	1998	–	15–54	10
Qatar	1995	–	30	–
Saudi Arabia	1996	21	5–57	4.30
Somalia	2006	25	54	12.6
Sudan	2000	36	44	22
Syria	2006	22	30–52	73
Tunisia	2000	22	41	4.3
UAE	1995	14	22–62	2.22
Yemen	2000	40	5–36	32

Source: Musaiger & Miladi (1997); FAOSTAT (2009); Mason et al (2005); UNICEF (2007).

the remaining countries have ongoing programs for universal salt iodization, and 16 have appropriate legislation. As a whole, about 51% of households currently consume iodized salt (Djazayery 2004). In severely affected countries and sub-regions such as Iraq, strong salt iodization programs with effective monitoring and evaluation are needed.

Table 2 summarizes the prevalence of micronutrient deficiencies. Completely missing data in some countries and outdated estimates in others indicate the need for better surveillance systems.

Public Health, Nutrition, and Food Security: Synergy, Policies, and Interventions

Traditionally, food security, nutrition, and public health belong to three distinct areas of work carried out by different groups with limited collaboration in the region. This must change if we want to see improvements in the aforementioned nutrition and food security situation and consequent gains for public health and well-being. Combining forces across the three areas, and the engagement of many other interested actors, including civil society, can increase the effectiveness of advocacy and the impact of interventions. This is especially true with regard to food insecurity, which especially threatens the poor and thus poses an equity challenge.

The complex nature of malnutrition and its determinants indicates the need for multi-sectoral programs and interventions that consider political, economic, social, agricultural, environmental, demographic, and public health factors. The misguided concept that the health sector alone is responsible for overcoming nutritional problems is widespread in Arab countries. However, coordination and cooperation between the health and other sectors is weak and does not exist in some countries.

Although many Arab countries have established a Nutrition Plan of Action, as recommended by WHO/FAO in 1992, no country has completely implemented its plan, raising issues about political and policy commitments to these plans. Several technical factors contribute to poor implementation: lack of or limited nutritional surveillance data and health information systems, inadequate training for medical and paramedical professionals, a focus on curative rather than preventive measures for nutrition-related health problems, lack of studies related to ecological factors associated with nutritional problems, and lack of work on assessing the cost-effectiveness of various nutrition interventions.

Among existing public health nutrition programs, food fortification, public nutrition education, school feeding, breastfeeding support, and food subsidies are the most common. Food fortification focuses on fortification of flour, mainly wheat, with iron and folic acid to prevent and control IDA. Some countries fortify salt with iodine to prevent IDDs. Studies to evaluate the effectiveness of food fortification in the prevention of nutritional deficiencies are few, and

existing studies have several methodological deficiencies (WHO EMRO 1998).

Nutrition education programs for the public are usually carried out through mass media especially television, booklets, and newspapers. Although studies that evaluate the impact of these programs are limited, available evidence suggests little impact. This is mainly due to the high rate of illiteracy in some countries, lack of specialized staff in nutrition education, incorrect selection of target groups, and inadequate information provision (Musaiger 2000).

School feeding programs rely on regulating foods provided by school canteens, especially nutritive values and portion sizes. Sweets and carbonated beverages are usually forbidden. Some countries forbid potato chips and foods high in salt and fat. Not all countries have such regulations. In countries that do, implementation varies from country to country and from school to school within the same country. A relatively high percentage of children bring their foods from home, and many of these foods are rich in energy, salt, and fat (Musaiger 2004).

Most Arab countries have food subsidy policies that keep the price of staple foods within the purchasing power of the majority of population. Subsidies commonly cover rice, wheat, sugar, vegetable oils, fat, and red meat. Some believe that subsidies may encourage over-consumption of these foods, which are high in dietary energy, and might contribute to increasing obesity or to NCDs, especially in relation to consumption of red meat and animal fat (WHO EMRO 1990). Some have suggested that governments should subsidize healthy foods such as fruit, vegetables, and fish. However, this suggestion faces the problem that prices of these foods are unstable and vary seasonally.

In 2007, the third Arab Conference on Nutrition, held in Abu Dhabi, UAE, released the Abu Dhabi declaration to promote healthy nutrition in Arab countries (Musaiger 2008). The declaration proposed activities to prevent and control nutritional disorders (Box 2). To achieve the same goal, the Bahrain-based Arab Center for Nutrition has established food-based dietary guidelines for the Arab Gulf countries, following FAO recommendations with special emphasis on protection against chronic diseases. These guidelines can be used in all Arab countries as they cover the main messages to prevent and control diet-related diseases.

The public health approach of primary prevention is considered the most cost-effective and sustainable

Box 2. Abu-Dhabi Declaration to Promote Healthy Nutrition in the Arab Countries

Recommendations of the Third Arab Conference on Nutrition, held in Abu Dhabi-UAE, 4–6 December, 2007. In order to promote healthy nutrition in the Arab countries the following activities should be taken into consideration:

1. Training of health workers and related fields in assessment, prevention, and control of nutritional problems with special emphases on training of physicians, nurses, school teachers, and social workers.
2. Reviewing and evaluating the current curricula in both government and private schools in order to update the information related to nutrition and linking this information with the local and Arab situation.
3. Encouraging university academic carriers to write text books in Arabic and translate related academic publications, through financial support from international and regional organizations, as well as private sectors with special emphases on multi-author publications.
4. Providing opportunity to young local nutrition specialists to participate in nutrition activities and programs in order to prepare them to take the leadership in the future.
5. Updating and developing the current academic curricula, especially in colleges of agriculture and home economics in the region.
6. Encouraging establishment of a nutrition unit or section in the preventive health or public health departments in the ministry of health to promote preventive health programs.
7. Integrating nutrition in a broad way in university curricula as well as in medical, health sciences, and nursing schools.
8. Establishing legislations and regulations for commercial advertisements in mass media, especially for those related to nutrition, health, and physical activity.
9. Working with both public and private sectors to develop and improve food products to provide nutritious foods.
10. Encouraging health and nutrition specialists to participate in workshops, training courses, conferences which are carried out in various Arab countries, to exchange knowledge and experiences. This can be done through providing short fellowships from public and private sectors.
11. Supporting awareness programs to promote healthy nutrition and healthy lifestyle through various mass media.
12. Encouraging studies and research in food and nutrition through financial and technical supports, with more focusing on joint research among several countries in the Arab region.
13. Conducting regional conferences on food, health, and nutrition on a regular basis, especially the Arab Nutrition Conference and the Arab Conference on Obesity and Physical Activity, which are carried out every 3 years in one of the Arab countries.
14. Preparing or updating the national nutrition plan of action which should be a part of the national health plan in each country.
15. Encouraging and establishing nutrition societies in each Arab country to support and coordinate the nutrition activities.
16. Supporting the therapeutic nutrition activities in all hospitals throughout the Arab region by preparing uniform food guidelines, portion size and food composition tables to suit the Arab food habits and culture.
17. Developing and improving the food control activities to provide safe foods for the public.

Source: Musaiger (2008)

course of action to cope with the growing chronic disease epidemic, but this is hindered by many factors in the Arab countries. These factors include underestimation of the effectiveness of interventions, the perceived delay in achieving measurable impact, institutional inertia, and inadequate resources (Khatib 2004).

Conclusions

Arab countries have experienced dramatic changes in the health and nutritional status over the past decades. A double nutritional burden exists today with both under-nutrition and over-nutrition posing important public health challenges. Food security is already an important challenge for the region, which promises to become more serious in the future. A broad set of determinants underlie the nutrition and food security situation calling for inter-sectoral action. Unfortunately, such action remains weak. Current scientific evidence linking broader determinants, including food security, and dietary patterns with nutritional diseases provide a strong base on which to launch future inter-sectoral action toward combating the increasing prevalence of these diseases in the Arab countries.

References

Abdeen Z, Greenough PG, Chandran A, Qasrawi R (2007) Assessment of the nutritional status of preschool-age children during the second intifada in Palestine. *Food and Nutrition Bulletin*, 28(3): 274–282

Abu-Ismail K, Moustafa A (2009) *Development challenges for the Arab region: Food security and agriculture. UNDP Regional Bureau for Arab States*. New York and League of Arab States, Cairo, Egypt

Al Saffa AJ (2009) Stunting among primary-school children: A sample from Baghdad, Iraq. *Eastern Mediterranean Health Journal*, 15: 322–329

Ali HI, Baynouna LM, Roos M, Bernsen RM (2010) Barriers and facilitators of weight management: Perspectives of Arab women at risk for type 2 diabetes. *Health and Social Care in the Community*, 18(2): 219–228

Allali F, El Aichaoui S, Khazani H, et al (2009) High prevalence of hypovitaminosis D in Morocco: Relationship to lifestyle, physical performance, bone markers, and bone mineral density. *Seminars in Arthritis and Rheumatism*, 38(6), 444–51

AOAD (Arab Organization for Agricultural Development) (2010) *Arab food security report*. Khartoum, Sudan: Arab Organization for Agricultural Development

Arab Center for Nutrition (2003) *Nutritional and health status in the Arab Gulf countries*. Manama, Bahrain: Arab Center for Nutrition

Ardawi MS, Maimany AA, Bahksh TM, Nasrat HA, Milaat WA, Al-Raddadi RM (2005) Bone mineral density of the spine and femur in healthy Saudis. *Osteoporosis International*, 16(1): 43–55

Ayoub AI (1995) Iron deficiency anemia in Dubai medical college for girls: A preliminary study. *Journal of the Egyptian Public Health Association*, 70(1–2): 213–228

Azizi F, Mehran L (2004) Experiences in the prevention, control and elimination of iodine deficiency disorders: A regional perspective. *Eastern Mediterranean Health Journal*, 10(6): 761–770

Baba N, Shaar K, Faour D, Musaiger AR, Al-Housani H, Adra N (1997) Nutritional status of school children aged 6–10 years in United Arab Emirates: Comparison with children from different ethnic origins. *Ecology of Food and Nutrition*, 36: 367–384

Bagchi K (2004) Iron deficiency anemia–an old enemy. *Eastern Mediterranean Health Journal*, 10(6): 754–760

Barlow R (1999) Health trends in the Middle East, 1950–95. *In:* J Brown, R Barlow (Eds.) *Studies in Middle Eastern health* (p. 1–28). Ann Arbor, MI: University of Michigan Press

Batal M, Boulghourjian C, Abdallah A, Afifi R (2006) Breast-feeding and feeding practices of infants in a developing country: A national survey in Lebanon. *Public Health Nutrition*, 9(3): 313–319

Bener A, Al-Ali M, Hoffmann GF (2009) High prevalence of vitamin D deficiency in young children in a highly sunny humid country: A global health problem. *Minerva Pediatrica*, 61(1): 15–22

COSIT (Central Organization for Statistics & Information Technology) *Ministry of Planning and Development Cooperation (Iraq), Kurdistan Region and Statistics Office (KRSO)*, Nutrition Research Institute, Ministry of Health (Iraq): United Nations World Food Programme

De Benoist B, Andersson M, Egli I, Takkouche B, Allen H (2004) *Iodine status worldwide. WHO Global Database on iodine deficiency.* Geneva, Switzerland: World Health Organization.

Djazayery A (2004) Regional review of maternal and child malnutrition: Trends, intervention and outcomes. *Eastern Mediterranean Health Journal*, 10(6): 731–736

Dougherty G, Al-Mazrouk N (2001) Bone density measured by dual-energy X absorptiometry in healthy Kuwaiti women. *Calcification of Tissue International*, 68: 225–229

Eapen V, Mabrouk AA, Bin-Othman S (2006) Disordered eating attitudes and symptomatology among adolescent girls in the United Arab Emirates. *Eating Behaviors*, 7(1): 53–60

El-Ghannam AR (2003) The global problems of child malnutrition and mortality in different world regions. *Journal of Health Social Policy*, 16(4): 1–26

El-Hajj Fuleihan G, Baddoura R, Awada H, Salam N, Salamoun M, Rizk P (2002) Low peak bone mineral density in healthy Lebanese subjects. *Bone*, 31(4): 520–528

El-Taguri A, Besmar F, Abdel Monem A, Betilmal I, Ricour C, Rolland-Cachera MF (2009) Stunting is a major risk factor for overweight: Results from national surveys in 5 Arab countries. *Eastern Mediterranean Health Journal*, 15(3): 549–562

FAO (Food and Agriculture Organization) 2009. *FAOSTAT*. Available from http://faostat.fao.org/ [Accessed 4 October 2010]

Fawzi WW, Herrera MG, Willett WC, Nestel P, El Amin A, Mohamed KA (1997a) Dietary vitamin A intake in relation to child growth. *Epidemiology*, 8(4): 402–407

Fawzi WW, Herrera MG, Willett WC, Nestel P, El Amin A, Mohamed KA (1997b) The effect of vitamin A supplementation on the growth of preschool children in the Sudan. *American Journal of Public Health*, 87(8): 1359–1362

FAO (Food and Agriculture Organization) (2010) 2008 *FAOSTAT*. Rome, Italy: FAO

Galal O (2003) Nutrition related health patterns in the middle east. *Asia Pacific Journal of Clinical Nutrition*, 12(3): 337–343

Gannage-Yared MH, Maalouf G, Khalife S, et al (2009) Prevalence and predictors of vitamin D inadequacy amongst Lebanese osteoporotic women. *British Journal of Nutrition*, 101(4): 487–491

Halileh S, Gordon NH (2006) Determinants of anemia in pre-school children in the Occupied Palestinian Territory. *Journal of Tropical Pediatrics*, 52(1): 12–18

Halileh S, Abu-Rmeileh N, Watt G, Spencer N, Gordon N (2008) Determinants of birthweight: Gender based analysis. *Maternal and Child Health Journal*, 12(5), 606–612

Khatib O (2004) Non-communicable diseases: Risk factors and regional strategies for prevention and care. *Eastern Mediterranean Health Journal*, 1(6): 778–788

Maalouf G, Gannage-Yared MH, Ezzedine J, et al (2007) Middle East and North Africa consensus on osteoporosis. *Journal of Musculoskeletal and Neuronal Interactions*, 7(2): 131–143

Mason J, Rivers J, Helwig C (2005) Recent trends in malnutrition in developing regions: Vitamin A deficiency, anemia, iodine deficiency, and child underweight. *Food and Nutrition Bulletin*, 26(1): 1–105

Meddeb N, Sahli H, Chahed M, et al (2005) Vitamin D deficiency in Tunisia. *Osteoporosis International*, 16(2): 180–183

Mehio Sibai A, Nasreddine L, Mokdad AH, Adra N, Tabet M, Hwalla N (2010) Nutrition transition and cardiovascular disease risk factors in Middle East and North Africa countries: Reviewing the evidence. *Annals of Nutrition & Metabolism*, 57(3–4): 193–203

Musaiger AO (2000) *Studies on nutrition and health education*. Bahrain: Bahrain Center for Studies and Research

Musaiger AO (2002a) Diet and prevention of coronary heart disease in the Arab middle east countries. *Medical Principles and Practice*, 11(Suppl. 2): 9–16

Musaiger AO (2002b) Iron deficiency anaemia in the Arab Gulf countries: The need for action. *Nutrition and Health*, 16: 161–171

Musaiger AO (2003) Recommendation of the First Conference on Obesity and Physical activity in the Arab Countries. *Nutrition and Health*, 17: 117–121

Musaiger AO (2004) *Proceedings of symposium on school nutrition in the Arab countries*. Bahrain: Bahrain Center for Studies and Research

Musaiger AO (2007) *Overweight and obesity in the Arab countries: The need for action. Technical report.* Manama: Bahrain Center for Studies and Research

Musaiger AO (Ed.) (2008) *Proceedings of the Third Arab Conference on Nutrition*, Bahrain: Arab Center for Nutrition. Available from http://www.acnut.com/images/stories/pdf/journals/food_and_nutrition_in_the_arab_world.pdf [Accessed 16 November 2010]

Musaiger AO, Miladi S (1997) *Nutrition situation in the Near East region*. Cairo, Egypt: FAO

Muwakkit S, Nuwayhid I, Naboulsi N, et al (2008) Iron deficiency in young Lebanese children: Associated with elevated blood lead levels. *Journal of Pediatric Hematology/Oncology*, 30: 382–386

Nasreddine L, Hwalla N, Sibai A, Hamze M, Parent-Massin D (2006) Food consumption patterns in an adult urban population in Beirut, Lebanon. *Public Health Nutrition*, 9(2): 194–203

Nasreddine L, Mehio-Sibai A, Mrayati M, Adra N, Hwalla N (2010) Adolescent obesity in

Syria: Prevalence and associated factors. *Child Care, Health and Development*, 36(3): 404–413

Ng SW, Zaghloul S, Ali HL, Harrison G, Popkin BM (2010) The prevalence and trends of overweight, obesity and nutrition-related non-communicable diseases in the Arabian Gulf States. *Obesity Reviews*, 12: 1–13

Oweis A, Tayem A, Froelicher ES (2009) Breastfeeding practices among Jordanian women. *International Journal of Nursing Practice*, 15(1): 32–40

Riely F, Mock N, Cogill B, Bailey L, Kenefick E (1999) *Food security indicators and framework for use in the monitoring and evaluation of food aid programs*. Washington, DC: Food and Nutrition Technical Assistance Project

Ross DA (1998) Vitamin A and public health: Challenges for the next decade. *Proceedings of the Nutrition Society*, 57(1): 159–165

Saadi HF, Dawodu A, Afandi BO, Zayed R, Benedict S, Nagelkerke N (2007) Efficacy of daily and monthly high-dose calciferol in vitamin D-deficient nulliparous and lactating women. *The American Journal for Clinical Nutrition*, 85: 1565–1571

Sharief NM, Margolis S, Townsend T (2001) Breastfeeding patterns in Fujeirah, United Arab Emirates. *Journal of Tropical Pediatrics*, 47(5): 304–306

UNDP (United Nations Development Programme) (2009) *Arab Human Development Report 2009. Challenges to human security in Arab countries.* New York, NY: UNDP

UNESCWA (Economic and Social Commission for Western Asia) (2007) *The millennium development goals in the Arab Region: A youth lens.* Beirut, Lebanon: ESCWA

UNICEF (United Nations Children's Fund) (2007) *The state of world's chidlren, 2008.* New York, NY: UNICEF

WFP (World Food Programme) (2008) *Comprehensive food security and vulnerability analysis in Iraq.* Available from http://cosit.gov.iq/english/pdf/e_food_iraq1.pdf [Accessed 15 November 2010]

WFP/FAO (2009) *Socio economic and food security survey. Report 1 (West Bank) and Report 2 (Gaza Strip).* Rome: Italy: WFO & FAO

WHO (World Health Organization) (2001) *Assessment of iodine deficiency disorders and monitoring their elimination: A guide for programme managers,* Geneva, Switzerland: WHO. Available from http://www.who.int/nutrition/publications/en/idd_assessment_monitoring_eliminination.pdf [Accessed 15 December 2010]

WHO (2008) *Worldwide prevalence of anemia (1993–2005). WHO global database on anaemia.* Geneva, Switzerland: World Health Organization

WHO (2010a) *Global database on body mass index.* Geneva, Switzerland: WHO

WHO (2010b) *Global database on child growth and malnutrition.* Geneva, Swtzerland: WHO

WHO EMRO (Eastern Mediterranean Regional Office) (1990) *Towards a national nutrition in the Arab countries. Proceedings of the third Arab Conference of Nutrition.* Bahrain: Arab Center for Nutrition, WHO EMRO

WHO EMRO (1998) *Fortification of flour with iron in countries of the Eastern Mediterranean, Middle East, and North Africa.* Alexandria, Egypt: WHO EMRO

Infectious Diseases: The Unfinished Agenda and Future Needs

Rana A. Hajjeh, Maha Talaat, and Aisha O. Jumaan

In the twenty-first century, infectious diseases continue to be a major public health problem in most countries across the national income spectrum. While the Arab world has seen substantial improvement of life expectancy and reduction of infant and child mortality since the 1950s, infectious diseases still account for a large proportion of the total disease burden. The WHO report on the global disease burden (WHO 2008a) estimates that almost one third of all deaths in the Eastern Mediterranean region is due to infectious diseases (1,315,000 out of 4,306,000 deaths or 30%); the most common infectious diseases causing deaths included respiratory infections, followed by diarrheal diseases, tuberculosis, and childhood vaccine preventable diseases. Over the past two decades, the Arab world has witnessed the emergence or re-emergence of various infectious diseases, including some that were thought to be almost eliminated. We review here a selected set of infectious diseases of particular public health importance, such as diseases of epidemic potential, vaccine preventable diseases, and health care-related infections, and the factors associated with their persistence. We explore infection control as well as surveillance programs and conclude with next steps for infectious disease control and prevention.

Socio-economic and Political Determinants of Infectious Diseases

Infectious diseases raise equity concerns because they often affect the poorer and socially disadvantaged groups disproportionately. Therefore, understanding the determinants of these diseases is necessary for achieving better health for all. Over the past two decades, the Arab world has witnessed the emergence or re-emergence of various infectious diseases, including some that were thought to be almost eliminated. Multiple factors are responsible for this re-emergence,

both globally (see a useful review in Institute of Medicine 2003) and in the Arab world, including ecological, environmental, climate-related, genetic, or political and socio-economic.

The Arab world is a center of international travel, with millions of international visitors each year from all over the world. One unique situation is the pilgrimage to Saudi Arabia where 2–3 million pilgrims are estimated to make the annual hajj to Mecca over a period of a few days each year. Such large gatherings can be associated with health risks (Ahmed et al 2006) as exemplified by the 2000 meningococcal meningitis outbreak due to a new strain (Lingappa et al 2003). Arab countries have experienced rapid urbanization and large urban migration, including migrant workers. Many live in crowded slums with poor infrastructure and hygiene. This has contributed to persistence of endemic diseases, such as typhoid and tuberculosis, and the re-emergence of others, such as dengue fever. Political instability whether due to war (Iraq, Lebanon), civil unrest (Sudan, Somalia), or occupation (Occupied Palestinian Territory-OPT) have displaced millions or contributed to breakdowns in basic infrastructure and health facilities (Wasfy et al 2005). In some settings, the limited resources, combined with poor infection control practices, have led to major infectious challenges, such as the hepatitis C epidemic in Egypt. Patchy availability, limited quality, and inadequate access to health care in some countries increase the risk of infectious disease. Cultural perceptions and stigmas around certain infections such as HIV/AIDS and tuberculosis continue to be major obstacles for their prevention and control.

Diseases of Epidemic Potential

Arab countries continue to experience many disease outbreaks (Figure 1). In addition to sickness and

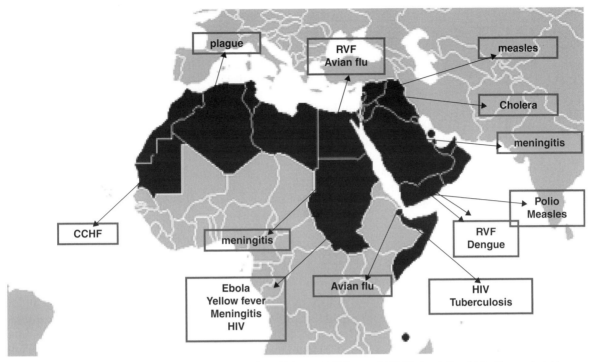

Figure 1. Selected infectious diseases outbreaks in the Arab world (2000–2010) Source: WHO "Outbreak News": http://www.who.int/csr/don/en/index.html. CCHF: Crimean-Congo haemorrhagic fever; RVF: Rift Valley fever.

death, such outbreaks disrupt routine public health services and have important economic consequences. The outbreaks of Rift Valley Fever (RVF) in Yemen and Sudan over the past decade, for example, affected the exports of cattle to Saudi Arabia, impoverishing many farmers. The recent alarms raised by cases of avian and H1N1 influenza in Egypt, each with pandemic potential, overwhelmed the public health staff and system.

The main outbreaks are those transmitted via respiratory routes (e.g., avian influenza, meningococcal meningitis), are water-borne (cholera, typhoid) or vector-borne (dengue, RVF). The re-emergence of viral hemorrhagic diseases such as dengue (Yemen, Saudi Arabia, Sudan, Djibouti, and Somalia), RVF (Yemen, Saudi Arabia, and Egypt), Ebola and yellow fever (Sudan), and Crimean-Congo Hemorrhagic Fever (CCHF, Mauritania) are of special concern given the associated high morbidity and mortality and difficulty of control. Dengue fever, transmitted by mosquito vectors such as *Aedes aegypti*, has been often associated with crowded urban and semi urban areas, where water is stored at home and solid waste

disposal is inadequate, conditions favorable for mosquito breeding. Breakdown of infrastructure and large population displacement during war, as in Sudan and Iraq, increase risk of outbreaks (Musani & Shaikh 2008). The re-emergence of cholera in over half of Iraqi provinces in 2007 provides one example (Al-Abbassi et al 2000). During the Israeli war on Lebanon in 2006 that resulted in displacement of almost a million people from South Lebanon, emergency measures were taken to protect the refugees from spread of diseases such as measles and typhoid.

Some enteric diseases are endemic. Srikantiah et al (2006) found a high rate of endemic typhoid (59/100,000 population) in Egypt during 2002. Another study by the same group found decreased risk with access to municipal water (Afifi 2005). In Ezbet El-Nawar, a Greater Cairo slum, child ill-health was related to lack of access to safe water and sanitation. When piped municipal water is in short supply, residents turn to well-water often contaminated by adjacent sewerage pipes (Nakashima et al 2004). In Israel, typhoid incidence was almost four times higher in Arabs compared to Jews, due to lower socio-economic status and suboptimal infrastructure in the Arab communities. Risk of other enteric diseases was related to parental education and crowding. Recent examples include an outbreak of bacillary dysentery due to *Shigella dysenteriae* in SW Saudi Arabia (El Bushra & Bin Saeed 1999); Giardiasis in Syria, (Almerie et al 2008), hepatitis A in Cairo (Salama et al 2007), *Helicobacter pylori* in Israeli Arab children (Muhsen et al 2006). Endemic foodborne infections, such as brucellosis, are associated with traditional consumption of unpasteurized milk and dairy products (Jennings et al 2007; Al-Shamahy et al 2000), indicating failure of public health education efforts. The cases of avian influenza in Egypt over the past 2 years were all linked to exposure to infected or dead poultry. In both urban slums and poor rural areas, extended families might live in small households that also shelter animals and poultry at night, conditions ripe for spread of zoonoses to humans.

Two epidemic diseases deserve special attention because of their chronicity and the associated cultural stigmas.

HIV/AIDS: An estimated 610,000 people live with HIV/AIDS in the Arab world, with three countries, Djibouti, Somalia, and Sudan, accounting for the majority. HIV/AIDS prevalence, seemingly low compared to other regions, may be underestimated due to under-reporting because of HIV/AIDS-associated stigma and inadequacy of surveillance, particularly among high-risk populations and pregnant women. Increasing high-risk practices, such as injection drug use in Libya, commercial sex in some Gulf countries, and men having sex with men increase HIV/AIDS spread (UNAIDS 2008). Such populations are usually marginalized in Arab societies and have little knowledge and understanding of their risks. But even college or high school students or health care workers at increased risk of exposure, display significant gaps in knowledge with respect to routes of HIV transmission as well as fear and intolerance toward HIV-infected people (Al-Serouri et al 2002; Chemtob & Srour 2005; Gańczak et al 2007). Much work is needed to prevent the spread of HIV, in particular education activities to increase awareness about the disease and measures to prevent it especially among high-risk groups, and to improve the quality of life of people living with HIV/AIDS.

Tuberculosis (TB): Historically associated with poverty and poor living conditions, TB continues to be an important public health problem. Six countries, Djibouti, Iraq, Morocco, Somalia, Sudan, and Yemen, shoulder high TB burden (incidence >100/100,000 population). Whereas Iraq, Morocco, and Yemen show a stable trend or even a decline in incidence, incidence is increasing in Somalia, Djibouti, and Sudan, likely exacerbated by the concurrent HIV/AIDS epidemic. Unless the latter epidemic is addressed, TB incidence could dramatically increase. Another concern is the development of multiple drug-resistant TB strains, which are difficult and costly to treat. Multidrug resistant tuberculosis is often fatal; its emergence is associated with inconsistent therapy due to poor education of patients and their access to medical services. Many countries have improved detection rates and increased the proportion of patients receiving "directly observed treatment, short-course" (DOTS), but many are short of reaching the target of 70% detection and 85% treatment rates: in 2006, only seven Arab countries reached these goals. A few studies described health care seeking behaviors of TB patients. In Syria, living far from the health facility, feeling a high degree of stigma, seeking initial care at a non-health care provider, and having more than one health care encounter before diagnosis were associated with delay in diagnosis (Maamari 2008). In Jordan, accessibility of health care was related to seeking care in a timely fashion; economic constraint was an obstacle in rural residents (Rumman et al 2008). A similar association was found between severe malaria in Yemen and distance to the nearest health station (Al-Taiar et al 2008). In Yemen, direct costs associated with TB diagnosis were burdensome, especially for patients from rural areas (Ramsay et al 2010). These studies illustrate the importance for Arab governments taking responsibility for making appropriate health care services accessible at affordable prices.

Vaccine Preventable Diseases (VPDs)

Infant and child mortality rates are among the best indicators of a country's health status. The Millennium Development Goal 4 (MDG 4) aims to reduce the under-5 year old mortality by two-thirds between 1990 and 2015. Addressing VPD is a key strategy to achieve this goal (the proportion of children under 1 immunized against measles is an indicator for MDG 4). In 2000, VPDs were still among the leading causes of under-5 mortality, accounting for about 1.4 million deaths (WHO EMRO 2001) with most deaths caused by measles, rotavirus, *Haemophilus influenzae* type b (Hib), and *Streptococcus pneumoniae*. It must be noted that reported cases of VPDs generally underestimate the true disease burden and vary from one country to another due to variations in case definitions, lack or inadequate reporting, surveillance performance, and outbreaks.

Arab countries have established successful national immunization programs leading to substantial improvements in child health (see also Chapter 17). Recently, the WHO Eastern Mediterranean Regional Office (EMRO), which provides technical assistance to most Arab countries, was recognized for achieving a United Nations goal of reducing measles deaths by a remarkable 90%, from 96,000 to 10,000 between 2004 and 2007, 3 years earlier than the target date. Polio cases fell by over 99%, (from 12,622 cases in 1980 to 107 in 2006). Between 1980 and 2006, vaccine coverage for measles increased from 15% to 83% and for diphtheria-pertussis-tetanus (DPT3) from 21% to 86% (WHO EMRO 2008). Hepatitis B vaccine coverage (three doses) increased from 3% in 1990 to 78% in 2006.

Despite the successes in most countries, many challenges remain. A few countries continue to struggle with VPDs; polio, targeted for eradication is still reported in Sudan and Somalia; and measles, targeted for elimination, is still a problem in Yemen, Sudan, Djibouti, and Somalia. There are significant discrepancies in vaccine coverage between rural and urban areas in some countries. While many countries have achieved a DTP3 coverage of over 90%, coverage hovers at < 70% in others, Sudan, Iraq, and Somalia (WHO, 2008b). Only four countries reported Tetanus Toxoid coverage of two or more doses to pregnant women over 70% (Tunisia, Iraq, Jordan, and Oman) with the remaining reporting coverage below 50% (WHO EMRO 2010).

Over the past decade, many upper- and middle-income Arab countries added Hib vaccines to their national immunization programs; low-income countries did the same between 2006 and 2008 as funding became available through the Global Alliance for Vaccines and Immunizations (GAVI). Only Egypt and Somalia have not yet introduced Hib vaccine, the former due mainly to financial difficulties, and the latter due to its low coverage of DTP3, which makes it ineligible for GAVI funding. By 2009, rotavirus vaccine was introduced in three of the Gulf countries, pneumococcal conjugate vaccine in six Gulf countries, and Yemen is planning introduction in 2010 (WHO EMRO 2010).

Many Arab countries need stronger immunization programs to increase and sustain vaccine coverage but this faces the challenge of weak health systems. In the Eastern Mediterranean region, 8 of the 10 countries that are considered high priorities for health system strengthening are Arab (Djibouti, Egypt, Iraq, Morocco, OPT, Somalia, Sudan, and Yemen). This is based on high adult and child mortality rates, non-satisfactory health indicators, low socio-economic status, and insecurity. Some of these countries still have far to go to achieve the MDG 4. In some countries, while national health indicators may be favorable, significant regional disparities exist. For example in Lebanon, while overall under-5 mortality is 30/1000 live births, it's 52 in the poorer North (WHO 2007)

Socio-economic status and access to health services impact immunization programs. For example, El-Sayed et al (2008) found that polio vaccination was less effective among children of under-educated mothers in Egypt, perhaps due to poorer hygiene interfering with the vaccine virus. Lack of security and collapse of infrastructure impact overall health status and vaccine coverage in particular. While the situation is improving in Iraq, it remains bleak in Somalia.

The Arab world has also experienced multiple health challenges due to insecurities and conflicts, especially in Yemen, Iraq, OPT, Somalia, and Sudan. These conflicts have resulted in displacement of over 200,000 people in northern Yemen; and about 350,000–400,000 people in southern Sudan (WHO-EMRO 2010). In addition, refugees from the horn of Africa who cross the border to Yemen contribute to spread of infectious diseases. In 2010, Yemen experienced multiple outbreaks including measles among the internally displaced population in the North due to low vaccine coverage in this population, and cholera and dengue outbreaks that originated with refugees from the horn of Africa.

In the next section, we will examine polio and measles in view of the global goals for eradication (no virus is left to circulate) and elimination (no further cases occur), respectively, and because they require significant resources and political country commitment.

Polio: In 1988, the World Health Assembly resolved to eradicate poliomyelitis globally by 2000. Although substantial progress has been achieved with elimination of circulating wild poliovirus in most of the world, some Arab countries had a setback with large polio outbreaks in Sudan, Somalia, and Yemen, and recent cases in Egypt. Since 2006, none of the

Arab countries had endemic polio transmission, and only Sudan reported cases in 2008, mainly imported from neighboring Chad.

Current polio-eradication efforts focus on two countries, Somalia and Sudan (out of nine countries worldwide), both suffering from armed conflict leading to disintegration of health systems and/or difficulties of access to populations (Tangermann et al 2000). Eradication requires maintenance of high vaccine coverage, conversion to inactivated polio vaccine (IPV) to prevent circulation of both wild and vaccine-derived polioviruses; and good surveillance.

Although eradication efforts have been expensive and labor intensive, they have led to strengthening surveillance and intervention capacities and have benefited the control of other important diseases, such as measles. A combined program of oral polio vaccine (OPV) and IPV in the OPT in 1978 resulted in a dramatic decline in the incidence of polio in both Gaza and the West Bank (in Gaza from 10.6 per 100,000 during 1968–1977 to 0.1 per 100,000 in 1983–1987, and the last case was reported in 1988). In Sudan, a large paralytic poliomyelitis outbreak in 1993 led to the implementation of National Immunization Days for poliomyelitis in 1994, 1996, and 1997 (Box 1) and to strengthening of overall routine immunization services (ElZein et al 1998).

Measles: Measles outbreaks continue to occur even among highly vaccinated populations, straining resources in most countries. Between 2000 and 2005, only three (Egypt, Morocco, and OPT) of the eight high priority countries crossed the MDG 4-related 95% vaccine coverage among children under 1. Coverage in Iraq and Somalia dropped from 90% to 85% and from 38% to 35%, respectively. Sudan has strengthened its immunizations system overall and managed to increase measles vaccine coverage from 47% to 73%. However, during the conflict in the Darfur region, in 2003, coverage was 46%, 57%, and 77% in North, West, and South Darfur, respectively (CDC, 2004). Ongoing measles transmission led to region-wide measles vaccination campaigns of children 9 months to 15 years. Despite the difficulties in accessing all the population, the campaigns vaccinated 93% of the accessible population and 77% of the overall targeted population. Recurrent wars, sanctions, and occupation in Iraq have damaged the health system, including the Expanded Program on Immunization (EPI). In 1990, the reported coverage for EPI routine immunizations was 90%. In Saladdin

Box 1. Controlling polio and strengthening the national immunizations program in Sudan

A large outbreak of paralytic poliomyelitis in 1993 in the Sudan prompted rapid rehabilitation of Sudan's Expanded Program on Immunization (EPI). A World Health Organization team visited Sudan in 1993, 1995, and 1996 to review such efforts and their impact. Measures taken to eradicate poliomyelitis, control measles, and eliminate neonatal tetanus included government financing of vaccine purchase, decentralization of EPI operations, a shift from a mobile to a less expensive fixed-site vaccine delivery strategy, installation of a solar cold chain network, resumption of managerial in-service training, and social mobilization. National immunization days were conducted in 1994, 1996, and 1997 throughout the country (during a ceasefire in the southern areas). From 1993 to 1996, reported infant immunization coverage increased for all antigens, with a concomitant decrease in the incidence of EPI target diseases. National coverage for the third dose of diphtheria-tetanus-pertussis increased from 51% in 1993 to 79% in 1996, while the proportion of immunizations delivered at fixed sites rose from 35% to 70%. By 1996, 19 of Sudan's 26 states were financing some of the operational costs for EPI.

Governorate, the percentage of children completely immunized declined in both urban and rural areas; Al-Sheikh et al (1999) reported that overall coverage declined from 65% in 1989 to 46% in 1993, followed by an increase to 73% in 1994 (Figure 2). The most common causes of incomplete immunization were lack of immunization knowledge among mothers, unavailability of vaccine, and distance from a health center.

Saudi Arabia's efforts to control measles and achieve elimination illustrate the importance of political commitment, well targeted intervention programs, and the importance of continuously evaluating public health programs and adjusting the interventions accordingly (Al-Mazrou et al 1999). In 1982, Saudi Arabia mandated a single dose of measles vaccine at age 9 months, leading to increased coverage from 8% in 1980 to 90% in 1990. Under this policy, 50% of cases were among children 6–8 months. In 1991, a two-dose policy was implemented, with a first dose given at 6 months and a second dose of the combined mumps-measles-rubella vaccine (MMR) at 12 months of age. Vaccine coverage for the second dose increased from less than 20% before 1991 to over 90% by 1993,

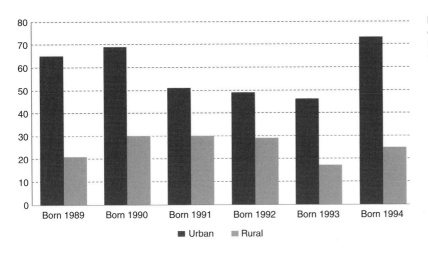

Figure 2. Percent of fully immunized children 0–2 years of age, by year of birth – Tikrit, Iraq. Source: Al-Sheikh et al (1999).

thus leading to a marked reduction in cases. In 1998, to initiate elimination efforts, an MMR campaign was launched in two phases, targeting secondary school children in 1998, and primary and intermediate schools in 2000 vaccinating over 4 million children and resulting in greater than 96% coverage in both groups.

Health Care-Associated Infections, Antimicrobial Resistance, and Infection Control

These infections have emerged as an important public health problem and a burden both for the patient and the health care system. Hospital acquired infections (HAIs) such as bloodstream infections, surgical site infections, urinary tract infections, ventilator-associated pneumonias, among others, lead to higher disease morbidity and mortality, longer hospital stays, and increased cost. Limited data exist on the burden, morbidity, mortality, and costs associated with HAIs in most Arab countries. Comprehensive infection control programs are quite limited and good surveillance programs to measure health care-associated infections are almost absent. In 1985, a WHO survey in 55 hospitals from 14 countries representing four regions (Europe, Eastern Mediterranean, Southeast Asia, and Western Pacific) revealed that an average of 8.7% of hospitalized patients developed HAIs. Hospitals in the Eastern Mediterranean region had the highest rates (11.8%) (see for example, Mayon-White et al 1988).

Most published studies of HAIs come from academic institutions and focus on high risk settings (see for example, Jroundi et al 2007; Atif et al 2008). A few studies observed a high frequency of bloodstream infections and high mortality among patients admitted to pediatric or neonatal intensive care units (NICUs). Two such studies from Egypt (El-Nawawy 2003; Moore et al 2005) prompted a cross-sectional survey of 22 NICUs from various Ministry of Health hospitals throughout Egypt. This study also documented a high rate of sepsis (54%). Most infections were due to highly drug-resistant, hospital-acquired pathogens, indicating they were preventable with adequate infection control measures. A prospective surveillance study in intensive care units at the Jordan University Hospital between 1993 and 1995 revealed overall infection rates much higher than reported rates in the United States in similar settings (Khuri-Bulos et al 1999). Most of these studies also found a low ratio of nurses/patients and very poor infection control practices due to inadequate education of health care workers. It is also known that HAIs are often found in crowded and poorly staffed public hospitals that cater to uninsured and socially disadvantaged populations. Despite the high prevalence of HAIs, many Arab countries have not taken initiatives to start nationwide infection control programs and strengthening surveillance to assess the burden of hospital infections.

Poor infection control practices in health care settings have led to outbreaks and spread of infectious diseases with significant long-term community impact. Several studies have documented blood-borne pathogen transmission in healthcare facilities in Egypt (Table 1). Between 1994 and 2000, there were two outbreaks of

Table 1. Studies Implicating Health Care-Related Transmission of Blood-Borne Pathogens in Egypt, 1996–2003

Author/year	Pathogen	Type of study and location	N	Risk factor/observed practice	Measure of association (odds ratio/relative risk)
El-Sayed et al 2000	HIV	Outbreak investigation in 2 dialysis centers	39	Reuse of syringes	NA
Hassan et al 1994	HIV	Outbreak investigation in 3 dialysis centers	82	Reuse of equipment	NA
El-Sayed 1996	HCV	Cross-sectional (Sinai)	740	Receipt of prior injection	**1.9** (1.04–3.5)
El-Sayed et al 1997	HBV HCV	Cross-sectional Reclaimed area, Sinai (same)	506 (same)	Parenteral therapy for schistosomiasis Surgery Parenteral therapy for schistosomiasis Surgery	**1.5** (0.5–4.1) **1.9** (0.9–4.0) **0.9** (0.5–1.8) **3.0** (1.4–6.9)
El-Zayadi 1999	HCV	Cross-sectional	354	Reuse of syringes, dental/invasive medical procedures	NA
Mohamed et al 1996	HCV	Cross-sectional Cairo, Lower and Upper Egypt	5071	Bilharzial injection Sharing syringes Injections for urography Blood transfusion Dental extraction Instrumental assisted delivery Cesarean delivery Stitches after delivery	**2.5** (2.1–3.0) **1.6** (1.4–1.8) **2.2** (1.6–3.1) **1.2** (0.8–1.9) **1.2** (1.06–1.4) **2.2** (1.3–3.7) **1.5** (0.7–3.0) **1.5** (0.9–2.7)
Habib et al 2001	HCV	HCV Cross-sectional Delta Region	3999	Schistosomiasis injections IV catheterization Blood transfusion Endoscopy Injections by informal provider Urinary catheterization Dental treatment Any delivery	**1.8** (1.3–2.4) **1.5** (1.2–1.9) **1.7** (1.1–2.7) **1.4** (0.6–3.3) **1.2** (1–1.4) **1.8** (1.2–2.7) **1.0** (0.9–1.3) **1.6** (1.1–2.4)
Medhat et al, 2002	HCV	Cross-sectional Upper Egypt	6031	Schistosomiasis injections IV catheterization Blood transfusion Endoscopy Injections by informal providers Urinary catheterization Dental treatment Any delivery Surgery	**4.6** (1.1–18.2) **1.4** (0.9–2.2) **5.7** (2.9–11.4) **6.2** (1.8–21.6) **0.9** (0.6–1.4) **3.0** (0.9–10.1) **1.5** (1.0–2.2) **1.1** (0.5–2.1) **1.6** (1.0–2.5)

Source: Talaat et al 2006.

HIV transmission in dialysis centers, related to poor adherence to standard infection control precautions, such as reuse of syringes and equipment (El-Sayed et al 2000; Hassan et al 1994). Hepatitis C virus (HCV) infection is highly prevalent in Egypt, with approximately 10% of the population having evidence of past or chronic infection. Wide-scale HCV transmission may have occurred in the 1960s and 1970s due to reuse of syringes in campaigns to treat schistosomiasis (Frank et al 2000). Ongoing HCV transmission is still happening and is associated with health care exposures, mainly unsafe procedures, and particularly reuse of injection needles and syringes (El-Sayed et al 1997, 2000; Habib et al 2001; Medhat et al 2002). Needle-stick injuries among health workers also play a role (Talaat et al 2003). This highlights the important role of the government in dealing with this national scourge and limiting the further spread of this infection through elimination of high risk practices.

Antimicrobial Resistance (AMR): Resistance to antimicrobial agents, especially related to infections acquired in hospital settings, is becoming a major problem worldwide. Some studies have suggested that AMR may be increasing in several Arab countries, but data from many countries is lacking, particularly in the absence of HAI surveillance systems. A recent study from an AMR surveillance network of Mediterranean countries (ARMed), most of which were Arab, revealed a high level of AMR among invasive *Escherichia coli* isolates collected from blood cultures and cerebrospinal fluid, the highest being reported from Egypt (Borg et al 2008). This corroborates the results of an earlier study which also found significant levels (El Kholy et al 2003). Therefore, there is an urgent need for infection control interventions to prevent further emergence of drug-resistant strains.

Unnecessary and inappropriate antibiotic use is often the principal driving force for the emergence and spread of bacterial resistance in the community. Insufficient physician training and poor infection control practices in hospitals may also play a role. In the Arab world, large scale and inappropriate use of antimicrobials is common. In most countries, people can buy antibiotics over the counter without a prescription or professional control (Abasaeed et al 2009). This practice must be eliminated if AMR is to be curbed at the community level.

Infection Control Programs: The aforementioned picture of HAI and AMR highlight the necessity of developing sound infection control programs at the

> **Box 2.** The National Infection Control Program in Egypt
>
> I. Creation of Organizational Structure at Central, Governorate and Facility Levels
> II. Development of National Guidelines
> III. Training and Capacity Building Activities
> IV. Promotion of Injection Safety (Hospital and Community-based)
> V. Ensure Availability of Critical IC Supplies and Equipment
> VI. Monitoring and Evaluation
> VII. Promotion of Occupational Safety
> VIII. Surveillance Programs to Measure Hospital-acquired Infections
> IX. Advocacy
> X. Partnership

country and hospital levels. Arab countries need to set up and/or strengthen infection control programs over the next decade to promote safety and quality of care and in particular to reduce the spread of HAI and AMR. All basic elements of infection control need to be strengthened, such as standard precautions, proper waste management programs, occupational safety, and HAI surveillance programs. Although, the political will is growing, most of the Arab countries are lagging behind. Implementing infection control programs faces many challenges. In the poorer countries, substantial deficiencies in health care quality and delivery are invariably the result of insufficient budgets, low salaries of health care personnel, and the diversion of resources to areas considered of higher priority, or thought to produce more tangible outcomes. In the richer countries, such as in the Gulf, national infection control programs are developing, and the discipline is rapidly growing (Memish 2002). However, the number of experts is still limited. Microbiologists or general practitioners manage most programs, unlike in northern nations where certified infection control nurses and hospital epidemiologists run most programs. As of 2007, only Lebanon, Saudi Arabia, and United Arab Emirates had certified infection control nurses (Memish et al 2007).

Egypt began a national infection control program in early 2000, with the help of various partners (Box 2), driven by high HCV prevalence. National guidelines and a 6-week training curriculum were developed for the first time and were endorsed by the WHO for use in the EMR (Talaat et al 2006). The Ministry of Health implemented the program in almost all large public hospitals and recently has made plans to expand their training activities to reach primary health care units and the private sector. Other Arab countries, such as Jordan and Oman, started to use the Egyptian model. Although Saudi Arabia has had a well-developed infection control program in some hospitals (Memish 2002; Memish et al 2007), it only recently started a new national department for infection control within the ministry of health. It is important for infection control initiatives to be coordinated by ministries of health, rather than by the individual hospitals as this may result in different policies and difficulties in monitoring compliance (Borg et al 2007).

Responding to the Challenges of Infectious Diseases

The previous discussion has highlighted many areas in which Arab governments have mobilized to address infectious diseases of public health concern, for example through immunization programs. We highlight here several additional issues that require attention and which can determine the long-term success of control and prevention efforts.

Strengthening Surveillance and Response Systems

Developing surveillance systems that provide quality data to local and national health authorities in a timely manner should be a high public health priority for decision makers as this can help assess disease burden, and detect and control outbreaks early. Surveillance requires adequate microbiologic laboratory capacity to confirm the diagnosis and ensure better data quality. Surveillance systems for disease in animals are also important to develop and link to surveillance among humans, and require additional attention as illustrated by the experience in Egypt (Hegazy et al 2009). Surveillance for adverse events after immunization is crucial for any strong national immunizations systems as shown by the experience in Oman (Al Awaidy et al 2010).

Most Arab countries rely on passive reporting for infectious diseases, resulting in substantial underestimates of the various reportable infections. Microbiologic capacity and other diagnostics for infectious diseases remain weak, which results in many of these diseases being reported based on

clinical case definitions that lack confirmation. Bacterial diseases are often under-diagnosed due to prior antibiotics use and poor laboratory practices. Hib, the most common cause of bacterial meningitis and a common cause of severe pneumonia in children, exemplifies the latter situation. Hib is difficult to culture in the laboratory and data on accurate disease burden are thus often lacking. This leads to a delay in adopting Hib vaccines, which are very safe and effective. Similar challenges for diagnosis and infection control are seen in hospitals as well as in TB and malaria control programs (Atta & Zamani 2008).

Governments should support surveillance and laboratory activities, especially in public hospitals, as the basis for monitoring various interventions. Surveillance has become particularly important as all Arab countries committed to international health regulations (IHRs) in 2005. These require countries to strengthen their surveillance and response systems by 2012. Countries need to evaluate their current systems and identify creative ways to improve them. In Egypt, such an evaluation led to the institution of a national electronic surveillance system requiring extensive training of health care personnel, both in the epidemiologic units and laboratories (Mahoney et al 2007) and the collaboration with multiple partners within the country. Because infectious diseases cross borders, there is obviously also a need for regional collaboration in surveillance and response efforts.

Building the Human Resource Capacity

Addressing infectious diseases requires strengthening the human capacity in countries within a broader regional strategy. This requires collaboration and coordination within and across countries. The involvement of academic institutions is especially important. In addition to training microbiologists and infectious disease specialists, epidemiologists and public health professionals with a focus on infectious diseases are needed. It is important to note that infectious disease epidemiology is not a major area of emphasis in existing academic public health programs and institutions. There is minimal interaction between these programs and institutions and communicable disease departments in the ministries of health. The region currently hosts three well-established Field Epidemiology Training Programs

(FETP) in Egypt, Jordan, and Saudi Arabia, based at the ministries of health. Newer programs are being developed/launched in Iraq, Morocco, and Yemen. Supported technically by the US Centers for Disease Control and Prevention, the FETP is a 2-year, full-time training and service program to develop national epidemiologists, with classroom instruction and field assignments. Efforts to link these programs are under way with the October 2009 launch of the Eastern Mediterranean Public Health Network (EMPHNET). EMPHNET hosted a regional meeting in 2010 focusing on health issues during mass gatherings. These programs could help to develop regional epidemiological capacity as well. Unfortunately, there is currently minimal interaction between these programs and academic institutions in the respective countries. Such an interaction can benefit both groups.

Addressing Social Determinant of Infectious Disease

The literature on social determinants of infectious diseases in the region remains limited and there is need for expanding and supporting research in this area. Nevertheless, there is enough evidence from this and other regions to support the need for structural and socio-economic interventions to reduce infectious diseases. This requires government commitment and resources and especially for disadvantaged populations. However, social determinants can also be used to target specific populations at risk and therefore provide more cost-effective interventions. In Egypt, Goldstein et al (2001) found that socio-economic factors were the only ones associated with participation in a school-based hepatitis B immunization campaign and recommended that strategies to increase immunization coverage should target children of low socio-economic status.

Strengthening Health Systems

Vertical programs focusing on immunization are important but not adequate; broader health system interventions are also needed. Strengthening health systems, particularly primary health care (PHC), can both contribute to controlling infectious diseases and to enhancing the capacity of these systems to address other health challenges. In areas with limited access to care, PHC offers a natural entry for infectious disease prevention and control. Incorporating immunization in PHC can be critical, and most cost-effective, for prevention of VPDs. More than 30 years after the Alma-Ata Declaration, this can also serve as a reminder that PHC was intended to deliver not only universal curative services, but preventive services as well. Doing so requires resources. Allocating a specific budget line for preventive services, such as vaccines, signals political commitment and allows tracking of resources. A recent analysis conducted by WHO and UNICEF, 2000–2006, reported a positive relationship between having a budget line and increased expenditure on routine vaccines and overall immunization (Lydon et al 2008), with only slight improvements reported in the EMR during the study period.

In recent years, providing expensive vaccines at affordable prices through GAVI support to low-income countries has made it possible for many of these countries to accelerate the introduction of new vaccines, such as hepatitis B and Hib vaccines, and in the near future, pneumococcal and rotavirus vaccines. Countries in the region that cannot benefit from such funding need to work together to identify alternative funding mechanisms; one suggested approach is to develop alliances to pool resources and increase purchasing and negotiation power for vaccines and medications similar to what the Gulf countries had done through the Gulf Countries Council.

Conclusions

For a region that is rich in natural and human resources, much more can be done to better control and prevent infectious diseases, which continue to extol a heavy burden especially on the disadvantaged. Preventing and controlling infectious diseases requires governments to commit resources to various interventions, especially those targeting the disadvantaged, beyond immunization. This includes improving surveillance capacity, training public health and laboratory personnel, developing infection control programs and supporting them, as well as improving primary preventive health care services, including immunizations, and accelerating the introduction of new vaccines. Countries need to do this not just to respond to pressures to meet global goals of disease control and international health regulations, but out of deep commitment to the well-being of all their populations.

References

Abasaeed A, Vlcek J, Abuelkhair M, Kubena A (2009) Self-medication with antibiotics by the community of Abu Dhabi Emirate, United Arab Emirates. *Journal of Infection in Developing Countries*, 3(7): 491–497

Afifi S, Earhart K, Azab MA, et al (2005) Hospital-based surveillance for acute febrile illness in Egypt: A focus on community-acquired bloodstream infections. *The American Journal of Tropical Medicine and Hygiene*, 73(2): 392–399

Ahmed QA, Arabi YM, Memish ZA (2006) Health risks at the Hajj. *The Lancet*, 367: 1008–1015

Al Awaidy S, Bawikar S, Prakash KR, Al Rawahi B, Mohammed AJ (2010) Surveillance of adverse events following immunization: 10 years' experience in Oman. *Eastern Mediterranean Health Journal*, 16(5): 474–480

Al-Abbassi AM, Ahmed S, Al-Hadithi T (2005) Cholera epidemic in Baghdad during 1999: Clinical and bacteriological profile of hospitalized cases. *Eastern Mediterranean Health Journal*, 11: 6–13

Al-Mazrou YY, al-Jeffri M, Ahmed OM, Aziz KM, Mishkas AH (1999) Measles immunization: Early two-doses policy experience. *Journal of Tropical Pediatrics*, 45(2): 98–104

Almerie MQ, Azzouz MS, Abdessamad MA, et al (2008) Prevalence and risk factors for giardiasis among primary school children in Damascus, Syria. *Saudi Medical Journal*, 29(2): 234–240

Al-Serouri AW, Takioldin M, Oshish H, Aldobaibi A, Abdelmajed A (2002) Knowledge, attitudes and beliefs about HIV/AIDS in Sana' a, Yemen. *Eastern Mediterranean Health Journal*, 8(6): 706–715

Al-Shamahy HA, Whitty CJ, Wright SG (2000) Risk factors for human brucellosis in Yemen: A case control study. *Epidemiology and Infection*, 125(2): 9–13

Al-Sheikh OG, al-Samarrai JI, al-Sumaidaie MM, Mohammad SA, al-Dujaily AA (1999) Immunization coverage among children born between 1989 and 1994 in Saladdin Governorate, Iraq. *Eastern Mediterranean Health Journal*, 5(5): 933–940

Al-Taiar A, Jaffar S, Assabri A, Al-Habori M, Azazy A, Al-Gabri A (2008) Who develops severe malaria? Impact of access to healthcare, socio-economic and environmental factors on children in Yemen: A case-control study. *Tropical Medicine & International Health*, 13(6): 762–770

Atif ML, Sadaoui F, Bezzaoucha A, et al (2008) Prolongation of hospital stay and additional costs due to nosocomial bloodstream infection in an Algerian neonatal care unit. *Infection Control and Hospital Epidemiology*, 29(11): 1066–1070

Atta H, Zamani G (2008) The progress of roll back malaria in the Eastern Mediterranean Region over the past decade. *Eastern Mediterranean Health Journal*, 14(Suppl.): S82–S89

Borg MA, Cookson BD, Scicluna E, ARMed Project Steering Group and Collaborators (2007) Survey of infection control infrastructure in selected southern and eastern Mediterranean hospitals. *Clinical Microbiology & Infection*, 13(3): 344–346

Borg MA, van de Sande-Bruinsma N, Scicluna E, et al (2008) Antimicrobial resistance in invasive strains of Escherichia coli from southern and eastern Mediterranean laboratories. *Clinical Microbiology & Infection*, 14(8): 789–796

CDC (Centers for Disease Control and Prevention) (2004) Emergency measles control activities, Darfur, Sudan. *Morbidity and Mortality Weekly Report*, 53(38): 897–899

Chemtob D, Srour SF (2005) Epidemiology of HIV infection among Israeli Arabs. *Public Health*, 119(2): 138–143

El-Bushra HE, Bin-Saeed AA (1999) Intrafamilial person-to-person spread of bacillary dysentery due to Shigella dysenteriae in southwestern Saudi Arabia. *East African Medical Journal*, 76(5): 255–259

El Kholy A, Baseem H, Hall GS, Procop GW, Longworth DL (2003) Antimicrobial resistance in Cairo, Egypt 1999–2000: A survey of five hospitals. *The Journal of Antimicrobial Chemotherapy*, 51(3): 625–630

El-Nawawy A (2003) Evaluation of the outcome of patients admitted to the pediatric intensive care unit in Alexandria using the pediatric risk of mortality (PRISM) score. *The Journal of Tropical Pediatrics*, 49(2): 109–114

El Sayed HF, Abaza SM, Mehanna S, Winch PJ (1997) The prevalence of hepatitis B and C infections among immigrants with a newly reclaimed area endemic for Schistosoma mansoni in Sinai, Egypt. *Acta Tropica*, 68(2): 229–237

El Sayed NM, Gomatos PJ, Beck-Sagué CM, et al (2000) Epidemic transmission of human immunodeficiency virus in renal dialysis centers in Egypt. *Journal of Infectious Diseases*, 181(1): 91–97

El-Sayed N, El-Gamal Y, Abbassy A, et al (2008) Monovalent type 1 oral poliovirus vaccine in newborns. *The New England Journal of Medicine*, 359(16): 1655–1665

El-Zayadi AR, Abe K, Selim O, Naito H, Hess G, Ahdy A (1999) Prevalence of GBV-C/hepatitis G virus viraemia among blood donors, health care personnel, chronic non-B non-C hepatitis, chronic hepatitis C and hemodialysis patients in Egypt. *Journal of Virological Methods*, 80(1): 53–58

ElZein HA, Birmingham ME, Karrar ZA, Elhassan AA, Omer A (1998) Rehabilitation of the expanded programme on immunization in Sudan following a poliomyelitis outbreak. *Bulletin* of the World Health Organization, 76(4): 335–341

Frank C, Mohamed MK, Strickland GT, et al (2000) The role of parenteral antischistosomal therapy in the spread of hepatitis C virus in Egypt. *The Lancet*, 355(9207): 887–891

Gańczak M, Barss P, Alfaresi F, Almazrouei S, Muraddad A, Al-Maskari F (2007) Break the silence: HIV/AIDS knowledge, attitudes, and educational needs among Arab university students in United Arab Emirates. *The Journal of Adolescent Health*, 40(6): 572

Goldstein ST, Cassidy WM, Hodgson W, Mahoney FJ (2001) Factors associated with student participation in a school-based hepatitis B immunization program. *The Journal of School Health*, 71(5): 184–187

Habib M, Mohamed MK, Abdel-Aziz F, et al (2001) Hepatitis C virus infection in a community in the Nile Delta: Risk factors for seropositivity. *Hepatology*, 33(1): 248–253

Hassan NF, El-Ghorab NM, Abdel-Rehim MS (1994) HIV infection in renal dialysis patients in Egypt. *AIDS*, 8(6): 853

Hegazy YM, Ridler AL, Guitian FJ (2009) Assessment and simulation of the implementation of brucellosis control programme in an endemic area of the Middle East. *Epidemiology and Infection*, 137(10): 1436–1448

Institute of Medicine (2003) *Microbial threats to health: Emergence. detection, and response.* Washington, DC: National Academies Press

Jennings GJ, Hajjeh RA, Girgis FY, Fadeel MA, Maksoud MA, Wasfy MO (2007) Brucellosis as a cause of acute febrile illness in Egypt. *Transactions of the Royal Society of Tropical Medicine and Hygiene*, 101(7): 707–713

Jroundi I, Khoudri I, Azzouzi A, et al (2007) Prevalence of

hospital-acquired infection in a Moroccan university hospital. *American Journal of Infection Control*, 35(6): 412–416.

Khuri-Bulos NA, Shennak M, Agabi S, et al (1999) Nosocomial infections in the intensive care units at a university hospital in a developing country: Comparison with national nosocomial infections surveillance intensive care unit rates. *The American Journal of Infection Control*, 27(6): 547–552

Lingappa JR, Al-Rabeah AM, Hajjeh R, et al (2003) Serogroup W-135 meningococcal disease during the Hajj, 2000. *Emerging Infectious Diseases*, 9(6): 665–671

Lydon P, Beyai P, Chaudhri I, Cakmak N, Satoulou A, Dumolard L (2008) Government financing for health and specific national budget lines: The case of vaccines and immunization. *Vaccine*, 26(51): 6727–6734

Maamari F (2008) Case-finding tuberculosis patients: Diagnostic and treatment delays and their determinants. *Eastern Mediterranean Health Journal*, 14(3): 531–545

Mahoney F, Hajjeh RA, Jones GF, Talaat M, Abdel Ghaffar ANM (2007) National notifiable disease surveillance in Egypt. *In*: NM M'ikanatha, R Lynfield, CA Van Beneden, H de Valk, (Eds.) *Infectious disease surveillance* (p. 318–332). London, UK: Blackwell Publishing

Mayon-White RT, Ducel G, Kereselidze T, Tikomirov E (1988) An international survey of the prevalence of hospital-acquired infection. *The Journal of Hospital Infection*, 11(Suppl. A): 43–48

Medhat A, Shehata M, Magder LS, et al (2002) Hepatitis C in a community in Upper Egypt: Risk factors for infection. *American Journal of Tropical Medicine and Hygiene*, 66(5): 633–638

Memish ZA (2002) Infection control in Saudi Arabia: Meeting the

challenge. *American Journal of Infection Control*, 30(1): 57–65

Memish ZA, Soule BM, Cunningham G (2007) Infection control certification: A global priority. *American Journal of Infection Control*, 35(3): 141–143

Mohamed MK, Hussein MH, Massoud AA, et al (1996) Study of the risk factors for viral hepatitis C infection among Egyptians applying for work abroad. *Journal of Egypt Public Health Association*, 71(1–2): 113–147

Moore KL, Kainer MA, Badrawi N, et al (2005) Neonatal sepsis in Egypt associated with bacterial contamination of glucose-containing intravenous fluids. *The Pediatric Infectious Diseases Journal*, 24(7): 590–594

Muhsen KH, Athamna A, Athamna M, Spungin-Bialik A, Cohen D (2006) Prevalence and risk factors of Helicobacter pylori infection among healthy 3- to 5-year-old Israeli Arab children. *Epidemiology and Infection*, 134(5), 990–996

Musani A, Shaikh I (2008) The humanitarian consequences and actions in the EMR over the last 60 years – a health perspective. *Eastern Mediterranean Health Journal*, 14(Suppl.): S150–S156

Nakashima RS, Zekrie Bisada G, Faheem Gergis O, Gawigati A, Hendrich JH (2004) *Making cities work. The Greater Cairo health neighborhood program: An urban environmental health initiative in Egypt.* Activity Report 142. Prepared for the USAID Mission to Egypt, Environmental Health Project. Available from http://www.ehproject.org/ PDF/ Activity_Reports/ AR142%20EGYP%20MCW%20Format.pdf [Accessed 15 January 2010]

Ramsay A, Al-Agbhari N, Scherchand J, et al (2010) Direct patient costs associated with tuberculosis diagnosis in Yemen and Nepal. *International Journal of Lung Diseases*, 14(2): 165–170

Rumman KA, Sabra NA, Bakri F, Seita A, Bassili A (2008) Prevalence of tuberculosis suspects and their healthcare-seeking behavior in urban and rural Jordan. *The American Journal of Tropical Medicine and Hygiene*, 79(4): 545–551

Salama II, Samy SM, Shaaban FA, Hassanin AI, Abou Ismail LA (2007) Seroprevalence of hepatitis A among children of different socioeconomic status in Cairo. *Eastern Mediterranean Health Journal*, 13(6): 1256–1264

Srikantiah P, Girgis FY, Luby SP, et al (2006) Population-based surveillance of typhoid fever in Egypt. *American Journal of Tropical Medicine and Hygiene*, 74(1): 114–119

Talaat M, Kandeel A, El-Shoubary W, et al (2003) Occupational exposure to needlstick injuries and hepatitis B vaccination coverage among healthcare workers in Egypt.

American Journal of Infection Control, 31(8): 469–474

Talaat M, Kandeel A, Rasslan O, et al (2006) Evolution of infection control in Egypt: Achievements and challenges. *American Journal of Infection Control*, 34(4): 193–200

Tangermann RH, Hull HF, Jafari H, Nkowane B, Everts H, Aylward RB (2000) Eradication of poliomyelitis in countries affected by conflict. *Bulletin of the World Health Organization*, 78(3): 330–338

UNAIDS (2008) *AIDS epidemic update. Regional Summary 07.* Middle East and North Africa.

Wasfy MO, Pimentel G, Abdel-Maksoud M, et al (2005) Antimicrobial susceptibility and serotype distribution of Streptococcus pneumoniae causing meningitis in Egypt, 1998–2003. *Journal of Antimicrobial Chemotherapy*, 55(6): 958–964

WHO (World Health Organization) (2007) *Health action in crises, Lebanon.* Geneva, Switzerland: WHO

WHO (2008a) *Global burden of disease report, 2004 update-2008.* Geneva, Switzerland: WHO

WHO (2008b) *Vaccine-preventable disease monitoring system. Global Summary 2007.* Geneva, Switzerland: WHO

WHO EMRO (World Health Organization, Eastern Mediterranean Regional Office) (2001) *Overview of child heath in Arab countries.* Cairo, Egypt: WHO/EMRO

WHO EMRO (2008) *The work of WHO in the Eastern Mediterranean region.* Annual report of the Regional Director, 2008

WHO EMRO (2010) *The work of WHO in the Eastern Mediterranean region.* Annual report of the Regional Director, 2010.

Chapter

12

Non-communicable Diseases – I: Burden and Approaches to Prevention

Ala Alwan, Nisreen Alwan, and Samer Jabbour

Non-communicable diseases (NCD), mainly cardio-vascular disease (CVD), cancer, diabetes, and chronic lung disease, are fast replacing the traditional enemies – infectious diseases, malnutrition, and maternal/child conditions – as the leading causes of disability and premature death in the Arab world. In 2005, NCD were responsible for approximately half of the disease burden in low- and middle-income countries (LMICs), a category that includes most Arab countries but whose characteristics apply to other Arab countries of high income due to oil rents. They caused an estimated 33 million deaths in 2005 (58% of all deaths globally) (WHO 2005). Eighty percent of all deaths caused by NCD occur in LMICs (WHO 2008d); NCD were responsible for half of the disease burden in 2004 (WHO 2008a). Death rates from NCD are 56% higher in men and 86% higher in women in LMICs than in high-income countries (Abegunde et al 2007). WHO estimates that there will be an overall 17% increase in mortality from NCD worldwide between 2006 and 2015 but the greatest increase is expected to

be seen in Africa (27%) and the Eastern Mediterranean Region (EMR) (25%), which includes all Arab countries except Algeria, Comoros, and Mauritania which are part of the WHO Africa region (Table 1). By 2020, NCD are expected to account for 60% increase in mortality in the EMR.

The four groups of NCD largely share the same risk factors, such as tobacco use, unhealthy diet, and physical inactivity, which are interconnected through the same lifecourse social, psychological, and material determinants (Marmot & Wilkinson 2006). In the next two decades, LMICs will be overwhelmed by strokes, heart disease, and diabetes in middle-aged adults. This chapter outlines the burden of NCD in the Arab world and explores strategies to address it, based on international experience and evidence-based policies. It reviews the concept of "integrated prevention" and the application of the recommendations of the Commission on Social Determinants of Health (CSDH 2008) as a key strategic approach to prevent NCD.

Table 1. Projected Global and Regional Mortality Trends: 2006–2015

Geographical regions (WHO classification)	2005		2006–2015 (cumulative)		
	Total deaths (millions)	NCD deaths (millions)	NCD deaths (millions)	Trend: Death from infectious disease	Trend: Death from NCD
Africa	10.8	2.5	28	6%	27%
Americas	6.2	4.8	53	−8%	17%
Eastern Mediterranean	4.3	2.2	25	−10%	25%
Europe	9.8	8.5	88	7%	4%
South-East Asia	14.7	8	89	−16%	21%
Western Pacific	12.4	9.7	105	1%	20%
Total	**58.2**	**35.7**	**388**	**−3%**	**17%**

Source: WHO 2005.

Public Health in the Arab World, ed. Samer Jabbour et al. Published by Cambridge University Press. © Samer Jabbour et al., 2012.

We use data from various sources including the Global Burden of Disease (GBD) estimates, population-based epidemiologic surveys, available data for nine countries (Bahrain, Egypt, Iraq, Jordan, Kuwait, Oman, Saudi Arabia, Sudan, and Syria) that have carried out the WHO-recommended STEPwise surveillance between 2003 and 2007 and, most recently, WHO estimates to be released in 2011 as part of the first Global Status Report on NCD as well as other individual studies.

NCD Burden and Epidemiological Trends

The Arab countries face increasing rates of NCD. Figure 1 provides mortality estimates in the different WHO regions including the EMR. The epidemiological transition and predominance is well advanced in the EMR.

Five of the ten most common killers are NCD, accounting for 47% of disease burden in 2004 (WHO 2008a). Figure 2 shows estimates based on further analysis of the 2004 updated GBD study. NCD are responsible for about 1.3 million deaths annually, representing 55% of deaths. The aforementioned four groups of diseases are responsible for over 80% of NCD deaths with cardiovascular diseases and cancer alone responsible for more than two thirds (Figure 3).

While recognizing the limitations of these estimates and the problems related to coverage, accuracy, and reporting of mortality data in some countries, there is no doubt that NCD are the major killers. A considerable proportion of NCD deaths are premature. Based on GBD estimates for 2004, over 61.5% of the 1.3 million NCD deaths occur under the age of 70 years, contributing to the negative impact of NCD on socio-economic development.

In the remainder of this section, we focus on selected NCD. We first examine CVD and cancer as top NCD killers before moving to discuss the burden of metabolic disorders, such as diabetes, and hypertension, themselves risk factors for other NCD.

Cardiovascular Disease

Figure 3 shows that CVD alone is responsible for more than 40% of NCD deaths in all countries; the proportion may be higher than 60% in some. Based on WHO's 2002 estimates, Ramahi (2010) shows that Egypt, Yemen, and Iraq, in this order, have the highest age-adjusted mortality rates, over 500 per 100,000 population, whereas Kuwait, Bahrain, and Algeria have the lowest rates, just over 300 per 100,000 population. Much of the CVD burden occurs prematurely. In an earlier study at Queen Alia Heart Centre in Jordan, almost half the patients with confirmed disease were below the age of 50 years and only 17% were above the age of 60 years (Doghmi 1989). In a more recent study from Aleppo, Syria, 49% of CVD deaths occurred before the age of 65 years (Maziak et al 2007). Chapter 13 explores CVD in more details.

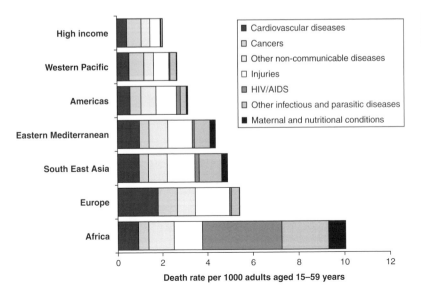

Figure 1. Mortality by major group and region (2004). Source: The Global Burden of Disease-2004 Update, WHO, 2008.

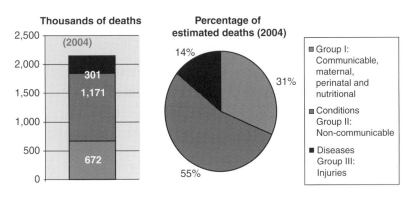

Data included:

Bahrain, Djibouti, Egypt, Iraq, Jordan, Kuwait, Lebanon, Libya, Morocco, Oman, Qatar, Saudi Arabia, Somalia, Sudan, Syria, Tunisia, UAE and Yemen

Figure 2. Estimated deaths by cause in Arab countries. Source: WHO Global Burden of Disease 2004.

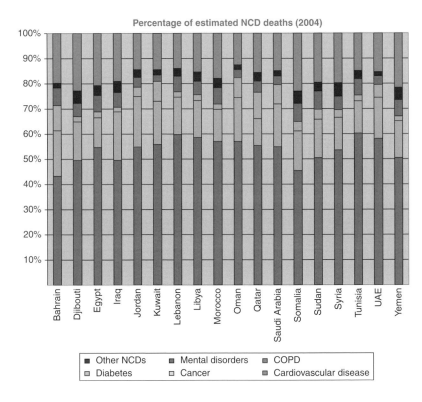

Figure 3. Estimated NCD deaths by cause in some Arab countries. Source: Who Global Burden of Disease 2004.

Cancer

According to the GBD study, cancer is already the fourth most common cause of death in the EMR after CVD, infectious diseases, and injuries (WHO 2005). Cancer is the second NCD killer in all countries after CVD (Figure 3) causing around 272,000 deaths yearly in the EMR, more than HIV/AIDS, tuberculosis, and malaria combined (241,000 deaths per year) (WHO 2002). The EMR will be the WHO region to see the greatest increase in cancer mortality by 2020

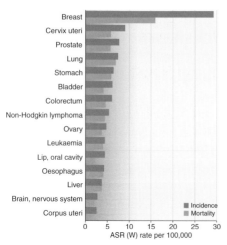

Figure 4. Most frequent cancers for both sexes in the East Mediterranean Region (EMR) – 2008. Source: Globocan 2008 (globocan.iarc.fr) – International Agency for Research on Cancer.

(Murray & Lopez 1996). Breast and lung cancers are the leading causes of cancer deaths; both are amenable to population-based prevention strategies or early detection/screening programs (Omar et al 2007).

Data from cancer registries, which are common across the region, provide useful insights. Overall incidence rates per 100,000 population range from 51 in Qatar to 183 in Palestine for males and from 58 in Saudi Arabia to 143 in Bahrain (Salim et al 2009). The most frequent cancers are breast in females, and lung and bladder cancers in males (Figure 4). Salim et al found time-trend incidence data for only Kuwait and Palestine and noted consistent increases in colon, prostate, endometrium, and breast cancers and non-Hodgkin's lymphomas. Childhood cancer is also important, most common being leukemia and non-Hodgkin's lymphoma. The observed increase in cancer can be attributed to population aging, better detection and registration, and most importantly increased exposure to risk factors. Among the latter, the most important are those shared with other NCD, mainly tobacco smoking, unhealthy diet, and reduced physical activity, as well as other behavioral lifestyle changes, pollution, and increased exposure to industrial and agricultural carcinogens.

It is estimated that half of the cancers occur before the age of 55, 10–20 years earlier than in industrial countries (WHO 2009b). In the case of breast cancer, the age at presentation is a decade earlier (Najjar & Easson 2010). Late stage at diagnosis and inadequate treatment may account for the high observed case-fatality rate. The mortality/incidence ratio (70%)

is much higher than in other regions (40% in the Americas and 55% in Europe) (WHO 2009b).

Metabolic Disorders: Diabetes, Metabolic Syndrome, and Dyslipidemia

While diabetes appears to account for a small proportion of NCD mortality in Figure 3, diabetes mortality may be underestimated because CVD is a leading cause of death among people with diabetes. Surveys over the past two decades have revealed very high prevalence rates. Of the 10 countries with the highest prevalence, 5 are Arab: United Arab Emirates (UAE), 18.7%; Saudi Arabia, 16.8%; Bahrain, 15.4%; Kuwait, 14.6%; Oman, 13.4% (International Diabetes Federation 2009). The Middle East and North Africa (MENA) region has the second highest prevalence rate (9.3%) after North America and Caribbean (10.2%). Expectedly, prevalence rates vary between studies. The STEPwise prevalence estimates range from 10.4% (Iraq) to 20.5% (Syria) (WHO 2010). Mehio Sibai et al (2010) reported rates ranging from 6.6% (Morocco) to over 20% in three countries (25.5%-Bahrain, 23.7%-Saudi Arabia, 23.3%-UAE). The summary estimate by Motlagh et al (2009) is 10.5%. New estimates of the first Global Status Report on NCD show overall prevalence of diabetes of around 11% in the EMR.

Time-trend studies suggest increasing diabetes prevalence reflecting ongoing epidemiologic transition. For example, in Jordan, Zindah et al (2008) reported that prevalence rates increased from 6.8% in 1996 to 17.9% in 2004 while Ajlouni et al (2008) reported a 31.5% increase in age-adjusted prevalence rates from 12% in 1994 to 17.1% in 2004.

One consistent finding of diabetes surveys is the high proportion of undiagnosed diabetes among people meeting criteria for diabetes. In recent studies, this proportion ranges from 19.2% in Kuwait (Al-Khalaf et al 2010), 25.1% in Jordan (Ajlouni et al 2008), 27.9% in Saudi Arabia (Al-Nozha et al 2004), 28.8% in Basrah, Iraq (Mansour et al 2008), about a third in Syria (Albache et al 2010), 35% in UAE (UnitedHealthGroup 2010), and over half in Yemen (Gunaid & Assabri 2008). Variations in prevalence, which may be explained by differences in the representativeness of the study samples, diagnostic criteria used and quality control issues, may affect the feasibility of time-trend and cross-country analysis. Among those under treatment, control rates, as measured by target hemoglobin A1C, are not satisfactory. For example, in studies in Jordan (Ajlouni et al 2008) and Yemen (Gunaid & Assabri 2008) less than a half and less than a quarter of diabetics, respectively, met targets.

Prevalence rates of the metabolic syndrome are also alarming. These range from 16.3% in Tunisia to 39.3% in Saudi Arabia and 39.6% in UAE (Mehio Sibai et al 2010). A UAE study estimated that the majority of cases of prediabetes are actually undiagnosed (UnitedHealthGroup 2010). Prevalence of the metabolic syndrome is higher among females in all countries, except in Lebanon and the West Bank, and among urban residents vs. rural ones. Hypercholesterolemia prevalence rates are quite variable across the region, ranging from 14.3% in Algeria and 17.1% in Yemen, to 50.6% in Oman and 54% in Saudi Arabia. Most studies report clustering of metabolic abnormalities (and other risk factors such as obesity and hypertension) especially in older age groups, which leads to increased risk.

Hypertension

In their review, Mehio Sibai et al (2010) reported hypertension prevalence rates ranging from 19.3% in Iraq to 40.5% in Syria and 42.1% in Bahrain. The summary estimate by Motlagh et al (2009) is 21.7%. The first Global Status Report on NCD estimates prevalence in adults aged 25+ years in the EMR at 40%, defined as systolic blood pressure (BP) 140+ mmHg and/or diastolic BP 90+ mmHg or using medication to lower BP. Recent studies show a higher prevalence rate than those reported from the 1990s (Alwan 1996), suggesting an increasing prevalence over time. Indeed, rates have increased by almost 20% in Tunisia between 1995 and 2004 and even higher in Lebanon in the last decade (Mehio Sibai et al 2010). The prevalence appears to be lower in rural than urban areas (Alwan 1982, 1995).

Region-wide reliable data for detection, treatment, and control rates are missing making this a crucial area for future research. Detection rates are very low in some studies: 20% in some areas in Iraq in an older study (Alwan 1982) but similarly low at 21.9% in Morocco recently (Tazi et al 2009). By contrast, detection rate in Oman was up to 60% (Oman Ministry of Health, 1996). Earlier studies from Saudi Arabia and Iraq showed that less than half of known hypertensives were under effective therapy (Abolfotouh et al 1996; Alwan 1982). In Algerian Sahara, treatment and control

rates were 30% and 25%, respectively (Temmar et al 2007), suggesting that much work needs to be done.

Risk Factors for Non-communicable Diseases

Much of the NCD burden is caused by avoidable risk factors. We focus here on the ones that cause the most attributable population fraction.

Tobacco Use

Data on the prevalence of tobacco use among adults is available only from about half of the Arab countries. However, there is clear evidence that tobacco consumption has considerably increased over the past three decades. The highest age-standardized prevalence rates of tobacco smoking are in Jordan and Tunisia (36% and 26%, respectively) and the lowest in Oman (11%) (WHO 2009c). Rates are much higher among adult males, up to 60% of whom are regular cigarette smokers in some countries (Figure 5). There is also an increase in other forms of tobacco consumption such as waterpipes (Rastam et al 2004). Table 5 provides tobacco use prevalence estimates.

Overweight and Obesity

Overweight and obesity are important health problems in the region (Figure 6) and are closely linked with the increasing NCD burden, especially diabetes (see also Chapter 10). Mehio Sibai et al (2010) reported obesity prevalence rates ranging from 19.1% in Algeria to 43.8% in Saudi Arabia. Motlagh et al (2009) based on 25 studies estimated regional prevalence of obesity at 24.5%. Overweight rates exceeding 70% have been reported in Egypt and Kuwait and exceeding 60% in Bahrain, Jordan, Qatar, and UAE in 2009 (WHO Global InfoBase). Prevalence rates are higher among women. In a systematic review of obesity prevalence in the Mediterranean region of 102 articles during a 10-year period (1997–2007), 25% of females versus 20% of males were reported as obese (Papandreou et al 2008).

Physical Inactivity

Estimates from the forthcoming WHO Global Status Report on NCD show that the prevalence of insufficient physical activity is highest in the EMR, where almost 50% of women and 36% of men are insufficiently

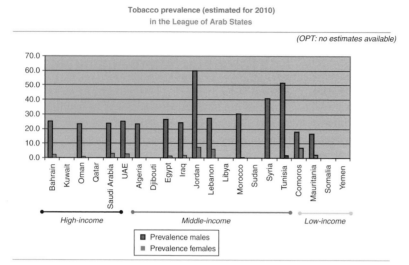

**Tobacco prevalence (estimated for 2010)
in the League of Arab States**

(OPT: no estimates available)

Figure 5. Tobacco prevalence estimates in some Arab countries. Source: WHO InfoBase-2009.

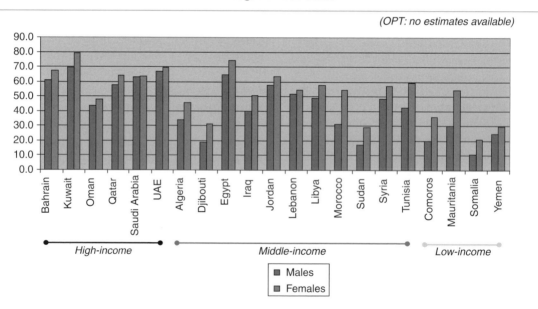

**Estimated prevalence of overweight in 2005
in the League of Arab States**

(OPT: no estimates available)

Figure 6. Prevalence of overweight in Arab countries. Source: WHO InfoBase.

physically active. Mehio Sibai et al (2010) report even higher rates of physical inactivity in many published studies; the rates in a few studies are astounding, for example, 86.8% in Sudan and 96.1% in Saudi Arabia. The STEPwise survey in seven countries (Egypt, Iraq, Jordan, Kuwait, Saudi Arabia, Sudan, and Syria) show that low physical activity among adults ranged from 32.9% in Syria to 86% in Sudan (WHO 2010). These findings are not surprising. With adoption of globalized lifestyles, urbanization with limited public space for physical activity, lack of effective pro-activity public policies, and other factors, the rates of physical activity during the past two decades have decreased steeply. Most studies indicate that women

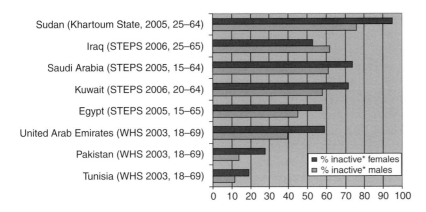

Figure 7. Reported level of physical inactivity in selected Arab countries. Source: WHO Global school-based student health survey (GSHS).

are less physically active. In their review of studies from Gulf countries, Mabry et al (2010) reported sufficient physical activity in only 39.0% to 42.1% of men and 26.3% to 28.4% of women. This is consistent with findings by Mehio Sibai et al (2010) of studies from a larger number of Arab countries. The studies that have explored reasons for gender differences emphasize gender roles whereby women spend more time at home, lack of spaces and facilities appropriate for women, and physiological conditions such as pregnancy and lactation.

NCD Risk Factors Among Children and Youth

The NCD challenge begins in early life reflecting the critical importance of good in utero nutrition, extended breastfeeding, and sound nutritional practices in infancy onward in preventing diet-related NCD later. Children are increasingly vulnerable to the inadequacies of diet and physical activity resulting in high levels of obesity, the unprecedented development of type 2 diabetes, and exposure to cardiovascular risks from an early age (Barker et al 2007; Godfrey & Barker 2007). As children and adolescents grow into adulthood, they will carry with them the risks accumulated in in utero, infancy, childhood, and youth.

Chapter 10 has discussed challenges of early nutrition in the region. As much of the population is relatively young (see Chapter 3), early exposure to NCD risk can have large public health consequences later. There is indeed strong evidence that rates of such early exposure are alarming. Smoking is particularly worrisome, and especially so in light of the waterpipe smoking epidemic. All Arab countries have participated in the Global Youth Tobacco Survey

among 13–15 year old pupils. Compiled data for the 20 countries in the EMR suggest not only high rates of current smoking but also considerable susceptibility to starting smoking among non-smokers and high rates of exposure to second hand smoke (WHO 2007). The latter finding was also documented based on ambient air and hair nicotine measurement in Syria (Maziak et al 2008). The situation in Lebanon is particularly alarming, reflecting weak tobacco control efforts: current use of any tobacco product was 60.1% with male and waterpipe predominance (Saade et al 2008).

Chapter 10 documented high rates of overweight and obesity among children and youth. Also common are metabolic abnormalities. For example, prevalence of the metabolic syndrome among 10–18 year olds was 7.4% and 9.4% in Egypt (Aboul-Ella et al 2010) and Saudi Arabia (Al-Daghri 2010), respectively, and was correlated with overweight/obesity. Prevalence rates of hypertension among school students vary between studies but are significant: 9.6% in Tunisia (Harrabi et al 2006), 5.1% in Kuwait (Saleh et al 2000), 3.6% in Jordan (Jaddou et al 2001), and 1.7% in Iraq (Subhi 2006). A common contributing factor to these problems is the well-documented low levels of physical activity (Figure 7). Just like the case for adults, various studies show clustering of NCD risk factors especially among obese children as documented in Tunisia (Ghannem et al 2003).

Social Determinants of NCD and Risk Factors

Most of the social and demographic transformations, such as population aging, rapid urbanization, and effects of globalization, that have led to rising NCD globally apply to the Arab world as well. These transformations have led to increased exposure to multiple NCD risk factors and generate the negative lifecourse developmental influences on heath. Beyond these broader transformations, the framework adopted by the Commission on Social Determinants of Health (CSDH 2008) denotes interactions among different levels of determinants, e.g., political, social, and economic, which can impact NCD and risk factors. However, there is very limited research on the multi-level links of NCD and risk factors with social determinants, beyond describing such determinants as merely "context" factors. This perhaps reflects the limitations of most available datasets. Instead, most epidemiologic prevalence studies of NCD and risk factors report at least demographic correlates such as age and gender, some report one or more social stratifiers such as education or urban/rural residence but very few report on other stratifiers such as income. Because of limited space, a concise evidence-based review focusing on CVD is provided in Chapter 13. Research on NCD social determinants that have been established in other settings such as income inequality, social class and exclusion, and economic hardship, is a priority for future action.

NCD Prevention and Control: The International Experience

The rapidly rising burden of NCD requires an urgent response from Arab countries. Available evidence, lessons learned from international experience, the clear directions of WHO's Global Strategy for the Prevention and Control of Non-communicable diseases (WHO 2000) and the recommendations of the Commission on Social Determinants of Health (CSDH 2008) provide strong foundations for action in the Arab world.

The Integrated Prevention Approach

Single-disease prevention approaches have failed because they do not address the complexity and the interconnectedness of biological, behavioral, and health systems-related risk factors and determinants. There is clear evidence that addressing the shared NCD risk factors in an integrated manner can make a major contribution in reducing the burden of NCD (WHO 2000; World Health Assembly 2008). Tobacco is the prime example. Killing up to half of its long-term

users, tobacco is a risk factor for six of the eight leading causes of death including NCD (WHO 2008d). Unfortunately, health authorities in many countries, including in this region, adopt a narrow focus on the prevention of one disease when the same interventions, targeted to specific risk factors and their determinants, are equally effective against other equally important health problems. This is neither feasible nor logical, particularly in under-funded health systems. Parallel planning, funding, and management, and duplication of intervention and training programs are not sustainable and result in unnecessary fragmentation particularly when programs compete for scarce financial and human resources.

The integrated approach emphasizes interventions at the levels of the society, community, and family because causal risk factors and determinants are deeply entrenched in the society and culture. Because, as discussed earlier, the root of NCD risk exposure begins early in life, interventions must likewise start early. Addressing the social determinants of health should be given the highest priority in an integrated approach to prevent NCD in the Arab world.

An integrated approach requires multi-disciplinary and inter-sectoral action at multiple levels that utilize a full range of health promotion and disease prevention strategies as well as appropriate clinical and rehabilitative services. As the World Health Report 2008 (WHO 2008c) recommends, an effective response to NCD, and other health challenges of today's world, must involve health system reforms that integrate public health actions with primary health care and ensure healthy public policies across all government sectors – Health in All Policies. The primary care setting is relied upon for planning and delivery of preventive programs targeted to individuals while the public health system is relied upon to provide leadership for developing and coordinating intersectoral programs and activities targeted at populations. This approach means that NCD prevention and control becomes a fundamental component in existing health systems, tailored to local community needs and capacity, as well as an integral part of socio-economic policies and programs.

Evidence for Effective Interventions and Lessons From International Experience

In principle, given that the majority of NCD have an early-origin, environmental or lifestyle etiology they can be prevented or treated by low-cost, high-impact, and evidence-based interventions. Investing in such interventions, particularly those related to primordial and primary prevention, provides the highest return in health and economic terms. There is good evidence that comprehensive public health and community-based interventions to reduce NCD and related risk factors are both effective and cost-effective in high-income countries and LMICs alike (Gaziano et al 2007; Puska et al 2009). The evidence is particularly strong for strategies directed at tobacco control and salt reduction. It is estimated that the implementation of these strategies in 23 countries, which represent 80% of the global NCD burden, would avert 13.8 million deaths between 2006 and 2015 at low and affordable cost (Abegunde et al 2007). A similar case can be made for the Arab world.

The WHO's Framework Convention on Tobacco Control (FCTC) is the first global health treaty negotiated under the auspices of WHO. This convention is an evidence-based treaty that reaffirms the right of all people to the highest standard of health. It represents a paradigm shift in developing regulatory strategies to address addictive substances; in contrast to previous drug control treaties, the FCTC asserts the importance of demand, not just supply, reduction strategies. To date, there are 168 parties, including most Arab countries, to the convention. Addressing the demand reduction component, WHO recommends six proven and cost-effective tobacco control measures that build on the core elements of the FCTC: effective policies, proven to reduce the prevalence of tobacco use; monitoring tobacco use and prevention; protecting people from tobacco smoke; offering help to quit tobacco use; warning people about the dangers of tobacco; enforcing bans on tobacco advertising, promotion, and sponsorship; and raising taxes on tobacco.

There are many examples of interventions on diet and physical activity that are effective and suitable for resource-constrained settings. In 1987, Mauritius introduced a regulatory policy to change the composition of general cooking oil, limiting the content of palm oil and replacing it with soya bean oil. Five years later, total cholesterol concentrations had fallen significantly in men and women. Consumption of saturated fatty acids had decreased by an estimated 3.5% of energy intake (Uusitalo et al 1996). Other interventions include laws and regulations, tax and price interventions, improving the built environment, advocacy, mass media, community-based

interventions, school- and workplace-based interventions, screening, and clinical prevention. Evidence indicates that multi-component interventions that are adapted to the local context are the most successful (WHO 2009a) and form the basis for WHO's Global Strategy on Diet, Physical Activity And Health launched in 2004.

Action on the Social Determinants of Health

In constructing a prevention strategy, Arab countries must consider the increasing global evidence that NCD are affecting poor and disadvantaged populations disproportionately, and contributing to widening health gaps between and within countries. NCD risk factors, especially tobacco use, are more common in deprived communities leading to widening health inequalities between and within countries caused by unequal distribution of power, income, goods, and services (CSDH 2008). The principle of equity thus lies at the core of NCD action.

A Global Strategy to Address NCD

The most important progress made in recent years in NCD action has been the development of a clear global vision on ways to address the NCD epidemic. This vision, shared by the WHO Member States, is the Global strategy for the Prevention and Control of Noncommunicable Diseases which was endorsed by the World Health Assembly in May 2000 (WHO 2000). The Strategy is based on the lessons and evidence from diverse settings, which can be summarized in six key points: preventing the emergence of risk factors in addition to addressing established risk factors, combining a high-risk strategy with a population-based approach, ensuring adequate intensity and sustainability of interventions, engaging other sectors, working with all stakeholders, and reforming health systems and emphasizing the role of primary health care.

The Global Strategy includes three key components: *a surveillance component* to map the epidemics of NCD, analyze their social, economic, behavioral, and political determinants with particular reference to poor and disadvantaged populations, guide policy and advocacy, and help monitor and evaluate intervention programs; *a primary prevention and health promotion component* to reduce the level of exposure of individuals and populations to shared risk factors through multi-sectoral policies and legislative and fiscal measures that develop an environment supportive of NCD control and through strengthening the capacity of individuals and populations to make healthier choices and follow lifestyle patterns that foster good health; and *a management component* to strengthen health care for people with NCD by developing evidence-based norms, standards, and guidelines for cost-effective interventions and by reorienting health systems to respond more effectively to the management needs of chronic conditions, with emphasis on primary health care.

NCD Prevention and Control: The Arab World Situation

How have the Arab countries integrated the vast international evidence and experience in NCD prevention and control? Despite the enormous magnitude of NCD, the rising mortality and disease burden, and the serious impact on socio-economic development, initiatives on NCD prevention and control are generally scarce and fragmented. On the regional level, an Eastern Mediterranean Approach to Non-communicable Diseases Network (EMAN) was launched, health ministers have passed joint resolutions on NCD, and countries have collectively endorsed the FCTC. There is wide recognition that the potential impact of common regional action on NCD is not yet exploited.

On the national level, a few countries have launched promising community-based initiatives (see a brief review in Chapter 13). However, NCD prevention is not yet regarded as a national priority. This situation is unfortunately a reflection of a wider, global environment in which development and donor agencies are missing in action. If the high mortality and heavy burden of disease experienced by Arab countries are to be tackled comprehensively and ultimately successfully, global and regional development initiatives need to take into account more seriously the prevention and control of NCD.

Action on social determinants of NCD is particularly weak and typically not on the radar screen of NCD prevention and control efforts. Few governments have policies aimed at providing equal health opportunities for all of their citizens. This is an opportunity for academic institutions to work with governments to generate, share, and apply actions to provide equal

opportunities for early child development; ensure decent employment and working conditions; provide healthy urban environments; tackle social exclusion, including gender inequality; and ensure fairness in local and national policy making (Rashad 2006).

As part of the implementation of the Global Strategy, WHO conducted an assessment of the capacity of Member States in NCD prevention and control in 2001 and repeated it in 2005 (Alwan et al 2001; Shao et al 2007). In 2001, 50% of countries in the EMR had no NCD policies or plans for diabetes, cancer, or tobacco control. Over half (56%) had no data on NCD risk factors in their annual health reports or regular health reporting systems. There were major gaps in the availability and skills of health professionals and in the availability and affordability of essential medicines, particularly in primary health care. For example, one third of countries reported problems in availing anti-neoplastic drugs and two thirds reported they were not affordable. Primary health care facilities for the early detection of common cancers like breast and cervical cancers were minimal. The 2005 survey suggested some improvements but there was no significant progress in a number of key areas (Shao et al 2007). These surveys show that while some countries designate NCD prevention as a priority, this is not translating into serious policy development and in dedication of more fiscal or human resources. Where there are policies and/or programs in place, the approach to policy development and program implementation is often fragmented and uncoordinated.

One area that deserves increased attention is tobacco, as Arab countries need to do much more in preventing its use. In 2008, no country had tobacco taxes reaching 75% of the retail price of cigarettes. The WHO Report on the Global Tobacco Epidemic (2008b) indicates that six countries have taxes between 51% and 75%, while 11 have taxes between 26% and 50%, and 3 have taxes below or equal to 25%. A small number of countries have national smoke-free legislation that covers all public places. Most of the other countries have smoke-free legislation that covers only certain public places such as health care, or educational facilities, while a small number are completely lacking national smoke-free legislation. Eight countries have legislation that bans all forms of tobacco advertising, promotion, and sponsorship, although compliance is variable. The rest have partial bans, no bans at all, or bans that do not cover national TV, radio, and print media. Only two countries have

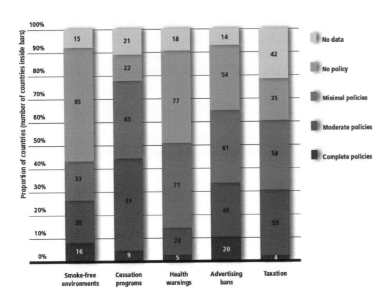

Figure 8. The state of demand-reduction tobacco control measures. Source: WHO Report on the Global Tobacco Epidemic, 2008.

large warnings (average of front and back of the cigarette pack is at least 50%) with all appropriate characteristics. Nine countries have no warnings at all, and eight others have warnings that cover less than 30% of the pack. Unless countries intensify their commitment and work to control tobacco through social, economic, and legislative actions, the tobacco epidemic will continue to increase, causing more avoidable and premature death. Figure 8 provides the baseline for the status of countries, in 2008, in implementing tobacco control measures. Regular reporting by countries will help in monitoring future implementation.

In many Arab countries, NCD management takes place within underfunded and weak health systems with grossly inadequate infrastructure and human resources. In many cases, health professionals, particularly doctors, are not committed to prevention, being more concerned and familiar with treatment. There is inadequate funding for preventive health interventions both at the professional and managerial levels. Health policy makers express the common view that, in many instances, there is no leadership with capacity and skills necessary for effective programs. Thus, capacity building in public health in general and in NCD prevention and policy development in particular is a central issue for most Arab countries. The development and implementation of a "national policy framework" and inter-country cooperation with regional networking and exchange of experience are key.

Weak surveillance and the lack of reliable data on which to base health policy and program decisions are major barriers to action on NCD. In many cases, there is limited availability of population-based cause-specific mortality data, as death certification by cause is unreliable and incomplete, or data on major risk factors. In some countries, information is often rudimentary, facility-based, and only available from previous cross-sectional surveys that lack standardization and comparability. In many cases, these surveys are not institutionalized as part of the national health information system. In recent years, some countries adopted the WHO STEPwise surveillance system on risk factors and conditions, which has partly addressed this gap. Even less available are data on NCD social determinants that are linked to mortality, morbidity, and risk factors. Despite the limitations, there is enough evidence, as discussed in this review, to make a strong case for urgent action on NCD.

The Way Forward for NCD Prevention in the Arab World

There is no reason to doubt that strategies for NCD prevention and control that have worked in established economies and in other LMICs would work in Arab countries too; however, the main challenge is in implementing these strategies and overcoming the gaps mentioned above (Alwan 2001).

Taking into account the needs of countries and in order to promote the implementation of the Global Strategy, the WHO in collaboration with Member States has developed a concrete 6-year Action Plan. The Plan, adopted at the 61st World Health Assembly in May 2008 (World Health Assembly 2008), has a specific focus on LMICs, and is based on current scientific knowledge, available evidence, and a review of international experience. To implement the Plan successfully, high-level political commitment and the concerted involvement of governments, communities, and health care providers are required. The Plan builds on the integrated prevention approach of the Global Strategy through supporting coordinated strategies and evidence-based interventions across individual diseases and risk factors, especially at the national level. The Plan identifies six objectives and key areas of work and specifies sets of actions to be implemented by countries, WHO, and the inter-national partners with clear performance indicators for monitoring and evaluation.

1. *Raising the priority accorded to NCD in development work at global and national level, and integrating the prevention and control of such diseases into policies across all government departments.* While Arab countries recognize the burden of NCD, they are yet to integrate prevention into their poverty reduction strategies and in relevant socio-economic policies. For this, a cross-sectoral response is essential.

2. *Establishing and strengthening national policies and plans for the prevention and control of NCD.* A multi-sectoral framework for prevention, risk factor reduction, and strengthening health systems are essential components of national programs. The lack of a clear and effective NCD prevention component in national health plans and the low priority given to risk reduction interventions are major gaps that most Arab countries should urgently address.

3. *Promoting interventions to reduce the main shared modifiable risk factors for NCD: tobacco use, unhealthy diets, physical inactivity, and harmful use of alcohol.* Higher levels of commitment and more work are needed to implement interventions for tobacco control, based on the WHO FCTC, and interventions recommended in the Global Strategy on Diet, Physical Activity and Health to support healthier composition of food. The latter focus on reducing salt levels; eliminating industrially produced trans-fatty acids; decreasing saturated fats; limiting free sugars; introducing transport policies that promote active and safe methods of travelling to and from schools and workplaces, such as walking or cycling; and

improving sports, recreation, and leisure facilities. National authorities should also ensure that marketing of food products, particularly for children, should not contribute to further dissemination of unhealthy dietary patterns.

4. *Promoting research for the prevention and control of cancer and other NCD.* A coordinated agenda for NCD research, important to both the global and national plans, aims to enhance international and regional inter-country collaboration, involving health-related research and public health institutions to promote and support the multidimensional and multisectoral research that is needed in order to generate or strengthen the evidence base for cost-effective prevention and control strategies. Collaboration within the Arab world is also needed to support countries in building capacity for epidemiological and health-systems research, including the analytical and operational research required for program implementation and evaluation.

5. *Promoting partnerships for the prevention and control of cancer and other NCD.* Effective public health responses to the global threats of NCD require strong international partnerships. Collaborative work and networking should include international and Arab world institutions, academia, research centers, nongovernmental organizations, consumer groups, and the business community. Since the major determinants of NCD lie outside the health sector, collaborative efforts must also be intersectoral and include sharing of experiences between countries in legislative actions, fiscal measures, and successful policies of the various non-health sectors. Efforts to strengthen networking of national NCD prevention programs should be encouraged.

6. *Monitoring NCD and their determinants and evaluate progress at the national, regional, and global levels.* Monitoring provides the foundation for advocacy, policy development, and action. Health policy makers in the region have consensus on the critical need for sustainable surveillance systems tailored to the local situation and stage of development. However, the core components should include reliable mortality statistics, data on exposure to major risk factors and a morbidity component, when feasible, such as a cancer registry. It is crucial for policy makers to

recognize that surveillance of NCD and their risk factors has to be institutionalized and integrated into the existing health information system. Beyond tracking trends in burden and risk factors, monitoring also includes assessing country progress in addressing the NCD challenge. WHO is currently developing a standardized tool to support countries in collecting comparable data and to support the implementation of this objective. A pilot step in this direction is the WHO Report on the Global Tobacco Epidemic which provides data on tobacco use trends and the status of countries in implementing tobacco control measures.

Conclusions

Evidence over the past two decades clearly documents the gathering global epidemic of NCD and in particular, the increasing magnitude of NCD burden in the Arab world. This reality has lain to rest many of the myths concerning NCD, particularly their implications. For most of the twentieth century, NCD were mistakenly considered in many health professional and policy arenas as problems primarily of high-income populations, or issues primarily affecting the elderly, especially men, for which there was little that could or should be done. Today, the evidence is clear that NCD are the leading causes of death and disease burden, with a major proportion of related deaths being premature. This evidence also clearly demonstrates the negative impact on socio-economic development. NCD contribute to poverty and are impeding initiatives at poverty reduction globally and in the Arab region.

Future projections point to considerable increases in NCD burden. Epidemiological analyses estimate that the greatest increase in LMICs will take place in Africa and in this region. This does not have to happen. Much has been learned over the past decades on how to address NCD, the bulk of which are preventable. NCD share many of the same risk factors and determinants and much of their burden can be avoided through an integrated prevention approach.

The Global Strategy for the Prevention and Control of Noncommunicable Diseases has put forward a clear vision on how to tackle the NCD epidemic. With the adoption of its Action Plan in 2008, the World Health Assembly has provided a comprehensive blueprint for going forward with implementation. To learn from the lessons elsewhere, Arab countries need to take action now before risk factors become more entrenched in their populations.

The global assault on NCD faces many challenges. This includes generating reliable data on a global scale to guide planning, priority setting, monitoring, and evaluation; intersectoral action based upon partnerships at all levels, particularly needed to address NCD determinants; and functioning health systems based on primary health care with an emphasis on prevention and community action. Addressing these challenges requires significant fiscal resources, appropriately trained human resources, and, perhaps most importantly, commitment to tackle NCD. These actions are within reach of the Arab countries today.

Acknowledgment

Ala Alwan is a staff member of the World Health Organization. The author alone is responsible for the views expressed in this publication and they do not necessarily represent the decisions or policies of the World Health Organization.

References

Abegunde D, Mathers C, Adam M, Ortegon K (2007) The burden and costs of chronic diseases in low-income and middle-income countries. *The Lancet*, 370: 1929–1938

Abolfotouh M, Abu-Zeid H, Aziz M, Alakija A (1996) Prevalence of hypertension in south-western Saudi Arabia. *Eastern Mediterranean Health Journal*, 2(2): 211–218

Aboul-Ella NA, Shehab DI, Ismail MA, Maksoud AA (2010) Prevalence of metabolic syndrome and insulin resistance among Egyptian adolescents 10 to 18 years of age. *Journal of Clinical Lipidology*, 4(3): 185–195

Ajlouni K, Khader YS, Batieha A, Ajlouni H, El-Khateeb M (2008) An increase in prevalence of diabetes mellitus in Jordan over 10 years. *Journal of Diabetes and its Complications*, 22(5): 317–324

Albache N, Al-Ali R, Rastam S, Fouad FM, Mzayek F, Maziak W (2010) Epidemiology of Type 2 diabetes mellitus in Aleppo, Syria. *Journal of Diabetes*, 2(2): 85–91

Al-Daghri NM (2010) Extremely high prevalence of metabolic syndrome manifestations among Arab youth: A call for early intervention. *European Journal of Clinical Investigation*, 40(12): 1063–1066

Al-Khalaf MM, Eid MM, Najjar HA, Alhajry KM, Doi SA, Thalib L (2010) Screening for diabetes in Kuwait and evaluation of risk scores. *Eastern Mediterranean Health Journal*, 16(7): 725–731

Al-Nozha MM, Al-Maatouq MA, Al-Mazrou YY, et al (2004) Diabetes mellitus in Saudi Arabia. *Saudi Medical Journal*, 25(11): 1603–1610

Alwan A (1982) Studies on the prevalence of hypertension in Iraqi rural and urban communities. *Iraqi Medical Journal*, 29: 99–104

Alwan A (1995) *Prevention and control of cardiovascular diseases*. Cairo, Egypt: WHO/EMRO

Alwan A (1996) *Prevention and management of hypertension*. Alexandria, Egypt: WHO/EMRO

Alwan A (2001) Prevention of cardiovascular disease is possible but a major challenge. *Bulletin of the World Health Organization*, 79(10): 980–987

Alwan A, Maclean D, Mandil A (2001) *Assessment of national capacity for the prevention and control of non-communicable diseases: The report of a global survey, Who/Mnc/01.2*. World Health Organization

Barker DJ, Osmond C, Forsen TJ, Kajantie E, Eriksson JG (2007) Maternal and social origins of hypertension. *Hypertension*, 50(3): 565–571

CSDH (Commission on the Social Determinants of Health) (2008) *Closing the gap in a generation: Health equity through action on the social determinants of health*. Geneva, Switzerland: World Health Organization

Doghmi F (1989) Fourteen years' experience with cardiac catheterization and angiography in Jordan. *Jordan Medical Journal*, 23: 21–37

Gaziano T, Gauden G, Reddy K (2007) Scaling up interventions for chronic disease prevention. The evidence. *The Lancet*, 370: 1939–1946

Ghannem H, Harrabi I, Ben Abdelaziz A, Gaha R, Mrizak N (2003) Clustering of cardiovascular risk factors among obese urban schoolchildren in Sousse, Tunisia. *Eastern Mediterranean Health Journal*, 9(1–2): 70–77

Godfrey KM, Barker DJP (2007) Fetal programming and adult health. *Public Health Nutrition*, 4(2b): 611–624

Gunaid AA, Assabri AM (2008) Prevalence of type 2 diabetes and other cardiovascular risk factors in a semirural area in Yemen. *Eastern Mediterranean Health Journal*, 14(1): 42–56

Harrabi I, Belarbia A, Gaha R, Essoussi AS, Ghannem H (2006) Epidemiology of hypertension among a population of school children in Sousse, Tunisia. *Canadian Journal of Cardiology*, 22(3): 212–216

International Diabetes Federation (2009) IDF Diabetes Atlas, available from http://www.eatlas.idf.org [Accessed 14 January 2011]

Jaddou HY, Bateiha AM, Khawaldeh AM, Goussous YM, Ajlouni KM (2001) Blood pressure profile in schoolchildren and adolescents in Jordan. *Annals of Saudi Medicine*, 21(1–2): 123–126

Mabry RM, Reeves MM, Eakin EG, Owen N (2010) Evidence of physical activity participation among men and women in the countries of the Gulf Cooperation Council: A review. *Obesity Reviews*, 11(6): 457–464

Mansour A, Wanoose H, Hanic I, Abed-Alzahread A, Wanoosee H (2008) Diabetes screening in Basrah, Iraq: A population-based cross-sectional study. *Diabetes Research And Clinical Practice*, 79(1): 147–150

Marmot M, Wilkinson R (2006) *Social determinants of health*. Oxford: Oxford University Press

Maziak W, Rastam S, Mzayek F, Ward KD, Eissenberg T, Keil U (2007) Cardiovascular health among adults in Syria: A model from developing countries. *Annals of Epidemiology*, 17(9): 713–720

Maziak W, Ali RA, Fouad MF, et al (2008) Exposure to secondhand smoke at home and in public places in Syria: A developing country's perspective. *Inhalation Toxicology*, 20(1): 17–24

Mehio Sibai A, Nasreddine L, Mokdad AH, Adra N, Tabet M, Hwalla N (2010) Nutrition transition and cardiovascular disease risk factors in Middle East and North Africa countries: Reviewing the evidence. *Annals of Nutrition & Metabolism*, 57(3–4): 193–203

Motlagh B, O'Donnell M, Yusuf S (2009) Prevalence of cardiovascular risk factors in the Middle East: A systematic review. *European Journal of Cardiovascular Prevention and Rehabilitation*, 16(3): 268–280

Murray CJL, Lopez A (1996) *Global burden of disease: A comprehensive assessment of mortality and disability from diseases, injuries, and risk factors in 1990 and projected to 2020* (1st edition). Boston: Harvard School Of Public Health

Najjar H, Easson A (2010) Age at diagnosis of breast cancer in Arab nations. *International Journal of Surgery*, 8: 448–452

Oman Ministry of Health (1996) *Manual on the management of hypertension in primary health care*. Muscat: Ministry of Health

Omar S, Alieldin NH, Khatib OM (2007) Cancer magnitude, challenges and control in the Eastern Mediterranean Region. *Eastern Mediterranean Health Journal*, 13(6): 1486–1496

Papandreou C, Mourad TA, Jildeh C, Abdeen Z, Philalithis A, Tzanakis N (2008) Obesity in Mediterranean region (1997–2007): A systematic review. *Obesity Reviews*, 9(5): 389–399

Puska P, Vartiainen E, Laatikainen T, Jousilahti P, Paavola M (Eds.) (2009) *The North Karelia Project: From North Karelia to national action*. Helsinki, Finland: Helsinki University Printing House

Ramahi TM (2010) Cardiovascular disease in the Asia Middle East region: Global trends and local implications. *Asia-Pacific Journal of Public Health*, 22(3): 83S–89S

Rashad H (2006). Promoting global action on the Social Determinants. *Diabetes' Voice*, 51(3): 33–35

Rastam S, Ward KD, Eissenberg T, Maziak W (2004) Estimating the beginning of the waterpipe epidemic in Syria. *BMC Public Health*, 4(1): 32

Saade G, Abou Jaoude S, Afifi R, Warren C, Jones N (2008) Patterns of tobacco use: Results from the 2005 Global Youth Tobacco Survey in Lebanon. *Eastern Mediterranean Health Journal*, 14(6): 1280–1289

Saleh EA, Mahfouz AA, Tayel KY, Naguib MK, Bin-al-Shaikh NM (2000) Hypertension and its determinants among primary-school children in Kuwait: An epidemiological study. *Eastern Mediterranean Health Journal*, 6(2/3): 333–337

Salim EI, Moore MA, Al-Lawati JA, et al (2009) Cancer epidemiology and control in the Arab world – past, present and future. *Asian Pacific Journal of Cancer Prevention*, 10(1): 3–16

Shao R, Liu B, Legowski B (2007) *Report of the Global Survey on the progress in national chronic diseases prevention and control*. Geneva: World Health Organization

Subhi MD (2006) Blood pressure profiles and hypertension in Iraqi primary school children. *Saudi Medical Journal*, 27(4): 482–486

Tazi MA, Abir-Khalil S, Lahmouz F, Arrach ML, Chaouki N (2009) Risk factors for hypertension among the adult Moroccan population. *Eastern Mediterranean Health Journal*, 15(4): 827–841

Temmar M, Labat C, Benkhedda S, et al (2007) Prevalence and determinants of hypertension in the Algerian Sahara. *Journal of Hypertension*, 25(11): 2218–2226

UnitedHealthGroup (2010) *Diabetes in the United Arab Emirates: Crisis or opportunity?* Abu Dhabi, UAE: UnitedHealthGroup/Ingenix

Uusitalo U, Feskens E, Tuomilehto T, et al (1996) Fall in total cholesterol concentration over five years in association with changes in fatty acid composition of cooking oil in Mauritius: Cross sectional survey. *British Medical Journal*, 313(7064): 1044–1046

World Health Assembly (2008) *Action plan for the global strategy for the prevention and control of noncommunicable diseases*. World Health Assembly, Document A61–8

WHO (World Health Organization) (2000) *Global strategy for the prevention and control of noncommunicable diseases*. WHA A53/14. Geneva: World Health Organization

WHO (2002) *WHO revised global burden of disease (GBD) 2002 estimates*. Geneva, Switzerland: WHO

WHO (2005) *Preventing chronic diseases: A vital investment*. Geneva, Switzerland: WHO

WHO (2007) *Trends in tobacco use among school students in the Eastern Mediterranean Region*. Cairo: WHO Regional Office for the Eastern Mediterranean

WHO (2008a) *The global burden of disease-2004 update*. Geneva, Switzerland: WHO

WHO (2008b) *WHO report on the global tobacco epidemic – The MPOWER package*. Geneva, Switzerland: WHO

WHO (2008c) *The world health report 2008: Primary health care – Now more than ever*. Geneva, Switzerland: WHO

WHO (2008d) *World health statistics*. Geneva, Switzerland: WHO

WHO (2009a) *Interventions on diet and physical activity: What works. Summary report*. Geneva, Switzerland: WHO

WHO (2009b) *Towards a strategy for cancer control in the Eastern Mediterranean Region: Technical paper*. Cairo, Egypt: WHO/EMRO

WHO (2009c) *WHO report on the global tobacco epidemic*. Geneva, Switzerland: WHO

WHO (2010) *STEPwise surveillance*, Cairo, Egypt: WHO Regional Office for the Eastern Mediterranean. Available from www.emro.who.int/ncd/stepwise.htm [Accessed 15 July 2010]

Zindah M, Belbeisi A, Walke H, Mokdad AH (2008) Obesity and diabetes in Jordan: Findings from the behavioral risk factor surveillance system, 2004. *Preventing Chronic Disease*, 5(1): 1–8

Chapter

13

Non-communicable Diseases – II: Focus on Cardiovascular Diseases

Habiba Ben Romdhane, Abdullatif Husseini, and Samer Jabbour

Chapter 12 has demonstrated the gathering epidemic of non-communicable diseases (NCD) in the Arab world and urged action based on evidence-based strategies and global and regional experiences. Largely focusing on cardiovascular diseases (CVD) as the NCD associated with the largest burden, this chapter first extends the review of the epidemiologic evidence and examines inequalities, identifies the main challenges in the largely neglected area of management of people with CVD and its risk factors, outlines regional examples of prevention and interventions, and discusses policy and research priorities.

The Epidemiological Evidence

Cardiovascular diseases include a variety of conditions, such as ischemic/coronary heart disease (IHD/CHD); hypertensive, rheumatic, and inflammatory heart diseases; cerebrovascular diseases; peripheral vascular diseases; and others. In this section, we review the evidence on mortality, morbidity, disability-adjusted burden, inequalities, and economic impact. Before doing so, it is useful to consider data sources and their limitations.

This region has long been recognized as a hot-spot for CVD with projections of its burden exceeding those of other regions, yet local data to inform health policy is inadequate (Murray & Lopez 1996). One challenge in comparing statistics is that reports and studies report data for either the Eastern Mediterranean Region (WHO), the Middle East, or the Middle East and North Africa (MENA). While countries included in these definitions overlap, they are not the same. To our knowledge, CVD data for the 22 countries of the Arab League has not been assembled. Considering the limitations of vital registration systems, especially in death certification, and limited population-based surveys in most countries, the

Global Burden of Disease (GBD) (WHO 2008) study estimated mortality, morbidity, and burden statistics for most countries based on estimates from Egypt, Bahrain, and Kuwait. We nevertheless report GBD data for CVD in this chapter and combine this with a review of research evidence and other estimates.

There are various sources for CVD event rates. The rigorous WHO-MONICA protocol (Tunstall-Pedoe et al 1994), which enables standardized international population-based comparisons to determine acute myocardial infarction events and coronary deaths, was applied only on two populations in the region: Palestinian residents of Jerusalem in 1997 (Jeremy et al 2006) and the Tunisian residents of Ariana district in 2001 (Ben Romdhane et al 2004). We do not review data on CVD risk factors, as this was covered in Chapter 12. It is encouraging that more and more countries have utilized the WHO-recommended STEPwise approach for risk factor surveillance with some countries using the opportunity to collect NCD and CVD data.

Cardiovascular Mortality

As discussed in Chapter 12, CVD are already the main causes of overall and NCD mortality in the region. The MENA registers the highest percentage of deaths due to CVD after Europe with IHD/CHD the leading cause. Reports have different but overlapping estimates of proportional mortality reflecting regional definition and data sources. The GBD study (WHO 2008) estimates that CVD causes almost 27% and 34.6% of all deaths in the EMR and MENA, respectively. Almost half of CVD deaths are due to IHD and 20.6% are due to cerebrovascular diseases while 11.0% are due to hypertensive disease. Inflammatory heart diseases represent 3.8% and rheumatic heart disease 2.1% of CVD deaths (Table 1). Gaziano et al (2010) estimated that CHD and cerebrovascular

Table 1. Cardiovascular Mortality

| | MENA | | | EMR | | | | | |
| | | | | Low- and middle-income countries | | | High-income countries | | |
	% of all deaths	% of CVD deaths	Deaths per 100,000 people	% of all deaths	% of CVD deaths	Deaths per 100,000 people	% of all deaths	% of CVD deaths	Deaths per 100,000 people
Cardiovascular diseases	34.6	100	226.0	26,7	100	229	37,2	100	135
Ischemic heart disease	16.7	48.1	108.7	13,3	50.0	114	17,7	50.0	65
Cerebrovascular disease	7.1	20.5	46.4	5,9	20.0	51	4,4	10.0	16
Hypertensive diseases	3.8	11.0	25.0	2.2	10.0	19	8,8	20.0	32
Rheumatic heart disease	0.5	1.3	3.0	0.6	2.1	5	0	0	0
Inflammatory heart disease	1.1	3.0	6.9	0.8	2.9	7	0	0	0

Notes: CVD: Cardiovascular diseases; EMR: Eastern Mediterranean Region; MENA: Middle East and North Africa.
Source: WHO (2008).

diseases account for about 16.9% and 6.8%, respectively, of total mortality and almost half and 19%, respectively, of CVD mortality.

Research evidence suggests that the picture is worse in some countries. For example, Maziak et al (2007) found that CVD accounted for 45% of all deaths with almost half of these occurring before 65 years of age. In the Occupied Palestinian Territory (OPT), Abu-Rmeileh et al (2008) also documented that circulatory conditions accounted for 45% of all deaths between 1999 and 2003 with myocardial infarction and cerebrovascular disease having the highest age-standardized mortality rates for both men and women. Also in OPT, Husseini et al (2009) reported that heart diseases and cerebrovascular diseases were the first and second leading causes of deaths (21% and 11%, respectively).

These observations are not new and have been long documented in some countries. For example, in Lebanon, Abou-Daoud (1967) documented that CVD accounted for 48.4% of all deaths in 1966. This percentage was 60.6% based on a verbal autopsy study between 1983 and 1993 (Sibai et al 2001a). Radovanovic (1994) showed that CVD accounted for 30–35% of all deaths in Kuwait between 1987 and 1992.

In terms of CVD death rate, the GBD estimates this at about 226 per 100,000 people, almost identical to rates in the Americas. However, estimates vary. Based on WHO data, Ramahi (2010) reported *age-standardized* CVD rates, per 100,000 people, ranging from the low 300s in Algeria, Bahrain, and Kuwait to the low 400s in Libya, Morocco, Syria, Tunisia, to over 500 in Egypt, Iraq, and Yemen. The determinants underlying these differences have not been studied. The study by Sibai et al (2001a) is unique in that it provides CVD mortality rates by sex for different age groups. Among the 50–59 age group, men had double the CVD mortality rate than women, but the rate was below 10 per 1000 person years in both. In the 90+ age groups, the mortality rate was almost identical, around 100 per 1000 person years. Husseini et al (2009) reported death rates for heart diseases, cerebrovascular diseases, and hypertension of 56.5, 29.8, and 13 per 100,000 people, respectively. Looking only at those aged 40 years and older, the *age-standardized* death rates per 100,000 people are much higher: for acute myocardial infarction 78.5 (not reported by sex group but twice as high for men), for stroke 41 among men and 35 among women, for heart failure 35 among men and 32 among women.

Table 2. Cardiovascular Morbidity

	MENA	EMR		
		Total	High-income countries	Low- & middle-income countries
	Per 100,000 inhabitants	Per 100,000 people	Per 100,000 people	Per 100,000 people
Stroke first ever (incidence)	80	87	32	87
Angina pectoris prevalence	800	784	681	790
Congestive heart disease prevalence	248	243	215	245
Cerebrovascular disease prevalence	210	205	157	213

Notes: EMR: Eastern Mediterranean Region; MENA: Middle East and North Africa.
Source: WHO (2008).

Cardiovascular Morbidity

As expected considering the level of cardiovascular mortality, CVD is also associated with high morbidity. Table 2 summarizes incidence and prevalence data for selected conditions from the GBD study.

In terms of research evidence, a few studies have reported incidence and prevalence rates. There was a stark contrast in coronary event rates in the Arab sites in the MONICA study. Jerusalem Palestinians had the highest incidence of CHD of all other 20 countries (Jeremy et al 2006) while the Ariana population had rates similar to those reported in other Mediterranean countries, Spain, Italy, and France, characterized by low incidence and low coronary mortality. Building on these data, Ben Romdhane et al (2004) reported CVD prevalence rates are substantial but vary across studies which may reflect actual rates or different definitions, conditions, and methods. Doctor-diagnosed "heart disease" was reported by 17.5% of 2487 Kuwaiti nationals aged 50 and above (Shah et al 2010). In Saudi Arabia among 17,232 subjects, 5.5% carried the diagnosis of CHD (Al-Nozha et al 2004). In Jordan, Nsour et al (2008) reported that 5.9% of 3083 subjects were told they had a prior myocardial infarction. In Lebanon, 7.5% of people in a large population-based survey reported cardiac disease (Ramahi et al 2010). In Aleppo, Syria, Maziak et al (2007) reported heart disease prevalence of 4.8% and stroke prevalence of 1%. In the OPT in 2006, heart disease was prevalent in 2.1% at age 40–49 years and 12·1% at 60 years and older (Husseini et al 2009). In a small Tunisian sample, 8.8% self-reported cardiovascular diseases (Méjean et al 2007). In a sample of 471 subjects in Saudi Arabia, Al-Sheikh et al (2007) found prevalence rate of peripheral arterial disease of 11.7% with 92.7% being asymptomatic.

Disability-Adjusted Burden of Cardiovascular Diseases

Disability adjustment can improve population summary measures as mortality estimates alone are inadequate. Expressed in disability-adjusted life year (DALY), the GBD estimates that, in the EMR, CVD causes 9.2% of lost DALYs with IHD accounting for 47.0%, while cerebrovascular diseases account for 20.6%. The years of life lost (YLL) is a measure of premature mortality and is an important input in the calculation of the DALYs for a disease or health condition. YLLs are calculated from the number of deaths at each age multiplied by a global standard life expectancy for the age at which death occurs. In the second biggest city of Tunisia, Hsairi et al (2003) recorded that out of a total of 52,316 YLL, 27,902 in men and 24,414 in women, CVDs caused 17.3% in men and 26.5% in women.

Economic Burden and Health Resource Utilization

The economic costs associated with the rise of CVDs and their risk factors are substantial but there is

Table 3. Burden of Cardiovascular Diseases in DALYs

	Total		High-income countries		Low- and middle-income countries	
	% of DALYs due to CVD	% of total DALYs	% of DALYs due to CVD	% of total DALYs	% of DALYs due to CVD	% of total DALYs
CVD	100	9.2	100	12.5	100	9.1
Ischemic heart disease	47.0	4.3	53.5	6.6	46.7	4.2
Cerebrovascular disease	20.6	1.89	9.6	1.2	21.1	1.9
Hypertensive diseases	7.1	0.66	16.4	2	6.7	0.6
Rheumatic heart disease	4.5	0.4	0.9	1	4.6	4.2
Inflammatory heart disease	4.0	0.3	2.0	0.2	4.1	3.8

Notes: CVD: Cardiovascular diseases; DALYs: Disability-adjusted life years.
Source: WHO (2008).

limited research evidence on such costs. Zhang et al (2010) recently estimated the health expenditures alone for diabetes in the "Eastern Mediterranean and Middle East" at $5.57–9.25 billion, or at 14% of total health expenditures. In 2030, it is projected that diabetes expenditures will rise to $11.4–19 billion. Abegunde et al (2007) estimated that forgone GDP due to CVD and diabetes in Egypt was $0.11 billion and that this would rise by 125% by 2015.

Resource use by people with CVD and its risk factors are substantial. Husseini et al (2009) reported cardiac diseases among the top five conditions for which Palestinian patients were referred for treatment by Palestinian Ministry of Health at tremendous costs. In a large multiregional study, diabetics in the Middle East had a mean (SD) of 2.5 (4.4) and 2.6 (13.5) general practitioner visits and inpatient days per year, respectively (Zhang et al 2010). The rates of hospitalization, inpatient days, ER visits and absenteeism were 4.4, 7.9, 3.9, and 9.9 times greater, respectively, in those with vs. without macrovascular complications. Diabetics with inadequate glycemic control, a common problem in the region, had higher rates of inpatient days and absenteeism.

Inequalities in Cardiovascular Disease and Risk

As in other regions, there are important inequalities in CVD. Despite the gaps in evidence, this is manifested in many areas.

National Income

There are marked inequalities in CVD mortality according to national income (Table 1). CVD cause proportionally more deaths in the high-income countries than in the low- and middle-income countries. This perhaps reflects more advanced epidemiological transition. CVD death rates, however, are higher in the latter group, including for the leading causes of IHD and cerebrovascular disease, probably reflecting worse outcomes. This is consistent with evidence from international comparisons suggesting shifting in cardiovascular risks to lower income countries (Ezzati et al 2005). Interestingly, hypertensive mortality rate is higher in high-income countries. The reason behind this needs further exploration.

There are also cross-country inequalities in CVD morbidity (Table 2). Incidence rates of first-ever stroke differ across countries, being 2.67 times higher in low- and middle-income countries. The corresponding rates in Europe and the Americas are 2.16 and 1.28, respectively. The prevalence of cerebrovascular diseases, angina, and congestive heart disease is also higher in the low- and middle-income countries. However, the difference is less important than observed in stroke incidence. Future research needs to confirm whether stroke incidence is a more sensitive marker of inequality in CVD morbidity than prevalence measures. As for disability-adjusted burden, the differences between high- and middle- and low-income countries are more difficult to interpret, with stroke being the area where the latter countries appear to be most disadvantaged (Table 3).

Conflict

There seems to be a link between occupation and conflict and CVD. In the MONICA study, Jerusalem Arabs exceeded all 20 countries both in coronary event rates and non-fatal infarction rates (Jeremy et al 2006). Higher incidence explains much of the excess CHD mortality in Jerusalem Arabs vs. Jews, although part is attributable to higher case fatality. Many factors could possibly contribute to this situation, among which undoubtedly are occupation and alienation of Arabs. Sibai et al (1989, 2001b) studied the conflict stress–heart disease link in a different context: the civil war in Lebanon. In a case-control design of angiographically confirmed coronary artery disease, exposure to acute war events was higher among cases compared with visitor controls (odds ratio [OR] 2.4) and angiographic controls (2.8). Crossing the "green lines" that separated the warring East and West Beirut, a very stressful event and an indicator of chronic stress, was associated with even higher risk (corresponding ORs 3.25 and 5.38, respectively). These associations persisted after adjustment for classic risk factors. Sibai et al (2007) also examined the association between marital status, intergenerational co-residence, and CVD mortality. Contrary to expectations, they found higher mortality among those residing with family members, thus raising the question whether traditionally known family support in the region can still hold during civil war.

Social Stratifiers

There are inequalities according to social stratifications within countries. CVD seem to be more prevalent in urban areas. For example, Al-Nozha et al (2004) documented 6.2% vs. 4% prevalence of CHD in urban vs. rural Saudis, respectively. The picture for gender differences is complex, and data are limited (Shara 2010). Mortality rates seem to be higher for CHD in men but for cerebrovascular disease in women, as demonstrated in Lebanon (Sibai et al 2001a) and Syria (Maziak et al 2007). Coronary event rates are also higher among men. In the Ariana population (Tunisia), the incidence of myocardial infarction was estimated at 161.9 per 100,000 men vs. 61.1 per 100,000 women (Ben Romdhane et al 2004). Heart disease prevalence also seems higher in men. In Syria (Maziak et al 2007), 6.2% of men vs. 3.7% of women reported heart disease. Stroke prevalence was closer, 1.0% in women and 0.9% in men.

A limited number of studies examine the links between CVD and socio-economic status. Ramahi et al (2010) examined this link, mainly between education and household income and self-reported heart disease and risk factors, in 7879 respondents above the age of 40 years in the 2004 Lebanese Survey of Family Health. Reported heart disease was inversely associated with education and household income. This association persisted after adjustment for classical risk factors. There was a clear gradient. In the case of education, the adjusted OR was 1.53, 1.34, and 1.27 for those with less than elementary, elementary, and preparatory education, respectively, as compared with secondary and higher education. As for household income, the adjusted OR was 1.42 and 1.17 for the low- and middle-income categories, respectively, as compared with high income. Interestingly, there was more reported heart disease in the two most affluent areas (Beirut and Mount Lebanon, adjusted OR 1.86 and 1.29, respectively) as compared with the less affluent North and South areas, but the authors did not comment on this finding.

Ramahi et al rightly note that the persistent association between self-reported heart disease and socio-economic status after adjustment for risk factors implies that socio-economic factors may work through mechanisms beyond classical risk factors. One candidate mechanism is psychological distress, shown in the INTERHEART study to be a strong risk factor for myocardial infarction in the Arab Middle Eastern countries, especially for females (Yusuf et al 2004). Stress, among other factors, may partially explain the finding of more heart disease in the more affluent areas of Beirut and North Lebanon. Stress or other mechanisms, for example a sense of relative deprivation or alienation associated with inequality, may operate through other intermediary factors measured incompletely in the study, such as duration and extent of smoking, or not available in the dataset at all, such as physical inactivity, dietary patterns, or alcohol consumption.

Ramahi et al also found a significant association between reported heart disease and currently and previously married (adjusted OR 3.01 and 3.91, respectively) as compared with never married and hypothesized this to be due to marital/parental stressors in the first, and stressors of separation/bereavement in the latter. These patterns need to be investigated further.

There is good evidence linking socio-economic factors and CVD risk factors with many patterns consistent with those reported from other settings, whereby the more disadvantaged have more risk factors. For example, in Lebanon, Ramahi et al (2010) reported that classical risk factors, smoking, diabetes, and hypertension, but not hypercholesterolemia, were more prevalent in the lower education and income groups. In neighboring Syria, Maziak et al (2007) reported that people with low education had the worst risk profile, mainly because of high prevalence of obesity and hypertension.

Inequalities are also evident in the need for and use of resources. As part of a global study, Zhang et al (2010) showed that, in the Eastern Mediterranean/ Middle East, hospitalization for diabetics with university or primary/secondary education were 66% and 50%, respectively, lower than in those who are illiterate. The corresponding rates for inpatient days were 83% and 60%. Evidence also suggests that the less-advantaged shoulder a proportionately higher economic burden of risk factors. In a large household survey in Morocco, smokers in the lowest income category (family income of less than 1000 dirhams) spent 50.9% of income on tobacco while those in the higher income category (6000 dirhams or higher) spent 13% (Tachfouti et al 2010). If such is the case for a risk factor, then the situation is likely to be also serious with regard to cost associated with CVD diagnosis and treatment.

Care for Cardiovascular Disease and Risk Factors

With the large burden of CVD and risk factors, the complexity and cost of managing these conditions, and the current limitations of health systems in the region (see chapters in Section 6), CVD care is one of the most difficult areas for public health.

Risk Factor Management in People Without Overt CVD

Many studies document major gaps in this area. We focus therefore on studies of management of people with multiple CVD risk factors, including diabetes, as these have high CVD risk. In Bahrain, Damanhori et al (2008) found poor BP and glycemic control (<10% and <13%, respectively) in diabetic hypertensives with high cardiovascular risk. Statins and aspirin were underused. Al-Mahroos & Al-Roomi (2007) found that uncontrolled glycemia, elevated blood pressure (BP), elevated lipids, and higher body mass index (BMI) were common among diabetics and correlated with higher prevalence of diabetic complications, including peripheral arterial disease. Al-Khaja et al (2005) also documented poor control of glycemia (<15%) and BP (≤10%) among high-risk diabetics attending either primary care diabetes clinics or general practice. In Saudi Arabia, a primary care study reported better control rates: 24% for glycemia, 32% for BP, and 50.5% for lipids. However, a substantial proportion of subjects without prior history of hypertension or dyslipidemia had levels well above targets. A review by Al-Ahmadi & Roland (2005) documented many challenges in diabetes and CVD risk factor management in primary care. In a study of Palestinian refugees in Lebanon, Yusef (2000) reported better control rates of diabetes and hypertension, and lipids in people with either condition. However, non-pharmacological approaches were markedly underutilized. In Egypt, El-Shazly et al (2000) reported many gaps in management of diabetes.

Various studies have documented high prevalence of risk factors among people presenting with CVD, indicating missed opportunities for primary prevention. For example, Lihioui et al (2007) and Jemaa et al (2004) in Tunisia, Zubaid et al (2004) in Kuwait, and Al-Suwaidi et al (2010) and Ali et al (2010) from a large Gulf-wide study, documented the persistence of high prevalence of risk factors in various populations with CVD. Such factors are also highly prevalent among young people with CVD, as documented in Saudi Arabia among those surviving acute myocardial infarction (Shatoor 2004). The importance of primary prevention is further highlighted by the findings in the INTERHEART study that Middle Easterners (mostly in the Gulf States and Egypt) ranked first among 10 regions in the population fraction attributable to smoking, second for dyslipidemia and psychosocial factors, and third for diabetes (Yusuf et al 2004).

Management of CVD

There is less research here as compared with risk factor management. Most studies are hospital-based and examine care characteristics and outcomes, especially for acute myocardial infarction and coronary syndromes. Of particular interest for public health is the finding that many people with acute coronary events present late. This is well documented in Gulf countries (Al-Mallah et al 2010), Jordan (Khraim et al 2009), and Lebanon (Noureddine et al 2010).

Lack of population-based data on ambulatory care of people with CVD in different settings, both primary and subspecialty, undermines public health actions. For the most serious condition, CHD, there is both anecdotal and research evidence that invasive and costly approaches are over-utilized in some settings where invasive facilities are widely available. Sibai et al (2008a, 2008b) documented this phenomenon in Lebanon, which has a density of cardiac catheterization laboratory three times that of France (9.32 vs. 2.92 per 1,000,000 people) and has the world's third highest utilization rates after the US and Germany (53 per 10,000 people). Appropriateness rate was only 54.7%. The majority of subjects (84.7%) did not have non-invasive testing prior to catheterization. Appropriateness decreased as density of cardiac catheterization laboratories increased raising the possibility of the role of financial interests. Ironically, the health system set-up increased over-utilization, as catheterization is publicly reimbursed while non-invasive testing is not.

Considering CVD prevalence rates, secondary prevention becomes crucial. Here, studies also suggest substantial gaps and missed opportunities. Al-Sheikh et al (2007) found substantial rates of CHD, cerebro-vascular disease, and CVD risk factors among subjects with peripheral artery disease, most previously undetected due to lack of symptoms, raising the need for early detection and management of disease and risk factors. In Jordan, among 300 people with CHD, only 29.7% quit smoking after occurrence of diagnosis (Abu-Baker et al 2010). Among 1534 subjects with CHD, there were high rates of smoking (45%-men, 11%-women) and abnormal lipids (LDL >240 mg/dl 19%-men and 27%-women; TG>150 mg/dl 55% for both; HDL-C<40 mg/dl 60%-men, 39%-women). Al-Nozha et al (2004) in Saudi Arabia also documented persistent smoking and metabolic abnormalities among community subjects with CAD. In the REACH registry of people with CVD (CHD, cerebrovascular disease, peripheral arterial disease) or three or more CVD risk factors, essentially being CVD equivalent, persistent smoking, elevated blood pressure ($\geq$140/90 mmHg), or elevated cholesterol were present in around 15%, 55%, and 35%, respectively, in the Middle East (the sample included Lebanon, Saudi Arabia, and UAE) (Bhatt et al 2006). Under-treatment with evidence-based therapies was common. These gaps were common across regions, including need for globally coordinated efforts.

The time of discharge from a CVD event is an especially opportune time for initiating secondary prevention. Gaps are also noted in the limited available research evidence. Zubaid et al (2004) in Kuwait documented that, among subjects with acute myocardial infarction, rates of prescribed aspirin, beta-blockers, angiotensin-converting enzyme inhibitors, and statins at discharge were 98%, 86%, 51%, and 50%, respectively. These rates represent improvements over an earlier study. In a more recent and larger study, Al-Suwaidi et al (2010) documented better rates of prescribing at discharge the latter two classes but lower rates of beta-blockers. One challenge to secondary prevention is access to essential cardio-vascular medicines. In a study of 36 countries, including eight Arab ones in different income categories, there were important challenges in the availability, especially in the public sector, and affordability of such medicines (van Mourik et al 2010). Even the purchase of generic atenolol, a form of beta-blocker, can impoverish as demonstrated in a multi-national study that included Jordan, Tunisia, and Yemen (Niëns et al 2010).

Cardiac rehabilitation is an important component of secondary prevention. We have found only one study, involving 168 coronary patients in Algeria (Adghar et al 2008). Cardiac rehabilitation improved functional capacity and quality of life.

Responding to the CVD Epidemic: Programs and Initiatives

How have the Arab countries responded to CVD? With the pressure to respond to public demands for treatment and lack of long-term visionary strategies, downstream approaches in the form of hi-tech medical and hospital services, in the public or private sectors, have probably been the earliest and most common. Many countries pride themselves on developing such services. However, these have been concentrated in urban areas with inequitable population access.

The public health response to CVD, within the broader scope of responding to the NCD challenge, has slowly emerged since the mid-1990s with increasing recognition of the burden of NCD in general and CVD in particular (Alwan 1997). Important credit is due to the WHO's Regional

Office for the Eastern Mediterranean (EMRO) for working with and pushing countries to recognize the NCD burden, the cost of inaction, and the imperatives of prevention. Examples of successful outcomes include the passing of regional resolutions on NCD; the establishment of NCD departments in many ministries of health; the launching of the Eastern Mediterranean Approach to Noncommunicable Diseases Network (EMAN), which aims to link and network countries to work collaboratively in capacity building, community-based programs, risk factor surveillance, and improving care for NCD at the PHC level; the implementation of STEPwise surveillance approach in several countries; and the engagement in and ratification by all countries of the WHO's Framework Convention on Tobacco Control (FCTC).

The Broader NCD Response: National Programs and Initiatives

The success of international and regional NCD resolutions and initiatives, and their translation in the area of CVD, comes down to how governments put these into force. In many countries, published information on programs for NCD prevention and control is scarce. About 10 years ago, fewer than half of the EMR countries had national policies or proper legislation addressing NCD (Alwan et al 2001). Since then more and more countries have established national NCD programs or departments. Some countries have launched community-based initiatives for NCD prevention based on a multisectoral approach, the most well-known being the Nizwa Healthy Lifestyle Project in Oman (Belal 2009) and the Ariana Project in Tunisia (Ben Romdhane & Grenier 2009).

There are several caveats in national NCD programs. It is commonly acknowledged that in many countries Ministry of Health (MOH)-based NCD departments are weak and underfunded and do not have strong mandates. Thus, having NCD departments and programs does not guarantee successful action. Lebanon, for example, is an FCTC-signatory and has had both a national NCD and tobacco control programs but the government has yet to pass a ban on smoking in public areas despite the pressure by the Ministry of Health, the local WHO office and anti-tobacco activists and academia, due to the powers of special interests. There is no regional data on how

Box 1. Nizwa Healthy Lifestyle Project (NHLP)

This is an action-oriented community-based intervention for NCD prevention and health promotion in the Wilayat (governorate) of Nizwa, Oman. The population of Nizwa is almost 70,000 people. The objectives of the project are to map the emerging epidemics of NCD and analyze their determinants; to reduce the exposure of individuals and populations to the major determinants of NCDs; to prevent the emergence of preventable common risk factors and to strengthen health care for people by supporting effective interventions. The project promotes healthy lifestyle through three subcommittees: (1) tobacco control & accident prevention, (2) promotion of physical activity, and (3) promotion of healthy nutrition. The project uses a community-based approach through multisectoral collaboration and public–private partnership. Interventions are applied in two approaches: Interventions in the population approach include school programs, community empowerment and public education. Interventions in the high-risk approach include a lifestyle Clinic, Health professional's education and involvement, Obesity screening and management at PHC centers and Tobacco cessation clinic.

During the year 2007, raising tobacco awareness in the community was a major target. A large variety of activities were carried out, involving over 3000 people, some in partnership with the public sector, the private sector and the Oman Society for Cancer Awareness. One unique activity was a social worker-based tobacco cessation project carried out in schools to support students to quit using tobacco, whereby social workers were trained in two workshops on counseling methods for tobacco cessation.

While NHLP is very promising, the full impact of the project is yet to be well documented and presented for peer review.

much attention is given to various NCDs, including CVD, within national NCD programs. However, it is well known that some "control" aspects do not fall within the mandates of NCD programs. For example, care for CVD may fall under curative or hospital services and is not integrated with CVD/NCD prevention, which might represent missed opportunities for secondary prevention. The effectiveness of NCD programs is difficult to establish as monitoring and evaluation is either not done or results are not publicly shared. Most importantly, many if not most NCD programs do not focus on structural and social determinants but rather on lifestyle risk factors, an approach that is demonstrated to have limited success in many other regions.

Examples of CVD Prevention Models

We highlight here three models from the region focused on CVD. The Together for Heart Health research intervention study (Nakkash et al 2003) carried out in Beirut, Lebanon, was innovative in that it was based on sound theoretical considerations of community organizing. The assessment phase focused on community resources, survey and physiologic measurements of risk factors, and physician survey. This led to a coalition building that enacted the intervention phase which focused on multifactorial interventions but with special focus on anti-smoking, physical activity, and healthy nutrition. Early evaluation results were encouraging but the long-term impact and sustainability of the interventions were limited by the depletion of funding.

Like the Lebanon study, the Abu Dhabi Cardiovascular Program (Hajat & Harrison 2010) also combined research and intervention, and did so innovatively in a simple, well-evidenced package delivered to all stakeholders, but the program was of much bigger scale. The whole population cardiovascular screening was a main achievement whereby more than 173,000 people were screened. Using the core Framingham indicators, with some expansion, a Framingham risk score was calculated for each participant who was referred to the Weqaya (meaning "prevention" in Arabic) program Web site (Weqaya 2010). The Web site provides clear information for each person on her/his own health situation, explanation of her/his health report and screening results, and links to available services and booking appointments with service providers in both Arabic and English languages. The claimed scalability and adaptability of such a model for low- and middle-income countries needs more investigation and further research due to the unique characteristics of Abu Dhabi and the UAE, and the commitment and resources provided for this program.

The third model is still in development. Med-CHAMPS (Mediterranean Studies of Cardiovascular disease and Hyperglycaemia: Analytical Modelling of Population Socio-economic transitions) is a multi-country project that aims to develop CVD and diabetes models for the region (MedCHAMPS 2010). The study involves four countries, OPT, Syria,

Tunisia, and Turkey. The aim is to "make recommendations about policy initiatives, both within and outside the health sector, likely to be the most effective and cost-effective in reducing the burden of cardiovascular diseases and diabetes" in MENA. The study will develop, test, and validate CVD and diabetes models using country data and utilize a combination of methodologies to assess the effectiveness and cost-effectiveness of interventions and policies. The project has several advantages. It relies on the IMPACT model that has been validated and used in other settings (Capewell et al 2010). It includes countries with similarities and differences in CVD burden, health services, and research and health information systems. Ongoing work has raised questions concerning the availability and quality of data in countries, and the adaptability of the "IMPACT" model to the region. None of the three models focus specifically on the social determinants of CVD.

Interventions to Improve Care for CVD and Risk Factors

We are not aware of national or large-scale interventions programs to upgrade ambulatory care for CVD and improve outcomes. There are several reports of interventions aimed at improving management of CVD risk factors, with most focusing on diabetes. In Dubai, UAE, Khattab et al (2007) reported that a quality improvement program to improve diabetes care in 16 governmental PHC centers improved clinical indicators and outcomes including BP reduction and low density lipoproteins (LDL) targets. In Saudi Arabia, Moharram & Farahat (2008) reported that using flow sheets improved quality of diabetes care while Al Mazroui et al (2009) reported that pharmaceutical care from a clinical pharmacist reduced cardiovascular risk scores. The World Diabetes Foundation (2010) reports ongoing projects to improve diabetes care in Egypt, Jordan, the West Bank, and Yemen.

Policy and Research Recommendations
Rationale

Addressing CVD must be done within a broader strategy for addressing NCD. The WHO's global strategy for NCD is well outlined in Chapter 12. Within such a broad approach, we can envision a special attention on CVD for several reasons. NCD remains a vague and poorly understood term for the public in this region, which undermines potential for broad mobilization. CVD may well serve as a useful entry to broader NCD prevention because of broad understanding among the public of at least some CVD manifestations, including the possibility for exploiting the known "scare factor" in public imagery of CVD, especially CHD, and the large menu of options for action that can be pursued including prevention. Furthermore, because the role of upstream factors is readily identifiable for CVD, for example the role of tobacco-friendly policies, action on social determinants is also possible, indeed imperative. Work on CVD and its NCD-shared determinants and risk factors will necessarily translate into broader NCD benefits.

Considering the burden of CVD, the policy response has therefore been inadequate. The international climate today, as manifested for example in the UN summit on NCD planned for September 2011, is favorable to implementing global NCD prevention and control strategies. It is the national will and high-level commitment, engagement of all potential stakeholders, and local innovation that will determine how well this will work in the Arab countries. We do not underestimate the challenges of adapting policy measures to country specific needs, converting generic strategies into feasible action plans, and providing the needed resources whether human or financial to implement them. We focus here on three priority areas.

The Social Determinants of CVD and Risk Factors

The evidence on social determinants of CVD and their risk factors is strong but still scant. From an equity perspective, governments have a moral imperative to collect, or support the collection of, data on the socio-economic dynamics of the CVD epidemic and to develop corresponding policies. Such policies must address inequalities in the incidence and prevalence of CVD and risk factors in population strata, CVD mortality, the provision and quality of care and access to essential cardiovascular medicines, the economic burden of CVD borne by families and individuals, and the benefits that different population groups receive from CVD interventions. The latter point is especially important considering the evidence

from other settings that the better-off benefit more from CVD prevention efforts (Capewell & Graham 2010). Interventions that are explicitly based on a consideration of structural and social determinants of CVD are sorely missing in the region but are indispensable if the root causes of the epidemic are to be addressed. Rather than being projected as a side effect of affluence, the CVD/NCD epidemic must be projected and addressed as it really is, a failure of development.

Health System Adaptation to the Epidemiological Transition

The health systems in Arab countries face many challenges today (see chapters in Section 6). NCD will invariably stress these systems further (see also Chapter 12) as in many other countries with similar levels of development (Samb et al 2010). CVD poses special challenges because of the need for action on the many levels spanning the spectrum from determinants to managing cardiovascular risk to costly care for people with chronic and debilitating cardiovascular conditions.

A two-pronged approach is needed (Joshi et al 2008). Population approaches focus on the upstream determinants and risk generators and are potentially more equitable than high-risk approaches (Capewell & Graham 2010). These include a diverse set of actions ranging from population and community-based prevention, to improving public response to cardiovascular symptoms to legislations, laws, and regulations. The highest priority is to meet the commitments already made. For example, it is no longer acceptable for countries not to put the FCTC into force. Pressure by the international community can add to local pressures to force governments into action. There are many other opportunities beyond tobacco but very few countries in the region have ventured into population-wide prevention.

The second approach relies on primary health care (PHC). Current primary care systems around the region were set up to address maternal–child health and infectious diseases (Al-Ahmadi & Roland 2005). A system transformation is needed to strengthen the abilities of such systems to deal with NCD. In addition to health promotion, PHC can improve detention, treatment, and control rates of CVD risk factors. But much more needs to be done to address CVD per se. If managing risk factors such as diabetes and hypertension is a challenge, as Al-Ahmadi and Roland found, early detection of CVD based on global risk assessment, assessing and triaging cardiovascular symptoms, and managing existing CVD and its advanced complications such as advanced heart failure in aging populations, will be far more difficult. Addressing this challenge requires a long-term vision, development of human resources, and devotion of appropriate funding and other forms of support. This is yet to happen in most countries.

Evidence supports the cost-effectiveness of CVD interventions in both approaches. For population-based approaches, the benefit is overwhelming, especially for tobacco and salt reduction (Gaziano et al 2007). However, there is also clear benefit for treatment. For example, Gaziano et al (2006) estimated that in MENA, secondary prevention with aspirin, angiotensin-converting enzyme inhibitors, beta-blockers, and statins would cost $341 while primary prevention with aspirin, angiotensin-converting enzyme inhibitors, calcium-channel blockers, and statins would cost $872 and $930 in medium and high-risk groups, respectively. These figures fall well within the cost-effectiveness range considering national incomes. More important than the cost-effectiveness is the right of people with CVD, or at risk of it, to prevention and treatment which include but are not limited to medicines.

A Public Health CVD Research Agenda

This review demonstrates that there is already plenty of evidence to support action on CVD/NCD. But weak health information and research systems in many Arab countries can undermine action. This calls for linking policy and action with strengthening health information systems and conducting priority research as this would inform the needed response.

The research agenda for CVD prevention and control is indeed vast as this review has highlighted, pointing to the need for a strong role for academia and researchers within NGOs and other settings. We prioritize three areas. The first concerns exploring and exposing inequalities and identifying vulnerable groups and elucidating the structural and social determinants. Demonstrating, for example, the link between weak tobacco control policies, poverty and CVD can build the momentum for public action on CVD. This requires new datasets that allow researchers to explore CVD inequalities in earnest. Another priority linked to this is examining the social differentials in cost of diagnosis and treatment of CVD, which are commonly acute and push families into catastrophic spending and potentially impoverishment. The third priority concerns care for CVD, whether in studying processes and outcomes in primary care, meeting targets for secondary prevention using evidence-based therapies, availability and affordability of essential cardiovascular medicines, or appropriateness of use of costly cardiac interventions. This agenda requires a multi-disciplinary approach beyond traditional medical and public health disciplines.

Conclusion

CVD are already the main causes of burden of mortality and ill-health in the Arab world. In some cases this has been the case for a long time, indicating poor action, if not inaction; this is a public health, health system, and social challenge. There are identifiable inequalities in CVDs and their burden on people and families; this is a social justice urgency. Arab countries have slowly developed national NCD prevention and control programs but these programs remain weak and attention to CVD is not well documented. A few demonstration projects have been carried out or are under way but are of limited scale. We have advocated a response strategy that is based on action on the social determinants, a combined approach of population strategy and primary health-care strengthening, and a public health research agenda. The international climate today is conducive to action on CVD and NCD. The years to come will show whether governments are ready to grasp the opportunity, with the aim of reducing the burden and human suffering. Researchers in the region have a major role to play in making this happen.

References

Abegunde DO, Mathers CD, Adam T, Ortegon M, Strong K (2007) The burden and costs of chronic diseases in low-income and middle-income countries. *Lancet*, 370(9603): 1929–1938

Abou-Daoud KT (1967) Mortality and cause of death in the city of Beirut. *Lebanese Medical Journal*, 20: 273–289

Abu-Baker NN, Haddad L, Mayyas O (2010) Smoking behavior among coronary heart disease patients in Jordan: A model from a developing country. *International Journal of Environmental Research and Public Health*, 7(3): 751–764

Abu-Rmeileh NM, Husseini A, Abu-Arqoub O, Hamad M, Giacaman R (2008) Mortality patterns in the West Bank, Palestinian Territories, 1999–2003. *Preventing Chronic Disease*, 5(4): 1–8

Adghar D, Bougherbal R, Hanifi R, Khellaf N (2008) [La réadaptation cardiaque du coronarien: première expérience en Algérie] (in French). *Annales de Cardiologie et d'Angéiologie*, 57(1): 44–47

Al-Ahmadi H, Roland M (2005) Quality of primary health care in Saudi Arabia: A comprehensive review. *International Journal for Quality in Health Care*, 17(4): 331–346

Ali WM, Zubaid M, El-Menyar A, et al (2010) The prevalence and outcome of hypertension in patients with acute coronary syndrome in six Middle-Eastern countries. *Blood Pressure*, 20(1): 20–26

Al-Khaja KA, Sequeira RP, Damanhori AH (2005) Comparison of the quality of diabetes care in primary care diabetic clinics and general practice clinics. *Diabetes Research and Clinical Practice*, 70(2): 174–182

Al-Mahroos F, Al-Roomi K (2007) Diabetic neuropathy, foot ulceration, peripheral vascular disease and potential risk factors among patients with diabetes in Bahrain: A nationwide primary care diabetes clinic-based study. *Annals of Saudi Medicine*, 27(1): 25–31

Al-Mallah MH, Alsheikh-Ali AA, Almahmeed W, et al (2010) Missed opportunities in the management of ST-segment elevation myocardial infarction in the Arab Middle East: Patient and physician impediments. *Clinical Cardiology*, 33(9): 565–571

Al Mazroui NR, Kamal MM, Ghabash NM, Yacout TA, Kole PL, McElnay JC (2009) Influence of pharmaceutical care on health outcomes in patients with Type 2 diabetes mellitus. *British Journal of Clinical Pharmacology*, 67(5): 547–557

Al-Nozha MM, Arafah MR, Al-Mazrou YY, et al (2004) Coronary artery disease in Saudi Arabia. *Saudi Medical Journal*, 25: 1165–1171

Al-Sheikh SO, Aljabri BA, Al-Ansary LA, Al-Khayal LA, Al-Salman MM, Al-Omran MA (2007) Prevalence of and risk factors for peripheral arterial disease in Saudi Arabia. A pilot cross-sectional study. *Saudi Medical Journal*, 28(3): 412–414

Al-Suwaidi J, Zubaid M, El-Menyar AA, et al (2010) Prevalence of the metabolic syndrome in patients with acute coronary syndrome in six middle eastern countries. *Journal of Clinical Hypertension*, 12(11): 890–899

Alwan A (1997) Noncommunicable diseases: A major challenge to public health in the region. *Eastern Mediterranean Health Journal*, 3: 6–16

Alwan A, Maclean D, Mandil A (2001) *Assessment of national capacity for noncommunicable disease prevention and control: The report of a global survey*. Geneva, Switzerland: WHO

Belal AM, Al-Hinai AG (2009) Community-based initiatives for prevention of non-communicable diseases: Nizwa Healthy Lifestyle Project planning and implementation experience in Oman. *Sudanese Journal of Public Health*, 4(1): 225–228

Ben Romdhane H, Bougatef S, Kafsi MN, et al (2004) Le registre des maladies coronaires en Tunisie: Organisation et premiers résultats. *Revue Epidemiologique de Santé Publique*, 52: 558–564

Ben Romdhane H, Grenier D (2009) Social determinants of health in Tunisia: The case-analysis of Ariana. *International Journal for Equity in Health*, 8: 9

Bhatt DL, Steg PG, Ohman EM, et al (2006) International prevalence, recognition, and treatment of cardiovascular risk factors in outpatients with atherothrombosis. *Journal of the American Medical Association*, 295(2): 180–189

Capewell S, Graham H (2010) Will cardiovascular disease prevention widen health inequalities? *PLoS Medicine*, 7: 8

Capewell S, Ford R, Croft J, et al (2010) Cardiovascular risk factor trends and potential for reducing coronary heart disease mortality in the United States of America. *Bulletin of the World Health Organization*, 88: 120–130

Damanhori A, Al Khaja K, Sequeira RP (2008) Gender-based treatment outcomes in diabetic hypertension. *Journal of Postgraduate Medicine*, 54(4): 252–258

El-Shazly M, Abdel-Fattah M, Zaki A, et al (2000) Health care for diabetic patients in developing countries: A case from Egypt. *Public Health*, 114(4): 276–281

Ezzati M, Vander Hoorn S, Lawes CMM, et al (2005) Rethinking the diseases of affluence paradigm: Global patterns of nutritional risks in relation to economic development. *PLoS Medicine*, 2(5): e133

Gaziano TA, Opie LH, Weinstein MC (2006) Cardiovascular disease prevention with a multidrug regimen in the developing world: A cost-effectiveness analysis. *Lancet*, 368: 679–686

Gaziano TA, Galea G, Reddy KS (2007) Scaling up interventions for chronic disease prevention: The evidence. *Lancet*, 370: 1939–1946

Gaziano TA, Bitton A, Anand S, Abrahams-Gessel S, Murphy A (2010) Growing epidemic of coronary heart disease in low- and middle-income countries. *Current Problems in Cardiology*, 35(2): 72–115

Hajat C, Harrison O (2010) The Abu Dhabi cardiovascular program: The continuation of Framingham. *Progress in Cardiovascular Diseases*, 53: 28–38

Hsairi M, Fki H, Fakhfakh R, et al (2003) [Années de vie perdues et transition épidémiologique dans le Gouvernorat de Sfax (Tunisie)] (in French). *Santé Publique*, 15: 25–27

Husseini A, Abu-Rmeileh NM, Mikki N, et al (2009) Cardiovascular diseases, diabetes mellitus, and cancer in the occupied Palestinian territory. *Lancet*, 373(9668): 1041–1049

Jemaa R, Kafsi MN, Kallel A, et al (2004) Distribution des facteurs de risque cardio-vasculaire chez une cohort tunisienne de 6901 coronariens. *Archives des Maladies du Cœur et des Vaisseaux*, 97(1): 20–24

Jeremy D, Kark R, Fink B, Goldman S (2006) The incidence of coronary heart disease among Palestinians and Israelis in Jerusalem. *International Journal of Epidemiology*, 35: 448–457

Joshi R, Jan S, Wu Y, MacMahon S (2008) Global inequalities in access to cardiovascular health care: Our greatest challenge. *Journal of American College of Cardiology*, 52: 1817–1825

Khattab MS, Swidan AM, Farghaly MN, et al (2007) Quality improvement programme for diabetes care in family practice settings in Dubai. *Eastern Mediterranean Health Journal*, 13(3): 492–504

Khraim FM, Scherer YK, Dorn JM, Carey MG (2009) Predictors of decision delay to seeking health care among Jordanians with acute myocardial infarction. *Journal of Nursing Scholarship*, 41(3): 260–267

Lihioui M, Boughzala E, Ben Farhat M, et al (2007) Distribution des facteurs de risque cardio-vasculaire chez des patients coronariens dans le Sahel tunisien. *Eastern Mediterranean Health Journal*, 13(3): 536–543

Maziak W, Rastam S, Mzayek F, et al (2007) Cardiovascular health among adults in Syria: A model from developing countries. *Annals of Epidemiology*, 17: 713–720

MedCHAMPS (2010) Project website. Available from http://research.ncl.ac.uk/medchamps/index.html [Accessed 16 October 2010]

Méjean C, Traissac P, Eymard-Duvernay S, El Ati J, Delpeuch F, Maire B (2007) Influence of socio-economic and lifestyle factors on overweight and nutrition-related diseases among Tunisian migrants versus non-migrant Tunisians and French. *BMC Public Health*, 7: 265

Moharram MM, Farahat FM (2008) Quality improvement of diabetes care using flow sheets in family health practice. *Saudi Medical Journal*, 29(1): 98–101

Murray C, Lopez A (eds.) (1996) *The global burden of disease: A comprehensive assessment of mortality and disability from diseases, injuries, and risk factors in 1990 and projected to 2020.* Cambridge, MA: Harvard University Press

Nakkash R, Afifi Soweid RA, Nehlawi MT, Shediac-Rizkallah MC, Hajjar TA, Khogali M (2003) The development of a feasible community-specific cardiovascular disease prevention program: Triangulation of methods and sources. *Health Education and Behavior*, 30(6): 723–739

Niëns LM, Cameron A, Van de Poel E, et al (2010) Quantifying the impoverishing effects of purchasing medicines: A cross-country comparison of the affordability of medicines in the developing world. *PLoS Med*, 7(8): e1000333

Noureddine S, Froelicher ES, Sibai AM, Dakik H (2010) Response to a cardiac event in relation to cardiac knowledge and risk perception in a Lebanese sample: A cross sectional survey. *International Journal of Nursing Studies*, 47(3): 332–341

Nsour M, Mahfoud Z, Kanaan MN, et al (2008) Prevalence and predictors of nonfatal myocardial infarction in Jordan. *Eastern Mediterranean Health Journal*, 14: 818–830

Radovanovic Z (1994) Mortality patterns in Kuwait: Inferences from death certificate data. *European Journal of Epidemiology*, 10(6): 733–736

Ramahi TM (2010) Cardiovascular disease in the Asia Middle East region: Global trends and local implications. *Asia Pacific Journal of Public Health*, 22(3 Suppl.): 83S–89S

Ramahi T, Khawaja M, Abu-Rmeileh N, et al (2010) Socio-economic disparities in heart disease in the Republic of Lebanon: Findings from a population-based study. *Heart Asia*, 2: 67–72

Samb B, Desai N, Nishtar S, et al (2010) Prevention and management of chronic disease: A litmus test for health-systems strengthening in low-income and middle-income countries. *Lancet*, 376(9754): 1785–1797

Shah NM, Behbehani J, Shah MA (2010) Prevalence and correlates of major chronic illnesses among older Kuwaiti nationals in two governorates. *Medical Principles and Practice*, 19(2): 105–112

Shara NM (2010) Cardiovascular disease in Middle Eastern women. *Nutrition, Metabolism & Cardiovascular Diseases*, 20: 412–418

Shatoor AS (2004) Prevalence of modifiable traditional coronary heart disease risk factors among young adult survivors of acute MI: A comparative study between Saudis and Non-Saudi patients. *Biomedical Research*, 15(1): 31–35

Sibai AM, Armenian HK, Alam S (1989) Wartime determinants of arteriographically confirmed coronary artery disease in Beirut. *American Journal of Epidemiology*, 130(4): 623–631

Sibai AM, Fletcher A, Hills M, Campbell O (2001a) Non-communicable disease mortality rates using the verbal autopsy in a cohort of middle aged and older populations in Beirut during wartime, 1983–93. *Journal of Epidemiology and Community Health*, 55(4): 271–276

Sibai AM, Fletcher A, Armenian HK (2001b) Variations in the impact of long-term wartime stressors on mortality among the middle-aged and older population in Beirut, Lebanon, 1983–1993. *American Journal of Epidemiology*, 154(2): 128–137

Sibai AM, Yount KM, Fletcher A (2007) Marital status, intergenerational co-residence and cardiovascular and all-cause mortality among middle-aged and older men and women during wartime in Beirut: Gains and liabilities. *Social Science and Medicine*, 64(1): 64–76

Sibai AM, Tohme RA, Saade GA, Lebanese Interventional Coronary Registry (LICOR) Working Group (2008a) Coronary angiography in Lebanon: Use and overuse. *International Journal of Cardiology*, 125(3): 422–424

Sibai AM, Tohme RA, Saade GA, Ghanem G, Alam S, Lebanese Interventional Coronary Registry Working Group (LICOR) (2008b) The appropriateness of use of coronary angiography in Lebanon: Implications for health policy. *Health Policy and Planning*, 23(3): 210–217

Tachfouti N, Berraho M, Elfakir S, Serhier Z, Elrhazi K, Slama K, Najjari C (2010) Socioeconomic status and tobacco expenditures among Moroccans: Results of

the "Maroc Tabagisme" survey. *Amercian Journal of Health Promotion*, 24(5): 334–339

The World Diabetes Foundation (2010) Projects: Middle East. Available from http://www.worlddiabetesfoundation.org/composite-166.htm [Accessed 15 December 2010]

Tunstall-Pedoe H, Kuulasmaa K, Amouyel P, et al (1994) Myocardial infarction and coronary deaths in the World Health Organization MONICA Project. Registration procedures, event rates and case fatality in 38 populations from 21 countries in four continents. *Circulation*, 90: 583–612

van Mourik MS, Cameron A, Ewen M, Laing RO (2010) Availability, price and affordability of cardiovascular medicines: A comparison across 36 countries using WHO/HAI data. *BMC Cardiovascular Disorders*, 10: 25

Weqaya (2010) The Weqaya Program. Available from http://www.weqaya.ae/en/index.php [Accessed 10 November 2010]

WHO (2008) *The Global Burden of Disease: 2004 update*. Geneva, Switzerland: WHO

Yusef JI (2000) Management of diabetes mellitus and hypertension at UNRWA primary health care facilities in Lebanon. *Eastern Mediterranean Health Journal*, 6(2–3): 378–390

Yusuf S, Hawken S, Ounpuu S, et al (2004) INTERHEART Study Investigators. Effect of potentially modifiable risk factors associated with myocardial infarction in 52 countries (the INTERHEART study): Case-control study. *Lancet*, 364: 937–952

Zhang P, Zhang X, Brown J, et al (2010) Global healthcare expenditure on diabetes for 2010 and 2030. *Diabetes Research & Clinical Practice*, 87(3): 293–301

Zubaid M, Rashed WA, Husain M, et al (2004) A registry of acute myocardial infarction in Kuwait: Patient characteristics and practice patterns. *Canadian Journal of Cardiology*, 20(8): 783–787

Chapter

14

An Overview of Mental Disorders

Elie G. Karam, Mariana M. Salamoun, Doris Jaalouk,
Olivia Shabb, and Driss Moussaoui

The domain of mental health is quite broad. This chapter intends to focus on one aspect: mental disorders (see also Chapter 15). Based on an evidence-based review, we show that mental disorders, including mood disorders, anxiety disorders, and others, are quite prevalent in countries where nationally representative data exist. We examine the various determinants of mental disorders, arguing that the profound changes that the Arab societies are witnessing are straining their traditional fabric and are paralleling an increase in mental disorders. Mental health services remain inadequate in the region and only limited studies have mapped the actual resources and gaps. The prevalence of mental disorders contrasts with limited mobilization and official policy in addressing mental disorders, and this is reflected in the limited resources to mental health (services and research). Building on identified barriers and challenges, we conclude with a discussion of next steps to address the rising burden of mental disorders.

The Burden and Prevalence of Mental Disorders

The Global Burden of Disease (GBD) study for the Eastern Mediterranean region, where most Arabs live, indicate that the burden of mental disorders is substantial: unipolar depression alone ranks as the seventh leading cause of burden and accounts for 3.7%; this percentage rises to 8.1% when considering eight other mental conditions (schizophrenia, bipolar affective disorder, alcohol use, drug use, post-traumatic stress disorder [PTSD], obsessive compulsive disorder [OCD], panic disorder, and insomnia) (WHO 2008).

Mental health research remains limited in the Arab world (Okasha & Karam 1998; Okasha 2003),

reflecting a broader problem of weaker national health research systems (Kennedy et al 2008). Most available studies of mental disorders are limited to single disorders, subpopulations, or specific cities and areas. To our knowledge, only two national studies have been published using comparable methodology, based on WHO's World Mental Health (WMH) Survey framework, to assess mental disorders: the Lebanese Evaluation of the Burden of Ailments and Needs Of the Nation (L.E.B.A.N.O.N.) (Karam et al 2006; Karam et al 2008a) and the Iraq Mental Health Survey (IMHS) (Alhasnawi et al 2009) (see Box 1). Two other national studies in Morocco (Kadri et al 2010) and Egypt (Ghanem et al 2009) use different methodologies, and are thus difficult to compare with the more established studies done within the WMH initiative. Some data from these two studies will still be presented.

Only results on the prevalence of mental disorders, but not burden, have been published from the L.E.B.A.N.O.N. and IMHS studies. Early analyses from the L.E.B.A.N.O.N study confirms the worldwide findings of the very important burden of mental disorders on the individual's life in the following domains: close relations, home, work, and social life. Data on what has been published on the burden of mental disorders in the Arab world show that mental disorders have a clear burden on several dimensions of human functioning. For example, alcohol and drug abuse were associated with fights (and sometimes physical fights) with parents and friends, drop out in school grades, losing a job, absenteeism from school/work, accidents, illegal problems, financial problems, and marital/family problems (Salamoun et al 2008). Post-traumatic stress disorder was associated with difficulties in school among children exposed to war and decreased self-confidence (Tanios et al 2009). People suffering from schizophrenia and related

Box 1. The L.E.B.A.N.O.N. and IMHS Studies

Both the Lebanese Evaluation of the Burden of Ailments and Needs Of the Nation (L.E.B.A.N.O.N.) and Iraqi Mental Health Survey (IMHS) are national studies conducted as part of the World Mental Health (WMH) Survey. The WMH surveys was coordinated by the World Health Organization (WHO, Geneva) and completed in more than 27 countries, including Lebanon, Iraq, and soon Saudi Arabia (www.hcp. med.harvard.edu/wmh). Teams from the three participating countries were trained by the Institute for Development Research Advocacy and Applied Care (IDRAAC), a WHO training center for the principal instrument, the Arabic Composite International Diagnostic Interview (CIDI).

L.E.B.A.N.O.N.'s objectives include assessment of prevalence of mental health disorders and their social burden, co-morbidity with other chronic medical conditions, treatment, and associated factors. The study also assessed information on the quality and intricacies of couple life (married, cohabited), on childhood and upbringing, and on the effect of stress on onset and course of mental disorders. Uniquely among other WMH studies, L.E.B.A.N.O.N. assessed temperament in the total population, its impact on productivity, quality, and enjoyment of life and on mental health problems (Karam et al 2006, 2008a).

The IMHS was conducted by the Ministry of Health of Iraq with the support of WHO. It has provided previously unavailable information regarding prevalence, including in different regions, of mental disorders in Iraq, the relation of trauma exposure and mental disorders, family burden, and treatment utilization by people with mental disorders. The response rate (95.2%) was remarkable considering the very challenging and insecure circumstances (Alhasnawi et al 2009).

Anxiety Disorders

In L.E.B.A.N.O.N., the lifetime prevalence of any DSM-IV anxiety disorder is 16.7% (11.2% prevalence in any 1 year): 0.5% panic disorder, 2.0% generalized anxiety disorder (GAD), 1.9% social phobia, 0.5% agoraphobia without panic, 3.4% post-traumatic stress disorder (PTSD), 6.1% separation anxiety disorder (Karam et al 2006, 2008a). In IMHS, lifetime prevalence is 13.8% (Alhasnawi et al 2009) with comparable results to the L.E.B.A.N.O.N. study by category. These rates are in the mid-range compared to non-Arab countries (Table 1) .

Using different methodologies than the WMH surveys, the point prevalence of GAD was 9.3% in Morocco (Kadri et al 2010) and 4.8% for anxiety disorders in Egypt (Ghanem et al 2009). In a study limited to the Al Ain region in the United Arab Emirates (UAE), and using a different diagnostic system (ICD-10), the lifetime prevalence of anxiety disorders was 0.9% for agoraphobia, 0.6% for GAD, 0.4% for social phobia, 0.1% for panic disorder, and 0.07% for OCD (Abou Saleh et al 2001). Other studies have reported lifetime prevalence of any anxiety disorder ranging from 10% to 28.2% (Tanios et al 2009).

Mood Disorders

The lifetime prevalence of any mood disorders in L.E.B.A.N.O.N. was 12.6%: 10% major depressive disorder (MDD), 1.1% dysthymia, and 2.4% bipolar disorders (Karam et al 2008a), with the 1-year prevalence of any mood disorder 6.6% (Karam et al 2006). In IMHS, the lifetime prevalence of mood disorders was 7.5% (7.2% MDD, 0.2% dysthymia, 0.2% bipolar disorders); the 1-year prevalence 4.1% (Alhasnawi et al 2009). Again, these rates are in the mid-range compared to non-Arab countries (Table 1). Using different methodologies than the WMH surveys, in Morocco, MDD point prevalence was 26.5% (Kadri et al 2010). In Egypt, the point prevalence of mood disorders was 6.4% (Ghanem et al 2009). Other studies, on non-national samples report lifetime prevalence of mood disorders with a wide variability (10%–28%), depending on the samples studied and methodology used. In Al Ain (UAE), the lifetime prevalence was 3.4% for MDD and 0.3% for bipolar disorders (Abou Saleh et al 2001).

disorders suffered from stigma, discrimination, negligence from caregivers and family members, and abuse. Children with attention deficit hyperactivity disorder (ADHD) had poorer school performance, were more likely to be aggressive and possibly engaged in stealing and lying behaviors. In adulthood, ADHD was associated with disability in cognition and social interactions (Farah et al 2009).

It is difficult to compare prevalence rates across studies due to the diversity of the samples studied, the instruments used, and differences in research procedures.

Table 1. Comparison of Lifetime Prevalence (in Percent of Population) of Mental Disorders Between Selected Countries

Country	Any disorder	Any anxiety disorder	Any mood disorder	Any impulse control disorder	Any substance abuse disorder
USA	47.4	31	21.4	25	14.6
Colombia	39.1	25.3	14.6	9.6	9.6
France	37.9	22.3	21	7.6	7.1
Ukraine	36.1	10.9	15.8	8.7	15
South Africa	30.3	15.8	9.8	–	13.3
Mexico	26.1	14.3	9.2	5.7	7.8
Lebanon*	**25.8**	**16.7**	**12.6**	**4.4**	**2.2**
Germany	25.2	14.6	9.9	3.1	6.5
Spain	19.4	9.9	10.6	2.3	3.6
Iraq**	**18.8**	**13.8**	**7.5**	**1.8**	**0.9**
Italy	18.1	11	9.9	1.7	1.3
Japan	18	6.9	7.6	2.8	4.8
China	13.2	4.8	3.6	4.3	4.9
Nigeria	12	6.5	3.3	0.3	3.7

Sources: *L.E.B.A.N.O.N. Study (Karam et al 2008a); **IMHS Study (Alhasnawi et al 2009); all other countries from Kessler et al 2007.

Substance Use Disorders

Reported prevalence of substance use might not reflect true rates, especially in countries where use is strictly prohibited. The lifetime prevalence of such use in L.E.B.A.N.O.N. was 2.2% (1.5% alcohol abuse, 0.4% alcohol dependence, 0.5% drug abuse, and 0.1% drug dependence) (Karam et al 2008a). In IMHS, the prevalence was about half of that reported in L.E.B.A.N.O.N.: 0.9% (0.7%, 0.2%, 0.2%, and 0.0%, respectively) (Alhasnawi et al 2009). Both Lebanon and Iraq report a lower prevalence of substance use than most other nations (Kessler et al 2007). In Morocco, a point prevalence of substance use disorders was 3%–6% (Kadri et al 2010). In Egypt, the point prevalence was 0.03% for alcohol abuse/dependence and 0.1% for drug abuse/dependence (Ghanem et al 2009). In Al-Ain (UAE) the lifetime prevalence of "substance misuse" was 0.4% (Abou Saleh et al 2001). Although illegal in some and shunned by the mostly Muslim Arab countries, alcohol is consistently shown to be the most commonly used mood altering substance across the Arab world (Salamoun et al 2008).

Three Arab countries, Yemen, Somalia, and Djibouti, face health and social challenges of the traditional khat chewing practice. Khat is not considered an addictive drug by WHO and Arab legislation and importing its leaves is legal. However, khat chewing has a proven mood altering effect, and researchers have associated it with mental disorders (Hassan et al 2002; Adam & Hasselot 1994; Odenwald et al 2005).

Impulse Control Disorders

These disorders typically manifest themselves first in childhood and extend into adulthood. They can impair educational attainment and thus influence productivity and economic status later in life. In L.E.B.A.N.O.N., the lifetime prevalence was 4.4% among adults aged 18–44 years: 1.0% for conduct disorder, 1.5% for attention deficit hyperactivity disorder (ADHD), and 1.7% for intermittent explosive disorder (IED) (Karam et al 2008a). In IMHS, the lifetime overall prevalence was lower than that of Lebanon (1.8%) largely due to the much lower rates of ADHD (0.1%), but an exactly equal rate of 1.7% for IED (Alhasnawi et al 2009). Lebanon had a prevalence of impulse control disorders in the upper range compared to Iraq and other countries across the world, but not as high as the United States (Kessler et al 2007).

Schizophrenia and Related Disorders

The Moroccan and Egyptian national studies assessed schizophrenia and psychotic disorders, reporting a point prevalence of 5.6% (Kadri et al 2010) and 0.2% (Ghanem et al 2009), respectively. In UAE, a community survey in Dubai reported that 0.3% of subjects were diagnosed with schizophrenia (Ghubash et al 2004), whereas the Al Ain study reported a 0.7% lifetime prevalence of psychotic disorders (Abou Saleh et al 2001).

Suicidality

Suicide is a leading cause of death worldwide and is consistently shown to be related to mental disorders. In L.E.B.A.N.O.N., lifetime rates for suicide ideation, plan, and attempt were 4.3%, 1.7%, and 2.0% respectively (Nock et al 2008). The IMHS reported lifetime suicide ideation only (2.92%) (Alhasnawi et al 2009). The lifetime prevalence of suicide attempt in Lebanon (2.0%) ranks it in the middle range of 17 other countries (mean 2.7%), which used the same methodology within WMH (Nock et al 2008). Few countries from the Arab world have assessed suicidality in the community. Lifetime prevalence of suicide ideation ranged from 2.09% to 13.9% with lifetime prevalence of attempts ranging from 0.72% to 6.3% (Karam et al 2007; Karam et al 2008b).

Somatoform Disorders

The Egyptian national study reported a point prevalence of 0.1% for somatization, 0.3% for hypochondriasis, 0.1% for body dysmorphic disorder, and 0.08% for pain (Ghanem et al 2009).

Mental Disorders in Non-adult Populations

Disorders in *childhood and adolescents* have tremendous life-long effects, highlighting the need for early screening, detection, and intervention, as well as prevention. Studies of such disorders in Arab countries have sampled mostly cities or regions within countries except for one school-based, nationally representative study (Jaju et al 2009). Most studies have used screening instruments to investigate general psychopathology or specific disorders. Given the different methodologies used, comparisons across various studies and countries are not possible. Most studies report substantial rates of disorders, within the range found in similar studies in some developed countries (Costello et al 2003). For example, in Al Ain, UAE, Eapen et al (1998, 2003) reported a prevalence of any psychiatric disorder of 10.4% and 14.3% in a school sample and in a community household study, respectively. In Yemen (Alyahri & Goodman 2008), prevalence was 15.7%. Studies using general screening instruments detected high levels of symptoms of childhood mental disorders. For example, in the Occupied Palestinian Territory, two studies (Zakrison et al 2004; Thabet & Vostanis, 1998) reported prevalence of 42.3% and 43.4%, respectively. As expected, studies from non-conflict settings report lower rates of symptoms. For example, in a large sample from Minia, Egypt (Elhamid et al 2009), emotional and behavioral symptoms were reported at 34.7% by teachers and 20.6% by parents, with the prevalence of probable psychiatric diagnoses being much lower.

Several impulsive psychiatric disorders such as ADHD have their onset in early childhood and persist into adulthood. A recent review (Farah et al 2009) found that rates in populations in the Arab region to be similar to those in other settings. ADHD symptom prevalence was 5.1% to 14.9%, while ADHD diagnosis using structured interviews ranged from 0.5% in the school setting to 0.9% in the community. Similar rates of ADHD symptoms were found in a study from OPT (Thabet et al 2006). Rates of persistence of ADHD from childhood into adulthood in surveys ranged from 32.8% to 84.1% with a rate of 52.4% in Lebanon (Lara et al 2009). As such, a study that includes a nationally representative sample of Lebanese adults found a prevalence of adult ADHD of 1.8% in Lebanon (3.4% cross nationally) (Fayyad et al 2007).

Mental disorders in *older adults* are common; progressive population aging highlights their public health importance. A national sample study in UAE (Ghubash et al 2004) reported the following rates: 20.2% depression, 5.6% anxiety, 0.7% schizophrenia, 4.4% hypochondriasis, and 3.6% cognitive impairment with or without dementia. A study from Egypt reported a point prevalence of 2.2% for Alzheimer's disease, 0.95% multi-infarct dementia, and 0.55% for mixed dementias (Farrag et al 1998). Both

L.E.B.A.N.O.N. and IMHS studies included age of onset and distributions of mental disorders to generate estimates of projected lifetime risk as of age 75 (Karam et al 2008a; Alhasnawi et al 2009). If all sample respondents reach the age of 75, the model estimates that 32.9% of the Lebanese, and 40.8% of Iraqi respondents will have a lifetime history of at least one mental disorder. However, both nationally representative studies excluded from their sample participants who were cognitively impaired, thus the prevalence of mental disorders may be underestimated.

In conclusion, although the reported studies (except for L.E.B.A.N.O.N. and IMHS) used different methods, the published literature clearly highlights that mental disorders are common and pose an important burden in various age groups.

Determinants of Mental Disorders

Some of the risk and protective factors affecting mental health in the Arab countries have been studied albeit with varying breadth. We review here data on a few sets of such factors.

Biological Factors

The role of genetics in mental illness is increasingly appreciated and regional research is beginning to tackle this area. Such research is of special importance because of the high rates of consanguineous marriages (Rashad et al 2005), which might favor the appearance of genetically based mental disorders. However, research has not specifically tackled this question yet. However, from the available literature, it seems that prevalence rates of schizophrenia, which is thought to have a genetic basis, do not always seem to exceed the global prevalence rates. A few studies have reported genetic variations linked to mental disorders (see for example, Mujaheed et al 2000) or response to treatment (see for example, Benmessaoud et al 2008). Research on metabolic factors affecting mental health in the region is rare. It is not clear whether genetic variations or metabolic abnormalities are of any particularity to this region.

Socio-economic and Demographic Factors

It is an important exercise to look at social context to understand increasing rates of mental disorders in this region knowing that this is also a world-wide phenomenon. Many factors are potentially relevant under this category, but this review focuses on a few variables because of their particular relevance to the region. Some authors (see for example, Mohit et al 2006) suggest that the economic and social changes under way in the region in the era of globalization are contributing to rising mental ill-health. They suggest that "rapid rate of urbanization... is placing stress on the social fabric of society. Massive internal migration from the countryside to the city is resulting in the break-up of the extended family system and social institutions, giving way to nuclear families, separation and higher divorce rates, single-parent families, children growing up without parent figure(s), older members of families being left on their own, lack of social cohesion, conflict of value systems, identity crises, increasing rates of unemployment, violence and abuse." (Mohit et al 2006 p.9) However, there is no evidence at present to support this interesting and thought-challenging possibility. An alternative explanation when looking closely is that some disorders which are identified readily by outsiders, such as bipolar, externalizing disorders, schizophrenia, do not seem to have lower rates in communities in the Arab world. On the other hand, rates of internalizing disorders, such as depression and anxiety, seem to be lower or equal to those reported in other settings. As we have noticed in the clinical setting, it is possible that cultural norms in the Arab world do not encourage voicing symptoms and the burden is carried in silence.

Mental disorders are not evenly distributed by age groups. For instance, anxiety disorders tend to be more prevalent in youth, and mood disorders in middle age groups in Lebanon (Karam et al 2006). Suicide attempt, closely linked to mental health dysfunction, is also reported to be highest in the young (15–25 years) (Karam et al 2008b). A report from Saudi Arabia has suggested that depression and other forms of psychopathology tend to increase with age (Al-Shammari et al 2000). Further confirmation of the latter will have to await the results of the WMH-Saudi study.

The majority of studies from the region confirm the global patterns in the gender distribution of mental illnesses with higher prevalence of mood and anxiety disorders among women (Tanios et al 2009; Ghanem et al 2009), more externalizing and substance use disorders among men (Seedat et al 2009). Women also had a higher rate of suicide ideation, plan, and attempts, in Lebanon, Iraq, and Egypt (Karam et al 2008b; Alhasnawi et al 2009). However, there were some exceptions to these observations. For example, in Iraq, females have fewer mood disorders than men (Alhasnawi et al 2009) while in Saudi Arabia, men had more anxiety disorders (El-Rufaie et al 1988).

Research on the role of educational attainment in mental illnesses has yielded mixed results. In L.E.B.A.N.O.N., low levels of education were associated with substance abuse only, and not with mood and anxiety disorders (Karam et al 2006). In IMHS, only anxiety disorders were associated with lower education. Studies from Egypt, Jordan, and Syria found illiteracy or poor education to be associated with psychiatric distress or morbidity (Ghanem et al 2009; Daradkeh et al 2006; Maziak et al 2002). In a primary care setting in Kuwait, higher levels of education predicted depression (Al-Otaibi et al 2007). This discrepancy in results may be due to the differences in the screening instruments used and indicates the need for valid and culturally sensitive instruments.

Marital status and family life have a major impact on mental disorders. In L.E.B.A.N.O.N, being single predicted mood, anxiety, and substance abuse disorders (Karam et al 2006). The same was observed in Egypt (Ghanem et al 2009), in Saudi Arabia (Al-Shammari et al 2000), in Jordan (Daradkeh et al 2006), in Syria (Maziak et al 2002), and in Iraq (Alhasnawi et al 2009). Only the study conducted in Kuwait deviated from this pattern, finding that depressive disorders correlate with married status (Al-Otaibi 2007).

Parenting styles may influence mental health in children and adolescents. Dwairy & Menshar (2006) found that authoritarian style was common in Egypt and claimed to be quite inoffensive "within an authoritarian culture." In a community intervention in poor suburbs in Lebanon, it was found that 40% of mothers had used corporal punishment and physical abuse in response to their children's disruptive behaviors (Fayyad et al 2010). Income and living conditions may play a significant role in the expression of psychological distress. Low socio-economic status was a risk factor for attempting suicide in Bahrain and Egypt, but not in Lebanon (Karam et al 2008b). Poor housing, low-income status, or dependence on charity or relatives, and living in a remote or rural area were reported as risk factors for anxiety and mood disorders in studies conducted on non-representative samples in Jordan (Daradkeh et al 2006), Kuwait (Malasi et al 1988), and Saudi Arabia (Al-Shammari et al 2000). However, in IMHS, higher income was

positively associated with behavioral disorders (Alhasnawi et al 2009).

Religiosity is generally a significant component of daily life in the Arab world and potentially an important factor in relation to mental health. Short of national data, regional research supports widely shared beliefs that a balanced spiritual life can buttress against life stressors (Karam et al 2007; Abdel-Khalek 2002). In Lebanon, faith and practice, among both Christians and Muslims, were protective against alcohol use, abuse, and dependence (Karam et al 2004). Whether faith and/or religious practice are expressions of other mediating factors remains to be seen. A study from Egypt found practicing religion to be a risk factor for suicide attempts (Okasha & Lotaif 1979). This result is unexpected as the major religions practiced in the Arab world condemn suicide. It is to be noted that "religiosity" includes various dimensions such as spirituality, rituals, cultural practices, and social networks. Future research in the region should explore the relative contribution of these dimensions.

Understanding the role of the individual's emotional reactivity, otherwise known as temperament, in affecting psychological well-being has been gaining attention recently, especially in psychoeducation and in a better understanding of individuals in their daily lives. Results from the L.E.B.A.N.O.N study found that Lebanese adults who are naturally anxious are more likely to develop mood and anxiety disorders than individuals who are hyperthymic (Karam et al 2010).

Social Support

The Arab world traditionally exhibits a high level of familial cohesiveness that stretches beyond the nuclear to the extended family. Social support commonly extends beyond the family to include the extensive web of friendship and community support that are highly valued. As such, solidarity with friends and neighbors are defining attitudes. Research suggests that social support does act as a protective factor against psychological distress in several settings and among different population groups including children and adolescents (Al-Otaibi et al 2007; Thabet et al 2009), adults (Daradkeh et al 2006; Maziak et al 2002), the elderly (Al-Shammari et al 2000), and pregnant women (El-Khoury et al 1999).

AbuMadini & Rahim (2002) report a positive correlation between family support, patient compliance, and reduction in re-hospitalization rates for mental disorders in Saudi Arabia. Obviously, the degree of adequate support a family affords a psychiatrically ill individual depends on its perception of and attitude toward the illness and on available family resources. Arab governments in general do not provide major support to mentally ill individuals beyond basic medical care. Family members are commonly left alone as the sole, and often inadequately equipped, providers of health, social, and economic support. This situation compromises the benefits of family support, favors the marginalization and the neglect of the mentally ill, and increases the social cost of mental disorders.

War

War, occupation, and violent conflicts have resounding impacts on the mental health of individuals and communities (see also Chapters 23 and 24). There is rich research on this issue in the region. L.E.B.A.N.O.N., conducted 10 years after the end of the civil war, still showed that war exposure predicted the first onset of mood, anxiety, and impulse control disorders and was significantly related to various mental disorders, and not only to post-traumatic stress disorder (PTSD): adults were about five times more likely to have mood disorders, and nine times more likely to have impulse control disorders if they were exposed to three or more war events (such as witnessing the death of a close one, witnessing atrocities, being a civilian in a war region, being a refugee, kidnapped, etc.) (Karam et al 2006, 2008a). Studies assessing mental illness in Lebanese post-war communities 1 month after war exposure found MDD rates to vary from 16.3% to 43.2% for adults and 23.6% for children; when these children were reassessed 1 year later the prevalence of MDD had dropped to 5.6% (Karam et al 2008c). Studies on Palestinian children and adolescents have reported the prevalence of PTSD to be as high as 37.1%. Similarly studies on Algerians living in areas exposed to massacres showed levels of PTSD of 37.2% (Tanios et al 2009).

The interplay between repeated exposure, social cohesion, perceived outcome of war, and other potential social, economic, and physical health effects remains a challenging area of study. Some researchers point to the possibility of emergence of resilience by political participation and identity reaffirmation (Nguyen-Gillham et al 2008), or by adopting a collective patriotic mission (Yamout & Chaaya, 2010).

Social support seems to be especially valuable in populations exposed to wars. Studies in Lebanon point to the role of social support in mediating individuals' response to psychological distress (Hourani et al 1986) and enhancing their cognitive coping skills (Farhood 1999). Such support buffers against post-traumatic stress disorder in wives of Kuwaiti war veterans (Al-Turkait & Ohaeri 2008). Similarly parental support was found to protect Palestinian children exposed to war from post-traumatic symptoms (Thabet et al 2009).

Mental Health Services

The Arab-Islamic civilization was a pioneer in developing services for mental disorders with *bimaristans* (hospitals) for the mentally ill operating in cities such as Aleppo, Baghdad, and Fes in the tenth and eleventh centuries. For our purpose, we use "services" to include legislations, policies, programs as well as clinical, preventive, and health promotion activities. We use the data from the WHO's Mental Health Atlas (2005) updated with data from the WHO's Assessment Instrument for Mental Health Systems (2009). There is only one comprehensive study modeled after the Atlas, in Saudi Arabia (Al-Habeeb & Qureshi 2010). An NGO, Arab Resource Collective, has published a survey of mental health resources and services, including those provided by NGOs, in nine Arab countries (Samuel et al 2008). These sources and many articles agree that there are major gaps in services (Okasha & Karam 1998; Okasha 2003). Nevertheless, there are many community-based resources and NGOs whose work concern mental health (see directory compiled by Kobeisy et al 2008).

Of 20 Arab countries, 14 have policies covering mental health, and 10 have passed specific legislation regarding mental health and its funding (WHO 2005, 2009), although the extent to which these policies and laws are implemented or effective is unknown. Many health ministries do not have well-structured mental health departments or units that can engage in long-term planning. Only Egypt and Qatar have provided proportionate figures on budgets for mental health: 9% and 1% of the total health budget, respectively (WHO recommends a minimum of 10%). Information is lacking on budget allocations to public vs. private sectors and to rural vs. urban populations. There is no research evidence on the equitable distribution or efficient use of available resources for mental health. The most important sources of financing are state funded payment followed by out of pocket payments, but this differs widely from one Arab country to another. Quite importantly, insurance groups do not cover mental health services in most Arab countries.

In terms of available services, the state's contribution in some Arab countries is limited to the provision of free inpatient, hospital or institutional, services. Outpatient services are mostly paid out of pocket. However, this varies from country to country. Services are commonly centralized in major cities and centers. Mental health is not well integrated into already weak primary care systems. There are important gaps in psychiatric care. For example, some have found that psychiatric staff may have negative attitudes toward care of the mentally ill (Hamdan-Mansour & Wardam 2009). There are no state-wide programs to prevent mental disorders or to promote mental health, these remain within the realm of individual institutions or organizations.

The number of reported psychiatric beds varies widely. Except for Lebanon, Arab countries fall short of the WHO recommendation of five to eight mental health beds per 10,000 people. There is mal-distribution of psychiatric beds between rural and urban settings, and between different population groups. Supply of mental health professionals shows wide disparities. Only five countries met or approached the WHO recommended figure of 2.5 to 10 psychiatrists per 100,000 citizens: Bahrain (5), Qatar (3.4), Kuwait (3.1), Lebanon and UAE (2); Libya (0.18) and Sudan (0.09) had the fewest. The overall number of professionals working in mental health (psychiatrists, neurologists, neurosurgeons, psychiatric nurses, psychologists, and social workers), including those in the private sector, is unknown. There is agreement about the inadequate skills of primary care practitioners to treat mental disorders.

These various deficiencies combined mean that families, already confronted with the social stigma and public neglect of mental disorders, find themselves alone in facing the financial, social, and psychological burden of caring for members with mental illnesses (Kadri et al 2004), adding to their other burdens and raising the possibility of neglect and abuse.

Challenges to Management and Interventions

Reliability of Data and Research Production

The aforementioned review indicates that there are plenty of unanswered questions for research in mental health. Research and data will assist decision and policy makers for future planning and should be based on comparable methodologies. Many instruments have been translated, and some adapted and validated for use on Arab samples, for example, the Arabic versions of WHO's Composite International Diagnostic Interview (CIDI) (Abou Saleh et al 2001; Karam et al 2006), Diagnostic Interview Schedule (DIS) (Karam et al 1991), and the Mini International Neuropsychiatric Interview (MINI) (Kadri et al 2010). Researchers are increasingly aware that instruments should be adapted further to each specific Arab country, even sub-national context, to take into account not only the particularities of language but also the social, cultural, and value constructs of different populations and groups.

A review of the corpus of mental health research for the period of 1966–1999 found a steady increase in the number of publications, in particular as of the mid-1990s, despite the scarce funding allocated for research by Arab governments (Karam & Maalouf, 2001). The average productivity rate was 28 articles per year, equivalent to 1.6 articles/country/year. Top ranking Arab countries were Egypt, Saudi Arabia, Lebanon, Kuwait, and Tunisia. When productivity rate was measured per population size, then leading countries were Kuwait, Lebanon, and UAE, followed by Saudi Arabia, Jordan, Tunisia, and Egypt. Mental health studies were more often published in local journals and not in international ones and, hence, were not indexed by international electronic databases. In a recent update of this data, the average productivity rate increased steeply to 117 articles per year for the period 1999 to mid-2007, which is equivalent to 8.4 articles/year/Arab country. In terms of publications per population size, top ranking countries were Kuwait, Bahrain, Lebanon, and UAE (Karam, 2009).

Stigma and Mental Illness

Stigmatizing the mentally ill is a worldwide reality, including in Arab countries (Alonso et al 2008). A recent review of anxiety disorders (Tanios et al 2009) pointed out that Arab men under-reported symptoms of mental illness probably due to their "fear of being vulnerable." Substance use is a particularly sensitive issue. Among UAE men, stigma is being compounded by criminalization as alcohol is prohibited in many Arab countries (Abou-Saleh 2006).

It would be interesting to speculate about the role of stigma in the low rates of treatment of mental disorders or in treatment seeking delays. In L.E.B.A. N.O.N., only 11% of adults with a mental disorder sought any treatment and there were major delays (ranging from 3 years for impulse control disorders to 28 years for anxiety disorders) (Karam et al 2008a). Respondents denied stigma as a major cause for this delay. L.E.B.A.N.O.N. may have under-estimated the importance of stigma. In IMHS, only a quarter of those with serious disorders have sought treatment. More studies on the relationship between stigma and care seeking are needed considering that there are potential explanatory variables other than stigma such as perceptions that treatment will not help, and not knowing where to go or whom to ask for help (Karam et al 2006, 2008a).

Some reports speculate that Arab women might seek mental health care less often than men because they worry that doing so might damage their prospect of getting married, or provide their husbands with justification for remarriage (Al-Krenawi et al 2000). This might explain how psychological problems might be expressed in physical symptoms, which may lead to misdiagnosis (Douki et al 2007).

Social stigma might extend to the family members of the mentally ill. In a Moroccan study, almost 30% of family members of schizophrenic patients experienced rejection, 40% were maltreated, and 30% felt contempt and neglect from relatives and neighbors (Kadri et al 2004). Parents of children with mental disorders can also be vulnerable to stigma and be less likely to seek care for their children (Eapen & Ghubash 2004).

International studies indicate that many people with mental disorders are unemployed because of disease and associated disability or stigma. This highlights another area for equity-oriented research and for government assessment and interventions. There are no published data on this subject in the region.

Mental Disorders and Medical Co-morbidities

International research suggests that people with mental disorders suffer from significant physical co-morbidities, receive less treatment, and have higher mortality. Corresponding research in the region is limited. In a population-based study in Aleppo, Syria, Kilzieh et al (2008) found that self-report of physician-diagnosed depression was significantly associated with several chronic non-communicable diseases and that the association between depression and physical impairment may be mediated through co-existing chronic diseases. However, on a global level, a cross-national publication on 17 countries from the WMH surveys including Lebanon, found that physical conditions such as diabetes, asthma, hypertension, arthritis, ulcer, heart disease, back/neck problems, chronic headache, and multiple pains were significantly associated with anxiety and/or depressive disorders albeit with variability (Scott et al 2007). We are not aware of comparative assessments of treatments and mortality in people with vs. without mental disorders.

Mobilizing for Mental Health

This review has identified many gaps and thus areas for action in mental health. Most required actions, for example, improving services, require financial resources and commitments by governments to a progressive mental health agenda. In turn, this depends on a proper legal framework that gives different parties clear mandates and responsibilities. Developing this framework often requires a push by mental health advocates. An experience in Lebanon of drafting the mental health act was instructive in this regard.

Only some of the Arab countries have a mental health act, but in Lebanon the last one, albeit not comprehensive, dates back to 1983 and did not address seriously the rights of mental health patients. Recognizing this serious deficiency, IDRAAC in association with the Department of Psychiatry and Clinical Psychology at St George Hospital University Medical Center and Balamand University have drawn up plans to develop and push for a mental health act in Lebanon and received a supporting grant from the European Commission for this purpose, which was managed by the Office of the Ministry of State for Administrative Reform (OMSAR) in Lebanon. Mental health acts were retrieved from six Arab countries (Egypt, Iraq, Jordan, Morocco, Saudi Arabia, and UAE) and six non-Arab countries (France, Italy, New Zealand, Spain, United Kingdom, and USA). The IDRAAC team reviewed the World Health Organization (WHO) Mental Act checklist and guidelines, as well as that of the United Nations, and drafted an extensive document that outlines what relevant laws already exist in Lebanon, what other Arab countries have, and what was missing in Lebanon. This helped to draft a mental health act document which served as a reference document to be used in the focus group discussions (FGD). Focus groups (psychiatrists, psychologists, lawyers, judges, psychiatric nurses, internal security forces, etc) received material to study in advance. Following each FGD, a committee from IDRAAC analyzed the data using the triangular approach to ensure validity and reliability of the data gathered. Then the updated version was circulated to the following FGD participants and the process was repeated.

Data compiled from the different sources were evaluated by the IDRAAC team, which drafted a culturally and contextually appropriate law proposal. This proposal was reviewed by all participating parties and then sent to policy makers for action. The proposed act was approved by the Ministry of Public Health and is currently awaiting the parliament approval. A follow-up committee of IDRAAC and governmental members are following the status of the law. As with any legal act, mobilization of important players (political, medical, and social) is essential in sustaining such long-term efforts especially when the government priorities do not coincide necessarily with such endeavors. Regular and constant lobbying, we believe, is essential to introduce changes. For example, we have kept a regular contact with law makers in providing them all along with research data that not only informs but also sensitizes these policy makers to the importance of mental health services and legislation.

Conclusions

There is enough evidence from national and subnational studies to suggest that mental disorders are prevalent. Nevertheless, there is a need to build the evidence base through epidemiological and cohort studies that develop and adapt instruments that are appropriate to the Arab world's dialects, contexts, and cultural norms but which are still uniform in methods to allow cross-country comparison. Studies are also needed on treatment, remissions and relapses, and cost-effectiveness. Risk factors and determinants of mental disorders need to be explored in more depth. Carrying out this ambitious research agenda requires allocation of budgets to support research that could draw on the many research talents available in the Arab world.

Much remains to be done to improve the challenges of mental health management, which includes different modalities ranging from public awareness, education, and school-based programs to individual psychotherapy and pharmacologic treatment. There is a clear need for advocacy to place mental health and disorders higher up on the political and public health agendas and build the institutional capacity to respond to identified challenges. Equally important is building the human resource capacity in mental health at various levels: primary care, specialist care, and the community. Systems need to be created to encourage public–private partnership and involve other sectors from the community to promote mental health.

Acknowledgment

We would like to thank Dr. John Fayyad (Lebanon) for contributing information about mental disorders of children and adolescents, Dr. George Karam (Lebanon) for contributing information about mental disorders of older adults, and Dr. Muhammad Lafta (Iraq) for contributing information about the Iraq Mental Health Survey.

References

Abdel-Khalek AM (2002) Age and sex differences for anxiety in relation to family size, birth order, and religiosity among Kuwaiti adolescents. *Psychological Reports*, 90(3): 1031–1036

Abou Saleh M, Ghubash R, Daradkeh TK (2001) Al Ain Community Psychiatric Survey I. Prevalence and socio-demographic correlates. *Social Psychiatry and Psychiatric Epidemiology*, 36: 20–28

Abou Saleh M (2006) Substance use disorders: Recent advances in treatment and models of care. *Journal of Psychosomatic Research*, 61: 305–310

AbuMadini MS, Rahim SI (2002) Psychiatric admission in a general hospital. Patients profile and patterns of service utilization over a decade. *Saudi Medical Journal*, 23(1): 44–50

Adam F, Hasselot N (1994) Khat: From traditional usage to risk of drug addiction. *Médecine Tropicale*, 54(2): 141–144

Al-Habeeb AA, Qureshi NA (2010) Mental and Social Health Atlas I in

Saudi Arabia: 2007–08. *Eastern Mediterranean Health Journal*, 16(5): 570–577

Alhasnawi S, Sadik S, Rasheed M, et al (2009) The prevalence and correlates of DSM-IV disorders in the Iraq Mental Health Survey (IMHS). *World Psychiatry*, 8, 2–14

Al-Krenawi A, Graham J, Kandah J (2000) Gendered utilization differences of mental health services in Jordan. *Community Mental Health Journal*, 36(5): 501–511

Alonso J, Buron A, Bruffaerts R, et al (2008) Association of perceived stigma and mood and anxiety disorders: Results from the World Mental Health Surveys. *Acta Psychiatrica Scandinavica*, 118: 305–314

Al-Otaibi B, Al-Weqayyan A, Taher H, et al (2007) Depressive symptoms among Kuwaiti population attending primary healthcare setting: Prevalence and influence of sociodemographic factors. *Medical Principles and Practice*. 16(5): 384–388

Al-Shammari SA, Al Mazrou Y, Jarallah JS, Al Ansary L, El Shabrawy AM, Bamgboye EA (2000) Appraisal of clinical, psychosocial, and environmental health of elderly in Saudi Arabia: A household survey. *International Journal of Aging and Human Development*, 50(1): 43–60

Al-Turkait FA, Ohaeri JU (2008) Post-traumatic stress disorder among wives of Kuwaiti veterans of the first Gulf War. *Journal of Anxiety Disorders*, 22(1): 18–31

Alyahri A, Goodman R (2008) The prevalence of DSM-IV psychiatric disorders among 7–10 year old Yemeni schoolchildren. *Social Psychiatry and Psychiatric Epidemiology*, 43(3): 224–230

Benmessaoud D, Hamdani N, Boni C, et al (2008) Excess of transmission of the G allele of the -1438A/G polymorphism of the 5-HT2A receptor gene in patients with schizophrenia responsive to

antipsychotics. *BMC Psychiatry*, 8: 40–46

Costello EJ, Mustillo S, Erkanli A, Keeler C, Angold A (2003) Prevalence and development of psychiatric disorders in childhood and adolescence. *Archives of General Psychiatry*, 60: 837–844

Daradkeh TK, Alawan A, Al Ma'aitah R, Otoom SA (2006) Psychiatric morbidity and its sociodemographic correlates among women in Irbid, Jordan. *Eastern Mediterranean Health Journal*, 12(Suppl. 2): S107–S117

Douki S, Ben Zineb S, Nacef F, Halbreich U (2007) Womens mental health in the Muslim world: Cultural, religious, and social issues. *Journal of Affective Disorders*, 102: 177–189

Dwairy M, Menshar KE (2006) Parenting style, individuation, and mental health of Egyptian adolescents. *Journal of Adolescence*, 29(1): 103–117

Eapen V, Al-Gazali L, Bin-Othman S, Abou-Saleh M (1998) Mental health problems among schoolchildren in United Arab Emirates: Prevalence and risk factors. *Journal of the American Academy of Child and Adolescent Psychiatry*, 37(8): 880–886

Eapen V, Essa JM, Abou-Saleh M (2003) Children with psychiatric disorders: The Al Ain community psychiatric survey. *Canadian Journal of Psychiatry*, 48(6): 402–407

Eapen V, Ghubash R (2004) Help-seeking for mental health problems of children: Preferences and attitudes in the United Arab Emirates. *Psychological Reports*, 94(2): 663–667

Elhamid AA, Howe A, Reading R (2009) Prevalence of emotional and behavioral problems among 6–12 year old children in Egypt. *Social Psychiatry and Psychiatric Epidemiology*, 44: 8–14

El-Khoury N, Karam E, Melhem NM (1999) Depression et grossesse (in

French). *Eastern Mediterranean Health Journal*, 47(3): 169–174

El-Rufaie OE, Albar AA, Al-Dabal BK (1988) Identifying anxiety and depressive disorders among primary care patients: A pilot study. *Acta Psychiatrica Scandinavica*, 77: 280–282

Farah L, Fayyad J, Eapen V, et al (2009) ADHD in the Arab world: A review of epidemiologic studies. *Journal of Attention Disorders*, 13(3): 211–222

Farhood LF (1999) Testing a model of family stress and coping based on war and non-war stressors, family resources and coping among Lebanese families. *Archives of Psychiatric Nursing*, 13(4): 192–203

Farrag A, Farwiz HM, Khedr EH, Mahfouz RM, Omran SM (1998) Prevalence of Alzheimer's disease and other dementing disorders: Assiut-Upper Egypt study. *Journal of Dementia and Geriatric Cognitive Disorders*, 9(6): 323–328

Fayyad J, de Graaf R, Kessler RC, et al (2007) The cross national prevalence and correlates of ADHD: Results from the WHO World Mental Health Surveys. *British Journal of Psychiatry*, 190: 402–409

Fayyad J, Farah L, Cassir Y, Salamoun M, Karam E (2010) Dissemination of an evidence based interview to parents and children with behavioral problems in a developing country. *European Child & Adolescent Psychiatry*, 19(8): 629–636

Ghanem M, Gadallah M, Meky FA, Mourad S, El-Kholy G (2009) National survey of prevalence of mental disorders in Egypt: Preliminary survey. *Eastern Mediterranean Health Journal*, 15: 65–75

Ghubash R, El-Rufaie O, Zoubeidi T, Al-Shboul QM, Sabri SM (2004) Profile of mental disorders among the elderly United Arab Emirates population: Sociodemographic correlates. *International Journal of Geriatric Psychiatry*, 19(4): 344–351

Ghubash R, Hamdi E, Bebbington P (1992) The Dubai psychiatric survey: I. Prevalence and socio-demographic correlates. *Social Psychiatry and Psychiatric Epidemiology*, 27: 53–61

Hamdan-Mansour AM, Wardam LA (2009) Attitudes of Jordanian mental health nurses toward mental illness and patients with mental illness. *Issues in Mental Health Nursing*, 30(11): 705–711

Hassan NA, Gunaid AA, El-Khally FM, Murray-Lyon IM (2002) The effect of chewing khat leaves on human mood. *Saudi Medical Journal*, 23(7): 850–853

Hourani LL, Armenian H, Zurayk H, Afifi L (1986) A population-based survey of loss and psychological distress during war. *Social Science & Medicine*, 23(3): 269–275

Jaju S, Al Adawi S, Al Kharusi H, Morsi M, Al Riyami A (2009) Prevalence and age-of-onset distributions of DSM IV mental disorders and their severity among school going Omani adolescents and youths: WMH-CIDI findings. *Child and Adolescent Psychiatry and Mental Health*, 3: 29–39

Kadri N, Agoub M, Assouab F, et al (2010) Moroccan national study on prevalence of mental disorders: A community-based epidemiological study. *Acta Psychiatrica Scandinavica*, 121: 71–74

Kadri N, Manoudi F, Berrada SM, Moussaoui D (2004) Stigma impact on Moroccan families of patients with schizophrenia. *Canadian Journal of Psychiatry*, 49(9): 625–629

Karam EG (2009) Mental Health Research in the Arab World. Presented at the Annual Psychiatric International Congress. Cairo, 3–5 June 2009.

Karam E, Barakeh M, Karam A, El-Khoury N (1991) The Arabic Diagnostic Interview Schedule. *Revue Medicale Libanaise*, 3: 28–30

Karam E, Maalouf W (2001). Mental Health Research in the Arab speaking countries. *In*: A. Okasha & PM. Maj (Eds), *Images in Phychiatry: An Arab Perspective* pp 329–336, Cairo, Egypt, Scientific Book House.

Karam E, Maalouf W, Ghandour L (2004) Alcohol use among university students in Lebanon: Prevalence, trends and covariates. *Drug and Alcohol Dependence*, 76: 273–286

Karam E, Mneimneh Z, Karam A, et al (2006) Prevalence and treatment of mental disorders in Lebanon: A national epidemiological survey. *The Lancet*, 367: 1000–1006

Karam E, Hajjar R, Salamoun M (2007) Suicidality in the Arab world part I: Community studies. *Arab Journal of Psychiatry*, 18(2): 99–107

Karam E, Mneimneh Z, Dimassi H, et al (2008a) Lifetime prevalence of mental disorders in Lebanon: First onset, treatment, and exposure to war. *PLoS Med*, 5(4): e61

Karam E, Hajjar R, Salamoun M (2008b) Suicidality in the Arab world Part II: Hospital and governmental studies. *Arab Journal of Psychiatry*, 19(2): 1–24

Karam E, Fayyad J, Karam AN, et al (2008c) Effectiveness and specificity of a classroom-based group intervention in children and adolescents exposed to war in Lebanon. *World Psychiatry*, 7(2): 103–109

Karam EG, Salamoun MM, Yeretzian JS, et al (2010) The role of anxious and hyperthymic temperaments in mental disorders: A national epidemiologic study. *World Psychiatry*, 9(2): 103–110

Kennedy A, Khoja TA, Abou-Zeid AH, Ghannem H, Jsselmuiden C, on behalf of the WHO EMRO/ COHRED/GCC NHRS Collaborative Group (2008) National health research system mapping in 10 Eastern Mediterranean countries. *Eastern Mediterranean Health Journal*, 14(3): 502–517

Kessler RC, Angermeyer M, Anthony JC, et al (2007) Lifetime prevalence and age-of-onset distributions of mental disorders in the WHO World Mental Health (WMH) Surveys. *World Psychiatry*, 6: 168–176

Kilzieh N, Rastam S, Maziak W, Ward KD (2008) Comorbidity of depression with chronic diseases: A population-based study in Aleppo, Syria. *International Journal of Psychiatry in Medicine*, 38(2): 169–184

Kobeisy A, Ataya O, Abou Ghazaleh S, Hachem T, Issa G (2008) *Directory of programs working in the field of mental and psychosocial health in nine Arab Countries.* Beirut: Arab Resource Collective.] (Arabic)

Lara C, Fayyad J, de Graaf R, et al (2009) Childhood predictors of adult ADHD: Results from the WHO World Mental Health (WMH) Survey Initiative. *Biological Psychiatry*, 65: 46–54

Malasi TH, El-Hilu SM, Mirza IA, El-Islam MF (1988) Some psycho-social aspects of old people living outside their families in Kuwait. *International Journal of Social Psychiatry*, 34(1): 13–24

Maziak W, Asfar T, Mzayek F, Fouad FM, Kilzieh N (2002) Socio-demographic correlates of psychiatric morbidity among low-income women in Aleppo, Syria. *Social Science & Medicine*, 54(9): 1419–1427

Mohit A, Murthy RS, Saraceno B, Wig NN, Saeed K (2006) Preface. In: *WHO EMRO. Mental health in the Eastern Mediterranean Region: Reaching the unreached.* Cairo, Egypt: WHO EMRO

Mujaheed M, Corbex M, Lichtenberg P, et al (2000) Evidence for linkage by transmission disequilibrium test analysis of a chromosome 22 microsatellite marker D22S278 and bipolar disorder in a Palestinian Arab population. *American Journal of Medical Genetics*, 96(6): 836–838

Nguyen-Gillham V, Giacaman R, Naser G, Boyce W (2008) Normalising the abnormal: Palestinian youth and the contradictions of resilience in protracted conflict. *Health & Social Care in the Community*, 16(3): 291–298

Nock MK, Borges G, Bromet EJ, et al (2008) Cross-national prevalence and risk factors for suicidal ideation, plans and attempts. *British Journal of Psychiatry*, 192(2): 98–105

Odenwald M, Neuner F, Schauer M, et al (2005) Khat use as risk factor for psychotic disorders: A cross-sectional and case-control study in Somalia. *BMC Medicine*, 3: 5

Okasha A, Lotaif F (1979) Attempted suicide: An Egyptian investigation. *Acta Psychiatrica Scandinavica*, 60: 69–75

Okasha A (2003) Mental health services in the Arab world. *Arab Studies Quarterly*, 25: 39–52

Okasha A, Karam E (1998) Mental health services and research in the Arab world. *Acta Psychiatrica Scandinavica*, 98: 406–413

Rashad H, Osman M, Roudi-Fahimi F (2005) *Marriage in the Arab world*. Washington, DC: Population Reference Bureau

Salamoun M, Karam A, Okasha T, Atassi L, Mneimneh Z, Karam E (2008) Epidemiologic assessment of substance use in the Arab world. *Arab Journal of Psychiatry*, 19(2): 100–125

Samuel M, Lakkis N, Ataya O, Issa G (2008) *A report on mental health in nine Arab countries*. Beirut: Arab Resource Collective (Arabic)

Scott, KM, Bruffaerts R, Tsang A, et al (2007) Depression-anxiety relationships with chronic physical conditions: Results from the World Mental Health surveys. *Journal of Affective Disorders*, 103: 113–120

Seedat S, Scott KM, Angermeyer MC, et al (2009) Cross-national associations between gender and mental disorders in the WHO World Mental Health Surveys. *Archives of General Psychiatry*, 66 (7): 785–795

Tanios C, Abou Saleh MT, Karam AN, Salamoun M, Mneimneh ZN, Karam EG (2009) The epidemiology of anxiety disorders in the Arab world: A review. *Journal of Anxiety Disorders*, 23(4): 409–419

Thabet AA, Abdulla T, El-Helou M, Vostanis P (2006) Prevalence of ADHD and PTSD among Palestinian children in the Gaza and West Bank. *Arabpsynet E Journal*, 12: 57–64

Thabet AA, Abu Nada I, Shivram R, Winter EW, Vostanis P (2009) Parenting support and PTSD in children of a war zone. *International Journal of Social Psychiatry*, 55: 226–237

Thabet AA, Vostanis P (1998) Social adversities and anxiety disorders in the Gaza strip. *Archives of Disease in Childhood*, 78: 439–442

WHO (World Health Organization) (2005) *Mental Health Atlas 2005*. Geneva, Switzerland: WHO

WHO (2008) *Global burden of disease: 2004 Update*. Geneva, Switzerland: WHO

WHO (2009) *Assessment instrument for mental health systems*. Geneva, Switzerland: WHO

Yamout R, Chaaya M (2011) Individual and collective determinants of mental health during wartime. A survey of displaced populations amidst the July-August 2006 war in Lebanon. *Global Public Health*, 6: 354–370

Zakrison TL, Shahen A, Mortaja S, Hamel PA (2004) The prevalence of psychological morbidity in West Bank Palestinian children. *Canadian Journal of Psychiatry*, 49(1): 60–63

Chapter

15

Recognizing Omitted Contexts and Implicit Paradigms: Toward a Valid Mental Health Discourse

Ghena A. Ismail

The relevance of the Western health model for the health needs of people in non-Western parts of the world is being increasingly criticized today (Blowers et al 2009; Gergen et al 1996; Giacaman et al 2010; Khaleefa, 1997; Moghaddam & Taylor, 1986; Paranjpe, 2002). Concerns are voiced about the appropriateness of global mental health care (Giacaman et al 2010; Summerfield 2001; Thomas et al 2005). Central to these concerns is that labels and constructs are not neutral, and misconstruing them as such could lead to hegemonic and possibly pathologizing interpretations of human responses (Raskin & Lewandowski, 2000). In this chapter, pathologizing is primarily discussed as a function of overlooking contextual factors necessary for understanding a given human response. Decontextualized trends of research and practice are examined against the realities and needs of individuals and communities in the Arab world with particular reference to the Occupied Palestinian Territory (OPT). Recommendations are made for developing a valid mental health discourse in the Arab world.

Background

More than half a century ago, Prothro and Melikian (1955) described research in Egypt and Lebanon in terms of adaptation of already existing Western tests to local use. Recently, Zebian et al (2007) showed that only 6% of regional authors discussed and/or challenged the appropriateness of applying mainstream measures that had been normed or piloted in another culture (i.e., the Western culture). Intelligence tests, such as the Wechsler Intelligence Scale for Children – fourth edition – WISC-IV, 2003, whose norms are based on the American population, are being administered in schools in the Arab world without attempting to at least establish locally relevant norms.

Concurrently in Canada, which shares many more similarities with the American culture, national norms have been established and used for interpreting the WISC scores. This is consistent with observations that most psychological tests in the Arab world were designed and constructed in the United States (US), translated with slight modifications, and used without standardization or norming (Khaleefa 1999). This phenomenon of passive or unreflective import is not exclusive to this region (Abou Hatab 1997; Gergen et al 1996; Moghaddam & Taylor 1986). While acknowledging the value of scientific knowledge and its technological application to the field of psychology, Paranjpe (2002) questioned its cross-cultural applicability and relevance and drew attention to the intellectual and economic cost of the application of a so-called psychological science.

The question of relevance and resources becomes more pressing when one considers current global strategies aimed at making governments more aware of mental health problems and urging them to invest more in psychiatric services. An example is the World Health Organization's (WHO) mental health Global Action Plan (mhGAP) (WHO 2002), which emphasizes the need for organized initiatives to counter the economic impact of psychiatric disorders. The WHO Project Atlas 2000–2001 (WHO 2001; 2005) surveyed 185 countries covering 99.3% of the world's population; more than 70% of the world's population had access to less than one psychiatrist per 100,000 people. To address the gap between costs of biomedical care and national resources, the mhGAP initiative proposed partnerships with other groups, including UN organizations, the World Bank, private industry, academic institutions, and NGOs. This would ensure that all governments develop strategies to augment the availability of psychiatric treatment in primary care, improve public awareness of psychiatric disorders,

Public Health in the Arab World, ed. Samer Jabbour et al. Published by Cambridge University Press. © Samer Jabbour et al., 2012.

and establish national policies and programs in mental health. Project Atlas occupies significant weight in the global community, and WHO continues to base much of its strategic planning on the survey (Thomas et al 2005).

These global strategies raise fundamental concerns and/or questions. The first is practical and pertains to implementation and resources. Technology has admittedly brought some benefits to health. However, it is expensive and possibly unsustainable and is likely to result in the dependence of Economically Disadvantaged countries on Economically Advantaged countries (Giacaman et al 2010; Nguyen-Gillham et al 2008; Paranjpe 2002; Summerfield 2000; Thomas et al 2005). The second pertains to the relationship between the construction of disorders and economic, social, and cultural factors. Are labels neutral categories that could be readily transported across the globe, or are labels fundamentally an extension to a given philosophical, historic, and developmental trajectory? Should the process of indigenizing knowledge not precede and inform the import of labels and instruments? The limits of treating culture as an additive variable is being increasingly criticized (Lewis-Fernandez & Kleinman 1994; Paranjpe 2002; Ratner 2008). Last, how could the requirements of indigenization be balanced against the immediate needs for relief and care?

It is my position that the process of importing mental health knowledge must be tempered by careful consideration and contemplation of indigenous resources; be they economic, cultural, intellectual, and/or historic. This implies examining indigenous values and definitions pertinent to progress, development, happiness, freedom, and well-being. Import of knowledge, if and when deemed necessary, needs to be mediated by considering that any health paradigm, even one that claims to be scientifically based, is not value free. Political, social, economic, and philosophical factors impact the shaping of any given knowledge system (Brown 2000; Cohen 1993; Greenberg 1997; Raskin & Lewandowski 2000). The field of mental health as taught and practiced in the West emerged in a given developmental trajectory whose origins can be traced back to the Enlightenment era. Permeating many of its constructs and defining parameters are values of progress and well-being that celebrate an emergent faith in technological advancement, individualism, autonomy, and control. These values run in sharp contrast to those held by many

people across the globe. In traditional societies, a vision of an interdependent existence of human beings and control that is distributed rather than individualized is what is commonly emphasized (Gergen et al 1996). Lack of awareness of culture-bound assumptions of modern mental health has biased the understanding of psychopathology (Lewis-Fernandez & Kleinman, 1994) and limited the scope of community based mental health interventions (Smith et al 2009). As a result of this unexplored bias, there has been a tendency to pathologize, if not stigmatize, the responses of oppressed and disadvantaged individuals and populations.

In this chapter, pathologizing is primarily discussed as a function of failing to appreciate the multiple contexts within which a given human experience occurs. To highlight the factors contributing to it, I will discuss first the global tendency to medicalize ordinary human pain (Cohen 1993; Horwitz & Wakefield 2007; Raskin & Lewandowski 2000). I will then focus on the tendency to essentialize the suffering of various non-Western groups as reflected in historic and contemporary research pertinent to colonized populations (Bhatia 2002; Clark et al 2010; Giacaman et al 2010; Pols 2007; Nguyen-Gillham et al 2008). I will highlight the continuum between contemporary development aid studies and mental health research to uncover the implicit paradigm governing the study of individuals and populations in the Arab world today. Finally I offer recommendations pertinent to developing a regionally valid mental health discourse.

Omission of Context and Medicalization of Ordinary Human Pain: A Global Trend

Every science is influenced by social factors. Human sciences are additionally impacted by ideological and evaluative considerations. The claim that biological psychiatry is totally objective cannot be substantiated. To diagnose someone as "paranoid," for instance, the clinician examines the behavior in its context and applies multiple cultural norms to assess its reasonableness. This means that classifications of human behavior, which may wear an outlook of neutrality, are rooted in everyday cultural understanding (Cohen 1993). Whereas the symptom-based approach in community epidemiological studies may appear as a neutral starting point for examining the complex phenomenon of human suffering, such an approach may be characterized in terms of imposing a medical context on symptoms that occur naturally; thus blurring the difference between suffering and pathology. According to Horwitz & Wakefield (2007), the prevailing decontextualized approach to mental illness resulted in inflating the rates of this mental illness. Note that "treatment of depression in the US increased by 300% between 1987 and 1997 ... Antidepressant medications, such as Prozac, Paxil, Zoloft, and Effexor, are now the largest selling prescription drugs of any sort. Their use among adults nearly tripled between 1988 and 2000 ... During the 1990s, spending on antidepressants increased by 600% in the United States, exceeding $7 billion annually by 2000" (p. 4–5).

These estimates could indicate an actual increase in the number of depressed people or an increased openness in the general population to seeking mental health services. While not necessarily negating these possibilities, Horwitz & Wakefield (2007) argue that the inflation in rates of depression is based on a relatively new definition of depression in particular and mental illness in general. This new definition is based on Diagnostic Statistical Manual of Mental Disorders (DSM) labels and studies which seem to ignore a previously placed emphasis on contextual factors prior to diagnosis. It is fair to argue that the DSM is not meant to substitute for clinical judgment. Horwitz & Wakefield (2007) stated "... in clinical practice contextual probes are usual, and all of the DSM manuals assume, with varying levels of explicitness, that clinicians will use their commonsense judgments in applying diagnostic criteria. Clinicians can, for example, reassure highly distressed people whose marriages are unraveling that their problems are mainly situational..." (p.133) People who seek help from clinicians "are by definition self-selected, and they use all sorts of contextual information to decide for themselves whether their conditions exceed ordinary and temporary response to stressors" (p. 132).

The problem of pathologizing what is normal, however, needs to be understood as a function of epidemiological community studies which affect mental health policy at national and global levels. The impact of such studies on shaping individual human experiences could be an area of study in and of itself. The main problem in such studies is that they seek to apply the DSM's symptom-based criteria to untreated samples in the community. It is true that a multi-axial system of diagnosis is used in the DSM whereby psycho-social contextual factors are placed

on a separate axis (Axis IV). However, the presence of social stressors does not mitigate the process of diagnosis. They are rather seen as mitigating factors of a condition that was already diagnosed. What this means is that symptoms that meet criteria for Major Depressive Disorder, (e.g., sadness, decreased appetite, lack of sleep) for example, would have already been defined as disordered before social context (e.g., loss of a job) would come into play. It is necessary here to outline the practical significance of incorporating contextual factors in the act of diagnosis itself. The argument by Horwitz & Wakefield (2007) is that the prognosis for people suffering seemingly similar symptoms is likely to differ depending on the circumstances (be they social or biological; communal or individual). Symptoms of non-disordered conditions are likely to gradually diminish without intervention, to disappear when circumstances change, and to be responsive to generic social support. Symptoms related to internal dysfunctions are likely to be recurrent and persist regardless of stressors. Furthermore, although medication or therapy can help ease the pain that arises from normal sadness, they are often unnecessary, and could be counterproductive.

What is being proposed by an increasing number of critics, including scholars from within the psychiatry tradition, is a framework that differentiates distress from pathology (Brown 2000; Giacaman et al 2010; Horwitz & Wakefield 2007). Horwitz & Wakefield (2007) argued that unless such a framework is developed, mental health professionals not only run the risk of pathologizing ordinary human responses to stressful situations; but also the risk of losing the scientific credibility of their own profession. The development of a framework that differentiates distress from pathology is expected to lead not only to a more precise and valid definition of mental health but also to the development of community-based interventions that draw upon local practices and experiences. By way of concluding this section and in order to point out some practical implications, it is relevant to note that even an economically advantaged country such as Britain is now revising its national health policy. Given the unsustainable costs of biomedical care, a fundamental shift in ethos, with a move away from disease-based models to preventive care has been proposed. An alternative approach is a public health model that recognizes the importance of building upon social capital and actively engaging community members. Several community programs have been developing, in Britain and elsewhere, over the past few years. One particularly innovative modality, which involves participatory drama, aims at enhancing collective identities and bonds and validating responses to injustice. It also encourages communities to consider ways of taking more responsibility for those who suffer rather than delegating this entirely to unknown professionals (Thomas et al 2005). Such alternative modalities are presented as a necessary complement rather than substitute of the biomedical health approach. Their importance lies in suggesting that there are forms of human suffering and pain that are better addressed via an interactive process that involves communal negotiation rather than expert care.

The key point I wish to emphasize is the importance of a thorough consideration of contextual factors when engaging in the import of mental health research tools and approaches into the Arab world. For scholars concerned with this region to contribute to proposed alternative frameworks it is necessary that they become increasingly aware of trends which foster existing global tendency to decontextualize human experience. In this section, I have discussed omission of context as a function of a global phenomenon of medicalizing pain. In the following section, I discuss an additional layer of pathologization that is more directly specific to studying individuals and communities in the Arab world.

Omission of Political Context and Essentializing the Experiences of the Other: A Function of Hegemonic Paradigms

A characteristic of studies of individuals and communities in the Arab world is a tendency to omit major macro-level political factors (see also Chapter 37). Okazaki et al (2007) noted that cross-cultural studies in psychology have long been criticized for being simplistic, ahistorical, and decontextualized with the culture and psychology approach suffering from "lack of attention to the historical and ideological sources of culture." This tendency to ignore macro-political factors is not specific to the psychology discipline but affects the broader field of mental health and is part of a larger well documented tendency of dominant forces to project their own understandings on the

experiences of marginalized groups. In compelling analyses, feminists and post-constructivists have exposed the systematic ways in which forces of hegemony shape and condition the paradigms and concepts of mental health (Smith et al 2000). Illuminating examples of how certain diagnoses were included and excluded from various editions of the DSM (currently in its fifth version) provide a powerful indication of the subjective element in the construction of disorders (Greenberg 1997; Raskin & Lewandowski 2000). Such examples shed light on the pre-emptive and foreclosed manner in which constructions are made leading to pathologizing the responses of certain groups. As Raskin and Lewandowski (2000) noted, each revision of the DSM seems to be a product of people with like-minded constructions about the definition and nature of disorder.

Examining historic practices of psychiatry in colonized countries offers a good starting point for illustrating how hegemonic paradigms and assumptions are likely to impact the study of individuals and communities in colonized populations in general and in the Arab world in particular. The emergent literature on mental health and colonialism suggests an unmistakable overlap between notions held by colonial regimes and those held by professionals about the psyche and behavior of natives. In his study of three prominent psychiatrists who practiced in countries subject to colonization during the early twentieth century, Pols (2007) observed that political ideas and values supporting inequality, colonialism, and imperialism were incorporated into medical and psychiatric theories. Bhatia (2002) examined the history of European and American psychology (citing pioneering figures in psychology such as Francis Galto, Herbert Spencer, and G. Stanley Hall following Darwin's evolutionary theory) to conclude that it played a central role in constructing the representations of the formerly colonized non-Western "others" as inferior and primitive (Okazaki et al 2007). It is now increasingly documented that colonialist psychiatrists referred to indigenous populations as possessing "a very different nature" not yet or ever equipped to rule themselves. Riots against occupation were perceived as a sign of emotionality and irrationality rather than a normal quest for freedom and self-rule (Pols 2007). Perhaps not surprisingly, psychiatrists practicing under colonial regimes failed to appreciate the pathological and disempowering effects of colonialist regimes themselves. This could be related to the passion many of them had to spread the ideals of "progress," albeit progress defined in their own terms. In imposing their definitions of progress and development, such psychiatrists invariably fell short of examining the traits of colonized people from the point of view of the indigenous people's own history, meaning making systems and ways of living. A direct negative result was pathologizing and stigmatizing not only ordinary human responses to stressful situations but possibly also positive coping strategies and strengths in the face of adversity.

Some may dismiss the above as an element of the past and that scientific progress made in the field of mental health limited the scope of hegemonic and one-sided interpretations of reality. However, trends of research in one of the most highly afflicted areas of the Arab world; namely the Occupied Palestinian Territories (OPT), suggests a recurrent trend to decontextualize the experiences of individuals and communities in colonized parts of the world. Echoing the observations made earlier about cross-cultural mental health studies failing to consider the impact of macro political and ideological factors on the constructions of the other, Giacaman et al (2010) commented on an academic trend to explain interpersonal violence in the OPT, among other places, via exclusively cultural/internal factors. Clark et al (2010) pointed out that few studies have investigated the link between intimate-partner violence and forms of collective violence in civilian populations despite evidence supporting this association. In the OPT, violence is everywhere, existing in the "weave of life." People face violence, brutality, and life chaos every day. Despite its pervasiveness, men are overwhelmingly the direct victims of political violence. By linking intimate-partner violence with exposure to direct and indirect forms of political violence and/or trauma, Clark et al highlighted some of the complexities entailed in the occurrence of intimate-partner violence. The result is a more accurate and realistic picture in which Palestinians are portrayed as human beings subject to many influences rather than demonic creatures whose violence can be explained exclusively via cultural/internal factors.

The tendency to stigmatize individuals in the Arab world should be understood at least partly as a function of a re-emergent colonialist paradigm being advanced by some Arab and Western scholars alike.

In fact, a key feature of different eras and forms of Western colonialism has been the central role played by the local educated (Blowers et al 2009) or powerful elites (Moghaddam & Taylor 2007), also referred to as transnational elites (Sukarieh 2011) in advancing the colonialist paradigm. Having observed that the September 11 events set the stage for the recolonization of the Arab world, Sukarieh (2011) reviewed different aid policies that have been targeting the Arab world in recent years. A common focus in many current policies is hope, a theme which is of particular relevance to mental health policy makers and professionals. Sukarieh (2011) pointed out that Culture of Hope, Culture of Optimism, Culture of Life and Culture of Development are some of the slogans that have lately dominated the public spaces in the Arab world. She commented that an underlying assumption in the conferences promoting those slogans is that individuals in Arab society lack hope, not due to structural injustices but rather due to cultural factors that promote pessimism. She observed that having divested the Arab culture from political, social, and historic factors, what follows then are claims of a "culture gap." In the Arab world, the West is portrayed as alive, modern, hopeful, and liberating while the native culture of the Arab world is portrayed as a dead tradition of despair, pessimism, and death (Sukarieh 2011). This trend in development aid studies undoubtedly highlights an emerging sociopolitical paradigm pertinent to the Arab world. To the extent that professionals overlook the biased assumptions of this paradigm, they may fail to question the validity of seemingly innocent questions such as, "Why are Jordanians pessimistic?" [or possibly "Why are Palestinian men violent?"] In a montage of expert opinion that was aired from a development conference on Al-Arabiya television, Sukarieh (2011) commented that none of the interviewed experts challenged the above question or the meaning of "culture of pessimism" (i.e., Is there such a culture? Are we pessimistic? And if yes, is it a culture?). Instead, the so-called experts began to give their opinions. These ranged from the idea that the Arab world is living in the past, to invoking the "religious mind," to lamenting the spread of fundamentalism that promotes a culture of fear in Arab people. No reference was made to the economic and political history of the Arab world, be it in the form of recent experiences of neo-colonization in Palestine or Iraq or previous eras of oppression and colonization.

Future Directions and Foreseen Obstacles

At the outset of this chapter, I expressed reservations on the dissemination of wholesale import of any given mental health model. The dissemination of biomedical care worldwide was introduced as an example of an import–export process that does not take into consideration the socio-economic and political realities of various societies. The experiences of some countries in trying to spread the benefits of the global biomedical care highlight important pragmatic limits which prompted even a country such as Britain to re-envision its public mental health policy. This coincides with scholarly calls worldwide (Horwitz & Wakefield 2007; Giacaman et al 2010) to redefine the parameters and limits of human problems that fall under the purview of mental health. In considering the proposed framework of differentiating suffering from pathology, scholars involved in the Arab world could play a pivotal role in directing national public health policies and associated expenditure. They also could contribute to a more effective use of already existing communal resources and healing practices. Before discussing the requirements and implications of working toward a framework that differentiates suffering from pathology, it is necessary to outline some of the foreseen obstacles.

Promoting a framework that differentiates suffering from pathology by definition limits the market that can be accessed by the pharmaceutical industry. The alliances that have emerged over the past decades between mental health professionals, government, and the pharmaceutical industry cannot be over-emphasized. These alliances constitute dual roles that defy commonly accepted norms of ethical practice. Despite promises to reduce conflicts of interest, 56% of DSM-V panel members reported industry ties, showing no improvement over the situation of DSM-IV members (CCHR 2010). Overlapping interests between governments, biomedical practitioners and the pharmaceutical industry constitutes only one obstacle in the face of de-pathologizing ordinary human experiences. This adds to obstacles discussed previously and is particularly relevant to the Arab world and other economically disadvantaged countries that have been subject to political, cultural, and socio-economic forms of Western colonialism, namely the tendency to construct the reality of the native culture in largely essentialized terms via the filter, values, and assumptions of the Western culture and the roles of the local educated and powerful elites in promoting those constructions.

The above obstacles cannot be addressed via a critical or reactive attitude. Some of the forwarded indigenous approaches have been criticized for advancing exoticizing portrayals of reality that only re-enact the essentialist hegemonic discourse contingent on binary categories (Okazaki et al 2007). Conducting contextualized research should be the first step in the direction of challenging the prevalent hegemonic discourse. To contribute to a framework that differentiates distress from pathology, we need to examine a given human response against the backdrop of existing stressors. We return to the example of Palestine.

Upon revisiting the research about interpersonal violence in the OPT in terms of possible clinical implications, one should consider the following questions: Is the violence seen among Palestinian men atypical given the violent political atmosphere men live in, or is it consistent with modes of interpersonal violence seen in other war zones? And if so, what mode of intervention is most suitable to help address interpersonal violence? Fortunately, some scholars are beginning to recognize the clinical value of considering multiple explanatory frameworks when examining a given human response. Clark et al (2010) sought to examine whether political violence was associated with male-to-female intimate-partner violence in the OPT. Using a nationally representative, cross-sectional survey done between December 2005 and January 2006, 4156 households were randomly selected. Exposure to political violence was defined as the husband's direct exposure, his indirect exposure via his family's experiences, and economic effects of exposure on the household. Findings indicated that political violence was significantly related to higher odds of intimate-partner violence. These findings are consistent with research conducted on military personnel in which exposure to war-zone stressors was shown to be associated with perpetration of domestic violence. More studies that examine the link between micro level problems and macro political factors in this region are needed. This could contribute to the development of valid mental health interventions, whether targeting individuals or the community. As suggested by feminist scholars, the person–situation must be the unit of analysis, even when only the individual her- or himself is the focus of assessment or treatment (Brown 2000).

Actively examining the usefulness of some of the imported diagnostic labels and frameworks is another step worth considering. Giacaman et al (2010) and Afana et al (2010) questioned the efficacy of the post-traumatic stress disorder (PTSD) framework that has been widely disseminated to many war-zone areas including the OPT. The question raised by Giacaman et al. is not whether Palestinians are subject to trauma but whether clinically based interventions are what is needed to address the collective political trauma. Regarding the injustices endured by Palestinians, Giacaman et al (2010) and Summerfield (2000) questioned whether an individualistic model of intervention would be helpful. Having described the collective trauma and political injustice to which Palestinians are subjected, Giacaman et al (2010) proposed a public health approach based on a quality of life model. This approach is proposed to facilitate a shift of focus from individual diagnosis and symptoms of depression and anxiety to the collective dimensions of suffering or distress. It is also said to encourage the development of social and political response to mass suffering with justice as its primary aim.

Giacaman's proposal is not inconsistent with the historic development of many of the diagnostic labels and frameworks used in mental health today. The PTSD construct itself developed at least partly in response to the experiences of former combatants and patients of the US Veterans Administration (Pedersen 2002). "Early proponents of the diagnosis of PTSD were part of the anti-war movement in the United States; they were angry that military psychiatry was being used to serve the interests of the military rather than those of the soldier-patients. The proponents lobbied hard for veterans to receive specialized medical care under the new diagnosis, which became the successor to the older diagnoses of "battle fatigue" and "war neurosis." The new diagnosis was meant to shift the focus of attention from the details of a soldier's psyche and background to the fundamentally traumatogenic nature of war. This was a powerful and essentially political transformation: Vietnam veterans were to be seen not as perpetrators or offenders but as people traumatized by roles thrust upon them by the US military. PTSD not only legitimized their "victimhood," giving them moral exculpation but also guaranteed them a disability pension because the diagnosis could be attested to by a doctor" (Summerfield, 2001, p.95).

If the PTSD model was deemed helpful to capture the plight of returning soldiers whose trauma (at least in terms of lived reality) had come to an end upon their return home, we may wish to follow Giacaman's footsteps in wondering about a framework that captures the plight and needs of a group of people whose trauma is protracted. This is not to infer that the PTSD framework is not effective for dealing with certain types of trauma lived by Palestinian individuals and which are likely to be similar to many other types of trauma existing elsewhere. The key point here is to emphasize the potential advocacy role that public health practitioners and clinicians may play via advancing possibly new constructs that address a given collective plight. The importance of the quality of life model proposed by Giacaman lies in acknowledging this potential role and responsibility. It also displays awareness that mental health constructs are human made. To capture different modes of human mental health, professionals may wish to experiment with advancing new labels that build upon indigenous concerns and aspirations which may include justice and peace.

Another future direction that could contribute to a valid mental health discourse in the Arab world pertains to the importance of establishing community-based criteria and norms pertinent to mental illness. To better use the scarce available clinical resources in the region, and particularly in highly afflicted areas such as the OPT, it is imperative to establish criteria by which to designate those cases that warrant clinical intervention. Ethnographic and participatory research could be a useful starting point. Community members may be directly asked about responses and behaviors considered expected in a given situation. Comparative research in which the responses of various individuals suffering similar modes of trauma could shed light on risk as well as protective factors. This brings us to the importance of exploring strengths and factors of resilience. In areas such as the OPT or Iraq, it may be easy to focus on problems and overlook, if not pathologize, strengths. A survey of the literature on Palestinian youth, for instance, reveals a population at risk for anxiety, depression, or PTSD. Alternatively, Palestinian youth are represented as pathological adolescents who resort to senseless acts of violence (Nguyen-Gillham et al 2008). The incessant focus on "what is wrong" as opposed to "what works" serves to objectify people.

A key to exploring "what is already working" in the Palestinian case possibly lies in tapping the collective indigenous construct of *sumud* (steadfastness).

The concept of *sumud*, which has no direct terminological equivalent in the English language, may be translated as a determination to exist through being steadfast and rooted to the land (Giacaman et al 2010). This construct goes beyond an individualistic interpretation: resilience is (re)constituted as a wider collective and social representation of what it means to endure. Its importance lies in offering an accurate collective response to occupation policies that target first and foremost the very existence of Palestinians as people with a unifying language, dialect, land, and history. A "dramatic" example of *sumud* would be the collective Palestinian response to the systematic killing of innocent civilians. The community members do a "wedding" to bury a *shahid* (martyr). They congratulate the mother. They dance and sing. By doing so, the feeling of helplessness is replaced by a sense of pride and perseverance. Palestinians choose to shift their status from "collateral victims" to dignified survivors. The tendency to accept and celebrate death in the face of war is not unique to Palestinians. It rather seems to be a common human response. However, similarly to what happens across various oppressive eras and regimes, responses of the victims are consistently pathologized. The Palestinian response to death imposed on them is largely depicted as a sign of an innately violent population that despises life and cherishes death. There are of course less dramatic examples of *sumud* worthy of further study as they pertain to everyday experiences and which warrant further study. Nguyen-Gillham et al (2008) provides an example of much needed research which poses questions about daily activities that help sustain normalcy in a largely abnormal living situation. Besides offering a contextualized mode of investigating the suffering of a given population, an exploration of strengths offers a good starting point for community-based interventions. Without awareness of existing healing practices, community-based interventions will fall short of offering a meaningful and constructive addition.

Conclusion

In this chapter, I have argued that the process of importing mental health knowledge needs to be tempered by careful consideration and contemplation of indigenous resources; be they economic, cultural, intellectual, and/or historic. To defend this argument, I have highlighted the inevitably constructionist aspect of the field of mental health. A tendency to pathologize human suffering was discussed as a function of omission of contextual factors. Some of the obstacles facing attempts to challenge the biomedically based paradigm were reviewed. I shall conclude that alternative models are not a substitute for biomedical care. A primary motive of such models is to make better use of available biomedical resources and also to facilitate the development of communal responses that may not and should not lend themselves to expert care. Contributing to an alternative paradigm requires moving beyond the exercise of validating existing mental health instruments. Perhaps a lesson can be derived from the path taken by feminist psychologists who not merely proposed adapting a given instrument and label but rather called for the necessity of re-envisioning aspects of the mainstream mental health paradigm to reflect structural and systemic socio-political inequities. Such calls translated later in interventions that were tested and whose efficacy was verified. Studies begin with questions and concerns. Mental health professionals concerned with advancing a valid mental health discourse in the Arab world may begin by deliberating on the questions that should direct future studies. Good research is evaluated not only in terms of the rigor of methodology but also the appropriateness of its governing question(s) and related concerns. Some promising examples of academic research and alternative frameworks proposed worldwide were reviewed in this chapter. Building upon those examples and frameworks could be a great starting point.

References

Abou Hatab F (1997) Psychology from Egyptian, Arab, and Islamic perspectives: Unfulfilled hopes and hopeful fulfillment. *European Psychologist*, 2: 356–365

Afana A, Pedersen D, Ronsbo H, Kirmayer LJ (2010) Endurance is to be shown at the first blow: Social representations and reactions to traumatic experiences in the Gaza Strip. *Traumatology*, 20(10): 1–12

Bhatia S (2002) Orientalism in Euro-American and Indian psychology: Historical representation of "natives" in colonial and postcolonial contexts. *History of Psychology*, 5(4): 376–398

Blowers G, Cheung BT, Ru H (2009) Emulation vs. indigenization in the reception of western psychology in Republican China: An analysis of the context of Chinese psychology journals (1922–1937). *Journal of the History of Behavioural Sciences*, 45(21): 21–33

Brown L (2000) Discomforts of the powerless: Feminist constructions of distress. *In:* R Neimeyer & J Raskin (Eds.) *Constructions of disorder: Meaning-making frameworks for psychotherapy.* (p. 287–308). San Antonio, TX: American Psychological Association

CCHR (Citizens Commission on Human Rights International) (2010) *DSM panel members still getting Pharma funds.* Available from http://www.cchrint.org/tag/lisa-cosgrove/ [Accessed 13 December 2010)

Clark CJ, Everson-Rose SA, Suglia SF, Btoush R, Alonso A, Haj-Yahia MM (2010) Association between exposure to political violence and intimate-partner violence in the Occupied Palestinian Territory: A cross-sectional study. *The Lancet*, 375: 310–316

Cohen C (1993) The biomedicalization of psychiatry: A critical overview. *The Community Mental Health Journal*, 29: 6

Gergen K, Gulerce A, Lock A, Misra G (1996) Psychological science in cultural context. *American Psychologist*, 51(5): 496–503

Giacaman R, Rabai'a Y, Nguyen-Gillham V, Batnijie R, Punamaki RL, Summerfield D (2010a) Mental health, social distress and political oppression: The case of the Occupied Palestinian Territory. *Global Public Health*, 23: 1–13

Giacaman R, Rabaia Y, Nguyen-Gillham V (2010b) Domestic and political violence: The Palestinian predicament. *The Lancet*, 375: 259–260

Greenberg G (1997) Right answers, wrong reasons: Revisiting the deletion of homosexuality from the DSM. *Review of General Psychology*, 1(3): 256–270

Horwitz A, Wakefield J (2007) *The loss of sadness: How psychiatry transformed normal sorrow into depressive disorder.* New York, NY: Oxford University Press

Khaleefa O (1997) The imperialism of Euro-American psychology in a non-Western culture: An attempt toward an ummatic psychology. *The American Journal of Islamic Social Sciences*, 14(1): 44–69

Khaleefa O (1999) Research on creativity, intelligene, and giftedness: The case of the Arab World. *Gifted and Talented International*, 14: 21–29

Lewis-Fernandez R, Kleinman A (1994) Culture, personality and psychopathology. *Journal of Abnormal Psychology*, 103(1): 67–71

Moghaddam F, Taylor D (2007) What constitutes an 'appropriate psychology' for the developed world. *International Journal of Psychology*, 21: 253–267

Nguyen-Gillham V, Giacaman R, Naser G, Boyce W (2008) Normalising the abnormal: Palestinian youth and the contradictions of resilience in protracted conflict. *Health and Social Care in the Community*, 16(3): 291–298

Okazaki S, David EJR, Abelmann N (2007) Colonialism and psychology of culture. *Social and Personality Psychology Compass*, 2(1): 90–106

Paranjpe A (2002) Indigenous psychology in the post-colonial context: An historical perspective. *Psychology and Developing Societies*, 14(1): 27–44

Pedersen D (2002) Political violence, ethnic conflict, and contemporary wars: Broad implications for health and social well-being. *Social Science and Medicine*, 55: 175–190

Pols H (2007) Psychological knowledge in a colonial context: Theories on the nature of the "native mind" in the former Dutch East Indies. *History of Psychology*, 2: 111–130

Prothro E, Melikian L (1955) Psychology in the Arab Near-East. *Psychological Bulletin*, 52(4): 303–310

Raskin J, Lewandowski A (2000) The construction of disorder as human enterprise. *In:* R Neimeyer & J Raskin (Eds.) *Constructions of disorder: Meaning-making frameworks for psychotherapy* (p. 15–40). San Antonio, TX: American Psychological Association

Ratner C (2008) *Cultural psychology, cross-cultural psychology and indigenous psychology.* New York, NY: Nova Science Publishers

Smith L, Chambers DA, Bratini L (2009) When oppression is the pathogen: The participatory development of socially just mental health practice. *American Journal of Orthopsychiatry*, 79(2): 159–168

Sukarieh M (2011) Hope crusades: Culturalism, and reform in the Arab World. Political legal Anthropology Review: Forthcoming

Summerfield D (2000) Conflict and health – war and mental health: A brief overview. *The Lancet*, 321: 232–235

Summerfield D (2001) The invention of Post-Traumatic Stress Disorder and the social usefulness of a psychiatric category. *British Medical Journal*, 322(7278): 95–98

Thomas P, Bracken P, Cutler P, May R, Yasmeen S (2005) Challenging the globalisation of biomedical psychiatry. *Public Health*, 4(3): 23–32

Zebian S, Alamuddin R, Maalouf M, Chatila Y (2007) Developing an appropriate psychology through culturally sensitive research practices in the Arabic-speaking World: A content analysis of psychological research published between 1950 and 2004. *Journal of Cross-Cultural Psychology*, 38(2): 91–122

Chapter 16

Injury Epidemiology and Prevention

Peter Barss

Injuries are a serious public health concern in the Arab world. This chapter reviews the evidence on injuries with the aim of identifying priorities for prevention and recommendations for public health research, training, and practice. Since understanding of injuries needs to be grounded in theoretical as well as practical knowledge, the chapter begins with a brief review of a public health approach to injury.

A Public Health Approach to Injuries

The theoretical basis, and corresponding evidence base, for understanding and preventing injuries has considerably advanced in the public health literature during the three decades since William Haddon first proposed his now classic injury matrix. The matrix cross classifies the three time phases of an injury incident with the three main categories of risk factors (Haddon 1980). The epidemiologic triad was modified by substituting vehicle, vector, or other equipment including safety devices risk factors for the agent. For most injuries, the agent is kinetic energy. Personal or host and environment factors are the other two categories (Barss et al 1998).

Although variations of the matrix include a subcategory of psychosocial environment, broad underlying political, structural, and socioeconomic determinants of injury are frequently not considered by injury practitioners and researchers. The study of injury and its prevention lie at the interface of many disciplines, ranging from public health and forensic medicine to engineering, anthropology, economics, justice, and politics, among others. While injuries are rarely considered so comprehensively and collaboratively, such an approach carries great promise for prevention.

Injury risk factors are considered in three phases: pre-event, event and post-event. Pre-event phase interventions are central to prevention of incidents, while event phase interventions minimize or control injuries during an incident. While there is limited evidence from the Arab world on the relative contribution of factors in the three phases for different injuries, the model can still help guide assessments of injury vulnerability and inform future research and prevention efforts. In the example of road traffic injuries (RTIs), pre-event phase factors range from chronic and often system-wide determinants such as poor road design and ineffective enforcement of laws to factors arising shortly before an injury such as non-functioning lighting. A frequent event phase factor includes non-use of vehicle restraint systems. Post-event determinants, such as communications and transport to hospitals and trauma centers and quality of care, contribute to or determine the outcomes for passengers who survive the immediate effects of a crash. Many factors operate across all three phases. Examples include ineffective policies, non-evidence based professional knowledge and attitudes regarding safety and feasibility of various approaches to injury prevention, and traditional cultural beliefs among the public regarding injury causality, destiny, and non-preventability.

The concept of intent is central to investigating injury whether from legal, medical or public health perspectives. While this framework for classification is fundamental to assignment of responsibility, it has limitations since assigning intent is complex and subject to manipulation. The proportion of injuries classified as intentional, undetermined or unintentional might differ, depending upon whether all relevant social determinants are considered. In illustration, unintentional deaths of migrant construction workers from falls or heat stroke could logically be reassigned to intentional negligent deaths resulting from conscious or ill-informed decisions by cost-cutting contractors (Rosenthal 2008). The term "accident" should be avoided since it is often used to describe physical damage of vehicles, is frequently

---

Public Health in the Arab World, ed. Samer Jabbour et al. Published by Cambridge University Press. © Samer Jabbour et al., 2012.

inappropriately applied to intentional injury, and can be a barrier to considering injuries in a public health model where health conditions are seen as non-random events and therefore subject to prevention. In many situations, this contradicts with public perceptions of causality, risk and preventability, which should be considered in the context of competing concepts such as destiny, the evil eye of jealousy, and jinns, which are beings invisible to humans. "Injury incident" is a less ambiguous alternative for accident, and can be combined with the appropriate term for intent. Both "incident" and "accident", however, do originate from the same Latin root *cid-*, meaning fall.

Injuries are classified not only by intent but also external cause. Many health records include only the nature of injury, such as a fractured bone, and not the cause, such as a fall or RTI. Such records are of limited value for prevention. Once causes are known and prioritized, the feasibility of active and passive countermeasures can be assessed. Active measures such as raising awareness of risk by public education about prevalent hazards require constant vigilance. They tend to be less effective over the long term than passive measures, which provide long-term automatic protection, often by design and engineering to permanently eliminate hazards in the built environment.

Magnitude of the Injury Problem

Several cautionary notes merit consideration in assessing the burden of injuries. First, one must carefully interpret published data as some researchers still confuse external cause and nature of injury codes. This leads to counting the cause and type of injury for the same individuals as separate incidents, thereby doubling the incidence. Second, official data quality for injury is generally poor, seriously understating the true burden of both unintentional and intentional (Al Belooshi et al 2007; Pritchard & Amanulla 2007; Barss et al 2009a). Third, choice of indicators can impact burden estimates. WHO uses life expectancy and some countries age 75 as endpoints for estimating loss of potential life; however, this tends to bias the indicator towards chronic diseases rather than injuries and conditions that kill during the working years (Barss et al 1998). If economic indicators are used, such as years of productive life lost prior to typical retirement age, the injury burden would appear much greater. In a random sample of deaths in one of the main cities of the United Arab Emirates (UAE), years of potential life lost prior to the formal retirement age of 55 was 450 years for injury compared with 10 for cardiovascular diseases (Al Belooshi et al 2007).

Mortality Official mortality data (WHO Statistics 2010) show all-cause injury mortality rates varying from a low of 35 per 100,000 population per year in Egypt to a high of 235 in Somalia (Table 1). As per capita income rises, these rates generally fall. As infant mortality rates fall the contribution of injury to under-five mortality rises. The positive effect of rising income in decreasing injury rates can be offset by consumption of alcohol as in Lebanon, and in Bahrain and Qatar where consumption by short-term visitors from neighboring countries is high. Similarly, costly items such as powerful vehicles, high speed highways, and home swimming pools, when used without essential safety devices, contribute to high mortality amongst the wealthy, while many poorly paid migrant workers die by falls at hazardous worksites and from suicide. In illustration, for the oil-rich Abu Dhabi emirate during 2007, injuries were the leading cause of mortality, accounting for 23% of all deaths (HAAD 2008).

The overall mortality rate for all injuries for the Eastern Mediterranean Region (EMR), which also includes Afghanistan, Iran, and Pakistan, was 109 per 100,000 in 2004, undoubtedly an underestimate of the true situation; it was greater than for Europe, the Americas, and the Western Pacific, less than for Southeast Asia and Africa (WHO 2009). For comparison, rates in Canada and Sweden were 33 and 32 respectively. Injuries accounted for 18% of years of life lost overall for the EMR, and as much as 34% in Iraq.

Injury mortality rates differ according to sub-regions, external cause and intent (Table 2). While some countries not in violent conflict have much lower crime rates than western countries, in others intentional injuries due to war, civil violence and occupation are the leading cause of injury death. In the 2004 Burden of Disease and Injury Report, WHO's Eastern Mediterranean Region had by far the highest proportion of disability adjusted life years (DALYs) in the world lost to war. This was the case in Somalia, Sudan, Algeria, Iraq, and Lebanon. Without this burden of war, the injury burden of DALYs would be considerably less than in Europe or the Americas, and comparable to Southeast Asia.

Table 1. Injury Mortality Data With Comparative Indicators, Arab Countries 2000–2006

Country	Age-standardized death rates/100,000 population/year			Injury deaths among ≤5 year olds (%)	IMR/ 1000 live births	Years life lost due to injury (%)	Pure alcohol consumed per person ≥15 years (liters)	Income ($) per capita (US$)	Registration of deaths (%)
	Injury	Cancer	CVD						
Algeria	85	103	314	5.0	33	20	0.15	5940	75–89
Bahrain	37	127	312	10.2	9	22	6.98	34310	75–89
Djibouti	92	116	533	1.8	86	8	1.79	2180	<25
Egypt	35	84	560	2.1	29	8	0.21	4940	75–89
Iraq	141	112	508	5.7	37	15	0.21		<25
Jordan	102	144	384	2.3	21	23	0.31	4820	25–49
Kuwait	34	78	309	7.9	9	22	0.03	48310	90–100
Lebanon	98	90	453	11.0	27	22	3.24	9600	<25
Libya	55	79	411	2.6	17	16	0.01	11630	<25
Morocco	48	67	411	4.0	34	12	0.45	3860	
Oman	41	105	409	4.1	10	19	0.26	19740	50–74
Qatar	40	75	340	5.2	9	21	4.40		75–89
Saudi Arabia	72	109	405	14.5	21	25	0.00	22300	25–49
Somalia	235	143	580	2.6	90	11	0.00		<25
Sudan	163	112	499	4.6	62	17	0.30	1780	<25
Syria	49	60	410	3.4	12	15	0.49	4110	90–100
Tunisia	72	78	417	9.7	19	19	1.23	6490	25–49
UAE	72	100	369	15.0	8	28	0.02	31190	50–74
Yemen	102	108	553	3.7	75	11	0.04	2090	<25
Sweden	30	116	176	3.4	3	11	5.96	34310	90–100
Year	2002	2002	2002	2000	2006	2002	2003	2006	2000–05

CVD = cardiovascular diseases; Age-standardized mortality rates (per 100,000 population); Deaths among children under five years of age due to injuries (%); Infant mortality rate (per 1000 live births) both sexes.
Source: Adapted from World Health Organization: http://www.who.int/whosis/indicators/compendium/2008.

In countries not immersed in war, road traffic tends to be the leading source of injury death, followed by immersion with drowning. Burns are more a problem in lower-income populations. In many countries road traffic accounted for the greatest burden of injury mortality, with the highest reported rates at about 50 per 100,000 in the UAE and Iraq, and 40 in Lebanon, Yemen, and Somalia. The highest reported immersion/drowning rates were at about 8 per 100,000 from Somalia and Yemen, followed by

Saudi Arabia, the UAE, Sudan and Iraq at about 6 to 7. In contrast, rates in Canada are 10 for traffic and 1 for immersion.

Adolescence is characterized by special vulnerability to injury, often attributed to but not necessarily a result of "risk taking". The reported rates of unintentional injury deaths among 10–14 and 15–19 year olds are about triple and double those for Europe, respectively (Table 3). More than a third of injury deaths result from traffic crashes, followed by drowning,

Table 2. Injury Mortality Rates/100,000 Population/Year by External Cause & Intent, Comparisons of Arab With Neighboring Countries, 2004

Region	GULF-GCC						Levant					North-east Africa				Northwest Africa-Maghreb				Other	For comparison		
Country	KSA	UAE	Oman	Kuwait	Qatar	Bahrain	Syria	Lebanon	OPT	Jordan	Iraq	Egypt	Sudan	Somalia	Djibouti	Libya	Algeria	Morocco	Tunisia	Yemen	Turkey	Iran	Sweden
Unintentional injuries																							
Road traffic	24.0	50.6	12.0	15.5	21.4	12.0	13.1	41.2	nd	nd	38.4	52.7	12.3	30.8	33.2	17.6	17.2	19.0	31.3	39.1	8.9	59.5	4.5
Poisoning	1.3	0.5	0.6	1.8	0.0	0.1	1.0	3.0	nd	nd		4.1	1.9	2.9	3.9	1.7	3.1	1.9	2.5	3.7	0.8	2.6	3.3
Falls	5.5	4.0	3.0	1.8	1.3	0.9	0.8	4.6	nd	nd		5.9	2.1	3.5	5.0	2.2	2.4	2.4	3.6	4.9	1.5	5.7	8.7
Burns	0.6	1.0	0.3	1.1	0.0	0.0	3.4	6.1	nd	nd		8.4	0.7	5.7	4.2	3.1	3.9	2.3	4.3	5.3	0.9	8.6	0.8
Immersion	6.7	5.7	3.9	0.8	2.3	0.9	1.8	3.5	nd	nd	8.7	6.5	4.4	6.1	9.6	2.4	3.7	3.5	3.1	8.4	1.0	3.3	1.1
Other	19.4	0.2	9.8	4.1	2.5	14.0	14.8	13.2	nd	nd		19.2	5.7	13.3	15.8	9.1	10.8	7.0	10.3	15.4	15.9	11.6	15.5
Total	57.5	62.0	29.6	23.9	27.5	27.9	34.9	71.6	nd	nd	79.7	96.8	27.1	60.7	71.7	36.1	41.1	36.1	55.1	76.8	29.0	91.3	35.5
Intentional injuries																							
Suicide	5.8	3.8	4.0	1.8	4.5	4.4	0.6	6.1	nd	nd	7.6	6.9	1.5	7.1	4.9	3.9	2.9	2.3	4.4	4.9	6.7	8.2	13.5
Homicide	3.0	1.0	2.0	1.4	1.1	1.1	2.7	2.6	nd	nd	33.1	2.9	1.2	30.4	3.5	2.5	12.0	1.1	1.9	2.1	3.4	3.8	0.9
War	0.0	0.0	0.0	1.1	0.0	0.0	0.0	5.8	nd	nd	72.2	7.6	0.0	46.4	0.2	0.0	16.1	0.0	0.0	0.0	0.2	0.1	0.0
Total	8.8	4.8	6.0	4.3	5.6	5.5	3.3	14.5	nd	nd	112.9	17.4	2.7	83.9	8.6	6.4	31.0	3.4	6.3	7.0	10.3	12.1	14.4
All Injuries	66.3	66.8	35.6	28.2	33.1	33.4	38.2	86.1	nd	nd	192.6	114.2	29.8	144.6	80.3	42.5	72.1	39.5	61.4	83.8	39.3	103.4	49.9
Unintent.: intentional	6.5	12.9	4.9	5.6	4.9	5.1	10.6	4.9	nd	nd	0.7	5.6	10.0	0.7	8.3	5.6	1.3	10.6	8.7	11.0	2.8	7.5	2.5

Source: Adapted from WHO December 2004: Estimated number of deaths by cause.

Table 3. Injury Deaths/100,000 Population/Year for Adolescents and Youth by Region, Europe and Eastern Mediterranean/Arab 2004

External cause of injury	Income level of countries	Region			
		European		East Mediterranean/Arab	
		Age group in years		Age group in years	
		10–14	15–19	10–14	15–19
All unintentional	High-income	4	19	23	52
	Low-middle	14	33	29	47
Road traffic	High-income	2	15	9	23
	Low-middle	5	16	12	20

Source: Adapted from WHO 2004, 2009.

burns and falls. Actual rates are undoubtedly higher due to underreporting. As demographics, lifestyle and the built environment change in a country falls can eventually overtake RTIs as the leading cause of death.

Morbidity, disability, consequences and costs For most types of injury, there tend to be several non-fatal incidents for each fatality. The main exception is immersion where, excluding small children who drown in or around the home, few victims survive to reach hospital and of those who do, a proportion are left with permanent brain injury. Little has been published regarding incidence of non-fatal injury. A community survey of 18–65-year-olds in Aleppo, Syria, provided self-reported estimates of injuries serious enough to require medical attention (Maziak et al 2006). There were 77 injuries per 1000 population overall, 93 for men and 64 for women. Traffic injuries and falls were most common. While infrequent, many burns had unfavorable outcomes.

The impact of non-fatal injury on individuals, family, and society can be overwhelming and costly, including both physical and psychological disability. While data are limited about acute non-fatal injuries and their long term impact, those reported are frequent and severe. In Aden, Yemen, prevalence of brain injury was 2.2 per 1000 population, varying from 4.8 among children to 1.6 in adults; traffic accounted for 40% and home injuries for 55% (Shukri et al 2006). In Saudi Arabia, 74% of spinal cord injury patients were 21 to 40 years of age, facing decades of severe impairment (Al-Jadid et al 2004).

There is an equity dimension to social costs of injuries. International research has shown widely varying results when correlating injury, injury prevention countermeasures, and socioeconomic status

(Laflamme et al 2010; Rodgers et al 2010). Certain categories of injuries and violence, particularly fatalities, are inversely associated with income in some settings (Cubbin et al 2000; Cubbin & Smith 2002; Mabrouk et al 2000). In Saudi Arabia, children with poor safety practices tended to have uneducated mothers and to come from families with many children (Jan et al 2000), suggesting that income alone is not the only social risk factor, and that education of mothers is protective. Egyptian wives living in poverty were more exposed to physical and sexual violence and more likely to maltreat their children including female genital cutting (Afifi 2009); low education of women and men associated with poverty explains at least part of the increased risk for wife beating, rather than poverty per se (Akmatov et al 2008).

In high income Arab countries with a large expatriate population, a growing prevalence of permanently disabled citizens from injury such as high-speed traffic crashes and non-fatal pool immersions impose an ever increasing burden of health and social costs. However, in such a context, the price of development in terms of morbidity and mortality is frequently paid by foreign workers, their impoverished families back home, and the health and social systems of their low-income countries of origin. The lifetime human capital costs for disability and death together with direct and indirect medical costs of permanently disabled workers are enormous and can ruin families.

Injuries, especially violence, can have serious psychological consequences (see also Chapter 14). In the Occupied Palestinian Territory (OPT), violence against Palestinian communities and families, frequent exposure to humiliation and risks of traumatic injury, punctuated by major bombardments and home demolitions, have led to an extremely high prevalence of post-traumatic stress disorder (PTSD), up to 90% including children and parents. PTSD often manifests as emotional problems, which may go unrecognized by health practitioners (Qouta & Odeb 2005, Elbedour et al 2007, Thabet et al 2002).

Psychological consequences also occur after unintentional injuries, including RTIs and others. In Casablanca, Morocco, 23% of patients in the burns department had PTSD and 55% major depression; PTSD and depression were associated (El Hamaoui et al 2002). Depression was also found in 36% of Moroccan mothers of burned children one month after the incident, and hence screening and treatment of both victims and mothers were recommended (El Hamaoui et al 2006). Mothers with several burned children, an only child, severe and complicated burns, and socioeconomic difficulties were at greatest risk. PTSD can be long-lasting after an earthquake. More than 40 years after the Agadir, Morocco earthquake survivors still had need of help (Kadri et al 2006).

Economic costs of non-fatal injuries are substantial. In high-income countries, lifetime costs of severe injuries, for example spinal cord lesions with paralysis, can amount to at least a few million dollars. Hence it is not surprising that for Saudi victims, main factors affecting quality of life were financial status, employment, necessary supplies, accessibility and social isolation (Al-Jadid et al 2004). Likewise, the cost of low bone strength and associated hip fractures from falls are serious in aging Arab populations with multiple risk factors. Cost of treatment in Saudi Arabia was estimated at one billion US dollars per year for about 9000 hip fractures among 1.5 million Saudis 50 years of age and older (Bubshait & Sadat-Ali 2007).

Specific Injury Issues

This section includes a brief summary of research on the main unintentional and intentional injury categories by intent and external cause.

Unintentional injuries

Road traffic injury Despite its large burden, traffic injury receives insufficient research attention. Some of the variability in injury rates among countries is real, and some due to differences in completeness of data collection and quality of analysis. The extent of the RTI problem is significant. In Saudi Arabia during 1971–1997, an estimated 565,000 persons

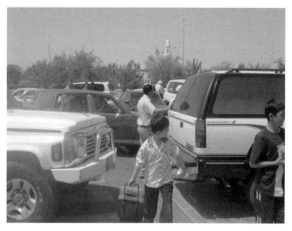

Photo 1. Unprotected traffic environment for children arriving at school, UAE.

(3.5% of the population) were injured on the roads, resulting in 67,000 deaths (Ansari et al 2000). In Ministry of Health hospitals, 81% of deaths were due to road crashes and 20% of beds occupied by crash victims, while nearly 80% of spinal cord injury patients admitted to the Armed Forces Hospital were there as a result of a crash.

Factors related to road design, law and enforcement are crucial for developing solutions (Photo 1). Travellers to different sub-regions observe the contrast between large well-lit high speed roads and expensive vehicles in high-income countries, and crowded mixes of road user types including heavy vehicles, cyclists, pedestrians and animals in others. However, better roads do not automatically translate to safety. In UAE, as roads improved, the number of crashes decreased but severity and fatalities per crash increased, probably due to increased speed combined with low wearing of safety restraints (El-Sadig et al 2002; Barss et al 2008a). Another factor is use of mobile phones while driving, which was reported by 60% of fathers in Saudi Arabia (Ali Aba Hussein and El-Zobeir 2007).

In lower-income countries many people travel by open-backed trucks (Photo 2), by two wheelers, animals, or on foot. In Tunisia, nearly 60% of children under 15 years of age presenting to emergency departments with traffic injuries in a rural agricultural area had been a passenger or driver of a two-wheeled vehicle (Ghribi et al 2003). Environmental hazards of the setting were reported for nearly half of such incidents.

Data on fatalities by road user type show that in most Arab countries, even the wealthiest, about

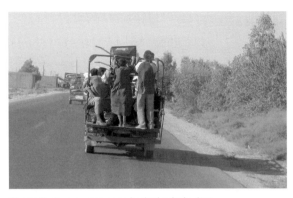

Photo 2. Transport in open-backed vehicle, Syria.

25–30% of victims are pedestrians (Table 4). In lower-income countries, frequent pedestrian victims are both children and the elderly (Abou-Raya & ElMeguid 2009). In high-income countries, many pedestrian victims are low-income male expatriate workers (Al-Shammari et al 2009) who cannot afford a car, as well as local children (Crankson 2006). Nevertheless, in Riyadh, Saudi Arabia, 71% of children were also injured as pedestrians, 27% as vehicle occupants, and only 2% on two-wheelers, in contrast to the situation with Tunisian children noted above (Crankson 2006). Nearly all pedestrian fatalities of the young, workers, and elderly resulted from head injuries; others were discharged with permanent impairment (Bahloul et al 2009, 2004, Abou-Raya & ElMeguid 2009). This leads one to wonder whether not just motorcyclists and bicyclists, but all vulnerable road users who need to cross busy streets with high energy traffic, should be wearing helmets.

Deaths by road user type vary among sub-regions, with a greater proportion of vehicle occupants in the Gulf countries and Jordan, more motorcyclists and bicyclists in the Maghreb, and a high proportion of pedestrians in all sub-regions, even wealthy Gulf countries with many vehicles relative to their population (Table 4). In some lower income countries such as Sudan with few vehicles per unit of population, death rates are also high, perhaps due to open trucks carrying many unprotected passengers. As for the motor vehicle mix, of note is the high proportion of minibuses in some countries and trucks in Jordan, the OPT, Egypt, Sudan and Morocco. In comparing traffic death rates by per capita income, it is evident that wealth is not necessarily protective, with rates in the UAE as much as 11 times higher than Sweden, and with citizens overrepresented among the victims.

As for vehicle occupant protection, few countries require use of restraints by all occupants in both front and rear seats. Reports from Oman and the UAE showed unacceptably low use of safety restraints for all, especially for rear occupants and children (McIlvenny et al 2004, Barss et al 2008a). Legislation for restraints had largely failed, possibly due to cultural and enforcement issues. In the UAE, wearing rates rose after legislation but subsequently fell to nearly zero among citizens. Enforcement is often difficult due to heavily tinted glass. In Saudi Arabia immediately after a safety belt law was implemented in 2000, promising results were observed; however, long-term follow-up was not available (Bendak 2005). Reduction of deaths and injuries was also seen in Kuwait subsequent to safety belt legislation in 1994 (Koushki et al 2003).

Non-use of safety restraints results in many hospitalizations as well as fatalities. Facial fractures from crashes with non-use of safety belts are frequent in UAE, with many complicated by blindness (Ashar et al 1998). In Kuwait, 55% of mandibular fractures were traffic-related, compared with 45% in Tunisia, 33% in Finland, and 7% in Canada (Oikarinen et al 2004, Bougila et al 2009). Many victims in Kuwait were young people; the researchers recommended increased use of safety belts and lower speeds. While most Arab countries mandate helmets for motorcyclists, helmet use among bicyclists is very low and head injuries frequent. Only 10% of child bicyclists in Jeddah used helmets, and 24% were allowed to play unsupervised in the street (Jan et al 2000). Families with poor safety practices more frequently had uneducated mothers (29% versus 5%) and were three times more likely to have four or more children.

The low use of primary safety restraints in the region is unfortunate since research both locally in Qatar and internationally has shown 50% or greater mortality reductions for vehicle occupants who wear safety belts (Munk et al 2008, NHTSA 1996). There is limited research evidence from the region on the multitude of other interventions to reduce RTI, such as public education, and post-event phase interventions to minimize consequences, such as basic or advanced life support training.

Immersion/drowning Drowning, resulting from the external cause immersion, is the second most common cause of unintentional injury fatalities in most Arab countries. In the UAE, clippings from a single major English-language newspaper documented nearly double the number of immersion deaths compared with Ministry of Health official

Table 4. Traffic injury Proportional Mortality by Road User Type, Vehicle Mix, Safety Legislation, Deaths/100,000 Population/Year, and Other Indicators, Arab Countries

Region	GULF-GCC						Levant					North-east Africa				Northwest Africa-Maghreb					Other	For comparison		
Country	KSA	UAE	Oma	Kwt	Qat	Bah	Syr	Leb	OPT	Jor	Ira	Egy	Sud	Som	Dji	Com	Lby	Alg	Mor	Tun	Yem	Turkey	Iran	Sweden
Proportional traffic-related mortality by road user type (%)																								
Vehicle occupants	70	nd	nd	nd	69	59	nd	nd	nd	75	nd	48	44			55	60		46	51		55	45	65
Motorcyclists	2	nd	nd	nd	4	5	nd	nd	nd	<1	nd	<1				8	2		16	14		8	11	16
Pedestrians	28	nd	nd	nd	27†	29	nd	nd	nd	25	nd	20				17	15		28	32		19	33	12
Bicyclists	nd	nd	nd	nd	nd	7	nd	nd	nd	nd	nd	2				nd	5		7	3		2	6	6
Other	0	nd	nd	nd	nd	0	nd	nd	nd	0	nd	30	56			nd	20		3	nd		16	11	1
Proportional motor vehicle mix (%)																								
Cars/SUVs	nd	86	72	55	nd	81	55	nd	76	65	35	60	64			86	76		72	62		50	48	77
Motorcycles	nd	1	1	<1	nd	1	9	nd	<1	<1	0	19	3			6	2		1	1		15	37	8
Minibuses	nd	2	12	35	nd	13	25	nd	6	12	53	nd	13			5	12		nd	24		18	<1	nd
Buses	nd	2	4	2	nd	2	3	nd	1	2	5	2	1			nd	5		1	1		2	<1	<1
Trucks	nd	7	6	7	nd	<1	7	nd	15	18	7	18	12			5	5		23	4		6	5	9
Others	nd	3	6	<1	nd	3	3	nd	1	3	0	1	7			nd	nd		3	1		9	9	6
Rates of traffic-related mortality/100,000 population/year and other indicators																								
Death rate/100,000 pop.	24.0	50.6	12.0	15.5	21.4	12.0	13.1	41.2	nd	nd	52.7	12.3	30.8	38.4	33.2	nd	17.6	17.2	19.0	31.3	39.1	8.9	59.5	4.5
Population in millions	25.0	4.4	2.6	3.0	0.8	nd	20.0	4.0	4.0	6.0	29.0	75.0	39.0	nd	nd	0.8	6.0	nd	31.0	10.0	22.0	75.0	71.0	9.1
People per vehicle	3.6	2.6	4.3	2.1	1.3	nd	14.3	2.9	5.0	7.5	13.2	18.8	32.5	nd	nd	4.0	3.3	nd	13.5	8.3	27.5	5.8	4.2	1.7
Vehicles in millions	7.0	1.7	0.6	1.4	0.6	nd	1.4	1.4	0.8	0.8	2.2	4.0	1.2	nd	nd	0.2	1.8	nd	2.3	1.2	0.8	13.0	17.0	5.5
GNI/capita in 1000 USD	15.0	41.0	11.0	40.0	66.0	nd	1.7	5.7	2.8	2.8	1.6	1.5	0.9	nd	nd	0.6	9.0	nd	2.2	3.2	0.8	8.0	3.5	34.3
Protective equipment legislation																								
Restraints all occupants*	yes	no	no	no	no	no	no	no	no	yes	yes	no	no			no	yes	yes	yes	no	no	yes	yes	yes
Helmets all** motorcyclists	no	yes	yes	yes	yes	yes	yes	yes	yes	yes	no	no	yes			no	no	yes	no	yes	no	yes	yes	yes

Source: Global Status Report on Road Safety, WHO 2009 and from WHO Statistical Data 2010 (Death rates are for 2002, Sweden 2005).

mortality reports (Barss et al 2009b). Furthermore, newspapers, unlike the reports, frequently included information about the location of drowning, the victim's activity, and swimming ability.

In some Gulf countries, prevalence of home pools is as high as 30%, almost none fitted with the only proven safety device, automatic self-closing and self-latching gates (Barss et al 2007, 2008c). In Riyadh, Saudi Arabia, most immersion injuries among children occurred in pools, none of which were equipped with appropriate safety equipment; in 87% supervision was deficient (Hijazi et al 2007). The incidents did not appear to have had any positive impact on water safety practices of the affected Saudi families. Measures shown to be effective in other settings, such as establishing and enforcing water safety standards and mandatory swimming programs for all children at school entry, are yet to be seriously considered in the region.

Falls Falls are often the most frequent cause of injuries seen in emergency departments and inpatients. In traditional homes, severe falls can occur from unenclosed stairs without safety barriers or hand rails and rooftops (Photo 3). In a retrospective home survey in urban, peri-urban, rural agricultural and non-agricultural areas in Damascus, Syria, falls accounted for 52% of injuries among preschool children (Bashour & Kharouf 2008). Nearly 75% of all injuries including falls occurred inside the home. The odds ratio (OR) for all injuries was 3.8 for rural non-agricultural areas compared with urban areas.

In a rural agricultural area of Tunisia, over 70% of injuries among 0–14-year-old children occurred at home; of these 35% were falls (Ghribi et al 2003). In the UAE, falls were the most frequent external cause of injury at emergency departments (Barss et al 2008b). The situation is probably similar in other countries. Most falls reaching hospital in the UAE occurred at home or work. Those at home tend to involve children and the elderly, whilst at work severe occupational falls from height mainly affect migrant workers at unsafe construction sites. In surveys of modern houses in the UAE, falls most frequently occurred on stairs, and were often associated with design deficiencies leading to missteps such as tripping and slipping. These included stair geometry such as irregular risers and shallow treads, inadequate difficult to grasp hand railings, slippery tread surfaces, and unsuitable lighting.

Another fall risk for children are babywalkers, a hazardous consumer product associated with severe falls on stairs and occasionally into swimming pools,

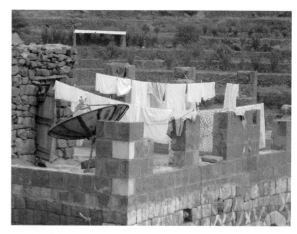

Photo 3. Open rooftop without barriers used by families, Yemen.

and a risk of death of about 1 per 1000 users in the UAE (Grivna et al 2008). These devices are now banned in Canada but are prevalent in as many as 90% of homes in the UAE, with injuries also reported from Iraq (Al-Nouri et al 2006). In poorer countries or populations, including Arab populations in the Galilee, severe falls at private homes in rural areas predominate, from stairs, balconies, roofs, and windows. Frequent causes included lack of protective barriers and use of roofs for play spaces due to insufficient playgrounds (Bar-Joseph et al 2007, Ittai et al 2000). Most severe falls affected Arabs, few Jews.

Among the wealthy elderly in GCC countries as well as the Maghreb and Levant, host factors such as an increasing lack of exercise and high body mass index (BMI), traditional clothing blocking sunlight, and hypovitaminosis D are prevalent (El Maghraoui et al 2010, Maalouf et al 2007) and contribute to higher rates of osteoporosis, which augments the risk of fractures with a fall. The adjusted OR for osteoporosis was 2.2 for veil versus no veil (Allali et al 2006). Bone density among Saudi males is lower than among Western males (Sadat-Ali & AlElq 2006). Cultural factors affecting mobility of women outside the home, hot climate, and modern lifestyle are potential barriers to weight bearing exercise. Furthermore, obesity is widespread and contributes to instability and osteoporosis, raising the risk of falling and associated fractures of the spine, hip, and wrist (Sellami et al 2006). Financial barriers, long working hours, and/or lack of transport to exercise facilities limit opportunities for exercise among sedentary low-income expatriates. In nearby Iran, poverty is associated with low bone density among women (Amiri et al 2008); this might not be the case in wealthy Arab countries and further study is needed. In Beirut, Lebanon, hip fracture patients were younger and mortality higher than in Western countries (Hreybe et al 2004).

Not surprisingly, in the Gulf countries hip fractures are as frequent or more so than in Western countries, with an incidence of about 3 per 1000 population per year for females 50 years and older and 2 per 1000 for their male counterparts among both Kuwaiti nationals and expatriates (Memon et al 1998). Such fractures were also more frequent than in nearby Asian countries such as Iran, where the incidence was about 1 per 1000 for both females and males (Moayyeri et al 2006). In Lebanon, incidence was about 1.7 per 1000 for females and 1.0 for males (Sibai et al 2011). In Rabat, Morocco, it was about 0.5 per 1000, greater than in Sub-Saharan Africa and less than Europe and North America (El Maghraoui et al 2005).

Occupational injuries (see also Chapter 22). Migrant workers in rapidly developing Gulf countries are at much greater risk of falls from considerable heights, falling objects, and machinery injuries than would be expected in more developed countries (Barss et al 2008b). Heat injury is another serious issue affecting migrant workers in the hotter countries. Some are recruited from cold mountainous regions, such as in Nepal, and may arrive un-acclimatized in the hot season. Risks of heat stroke are exacerbated by insufficient drinking water and lack of air-conditioned cool-down shacks at construction sites. In Lebanon, costs per occupational injury were highest for falls and vehicle crashes (Fayad et al 2003). Falls and falling objects were of concern; differences in epidemiology and limitations of access to care by nationality were observed (Nuwayhid et al 2003). Safety inspectors are few in number and hence consistent enforcement of penalties for violations is not feasible, except perhaps for the most egregious incidents with many casualties.

Child labor and associated injuries are an issue in many low- and middle-income countries. In Yemen, according to a 1999 labor force survey, there were over 300,000 unpaid and paid child workers 6–14 years old, mainly in agriculture but also in various workshops and other sites (Central Statistical Organization 2004). In Morocco, the prevalence of child workers ranged from 2% in the richest families to 17% in the poorest (Ministère de la Santé 2008). Even in Lebanon, working children 10–17 years old sustain brain damage by toxic solvents in workshops for spray painting and mechanical work (Saddik et al 2009, 2005).

Intentional Injury

Intentional injury includes political violence both structural and reactive, war, torture, and so-called "honor" killings as well as abuse, homicide, and self-harm in the form of suicide and parasuicide. It should also include injury of workers if employers knowingly neglect elemental safety precautions to protect the vulnerable. The greatest number of publications on all unintentional and intentional injuries in the Arab World concern self-harm, post-traumatic stress disorder (PTSD), and estimates of war, invasion, and occupation related injuries, especially in Iraq and Palestine. Elsewhere, even when war was absent, the effects of political violence such as torture were evident in publications on refugees living in foreign countries. Evidence is reviewed in three categories.

War and political violence. Chapters in Section V examine the tragic consequences of political violence in Iraq, Lebanon, and the OPT. A focused overview is provided here to complete the portrait of injury epidemiology in the Arab world.

Although the high burden of war and violence is well-acknowledged in the region, true injury mortality could be much worse than reported by official sources, sometimes by a factor of 10 to 1 or greater (Garfield & Diaz 2007, Tapp et al 2008). Field surveys with widely disparate estimates illustrate difficulties in choosing appropriate cluster sampling methodology when data collectors face extreme risks. Following the 2003 Iraq invasion and occupation, Burnham et al (2006) estimated a violence mortality rate of about 700 per 100,000 per year, about 2.5% of the population in study areas. In contrast the Iraq Family Health Survey Study Group (2008) estimated the figure at 170 per 100,000. Differences between these rates have been discussed extensively, with politics sometimes dictating science. It has been stated that the total mortality is similar for the two surveys. The Burnham survey reportedly determined a much greater proportion of deaths to be due to violence and the IFHSS survey more to other causes including unintentional injuries such as RTIs. Fearing reprisal, families were allegedly reluctant to declare deaths as violent. In any event, the high level of casualties, especially women and children, during the post-invasion occupation was unprecedented for US occupations, with killing reportedly at greater levels than in any other conflict during the past century (Garfield & Diaz 2007). The large number of deaths of women and child civilians was attributed mainly to targeting of air attacks and mortars to residential neighborhoods. The data support that these civilian lethal weapons should be prohibited in such locations under international humanitarian law (Hicks et al 2009). War and occupation have not been the only killers of civilians. Between the 1991 and 2003 invasions of Iraq, about 500,000 excess deaths of Iraqi children were attributed to economic sanctions.

In Darfur, Sudan, mortality field surveys estimated about 9000 violent deaths per 100,000 per year during a seven-month period of 2003–2004, with an additional 4500 per 100,000 mainly from other related causes (Degomme & Guha-Sapir 2010). This equates to more than 1 death for every 10 people, compared with the 1 per 40 noted above for Iraq.

War and occupation leave physical and psychological impairments, disabilities, and handicaps, sowing the seeds of future conflict. Deeply disturbed children and adults live on with long term chronic effects such as PTSD, domestic violence, and suicide (Al-Adili et al 2008, Thabet et al 2009, Elbedour et al 2007, Masmas et al 2008, Montgomery 2010, 1998). In the OPT, the odds ratio for PTSD in persons exposed to armed conflict, compared with the unexposed, was 10, while in Algeria the odds ratio for anxiety disorders was 2 (de Jong et al 2003).

Although less frequent than mental trauma, the impact of physical injuries is nonetheless severe on children, women, and older people, not to mention many young men. The leading cause of fatal injury in children and youth 0–19 in the OPT during 2001–2003 was firearms, with an annual incidence of 10 deaths per 100,000 population (Shaheen & Edwards 2008). Prior to the start of the intifada uprising against occupation in 2000, most violent injuries involved blunt trauma to men. However, during the intifada period, 12–25% of victims were school children, 10% persons over 50, and 5–9% women; 65% resulted from firearms or explosives (Helweg-Larsen et al 2004, Halileh 2002). Among children, most wounds were from firearms and involved the head, including brain and eye. Hospital contacts for intentional injury rose from 23 during 3 months prior to the intifada to 740 and 199 during the first and second phases of the uprising. During the 1996 attack by the occupiers on southern Lebanon, many young people were injured in the streets or hiding in open shelters, and about 50% of injuries, especially of lower limbs, resulted in impairments (Mehio Sibai et al 2000). Among injured students, 29% failed to complete their schooling, and among the employed, 42% lost their jobs with no possibility of return for 34%. Moreover, many children have been affected by physical violence during the post-war occupation of Iraq. In Baghdad, among children 16 and under presenting to hospital with such trauma, 54% were 11 or less years of age and 24% were girls (Al-Anbaki et al 2008). Fragmentation weapons causing blast injuries accounted for 80% of the injured and gunshot wounds 20%.

It is noteworthy that with political violence at extreme levels in some countries, it is not always feasible to separate the effects of war from those of other intentional injuries such as spousal and child abuse. High levels of financial stress, structural violence, and disruption of families by war have created refugees on a massive scale and extensive trafficking of women. Since humiliation of children and families under occupation causes severe health effects (Giacaman et al, 2007), it should fall under the category of intentional injury. Similarly, political violence in the OPT doubled the frequency of physical and sexual abuse of domestic partners (Clark et al 2010, Giacaman et al 2010) while the 2006 war in southern Lebanon was associated with an increase in child sexual abuse (Usta & Farver 2010). Such effects should be considered in assessing the overall impact of structural violence.

Although investigation and reporting of torture is seldom feasible, it is believed to be widespread in at least some countries (Abdel Aziz 2007, Afana 2009). Research with refugees from the region casts light upon practices and consequences (Masmas et al 2008, Moisander & Edston 2003). Imprisonment can range from months to years. Reported practices included sensory deprivation, beating, whipping, suspension, electric shock, and falanga or beating of the soles of the feet, sometimes while the victim is immobilized by being pressed into a tyre. Long term disability is prevalent in a majority of survivors, ranging from mental, such as post-traumatic stress and anxiety disorders in 70–90%, to physical, such as chronic pain and difficulty walking in 70% of falanga victims (Amris et al 2009, Edston 2009, Prip and Persson 2008).

Suicide and parasuicide Since suicide is forbidden by Islam, there is undoubtedly underreporting or misreporting as undetermined intent or other violence (Pritchard & Amanullah 2007). Nonetheless a number of reports suggest that completed suicide is less frequent among Muslims. This may not be the case for parasuicide (attempted suicide) (Lester 2006), which deserves greater attention (Daradkeh & Al-Zayer 1988). Intentional burns of women as punishment by husbands have been described from Egypt; when fatal, they may be misreported as suicide (Smith 1998). On the other hand, in Port Said, Egypt, 68% of completed suicides involved males, mainly between 20–30 years of age (Gad ElHak et al 2009). Rodenticide ingestion, drowning, burns, firearms, jumping, drugs, and hanging occurred in decreasing frequency from 25 to 8%.

In the UAE, and likely other Gulf states, completed suicide predominantly occurs among expatriate male workers, although expatriate females are also affected (Ministry of Health, Biannual Reports; Koronfel 2002, Suleiman et al 1986) as a result of disrespect for their basic human rights (Human Rights Watch 2006). Suicidal ideation among such workers is reportedly associated with family and financial problems and lack of a regular annual vacation (Al Haj et al 2008). The profile for nationals tends to be parasuicide among females, often involving overdoses of pharmaceuticals, as reported in Saudi Arabia (Al-Jahdali 2004, Daradkeh & Al-Zayer 1988). In Kuwait, repeaters were found to be less successful in social readjustment with levels of repeated attempts similar to those in Western Europe (Suleiman et al 1989).

In the Gulf, many suicides and parasuicides may be predominantly a response to acute and/or chronic situational difficulties, rather than from mental illness or long-term depression (Al Ansari et al 2001). The relation to dangerous and adverse working conditions, including violations of human rights, means that suicide/parasuicide in such cases cannot simply be attributed to mental illness. Prevention must be considered as an integral element of occupational health and safety.

Acute social/political pressures leading to more suicide may have also prevailed in the OPT during the intifada. Deaths from suicide and other violence were twice as frequent among unmarried women, mainly below 25 years of age, than among the married (Al-Adili et al 2008).

The situation in the Gulf and OPT contrasts with Morocco, where mental disorders were reportedly prevalent among persons with suicidal ideation (Agoub et al 2006). Population based studies are needed, since in Egypt suicidal ideation was reported

among nearly a third of adolescents and parasuicide has increased substantially (Afifi 2004).

Abuse and homicide Chapter 7 examines the issue of gender-based violence in more detail and highlights the importance of domestic abuse in women and political violence in men.

In non-Islamic countries, consumption of alcohol and other drugs by both victims and perpetrators is frequently associated with domestic abuse and other violence. In the Arab world, alcohol and other drugs appear to be a relatively uncommon determinant for interpersonal violence and suicide (Al Madni et al 2008, Shotar & Jaradat 2007).

Population surveys in Egypt found that 18% of married women in 1995 and 19% in 2005 had been physically beaten during the preceding 12 months (Akmatov et al 2008). Of these beatings, 2% were extreme, including strangling/burning or being attacked or threatened with a weapon, and 27% both strong (kicked, dragged, punched) and moderate (pushed, slapped, twisted), 19% mainly moderate, and 52% low. Education among the women was protective, higher greater than secondary, as compared with elementary, but only when the husband was educated. Among low-income married women in Syria, 26% had been physically abused at least three times in the past year (Maziak & Asfar 2003). Education was protective. In the West Bank, Palestinian women with less education were more accepting of wife beating (Dhaher et al 2010). In Lebanon, domestic violence was reported by 35% of women attending primary health centers; 88% was verbal and 66% physical (Usta et al 2007). Familial violence of a parent(s) was a predictor of domestic violence. Exposed women had more physical symptoms. Both women and men were open to speaking about such violence; another study in Lebanon found similar results with the exception of young men recently violent (Khawaja & Tewtel-Salem 2004). Pregnancy is a special time of vulnerability to violence. Among pregnant Palestinian refugees in Lebanon, university but not secondary education was protective against domestic violence (Hammoury et al 2009). In Jordan, pregnant women reported 6 to 24% of violence by husbands and 2 to 14% by other family members, mainly mothers in law (Oweis et al 2010). Unplanned pregnancy and low self-esteem of the woman were predictors. While many studies report the details of violence such as kicking, punching, and burning, few document the actual nature of the resulting injuries.

Fatal beatings would be expected to be underreported in surveys due to absence of the deceased, and a proportion misreported to authorities by the assailant. In a Jordanian refugee camp, actual injuries were more frequently reported by women than their husbands (Khawaja & Barazi 2005). With a lifetime wife beating prevalence of 45%, 10% of women and 3% of men recalled physical injury, with 7% bruises, cuts, scratches, or burns, and 2% miscarriage.

Honor killings are specific crimes against women. While there is much discussion in the media, far too little has been published on the epidemiology and prevention in the public health and medical literature. Researchers may hesitate to work on this sensitive topic. A small study of 16 such deaths in Jordan found that over 60% resulted from multiple gunshot wounds, mainly by a brother of the victim (Hadidi et al 2001). Sentencing varied considerably in severity. In the case of murdered single pregnant females, acquittal or a reduced sentence was usual, whereas for killers of women who had married without family consent, punishment was more severe, up to life imprisonment with hard labor.

Publications on child abuse are also somewhat scarce. Community surveys in Yemen documented that harsh physical punishment was used on more than half of rural and one-quarter of urban school children, with serious negative impact on school performance and psychopathology (Alyahri & Goodman 2008). Risk factors included being a male child, low maternal education, and large family size. The researchers advocated the need for changing prevalent beliefs that children who do wrong must be beaten. In the Gulf, a review based upon case reports suggested that physical abuse of children was more frequent than sexual abuse or neglect in most countries, excepting Bahrain (Al-Mahroos 2007). In the Egyptian city of Mansoura, 76% of deaths from child abuse were perpetrated by males, including 60% who were the father of the victim; 76% of fathers were from rural areas. The other 24% of abusers were women, including 7% who were mothers of victims (El Hak et al 2009). Among victims, 51% had separated parents, 22% married parents, and 27% polygamous families.

Public Health Training and Research Needs for Injury

What is not measured may not attract sufficient attention or resources. Although there are no available staff inventories, anecdotal evidence suggests that public health injury researchers such as injury epidemiologists and practitioners are scarce and do not constitute a necessary critical mass to inform, guide, and advance the injury agenda. Filling such gaps necessitates public funding for capacity building, including educating and training injury research and prevention professionals as well as supporting their work in surveillance, research, and evaluation on priority issues.

Action oriented public health epidemiology and surveillance are essential. Staff and costs should be shared by governments and universities, and especially by organisations with injury prevention programs, all of which require a research basis. Ecological studies comparing countries or regions within a country can shed light on social determinants of injuries, and on whether interventions are effective, or not, in different populations. Such research together with results from outcome based interventions can inform best practices in injury prevention and motivate national and regional governments to address inequities in vulnerability and to adopt proven country wide prevention. Small-scale local and community research can prevent hospitalizations and deaths by environmental study of vehicular hazards around schools, leading to alternative safer traffic environments. Trauma registries, generally oriented to evaluation of treatment, can be enhanced to document external causes including the injury matrix risk factors by pre-event, event and post-event time phases. As for scientific evaluation of specific interventions, the list of Cochrane reviews on injury is growing and should be consulted prior to undertaking new research and when considering interventions. The long-term impact of injuries in terms of impairments, disabilities, handicaps, quality of life, and costs are seldom studied and such research is greatly needed. Cultural issues in understanding traditional beliefs about causality and preventability can be elucidated by social science survey research. The results can guide and promote effective education of the public and of policymakers.

Injury Prevention: From Pre-Event to Post-Event Phases

Since many injuries have a multifactorial etiology, a multisectoral approach to prevention is frequently appropriate. More so for injury than for many other health conditions, prevention depends upon collaborations among public health specialists, governments, education, architects, engineers, economists, politicians, legislators, social scientists, civil society activists, and justice, including police and forensic investigators. Effective and sustainable working networks to bring such diverse constituents together are scarce. Various combinations of countermeasures including design (Pauls 2011), building code revisions, engineering, legislation, enforcement, education, social marketing, and post-trauma systems are needed for specific external causes.

Prevention should be surveillance- and evidence-based, comprehensive in structure, and targeted to personal, vehicle/safety equipment, and environment factors. As for the art and politics of a comprehensive injury policy, it is worth reviewing WHO's Ottawa Charter for Health Promotion as guidance. The approach of promoting safety measures that protect the most vulnerable by minimizing unprotected exposure to kinetic energy, as in school road design with drop-off and pick-up of students directly from sidewalks with safety barriers, is effective because it should protect all – provided that a safe built environment is a funded priority for all schools. In the case of RTI, there is strong research evidence for many interventions as synthesized and summarized in Cochrane injury reviews and in WHO documents from the Injuries and Violence section. Measures to increase the use of safety restraints to above 90% among all vehicle occupants, front and rear, adults and children, could immediately avert 50% of all motor vehicle fatalities and 80% of severe and moderate brain injuries in many Arab countries. As for other priorities such as falls, universal design incorporating safety for homes, public places, and walkways for disadvantaged as well as wealthy neighborhoods offers the possibility of equitable and long-term solutions. Evidence-based safe building codes help to meet this goal. Arab countries need to adopt proven measures, adapting them to local needs while collecting the evidence-base for their effectiveness in national and local contexts. Because the regulatory and enforcement capacities remain weak in most Arab nations, this is a key target for advocacy by public health researchers and practitioners, non-governmental organizations, civil activists, the media, concerned international agencies, donors, and other stakeholders.

The greatest potential for education would be ensuring equitable access to middle and high schools and to higher education for all women as well as men.

The evidence indicates that this would do much to reduce domestic violence, as well as help to protect children from unintentional injuries. Universal national programs of practical swimming training and water safety instruction would help to protect all from immersion deaths. On the other hand, educational measures such as poster campaigns in isolation are short-lived and may not effectively reach those at greatest risk. If used, such campaigns should be carefully piloted and evaluated. Because of the importance of cultural beliefs about vulnerability and preventability, evidence-based education directed to the general public or specific target populations should be carefully developed with local focus groups. The right to safety is especially attractive as a focus for education and mobilization campaigns by non-governmental organizations, civil society and academia. However, such campaigns should always be accompanied by equitable passive measures that ensure long-term safety for all, especially the most vulnerable.

National capacity building should focus on improving the quality of basic injury data, including routine reporting. This will require allocation of resources proportionate to the true burden of injury as assessed not only by valid crude mortality rates, but also by economic indicators of the true costs to communities and countries. Since some of the highest income countries in the world, including the Arab world, have low quality health and injury data, it is not necessarily more resources that are needed but rather reallocation together with capacity building of skilled national and international professionals to use the funds with skill and wisdom for epidemiology and prevention of injury.

International laws and insurance should be developed in such a way as to redress the unjust burden of injury borne by low-income expatriate workers, their families, and countries by ensuring that cost burdens are fairly and humanely met by wealthy employing countries where unsafe worksites and working conditions result in disability or death. Greater respect for international humanitarian law, including holding occupiers financially accountable for loss of life and property is overdue, in order to shift the enormous burden of being occupied from resident populations back to the occupiers. Measures such as safety-oriented legislation, regulations, and enforcement that impose minimum standards, together with passive safety measures to "level up" the safety of the physical environment have the potential to improve the equity of safety (Laflamme et al 2010). For children, this includes provision of secure off-street recreational areas. For adults, safe and enjoyable walking help to ensure adequate bone strength and balance, increasing personal resistance to falls.

On a broader scale, an end to the most egregious exploitations of inequitable societies, including occupations and national governments mainly sustained to serve foreign interests, is essential to deliver safety and indeed health to all, including the most vulnerable. A prevention approach that considers broader determinants such as failures of state agencies and contractors in the case of RTI is essential. Identifying structural determinants can be a means of discerning accountability of responsible parties by all available measures, including litigation, and provides a key to injury prevention. The very word "injury" hails from its early Latin roots *in juris*, i.e., "not right", "not lawful", "not just". Empowered by open communication networks, the combined pressures of public health researchers and practitioners, other professionals, activists, and most of all concerned citizens are driving long overdue change.

Acknowledgments

Thanks to Terri Everest, English lecturer, for expert review of drafts of this chapter.

References

Abdel Aziz BM (2007) Torture in Egypt. *Torture*, 17(1): 48–52

Abou-Raya S, ElMeguid LA (2009) Road traffic accidents and the elderly. *Geriatrics & Gerontology International*, 9(3): 290–297

Afana AH (2009) Weeping in silence: The secret sham of torture among Palestinian children. *Torture*, 19: 167–175

Afifi M (2004) Depression, aggression and suicidal ideation among adolescents in Alexandria. *Neurosciences*, 9: 207–213

Afifi M (2009) Wealth index association with gender issues and the reproductive health of Egyptian women. *Nursing & Health Sciences*, 11(1): 29–36

Agoub M, Moussaoui D, Kadri N (2006) Assessment of suicidality in a Moroccan metropolitan area. *Journal of Affective Disorders*, 90: 223–226

Akmatov MK, Mikolajczyk RT, Labeeb S, Dhaher E, Khan MM (2008) Factors associated with wife beating in Egypt: Analysis of two surveys (1995 and 2005). *BMC Women's Health*, 18: 15

Al-Adili N, Shaheen M, Bergström S, Johansson A (2008) Deaths among young, single women in 2000–2001 in the West Bank, Palestinian Occupied Territories. *Reproductive Health Matters*, 16(31): 112–121

Al-Anbaki D, Meyer F, Edan A, Lippert H (2008) The spectrum of war-like injuries in children and teenagers during a post-war wave of violence in Iraq (in German). *Zentralblatt für Chirurgie*, 133(3): 306–309

Al Ansari AM, Hamadeh RR, Matar AM, Marhoon H, Buzaboon BY, Raees AG (2001) Risk factors associated with overdose among Bahraini youth. *Suicide & Life-Threatening Behavior*, 2001; 31: 197–206

Al Belooshi SH, Al-Hosani SM, Al-Yamahi AR, Al-Zaabi MR, Barss P, Grivna M (2006) What are the real causes of death in the United Arab Emirates? *Emirates Medical Journal*, 24: 181–182

Al Haj EA, Al-Sharahan RY, Al-Kaabi KS, Khonji DM (2008) Prevalence of anxiety, depression, and suicidal behaviour among residents of labor camps in Al Ain city, UAE (Community Medicine Clerkship Report). Al Ain, UAE: Department of Community Medicine, Faculty of Medicine & Health Sciences, pp. 1–10.

Ali Aba Hussein N, El-Zobeir AK (2007) Road traffic knowledge and behaviour of drivers in the Eastern Province of Saudi Arabia (in Arabic). *Eastern Mediterranean Health Journal*, 13(2): 364–375

Al-Jadid MS, Al-Asmari AK, Al-Moutaery KR (2004) Quality of life in males with spinal cord injury in Saudi Arabia. *Saudi Medical Journal*, 25(12): 1979–1985

Al-Jahdali H, Al-Johani A, Al-Hakawi A, et al (2004) Pattern and risk factors for intentional drug overdose in Saudi Arabia. *Canadian Journal of Psychiatry*, 49: 331–334

Allali F, El Aichaoui S, Saoud B, Maaroufi H, Abouqal R, Hajjaj-Hassouni N (2006) The impact of clothing style on bone mineral density among post menopausal women in Morocco: a case-control study. *BMC Public Health*, 19:6: 135

Al Madni OM, Kharoshah MA, Zaki MK, Ghaleb SS (2010) Hanging deaths in Dammam, Kingdom of Saudi Arabia. *Journal of Forensic and Legal Medicine*, 17: 265–8

Al Madni O, Kharosha MA, Shotar AM (2008) Firearm fatalities in Dammam, Saudi Arabia. *Medicine, Science and the Law*, 48: 237–40

Al-Mahroos FT (2007) Child abuse and neglect in the Arab Peninsula. *Saudi Medical Journal*, 28(2): 241–248

Al-Nouri L, Al-Isami S (2006) Baby walker injuries. *Annals of Tropical Paediatrics*, 26(1): 67–71

Al-Shammari N, Bendak S, Al-Gadhi S (2009) In-depth analysis of pedestrian crashes in Riyadh. *Traffic Injury Prevention*, 10(6): 552–559

Alyahri A, Goodman R (2008) Harsh corporal punishment of Yemeni children: occurrence, type and associations. *Child Abuse & Neglect*, 32(8): 766–73

Amiri M, Nabipour I, Larijani B, et al (2008) The relationship of absolute poverty and bone mineral density in postmenopausal Iranian women. *International Journal of Public Health*, 53(6): 290–296

Amris K, Torp-Pedersen S, Rasmussen OV (2009) Long-term consequences of falanga torture. What do we know and what do we need to know? *Torture*, 19(1): 33–40

Ansari S, Akhdar F, Mandoorah M, Moutaery K (2000) Causes and effects of road traffic accidents in Saudi Arabia. *Public Health*, 114(1): 37–9

Ashar A, Kovacs A, Khan S, Hakim J (1998) Blindness associated with midfacial fractures. *Journal of Oral Maxillofacial Surgery*, 56(10): 1146–50; discussion 1151

Bahloul M, Chelly H, Gargouri R, et al (2009) Traumatic head injury in children in south Tunisia epidemiology, clinical manifestations and evolution. 454 cases (in French). La Tunisie Medicale, 87(1): 28–37

Bahloul M, Chelly H, Ben Hmida M, et al (2004) Prognosis of traumatic head injury in South Tunisia: a multivariate analysis of 437 cases. *Journal of Trauma*, 57(2): 255–61

Bar-Joseph N, Rennert G, Tamir A, Ore L, Bar-Joseph G (2007) Ethnic differences in the epidemiological characteristics of severe trauma due to falls from heights among children in northern Israel. *Israel Medical Association Journal*, 9: 603–606

Barss P, Addley K, Grivna M, Stanculescu C, Abu-Zidan F (2009a) Occupational Injury in the United Arab Emirates: Epidemiology and Prevention. *Occupational Medicine*, 59(7): 493–8

Barss P, Al-Darmaki MH, Al-Saqqaf AM, Al-Jenaibi, Grivna M, Al Maskari F (2007) Knowledge of swimming pool safety among vendors and home pool owners and provision of safety devices and

information by vendors in United Arab Emirates. World Water Safety Conference, Porto, Portugal, Conference Abstract Book, September 2007

Barss P, Al-Obthani M, Al-Hammadi A, Al-Shamsi H, El-Sadig M, Grivna M (2008a) Prevalence and Issues in Non-Use of Safety Belts and Child Restraints in a Desert City in the United Arab Emirates. *Traffic Injury Prevention*, 9: 256–263

Barss P, Grivna M, Subait O, Al-Kuwaiti A, Al-Kuwaiti M, Al-Rahoomi A (2008b) Epidemiology of Falls In a High-Income Middle Eastern Country: An Emergency Department Interview Survey. 3rd Australian & New Zealand Falls Prevention Conference Program and Abstracts. Melbourne, October 2008, p. 54

Barss P, Musaab A, Nassar A, Helal I, Karami A. Grivna M (2008c) Epidemiology and Prevention of Drowning in Coastal Cities of a High-Income Middle Eastern Country. Hanoi, Vietnam: 2nd Asia-Pacific Conference on Injury Prevention, November 2008, Ministry of Health of Vietnam, Conference Abstract Book, p. 62

Barss P, Smith GS, Baker SP, Mohan D (1998) Injury Prevention: An International Perspective. Epidemiology, Surveillance, & Policy. New York: Oxford University Press, pp. 12–25, 26–49, 219–232, 245–264

Barss P, Subait OM, Al Ali MH, Grivna M (2009b) Drowning in a high-income developing country: newspapers as an essential resource for injury surveillance. *Journal of Science & Medicine in Sport*, 12: 164–170

Bashour H, Kharouf M (2008) Community-based study of unintentional injuries among preschool children in Damascus. *Eastern Mediterranean Health Journal*, 14: 398–405

Bendak S (2005) Seat belt utilization in Saudi Arabia and its impact on road

accident injuries. *Accident, Analysis & Prevention*, 37: 367–71

Bouguila J, Zairi I, Khonsari RH, Lankriet C, Mokhtar M, Adouani A (2009) Mandibular fracture: a 10-year review of 685 cases treated in Charles-Nicolle Hospital (Tunis-Tunisia) (in French). *Revue de stomatologie et de chirurgie maxillo-faciale*, 110(2): 81–5

Bubshait D, Sadat-Ali M (2007) Economic implications of osteoporosis-related femoral fractures in Saudi Arabian Society. *Calcified Tissue International*, 81: 455–458

Burnham G, Lafta R, Doocy S, Roberts L (2006) Mortality after the 2003 invasion of Iraq: a cross-sectional cluster sample survey. *Lancet*, 368 (9545): 1421–1428

Central Statistical Organisation (2004) Statistical Year Book 2003, Tables 11, 12, pp. 78–79. Available at http://www.cso-yemen.org/books/stat_book_2003.pdf (Accessed 18 May 2010)

Clark CJ, Everson-Rose SA, Suglia SF, Btoush R, Alonso A, Haj-Yahia MM (2010) Association between exposure to political violence and intimate-partner violence in the occupied Palestinian territory: a cross-sectional study. *Lancet*, 375: 310–16

Crankson SJ (2006) Motor vehicle injuries in childhood: a hospital-based study in Saudi Arabia. *Pediatric Surgery International*, 22 (8): 641–5

Cubbin C, Smith GS (2002) Socioeconomic inequalities in injury: critical issues in design and analysis. *Annual Review of Public Health*, 23: 349–75

Cubbin C, LeClere FB, Smith GS (2000) Socioeconomic status and the occurrence of fatal and nonfatal injury in the United States. *American Journal of Public Health*, 90(1): 70–7

Daradkeh TK, Al-Zayer N (1988) Parasuicide in an Arab industrial community: the Arabian-American Oil Company experience, Saudi Arabia. *Acta psychiatrica Scandinavica*, 77: 707–711

Degomme O, Guha-Sapir D (2010) Patterns of mortality rates in Darfur conflict. *Lancet*, 375: 294–300

de Jong JT, Komproe IH, Van Ommeren M (2003) Common mental disorders in postconflict settings. *Lancet*, 361(9375): 2128–30

Dhaher EA, Mikolajczyk RT, Maxwell AE, Krämer A (2010) Attitudes Toward Wife Beating Among Palestinian Women of Reproductive Age From Three Cities in West Bank. *Journal of Interpersonal Violence*, 25: 518–537

Edston E (2009) The epidemiology of falanga–incidence among Swedish asylum seekers. *Torture*, 19: 27–32

Elbedour S, Onwuegbuzie AJ, Ghannam J, Whitcome JA, Abu Hein F (2007) Post-traumatic stress disorder, depression, and anxiety among Gaza Strip adolescents in the wake of the second Uprising (Intifada). *Child Abuse and Neglect*, 31(7): 719–29

El-Hak SA, Ali MA, El-Atta HM (2009) Child deaths from family violence in Dakahlia and Damiatta Governorates, Egypt. *Journal of Forensic and Legal Medicine*, 16(7): 388–91

El Hamaoui Y, Yaalaoui S, Chihabeddine K, Boukind E, Moussaoui D (2002) Post-traumatic stress disorder in burned patients. *Burns*, 28(7): 647–50

El Hamaoui Y, Yaalaoui S, Chihabeddine K, Boukind E, Moussaoui D (2006) Depression in mothers of burned children. *Archives of Women's Mental Health*, 9(3): 117–9

El Maghraoui A, Ghazi M, Gassim S, et al (2010) Risk factors of osteoporosis in healthy Moroccan men. *BMC Musculoskeletal Disorders*, 11: 148

El Maghraoui A, Koumba BA, Jroundi I, Achemlal L, Bezza A, Tazi MA (2005) Epidemiology of hip fractures in 2002 in Rabat, Morocco. *Osteoporosis International*, 16(6): 597–602

El-Sadig M, Norman JN, Lloyd OL, Romilly P, Bener A (2002) Road traffic accidents in United Arab Emirates: trends of morbidity and mortality during 1977–1998. *Accident, Analysis & Prevention*, 34: 465–476

Fayad R, Nuwayhid I, Tamim H, Kassak K, Khogali M (2003) Cost of work-related injuries in insured workplaces in Lebanon. *Bulletin of the World Health Organization*, 81(7): 509–16

Gad ElHak SA, El-Ghazali AM, Salama MM, Aboelyazeed AY (2009) Fatal suicide cases in Port Said city, Egypt. *Journal of Forensic and Legal Medicine*, 16(5): 266–8

Garfield R, Diaz J (2007) Epidemiologic impact of invasion and post-invasion conflict in Iraq. *Bioscience Trends*, 1(1): 10–5

Ghribi F, Ouali F, Bouchaala H (2003) Children's accidents in rural environment: study of 324 cases (in French). *La Tunisie Medicale*, 81(2): 86–93

Giacaman R, Abu-Rmeileh NME, Husseini A, Saab H, Boyce W (2007) Humiliation: the invisible trauma of war for Palestinian youth. *Public Health*, 121: 563–571

Giacaman R, Rabaia Y, Nguyen-Gillham V (2010) Domestic and political violence: the Palestinian predicament. *Lancet*, 375: 259–260

Grivna M, Barss P, Al-Dhabab A, Hanaee A, Al-Kaabi F, Al-Muhairi S (2008) Babywalkers in the United Arab Emirates: A survey among female high school students of prevalence, injuries, and knowledge. 9th World Conference on Injury Prevention and Safety Promotion, Merida, Mexico, March 2008, Conference Abstract Book, Abstract number 592, pp. 216–217

Haddon W (1980) Advances in the epidemiology of injuries as a basis for public policy. *Public Health Reports*, 95: 411–21

Hadidi M, Kulwicki A, Jahshan H (2001) A review of 16 cases of honour killings in Jordan in 1995. *International Journal of Legal Medicine*, 114(6): 357–9

Halileh SO, Daoud AR, Khatib RA, Mikki-Samarah NS (2002) The impact of the intifada on the health of a nation. *Medicine Conflict and Survival*, 18(3): 239–48

HAAD (Health Authority of Abu Dhabi) (2008) Causes of death 2007. In: Annual statistical report. Abu Dhabi, UAE, 2008, pp. 8, 12

Hammoury N, Khawaja M, Mahfoud Z, Afifi RA, Madi H (2009) Domestic violence against women during pregnancy: the case of Palestinian refugees attending an antenatal clinic in Lebanon. *Journal of Women's Health*, 18: 337–45

Helweg-Larsen K, Abdel-Jabbar Al-Qadi AH, Al-Jabriri J, Brønnum-Hansen H (2004) Systematic medical data collection of intentional injuries during armed conflicts: a pilot study conducted in West Bank, Palestine. *Scandinavian Journal of Public Health*, 32(1): 17–23

Hicks MH, Dardagan H, Guerrero Serdán G, Bagnall PM, Sloboda JA, Spagat M (2009) The weapons that kill civilians–deaths of children and noncombatants in Iraq, 2003–2008. *New England Journal of Medicine*, 360(16): 1585–8

Hijazi OM, Shahin AA, Haidar NA, Sarwi MF, Musawa ES (2007) Effect of submersion injury on water safety practice after the event in children, Saudi Arabia. *Saudi Medical Journal*, 28: 100–104

Hreybe H, Salamoun M, Badra M, et al (2004) Hip fractures in Lebanese patients: determinants and prognosis. *Journal of Clinical Densitometry*, 7(4): 368–75

Human Rights Watch (2006) United Arab Emirates. Building Towers, Cheating Workers. Exploitation of Migrant Construction

Workers in the United Arab Emirates. 18(8E): 1–71

Iraq Family Health Survey Study Group (2008) Violence-Related Mortality in Iraq from 2002 to 2006. *New England Journal of Medicine*, 358: 484–493

Ittai S, Gad B, Naim S, Davi F, Vardit J, Moshe R (2000) Hospitalizations due to falls in Jewish and Arab children in northern Israel. *European Journal of Epidemiology*, 16: 47–52

Jan MM, Hasanain FH, Al-Dabbagh AA (2000) Infant and child safety practices of parents. *Saudi Medical Journal*, 21: 1142–6

Kadri N, Berrada S, Douab S, Tazi I, Moussaoui D (2006) Post-traumatic stress disorder in survivors of the Agadir earthquake (Morocco) in 1960 (in French). *L' Encéphale*, 32: 215–221

Khawaja M, Barazi R (2005) Prevalence of wife beating in Jordanian refugee camps: reports by men and women. *Journal of Epidemiology & Community Health*, 59(10): 840–1

Khawaja M, Tewtel-Salem M (2004) Agreement between husband and wife reports of domestic violence: evidence from poor refugee communities in Lebanon. *International Journal of Epidemiology*, 33(3): 526–33

Koronfel AA (2002) Suicide in Dubai, United Arab Emirates. *Journal of Clinical Forensic Medicine*, 9: 5–11

Koushki PA, Bustan MA, Kartam N (2003) Impact of safety belt use on road accident injury and injury type in Kuwait. *Accident; Analysis & Prevention*, 35(2): 237–41

Laflamme L, Hasselberg M, Burrows S (2010) 20 Years of Research on Socioeconomic Inequality and Children's Unintentional Injuries – Understanding the Cause-Specific Evidence at Hand. *International Journal of Pediatrics*, pii: 819687. Epub 2010 Jul 25

Lester D. (2006) Suicide and Islam. *Archives of Suicide Research*, 10(1): 77–97

Maalouf G, Gannagé-Yared MH, Ezzedine J, et al (2007) Middle East and North Africa consensus on osteoporosis. *Journal of musculoskeletak Neuronal Interactions*. 7(2): 131–43

Mabrouk A, El Badawy A, Sherif M (2000) Kerosene stove as a cause of burns admitted to the Ain Shams burn unit. *Burns*, 26(5): 474–7

Masmas TN, Møller E, Buhmannr C, et al (2008) Asylum seekers in Denmark–a study of health status and grade of traumatization of newly arrived asylum seekers. *Torture*, 18(2): 77–86

Maziak W, Asfar T (2003) Physical abuse in low-income women in Aleppo, Syria. *Health Care for Women International*, 24: 313–26

Maziak W, Ward KD, Rastam S (2006) Injuries in Aleppo, Syria; first population-based estimates and characterization of predominant types. *BMC Public Health*, 6: 63

McIlvenny S, Al Mahrouqi F, Al Busaidi T, et al (2004) Rear seat belt use as an indicator of safe road behaviour in a rapidly developing country. *Journal of the Royal Society for the promotion of Health*, 124: 280–3

Mehio Sibai A, Sameer Shaar N, el-Yassir S (2000) Impairments, disabilities and needs assessment among non-fatal war injuries in south Lebanon, Grapes of Wrath, 1996. *Journal of Epidemiology & Community Health*, 54(1): 35–39

Memon A, Pospula WM, Tantawy AY, Abdul-Ghafar S, Suresh A, Al-Rowaih A (1998) Incidence of hip fracture in Kuwait. *International Journal of Epidemiology*, 27: 860–865

Ministère de la Santé (2008) Le travail des enfants, Tableau 5.4. In: Ministère de la Santé, Royaume du Maroc. Enquête Nationale à Indicateurs Multiples et Santé des Jeunes (ENIMSJ) 2006–2007, 2008, p 48. At URL: http://www.childinfo.org/files/ENIMSJ__Morocco_FinalReport_2006_Fr.pdf (Accessed 18 May 2010)

Ministry of Health. Annual Report 2002. Abu Dhabi, UAE: 2004, pp. 38–39.

Moayyeri A, Soltani A, Larijani B, Naghavi M, Alaeddini F, Abolhassani F (2006) Epidemiology of hip fracture in Iran; results from the Iranian Multicenter Study on Accidental Injuries. *Osteoporosis International*, 17: 1252–1257

Moisander PA, Edston E (2003) Torture and its sequel–a comparison between victims from six countries. *Forensic Science International*, 26; 137(2–3): 133–40

Montgomery E (2010) Trauma and resilience in young refugees: A 9-year follow-up study. *Development and Psychopathology*,22: 477–489

Montgomery E (1998) Refugee children from the Middle East. *Scandinavian Journal of Social Medicine*, 54 (supplement): 1–152

Munk MD, Carboneau DM, Hardan M, Ali FM (2008) Seatbelt use in Qatar in association with severe injuries and death in the prehospital setting. *Prehospital & Disaster Medicine*, 23(6): 547–52

NHTSA (National Highway Traffic Safety Administration) (1996) Third Report to Congress: Effectiveness of Occupant Protection Systems and Their Use. Washington, D. C. 20590 U.S. from www.nhtsa.dot.gov/people/injury/airbags/208con2e.html. (Accessed June 2010)

Nuwayhid I, Fayad R, Tamim H, Kassak K, Khogali M (2003) Work-related injuries in Lebanon: does nationality make a difference? *American Journal of Industrial Medicine*, 44(2): 172–81

Oikarinen K, Schutz P, Thalib L, et al (2004) Differences in the etiology of mandibular fractures in Kuwait, Canada, and Finland. *Dental Traumatology*, 20(5): 241–245

Oweis A, Gharaibeh M, Alhourani R (2010) Prevalence of violence during pregnancy: Findings from a Jordanian survey. *Maternal and Child Health Journal*, 14(3): 437–445

Pauls JL (2011) Checklist for Stairways, Especially for Homes. At URL: http://web.me.com/bldguse/Site/Checklist_for_Stairways.html (Accessed 2 February 2011)

Peltonen K, Punamäki RL (2010) Preventive interventions among children exposed to trauma of armed conflict: a literature review. *Aggressive Behavior*, 36(2): 95–116

Prip K, Persson AL (2008) Clinical findings in men with chronic pain after falanga torture. *Clinical Journal of Pain*, 24(2): 135–41

Pritchard C, Amanulla S (2007) An analysis of suicide and undetermined death in 17 predominantly Islamic countries contrasted with the UK. *Psychological Medicine*, 37: 421–30

Punamäki RL, Qouta SR, El Sarraj E (2010) Nature of torture, PTSD, and somatic symptoms among political ex-prisoners. *Journal of Traumatic Stress*, 23(4): 532–6

Qouta S, Odeb J (2005) The impact of conflict on children: the Palestinian experience. *Journal of Ambulatory Care Management*, 28: 75–79

Qouta S, Punamäki RL, Miller T, El-Sarraj E (2008) Does war beget child aggression? Military violence, gender, age and aggressive behavior in two Palestinian samples. *Aggressive Behavior*, 34(3): 231–44

Rodgers SE, Jones SJ, Macey SM, Lyons RA (2010) Using geographical information systems to assess the equitable distribution of traffic-calming measures: translational research. *Injury Prevention*, 16(1): 7–11

Rosenthal S (2008) Engels and the WHO Report. Dissident Voice 2008; September 2nd:1–7. Available at http://dissidentvoice.org/2008/09/engels-and-the-who-report. (Accessed 26 April 2010)

Sadat-Ali M, AlElq A (2006) Osteoporosis among male Saudi Arabs: A pilot study. *Annals of Saudi Medicine*, 26: 450–4

Saddik B, Williamson A, Black D, Nuwayhid I (2009)

Neurobehavioral impairment in children occupationally exposed to mixed organic solvents. *Neurotoxicology*, 30(6): 1166–71

Sellami S, Sahli H, Meddeb N, et al (2006) Prevalence of osteoporotic fractures in Tunisian women (in French). *Revue de chirurgie orthopédique et réparatrice de l'appareil moteur*, 92(5): 490–4

Shaheen A, Edwards P (2008) Flying bullets and speeding cars: analysis of child injury deaths in the Palestinian Territory. *Eastern Mediterranean Health Journal*, 14(2): 406–14

Shotar AM, Jaradat S (2007) A study of wound fatalities in the north of Jordan. *Medicine, Science, and the Law*, 47(3): 239–43

Shukri AA, Bersnev VP, Riabukha NP (2006) The epidemiology of brain injury and the organization of health care to victims in Aden (Yemen) (in Russian). *Zhurnal voprosy neĭrokhirurgii imeni N. N. Burdenko*, (2): 40–2; discussion 42

Sibai AM, Nasser W, Ammar W, Khalife MJ, Harb H, Fuleihan GE (2011) Hip fracture incidence in Lebanon: a national registry-based study with reference to standardized rates worldwide. *Osteoporosis International*, 22(9): 2499–506

Smith S (1998) Treating burns as if gender mattered. *Links*, 3

Suleiman MA, Moussa MA, el-Islam MF (1989) The profile of parasuicide repeaters in Kuwait. *International Journal of Social Psychiatry*, 35: 146–155

Suleiman MA, Nashef AA, Moussa MA, el-Islam MF (1986) Psychosocial profile of the parasuicidal patient in Kuwait. *International Journal of Social Psychiatry*, 32: 16–22

Talaat M, Kandeel A, El-Shoubary W, et al (2003) Occupational exposure to needlestick injuries and hepatitis B vaccination coverage among health care workers in Egypt. *American Journal of Infection Control*, 31(8): 469–74

Tapp C, Burkle FM Jr, Wilson K, et al (2008) Iraq War mortality

estimates: a systematic review. *Conflict & Health*, 2: 1

Thabet AA, Abed Y, Vostanis P (2002) Emotional problems in Palestinian children living in a war zone: a cross-sectional study. *Lancet*, 359: 1801–1804

Thabet AA, Ibraheem AN, Shivram R, Winter EA, Vostanis P (2009) Parenting support and PTSD in children of a war zone. *International Journal of Social Psychiatry*, 55(3): 226–37

Thabet AA, Matar S, Carpintero A, Bankart J, Vostanis P (2011) Mental health problems among labour children in the Gaza Strip. *Child Care Health and Development*, 37(1): 89–95

Usta J, Farver J (2010) Child sexual abuse in Lebanon during war and peace. *Child: Care, Health, & Development*, 36(3): 361–8

Usta J, Farver JA, Pashayan N (2007) Domestic violence: the Lebanese experience. *Public Health*, 121: 208–19

WHO (World Health Organization) (1986) Ottawa charter for health promotion. *Canadian Journal of Public Health*, 77: 425–430 (see also 384–443)

WHO (2008) The Global Burden of Disease – 2004 update. Geneva: WHO

WHO (2008) Global Burden of Disease and Injury. Country Specific Data 2004 update. 2008. At URL: http://www.who.int/healthinfo/global_burden_disease/estimates_country/en/index.html (Accessed 09/2010)

WHO (2008) World report on child injury prevention. Geneva: WHO, pp 164–167

WHO (2009) Global status report on road safety. Geneva: WHO

WHO (2009) World Health Statistics 2009. Geneva: WHO, pp 47–57

WHO EMRO (World Health Organization Regional Office for the Eastern Mediterranean) (2010) Eastern Mediterranean Status Report on Road Safety. Cairo, Egypt: WHO EMRO

Chapter

17

Child Health: Caring for the Future

Sherine Shawky, Rouham Yamout, Samia Halileh, and Mohamed E. Salem

Child health and early development are crucial for health across the lifespan, with social and economic circumstances playing an important role as emphasized by WHO's Commission on the Social Determinants of Health (CSDH 2008). There is strong evidence from the Arab world, as from other regions, that factors such as poverty (Jahan 2008), parental education (Gakidou et al 2010), place of residence (El-Mouzan et al 2010), social support, and mothers' empowerment (Myntti 1993) greatly influence child well-being. These factors operate long before the child comes to the world, and their consequences extend beyond childhood, as the person's physical and mental well-being take roots in the conditions of his/her childhood (Irwin et al 2007). Therefore, healthy and thriving children are signs of a nation's development. This explains why, of the eight Millennium Development Goals (MDGs), six have targets concerning child health.

Children comprise a large proportion of the population in the region. In the 1980s, more than 77 million were under the age of 15; this number has increased to over 100 million in the 1990s and around 130 million in 2010 (UNICEF 2009a). The harmonious development of children is an important stake for the future. However, governments and international donors mostly focus on MDG indicators with scattered attention to other components of child development. Where child health programs exist, they tend to be bio-medical in focus, with scant attention to social determinants and do not seem to decrease the disparities in child health between and within countries. In several countries, political tensions and violent conflicts hinder the implementation of child health policies and undermine children's future opportunities.

In this chapter, we present a comparative overview of child health status, using widely available indicators.

We then consider some of the key intermediate and structural determinants of children's health with special attention to child health systems and policies. We conclude by suggesting options for addressing current challenges and shaping future public health action.

Child Health Status

Child health-specific MDGs targets include reducing under-5 mortality rate (U5MR) and infant mortality rate (IMR) (MDG 4), increasing measles immunization coverage (MDG 4), and reducing child underweight as part of poverty reduction (MDG 1). In this section, we review corresponding indicators and supplement this with a review of child morbidity and mental health, while focusing on exploring the dynamics of cross-country health inequities. We use data from the UNICEF State of the World's Children report (2009a) unless indicated otherwise.

Child Survival

The U5MR is the most important indicator of the state of a nation's children; its reduction is the measure of progress toward the satisfaction of populations' essential needs. Notwithstanding the known under-reporting of child deaths in the region, countries have made important progress in reducing U5MR. The regional average U5MR decreased from 243 per 1000 live births in 1960 to 69 in 1990 and 47 in 2008. Nevertheless, this average remains seven-fold higher than the corresponding rate in industrialized countries. This unacceptable regional underachievement is partly due to large disparities between countries; U5MR ranges from 200/1000 live births in Somalia to 8/1000 live births in United Arab Emirates (UAE). While Somalia, Mauritania, Sudan, Comoros, and Djibouti are among the 20% worst achievers in the world, the wealthiest countries compete with

---

industrialized ones. Much of the regional improvement seems to be due to spectacular declines in some countries, such as the 74% decline in U5MR in Egypt between 1990 and 2008 while the lowest-income countries display the least progress (Table 1). Infant mortality accounts for 70% of under-5 mortality, with the poorest countries bearing the largest burdens; in Somalia almost 12% of infants die as compared with 0.7% in UAE.

Infectious diseases and neonatal conditions account for most of the under-5 mortality, with the first especially prominent in the poorest countries and after the age of 1 when children lose their innate immunity while the latter reflect pre-natal and perinatal causes (Black et al 2010) (Table 2; Figure 1). Illustratively, diarrhea and pneumonia account for 36.6% of under-5 deaths in the poorest countries. Many of the under-5 killers are preventable by preventive and hygienic measures and early detection. That is why factors such as socio-economic status, parental education, and access to drinking water largely determine the chances of a child's survival, whereas accessibility to quality antenatal and postnatal care and skilled delivery attendance increase neonatal survival and receive the attention of policy makers.

Child Nutritional Status

Child under-nutrition remains an important public health problem with profound consequences including increased mortality and morbidity in childhood and obesity in adulthood (El-Taguri et al 2009). Several indicators are commonly used to describe under-nutrition. *Low birth weight* (LBW) (less than 2.5 kilograms) at full term or due to premature birth is related to maternal malnutrition, infection, smoking, or complications of pregnancy and is an important determinant of neonatal and infant mortality (Hong & Ruiz-Beltran 2008). *Under-weight*, i.e., weight-for-age below two standard deviations from the mean, is an MDG target. *Wasting*, a weight-for-height below two negative standard deviations from the mean, is a consequence of acute food deprivation due generally to acute childhood diseases such as diarrhea. *Stunting*, a height-for-age below two negative standard deviations from the mean, expresses chronic food deprivation, and is generally related to poverty, chronic or repeated infections.

While nutrition has improved since 1980 (see Chapter 10), recent data still show high rates of under-weight children (Table 1). As most LBW is preventable through antenatal care, countries with strong maternal and child care such as Algeria, Tunisia, Occupied Palestinian Territory (OPT), and Syria perform equally or better than the highest income countries. After birth, children fail to thrive mostly by suffering chronic and repetitive infections, especially diarrheas. Similar to the case for mortality indicators, under-nutrition rates vary greatly across the region, ranging from almost one in two children (46%) in Yemen to 3% in OPT. The six poorest countries again show the highest rates. For instance, in Djibouti, 5.2% of under-5 children are at risk of dying because of severe under-nutrition (UNICEF 2010a). Interestingly, the highest income countries do not show the lowest rates of under-weight, rather the middle-income countries do (Table 1). This is an area for future research that explores child rearing and nutrition practices and health care usage as possible explanations.

Besides general under-nutrition, children may suffer from deficiencies of specific micro-nutrients, such as vitamin A and iron, which are attributed to undiversified diet and infectious illnesses. Chapter 10 explores this issue in more detail.

Child Immunization

Infections, many of which have become vaccine-preventable, were historically the major causes of morbidity and mortality during childhood. Measles is especially important because of its high incidence and life-threatening complications. Universal coverage of children with basic vaccines, including measles, is among the most effective ways to reduce child mortality. It is estimated that currently 2.5 million under-5 deaths are prevented annually around the globe by immunization (UNICEF 2010b). In the region (Table 1), high-income countries and middle-income countries with good public child care programs such as Tunisia and OPT, have near universal coverage while the others lag behind. For example, only one in four children are immunized against measles in Somalia. Lebanon is unique as it falls behind other middle-income countries (with only 53% of children immunized against measles). This is thought to reflect its health system characteristics (see Chapter 31). Hepatitis B and *Haemophilus influenzae* type B vaccines have been adopted in the national schemes of many countries (UNICEF 2010b). The pneumococcal conjugate vaccine and

Table 1. Millennium Development Goals Child Health Indicators by Country

Countries	GNI per capita (US$)	Survival U5MR per 1000 LB 1990	Survival U5MR per 1000 LB 2008	Reduction (%)	IMR per 1000 LB 1990	IMR per 1000 LB 2008	Nutrition % LBW <2.5kg	Nutrition % UW1 <=-2sd	Nutrition % Stunt <-2sd	Nutrition % Wast <-2sd	Immunization BCG	Immunization DPT1	Immunization DPT3	Immunization polio3	Immunization Measles	Immunization HepB	Immunization Hib3
Low-income countries																	
Somalia	140	200	200	0	119	119	11	36	13	42	36	40	31	24	24	–	–
Mauritania	840	129	118	9	81	75	34	31	12	32	89	88	74	73	65	74	–
Sudan	1,130	124	109	12	78	70	31	31	16	40	83	96	86	85	79	86	86
Comoros	750	128	105	18	90	75	25	25	8	44	81	85	81	81	76	81	–
Djibouti	1,130	123	95	23	95	76	10	33	17	33	90	90	89	89	73	88	89
Yemen	950	127	69	46	90	53	32	46	15	58	60	79	69	67	62	69	69
Middle-income countries																	
Iraq	2,170	53	44	17	42	36	15	8	6	26	92	84	62	66	69	58	–
Algeria	4,260	64	41	36	52	36	6	4	4	15	99	97	93	92	88	91	93
Morocco	2,580	88	36	59	68	32	15	10	10	23	99	99	99	99	96	97	99
OPT	1,230	38	27	29	33	24	7	3	1	10	99	99	96	97	96	96	96
Egypt	1,800	90	23	74	66	20	13	8	7	29	98	98	97	97	92	97	–
Tunisia	3,290	50	21	58	40	18	5	3	2	6	99	98	99	99	98	99	–
Jordan	3,310	38	20	47	31	17	13	4	3	12	95	98	97	98	95	97	97
Libya	11,590	38	17	55	33	15	7	5	4	21	99	98	98	98	98	98	98
Syria	2,090	37	16	57	30	14	9	10	10	28	90	88	82	82	81	82	82
Lebanon	6,350	40	13	68	33	12	6	4	5	11	–	90	74	74	53	74	74
High-income countries																	
KSA	15,500	43	21	51	35	18	11	14	11	20	98	98	98	98	97	98	98
Oman	12,270	31	12	61	23	10	9	18	7	13	99	97	92	99	99	92	92
Bahrain	19,350	16	12	25	14	10	8	9	5	10	–	99	97	97	99	97	97
Kuwait	38,420	15	11	27	13	9	7	10	11	24	–	99	99	99	99	99	99
Qatar	12,000	20	10	50	17	9	10	6	2	8	96	96	94	97	92	94	94
UAE	26,210	17	8	53	15	7	15	14	15	17	98	97	92	94	92	92	92
Arab countries	–	69	47	40	50	34	14	15	8	24	89	92	86	87	83	89	91
MENA	–	77	43	44	57	33	11	14	10	32	92	94	89	89	86	88	48
Industrialized countries	–	10	6	40	8	5	–	–	–	–	–	98	96	94	93	66	84
World	–	90	65	28	62	45	16	26	13	34	89	90	82	83	83	69	28

Notes: GNI = gross national income; U5MR = under-5 mortality rate; IMR = Infant mortality rate; LB = live-birth; LBW = Low birth weight; UW = under-weight children; Stunt = stunted; Wast = Wasted; DPT1&DPT3 = 1 & 3 doses of Diphteria/Tetanus/Pertussis vaccine; polio3 = 3 doses of poliomyelitis vaccine; HepB3 = 3 doses of hepatitis B vaccine; Hib3 = 3 doses of *haemophilus influenza* vaccine; sd = standard deviation. Source: UNICEF, State of the World's children 2009.

Table 2. Causes of Under-5 Mortality by Country

Country	AIDS (%)	Diarrhea (%)	Pertussis (%)	Tetanus (%)	Measles (%)	Meningitis (%)	Malaria (%)	Pneumonia (%)	Other infections (%)	Complicated preterm birth (%)	Birth asphyxia (%)	NN sepsis (%)	Congenital abnormalities (%)	NCD (%)	Injury (%)
Somalia	0.22	21.83	3.94	2.72	5.07	1.73	5.85	18.99	10.12	8.12	8.45	5.45	2.84	2.17	2.50
Mauritania	0.54	15.68	1.20	0.68	0.00	2.22	13.33	19.55	10.59	12.68	9.47	6.39	3.05	2.13	2.50
Sudan	2.42	10.64	0.86	0.39	0.01	1.79	24.89	15.56	8.49	18.06	6.92	1.81	3.60	1.78	2.77
Comoros	0.00	20.10	1.14	0.26	0.00	3.91	0.00	21.94	14.03	16.18	9.50	5.67	2.81	2.59	1.89
Djibouti	6.07	18.65	0.94	0.40	0.22	1.56	0.18	18.61	13.65	11.24	9.01	6.29	7.23	3.61	2.32
Yemen	0.00	20.20	5.99	2.42	0.78	1.98	0.46	18.04	6.83	16.77	11.67	5.28	4.90	2.14	2.54
Low-income	**1.54**	**17.85**	**2.35**	**1.15**	**1.01**	**2.20**	**7.45**	**18.78**	**10.62**	**13.84**	**9.17**	**5.15**	**4.07**	**2.40**	**1.54**
Iraq	0.00	11.55	5.51	0.83	0.23	2.31	0.00	20.33	5.55	22.61	11.70	4.63	8.21	1.46	5.08
Algeria	0.13	12.84	1.39	0.62	0.73	1.05	0.00	19.42	11.44	21.93	12.67	5.66	7.55	2.25	2.32
Morocco	0.09	12.36	0.85	1.18	0.01	1.35	0.00	17.22	9.29	20.57	14.58	8.10	9.99	1.74	2.65
Egypt	0.07	4.79	0.35	1.16	0.35	4.11	0.00	10.60	8.60	33.04	5.62	1.33	18.18	7.26	4.55
Tunisia	0.00	4.79	0.00	0.49	0.00	4.36	0.00	10.40	7.54	30.43	5.87	1.23	20.46	8.54	5.90
Jordan	0.00	3.88	0.00	0.36	0.00	1.47	0.00	10.72	8.57	35.24	6.19	1.56	19.48	7.95	4.56
Libya	0.00	3.66	0.00	0.00	0.00	0.41	0.00	8.79	8.67	29.86	6.04	1.11	21.89	12.20	7.35
Syria	0.00	4.66	0.01	0.62	0.01	1.33	0.00	10.94	9.21	26.22	5.44	0.94	21.56	11.81	7.26
Lebanon	0.70	2.44	0.47	0.00	0.47	2.91	0.00	7.67	7.21	30.23	5.93	1.05	23.49	9.77	7.56
Middle-income	**0.11**	**6.77**	**0.95**	**0.58**	**0.20**	**2.14**	**0.00**	**12.90**	**8.45**	**27.79**	**8.23**	**2.85**	**16.76**	**7.00**	**5.25**
KSA	0.00	4.79	0.00	0.00	0.00	0.38	0.00	9.84	7.27	31.47	5.89	1.29	18.88	11.71	8.48
Oman	0.00	1.86	0.00	1.00	0.00	0.57	0.00	6.72	5.87	32.19	6.29	1.14	25.46	11.87	7.01
Bahrain	0.00	0.58	0.00	0.00	0.00	0.00	0.00	1.17	7.60	23.39	6.43	1.17	42.69	7.02	9.94
Kuwait	0.00	0.54	0.00	0.00	0.00	0.00	0.00	3.77	5.03	28.19	3.23	1.62	47.58	5.57	4.49
Qatar	0.00	1.64	0.00	0.00	0.00	0.00	0.00	5.74	5.74	24.59	4.92	0.82	26.23	18.85	11.48
UAE	0.00	0.87	0.00	0.00	0.00	0.87	0.00	4.99	5.64	31.45	5.64	1.08	29.07	13.23	7.38
High-income	**0.00**	**1.71**	**0.00**	**0.17**	**0.00**	**0.30**	**0.00**	**5.37**	**6.19**	**28.55**	**5.40**	**1.19**	**31.65**	**11.38**	**8.13**
Average	*0.49*	*8.49*	*1.08*	*0.63*	*0.38*	*1.63*	*2.13*	*12.43*	*8.43*	*24.02*	*7.69*	*3.03*	*17.39*	*6.94*	*5.26*

Source: Black et al 2010.

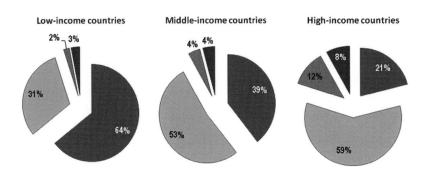

Figure 1. Causes of under-5 mortality in Arab countries grouped by income level. Source: Black et al 2010.

Low-income countries — 2%, 3%, 31%, 64%

Middle-income countries — 4%, 4%, 53%, 39%

High-income countries — 8%, 12%, 21%, 59%

■ Infectious diseases   ▨ Neonatal complications   ◼ NCD   ■ Injuries

rotavirus vaccine protecting children against pneumonia and diarrhea, respectively, are subsidized in the highest income countries but remain unaffordable in low-income countries and for the low-income categories of the middle-income countries.

Child Morbidity

The general picture of child morbidity is that of epidemiologic transition; like their parents and grandparents, children bear a double burden as diseases of poverty such as infectious diseases, epidemics, and under-nutrition, continue to exact their toll while non-communicable diseases (NCDs) and mental conditions become increasingly more prevalent. In addition, children in countries caught in violent conflicts suffer additional burden, both physical and mental.

Infectious Diseases

Thanks to immunization campaigns, mortality and morbidity due to classic infectious diseases have declined. Nevertheless, acute respiratory tract infections, and diarrheal diseases still persist, particularly in the poorest countries and among the poor in middle-income countries. Vaccine preventable diseases still occur, despite numerous vaccination campaigns. For example, cases of poliomyelitis are still reported in Sudan and Djibouti.

Mauritania, Comoros, Djibouti, Somalia, Sudan, and areas of Yemen, Syria, Iraq, and Saudi Arabia are endemic for malaria. The proportion of children sleeping under insecticide-treated nets, the prevention of choice against contracting malaria, is suboptimal in the poorest countries, not exceeding 1% in Southern Sudan, 2% in Djibouti, and 3% in Mauritania (UNICEF 2009a). Additionally, new threats are emerging such as resistant strains of bacteria due to misuse of antibiotics

(see Chapter 11). While HIV prevalence remains low, except in Djibouti and southern Sudan, treatment rates are low. Only 6% of the estimated 10,000 children with HIV in the Middle East and North Africa region (which includes Iran and Turkey) are covered by antiretroviral therapy (WHO 2010).

Non-communicable Diseases and Their Risk Factors

Urbanization, globalization of food consumption toward higher sugar and higher calorie intake, and change of childhood lifestyles toward more sedentary activities such as television watching at the expense of social and physical activity (Khader et al 2009) have led to increasing prevalence of over-weight and obesity among children.

A "nutrition transition" is under way, whereby persisting under-nutrition coexists with over-weight and obesity (Galal 2003). Childhood over-weight has increased over the past two decades to reach alarming levels in high-income countries with Bahrain reporting 38.5% of over-weight children, followed by Kuwait, with 31.8% over-weight among girls (Mirmiran et al 2010). Studies stratifying the prevalence of over-weight by socio-economic status showed that the phenomenon tended to be more prevalent in urban areas and among children of the higher socio-economic classes, as opposed to the tendency in the developed world where the contrary is true (Mirmiran et al 2010). Chapter 10 provides more details about this phenomenon.

Early over-weight predisposes children to type 2 diabetes, dyslipidemia, and cardiovascular diseases already in childhood and later in life (Taha et al 2009). The increased and earlier incidence of type I diabetes has also been linked with the nutritional transition (Abdullah 2005). Additionally, over-weight children have lower self-esteem and are at risk of growing up

Table 3. Prevalence of Dental Caries in Recent Studies From the Arab Region

Country	Year	Sample characteristics	Sample size	Age	Prevalence of dental caries (%)	Reference
Lebanon	2002	National	1,595	12	93	Doumit M & Doughan B (2002) La santé bucco-dentaire des écoliers au Liban. *Santé*, 12(2): 223–228 [in French]
Jordan	2002	Preschool	1,140	4–5	67.5	Sayegh A, Dini EL, Holt RD, Bedi R (2002) Caries in preschool children in Amman, Jordan and the relationship to socio-demographic factors. *International Dental Journal* 52(2): 87–93.
Tunisia	2004	School	600	6/12	57/48	Monastir AA (2004). Oral health in Tunisia. *International Dental Journal* 54 (6 Suppl 1): 389–94.
KSA	2008	Preschool	789	4–6	75	Wyne AH (2008) Caries prevalence, severity, and pattern in preschool children. *Journal of Contemporary Dental Practice* 9(3): 24–31.
UAE	2009	National	1,323	12	54	El-Nadeef MAI, Al Hussani E, Hassab H, Arab IA (2009) National survey of the oral health of 12- and 15-year-old schoolchildren in the United Arab Emirates. *Mediterranean Health Journal* 15(4): 993–1005.
Yemen	2010	school	1,489	6–14	95	Al-Haddad KA, Al-HebshiNN, Al-Ak'hali MS (2010) Oral health status and treatment needs among school children in Sana'a City, Yemen. *International Journal of Dentistry & Hygiene* 8; 80–85.

into obese adults and bear over-increasing health hazards later in their life (Mirmiran et al 2010).

Linked with the changing food consumption patterns, higher prevalence of dental caries emerges as one of the earliest consequences of urbanization and nutritional transition. This is attributed to exposure to cariogenic diet, insufficient water fluoridation, and poor oral hygiene. Prevalence rates range from 57% in Tunisia to 95% in Yemen (Table 3) with higher prevalence in children of lower socio-economic status.

Unchecked economic development in both high- and middle-income countries with limited environmental regulation have dramatically increased environmental pollution and deteriorated the quality of air, water, and food (Al-Sayed 2004). This has resulted in increasing prevalence of such diseases as childhood asthma, especially in urban populations, potentially damaging children's educational performance and social life (Al-Thamiri et al 2005).

Genetic Blood Disorders

Sickle cell anemia and thalassemia traits are endemic in some areas, specifically those that have been endemic for malaria for centuries. For example United Arab Emirates report 1% and 2% prevalence of sickle cell anemia and thalassemia, respectively, in schoolchildren (Al Hosani et al 2005). The biggest challenges in reducing the morbidity and mortality due to genetic blood disorders are the implementation of culturally acceptable prenatal measures to prevent emergence of disease and the prospective detection of carriers to reduce infectious complications.

Injuries

Unintentional injuries are the biggest threat to children's survival and a major cause of disabilities after 5 years of age. Children in poverty shoulder the highest burden as they are less protected and cared for (Peden 2008). There is limited population-based or nationally representative data on injuries. In Iraq, Awqati et al (2009) attributed 19.3% of deaths among 12- to 59-month-olds to accidents, injuries, and poisoning. In the West Bank and Gaza, flying bullets were a major cause of injury mortality (Shaheen & Edwards 2008). In the Gulf countries car accidents and drowning are designated as responsible for most deaths and disabilities due to injuries (Nour 2005; Chapter 16).

Disabilities

Childhood disability is a major public health problem. Besides injuries, a substantial part of disability, particularly mental disabilities, is due to delayed detection of disabling conditions in childhood or delayed treatment of disabling diseases (Nour 2005). In countries undergoing rapid economic development, the number of disabilities due to birth trauma is increasing (Fida et al 2007), probably due to the increased affordability and use of neonatal intensive care. Disabilities in older children are mainly the outcome of injuries due to road traffic and home accidents (Bashour & Kharouf 2008). Lack of appropriate rehabilitative, social, and educational services aggravates the situation, even when the disability is only physical. Except in higher income countries such as Saudi Arabia, which has achieved notable progress in integrating disabled children, a large proportion of children with disabilities do not enroll in any educational activity (Nour 2005). This puts such children at risk of growing up marginalized and dependent, which may also impair their psychosocial health.

Child Mental Health

There is now increasing recognition of the importance of child mental health. There is clearly a need for comprehensive assessment of disorder prevalence and unified and culturally sensitive screening tools to permit sound comparisons (see Chapters 14 & 15). Nevertheless, available studies suggest that mental disorders are as concerning in this region as in others (El-Gilany & Amr 2010). For instance, prevalence rates of child anxiety and depression are, respectively, 14% and 4% in Oman (Al-Sharbati et al 2003), and 4.3% and 1.5% in Iraq (Al-Obaidi et al 2010).

Similarly to what is happening in Western countries, children showing signs of aggressiveness, learning difficulties, and academic under-achievement are labeled as suffering from attention deficit disorders (ADHD). This group of disorders is gaining attention in the region; however, research is missing on the true meanings of ADHD in this regional context and accuracy of its medicalization. Social correlates of ADHD have been identified, with Bener et al (2006), for example, identifying low socio-economic conditions, problematic family relations, and low parental education as main contributors. Unfortunately, the rising interest in child mental health has not translated into development of corresponding research or services (see also Chapter 14).

Although ongoing cultural globalization is increasingly exposing families to a liberal-individualistic value system, the authoritarian parenting style remains prevalent, if not dominant. In a pioneering cross-regional study in eight countries Dwairy & Achoui (2006) explored the link between parenting styles and psychosocial development of children. They found that authoritarian parenting does not cause the expected harm on children's psychosocial development; it is the inconsistency between parenting styles and the ambient culture that does.

Intermediate Determinants of Child Health

In this part, we explore the intermediate social determinants that influence child health and development while we focus on the structural determinants in the following section.

Prenatal Factors

The prenatal period is crucial not just for newborn health but across the lifespan. Many factors are at play in this period. The genetic make-up of the newborn affects risk of stillbirths, neonatal mortality, congenital anomalies, and other genetically determined conditions. Since inbreeding of recessive and co-dominant alleles increases the risk of genetically determined traits, the practice of consanguineous marriages which enables the union of asymptomatic carriers, is of particular interest. Rates of consanguineous marriage in this region are among the highest in the world, about 20–25% of marriages (Tadmouri et al 2009). In their review of health impact, Saggar & Bittles (2008) noted an increase in conditions due to genetic defects in areas where consanguineous marriages are prevalent.

A multitude of health conditions in children depends on maternal health, especially in the earliest life period (Ben Hamida et al 2010). The continued high prevalence in the region of adverse maternal conditions, such as anemia and malnutrition, persistent practices of multiparity and early/late pregnancies, coupled with inadequate perinatal care affect child health especially those of the poorer women. Some practices such as smoking during pregnancy are especially problematic in some countries such as Lebanon where it is reported in 27% of pregnancies in Beirut (Chaaya et al 2004). Similarly, Qat chewing during pregnancy, which is common in Yemen and Djibouti, has been associated with a baby's lower birth weight (Greiner 1988).

Feeding Practices

The importance of breastfeeding, whose physical and psychosocial benefits for children are well established, cannot be overstated. Countries with relatively high rates of exclusive breastfeeding such as Egypt (53%) have lower prevalence of under-nutrition, whereas countries such as Yemen with low exclusive breastfeeding rates, not exceeding 12%, have high child undernutrition rates (UNICEF 2009a). While cultural norms and religious requirements encourage breastfeeding (Shaikh & Ahmed 2006), which explains the acceptable rates of initiating breastfeeding at birth, exceeding 95% in some surveys, continued exclusivity rates for six months is low: 2% in Djibouti, 7% in Tunisia, 14% in Algeria (UNICEF 2009a). Many factors contribute to this phenomenon, such as hospital policies discouraging early suckling, poor assistance, and poor knowledge of novel mothers, insufficient maternity leaves, and early introduction of supplementary food (Dashti et al 2010; Ben-Slama et al 2010).

Supplementing and weaning feeding patterns are also concerning. Practitioners observe the common practice of offering imported foods high in sugar content or traditional baby food often poor in iron as supplements for infants. In older ages, feeding and eating practices remain problematic. For example, unfortified cow milk is still widely offered as a main meal for toddlers, especially in lower-income groups, and sometimes until late childhood. Older children tend to opt for unhealthy eating habits, such as skipping breakfast and consuming junk snacks, which favors weight gain.

Feeding and eating practices are not merely family and individual matters. As elsewhere in the world, governmental policies do not counteract aggressive promotion by the food industry of an "obesogenic"

environment that would guarantee profits (Silink 2010). A quick glance at TV programs shown across the region demonstrates the extent of parents' and children's exposure to the commercial appeal of high-calorie, high-sugar and low-fiber food.

Housing Conditions

Many health conditions are directly affected by the housing conditions of children. Among these, access to safe drinking water and hygienic sanitation disposal is most important. Although Arab countries have markedly improved such access, a proportion of children still live in inadequate housing and are exposed to various risks including water-borne infections. In 2006, access of population to safe drinking water was comprehensive only in Gulf countries and Lebanon, and quasi-comprehensive in Jordan and Egypt (UNICEF 2009a). The proportion of population with access to safe drinking water in other countries varied from 60% in Mauritania and 66% in Yemen to 92% in Djibouti and 94% in Tunisia. The proportion of population with access to improved drinking water is unacceptably low in Somalia, with only 29% (only 10% of rural population). Disparities in access to drinking water favor urban areas, especially in the low-income countries and in the middle-income countries with vast rural zones, such as Morocco. As for access to improved sanitation, the lowest-income countries, except Djibouti, have the poorest rates, ranging from 23% in Somalia to 35% in Sudan. The situation in Egypt is concerning, with only two thirds of its population using improved sanitation facilities (UNICEF 2009a).

Parental Education

The relationship between parents', especially mother's, education and child health is well known. The combined effect of improved maternal knowledge and higher family income is a decisive determinant not only for early child development and school achievement but also for health indicators including mortality. Many regional studies have demonstrated this (Myntti 1993; Khawaja et al 2008).

Structural Determinants of Child Health

The socio-economic and political context, as well as the pattern distribution of wealth, power, and resources that are available to parents and families influence

Table 4. Disparities by Wealth and Residence in Four Selected Countries

Country/year	IMR	U5MR	Stunting	Wasting	Immunization	Treatment of fever	Antenatal care
Low/high wealth quartile ratio							
Egypt – 1995	3.45	3.77	2.07	2.95	0.70	0.55	0.23
Egypt – 2000	2.55	2.91	3.26	12.00	0.99	0.75	0.37
Jordan – 1997	1.51	1.67	6.80	14.00	1.25	0.96	0.95
Morocco – 1992	2.27	2.85	11.36	10.25	0.56	0.27	0.13
Morocco – 2004/05	2.59	2.98	3.52	3.66	0.83	0.37	0.43
Yemen – 1997	1.81	2.23	2.43	3.14	0.14	0.44	0.25
Rural/urban ratio							
Egypt – 1995	1.70	1.80	1.71	1.94	0.85	0.79	0.49
Egypt – 2000	1.43	1.50	1.93	1.50	0.99	0.82	0.62
Jordan – 1997	1.46	1.46	2.67	2.50	0.30	0.95	0.96
Morocco – 1992	1.34	1.67	3.74	4.67	0.71	0.45	0.33
Morocco – 2004/05	1.68	1.82	2.28	2.55	0.90	0.59	0.54
Yemen – 1997	1.24	1.34	1.59	1.80	0.35	0.60	0.45

Notes: IMR= infant mortality rate; U5MR= under-5 mortality rate.
Source: Gwatkin et al 2007- World Bank Country reports.

better or worse health of children (Tekce 1990). Below we review some of those determinants of health and health inequities.

Economic Factors

There are important within-country inequities in child health by socio-economic status (Table 4). Gwatkin et al (2007) demonstrated pervasive inequalities in health outcomes, quality of care, and service utilization according to family wealth and place of residence in Egypt, Jordan, Morocco, and Yemen with poorer and rural children worse off. Some inequities seem to have increased over the study period. In a meta-analysis that included Egypt, Saudi Arabia, and United Arab Emirates, Jahan (2008) found poverty, as indicated by mother illiteracy and low socio-economic status, was strongly associated with infant mortality. Even high-income countries, such as Saudi Arabia, still face significant disparities in child health indicators between their extreme socio-economic categories (Al-Mazrou et al 2008). In other countries, income inequality has emerged as an important correlate of child health outcomes. Studies are needed to examine this relationship in this region.

The link between wealth and child mortality is as true at the country level as it is at the household level with higher income countries faring better. Illustratively, the 13-fold lower gross national income per capita in Yemen vs. neighboring Oman is reflected in a five-fold increased risk of under-5 death (Table 1).

Child poverty is a specific form of poverty, which goes beyond what is classically measured in indicators of household socio-economic status such as family income and parental education, and is a key determinant of child well-being. Several factors explain the importance of this construct. Given the child's requirements for learning and growing, deprivation can occur at lower levels of household poverty. As children are more dependent on social policies, especially those concerning health and education, they pay the highest price of poor policies. Furthermore, the consequences of child deprivation are drastic and often life-long. Children deprived from adequate opportunities for education are likely to become poor parents and perpetuate poverty into their own future families (UNICEF 2010d). Based on surveys collected over the period 1991–2001, and using an approach tailored to measure child poverty, it seems that 40% of children in the region have been in absolute poverty during that decade, which is more than the average for the developing world (Ali 2007). Particularly grave are the rates of shelter, water, and education deprivation (Ali 2007). Considering the tremendous cost of child poverty on both individuals and societies, these numbers are daunting. In this context, poor urban slums have witnessed the appearance of the phenomenon of street children, as documented in Cairo and Alexandria. Besides impaired development due to poverty, street children are subject to abuse, exploitation, malnourishment, illiteracy, and mental ill-health (Salem & Abd El-Latif 2002).

Rapid regional and global economic developments affect children from non-poor social categories as well. Recurrent economic crises deplete family resources and consequently restrict children's access to health care, proper education, and other resources for development. With fewer job opportunities at home in low- and middle-income countries, many fathers seek work abroad, especially in Gulf States, with adverse consequences for family life. Better-off families in many Arab countries increasingly rely on foreign domestic workers for child rearing. The long-term impacts of this practice on child health and development have not yet captured the attention of public health researchers.

Factors Related to Cultural Norms and Traditional Practices

The culture of son preference which is common in most societies (El-Gilany 2007) is thought to contribute to gender differences in health. A gender dimension is present in many if not all aspects of child health (see Chapter 7). Yount (2001) reported that boys receive preferential treatment in seeking health care and food allocation. Some have argued that son preference might explain excess female mortality (see for example Ahmed 1990), gender differences in birth weight, or frequency of prenatal visits (Al-Akour 2009).

To exemplify the gender dynamics in child health we study IMR and mortality rates among infants and 1- to 4-year-olds (1–4 mortality), stratified by gender. Boys are biologically more vulnerable than girls to various congenital and environmental factors and this is reflected in higher mortality, especially during the first year of life. Therefore, equality in child mortality and morbidity indicators between sexes does not reflect gender parity. To understand gender dynamics in child survival, researchers use age-specific standard female/male (F/M) mortality

ratio, indexes of female excess mortality, or comparisons of F/M ratios with other world regions, assumed to be free from gender discrimination in childhood. Based on the latter approach, Khawaja et al (2008) showed that, in the 1990s, "only the UAE had a real female advantage... Twelve countries showed an excess female mortality in both IMR and U5MR". We use the WHO life tables (WHO 2009) to compare the F/M mortality ratios of 20 Arab countries with the average F/M mortality ratios of 39 European countries. As shown in Table 5, only Bahrain, Tunisia, Djibouti, and UAE show gender equality for 1–4 mortality. Lebanon, Syria, Qatar, Algeria, and Iraq show excess male mortality, raising the possibility of deteriorated environmental conditions. All the other countries show excess female mortality, ranging from 8% in Comoros, to a whopping 115% in Morocco. The regional average F/M mortality ratios show that excess female mortality increases from 6% for infants to 17% in the 1–4 year old, where the role of social determinants is stronger (see also Chapter 7).

Expanding from the lens of gender, cultural practices and norms in general impact virtually all aspects of child well-being and development. Traditional marital patterns such as early marriage, widespread consanguinity, early and late pregnancy, coupled with multiparity and inadequately spaced births are still common in many areas. However, these "cultural" practices also have economic and social bases, some of which are beneficial to child development and family life, that must be considered while designing interventions to limit the negative health effects of traditional marital patterns.

The family psychosocial environment has repercussion not only on child mental health (Dwairy & Achoui 2006) but also on their physical health (Al-Adili et al 2009). Family norms in the region promote a supportive environment for children. Families are generally cohesive, devote much time and energy to children, and willingly compensate for lack of public services for children. However, to inculcate social norms and behavioral manners, punishment, including corporal punishment, is still practiced widely in the family context (Achoui 2003) and is still tolerated in schools.

Some traditional practices have important health implications. Female genital cutting (FGC) is widely practiced in Egypt, Sudan, Somalia, and Djibouti and reported in Yemen, Jordan, Gaza Strip, Oman, and Iraqi Kurdistan. The possible immediate complications

Table 5. Mortality Rates by Sexes and F/M Ratio With Calculated Excess Gender Mortality

Infant mortality < 1 year

	Country	Boys/1000LB	Girls/1000LB	F/M Ratio	Excess (%)
Excess Male Mortality b/w Genders	Syria	1.74	1.15	0.66	−15
	Morocco	3.83	2.77	0.72	−9
	Djibouti	9.14	6.87	0.75	−6
	Tunisia	2.11	1.60	0.76	−5
Equal Mortality b/w Genders	Comoros	8.84	7.07	0.8	−1
	UAE	0.78	0.63	0.81	0
	Lebanon	1.31	1.08	0.82	1
	Algeria	4.03	3.40	0.84	3
	Egypt	2.17	1.85	0.85	4
Excess Female Mortality	Mauritania	8.44	7.27	0.86	5
	Iraq	3.95	3.41	0.86	5
	Kuwait	1.00	0.86	0.86	5
	Yemen	5.85	5.07	0.87	6
	Oman	1.10	0.98	0.89	8
	Qatar	0.68	0.63	0.93	12
	Somalia	13.21	12.78	0.97	16
	Libya	1.55	1.55	1.00	19
	Jordan	1.72	1.72	1.00	19
	Bahrain	0.95	0.99	1.04	23
	Sudan	7.04	7.61	1.08	27
	Average	**3.97**	**3.46**	**0.87**	**6**

Child 1–4 years mortality

	Country	Boys/ 1000 LB	Girls/ 1000LB	F/M Ratio	Excess (%)
Excess Male Mortality b/w Genders	Lebanon	0.05	0.03	0.6	−25
	Syria	0.06	0.04	0.67	−18
	Qatar	0.06	0.04	0.67	−18
	Algeria	0.15	0.11	0.73	−12
	Iraq	0.28	0.22	0.79	−6
Equal Mortality b/w Genders	Bahrain	0.07	0.06	0.86	1
	Tunisia	0.08	0.07	0.88	3
	Djibouti	0.55	0.49	0.89	4
Excess Female Mortality	Comoros	0.85	0.79	0.93	8
	Mauritania	1.23	1.16	0.94	9
	UAE	0.02	0.02	1.00	15
	Libya	0.04	0.04	1.00	15
	Kuwait	0.04	0.04	1.00	15
	Somalia	2.29	2.57	1.12	27
	Egypt	0.08	0.09	1.13	28
	Sudan	0.98	1.19	1.21	36
	Yemen	0.40	0.49	1.23	38
	Oman	0.03	0.04	1.33	48
	Jordan	0.06	0.08	1.33	48
	Morocco	0.07	0.14	2.00	115
	Average	**0.37**	**0.39**	**1.02**	**17**

Notes: F/M Ratio = female male ratio; Excess % = excess mortality (expressed in percentages) calculated by subtracting the average European F/M mortality ratio from each national F/M ratios. The European F/M ratio corresponds to 0.81 for Infant Mortality <1 mortality and 0.85 for 1–4 mortality. LB = live births (The life table of OPT is not available, and Saudi Arabia's rates showed aberrant reversion of excess mortality between the <1 mortality and the 1–4 mortality thus was withdrawn from analysis).
Source: WHO 2009 – life tables 2008.

of FGC, such as bleeding, wound infection, and psychological trauma seem obvious (UNICEF 2010c), while the long-term impacts on reproductive health, including sexual function of adult women is still debated (Makhlouf-Obermeyer 2003). The issue of FGC now receives increasing attention of national and international agencies with the aim of curbing the practice.

Violent Conflicts

In the past three decades, Algeria, Iraq, Lebanon, OPT, Somalia, Sudan, and Yemen have endured, or continue to endure, situations such as occupation, repeated wars, civil conflict, sporadic violence, international sanctions, large population displacement, or chronic political turmoil (see chapters in Section 5). These situations affect all aspects of child well-being and development, and exacerbate social vulnerabilities and health inequities (Watts et al 2009). Infant mortality has dramatically increased in Iraq because of sanctions, wars, and civil unrest (Ali & Shah 2000; Chapter 25). During the July-August 2006 Israeli war in Lebanon, approximately 400 children were killed and 1500 injured (HRC 2006); During the Israeli attack on Gaza in January 2008, approximately 400 children were killed and 1800 injured (WAM 2009).

Besides direct harm, children caught up in war suffer illnesses, malnutrition, neglect, and post-traumatic stress, as well as disrupted schooling and social and family ties. During armed conflicts the social and political infrastructure often breaks down leading to the loss of even basic health care services such as immunization. For example, in the OPT, after the Intifada of September 2000, fetal death, home deliveries, and LBW increased by 47%, 41%, and 22%, respectively, while immunization against measles, polio, hepatitis, skilled birth attendance and antenatal care dropped by 10%, 7%, and 4% respectively (UNRWA 2001).

Many studies have documented deterioration of child mental health during and in the aftermath of wars (Clark 2003). The traumatic effect of fear in life-threatening situations, disorientation in displacement, and the hardship in the after-war restitution of destroyed livelihood may accompany the child into adulthood. On the other hand, social support available in family, peer, and extended social networks, as well as the perceived meaning of war experiences are emerging as protective factors (Betancourt & Khan 2008), suggesting the need for a resilience-based approach in addressing the psychosocial needs of children affected by war (see Chapter 26).

Threats to children's lives continue after war's end. Unexploded cluster bombs and other ordinances still threaten the playgrounds of thousands of children in South Lebanon 4 years after the end of the war. Studies have reported an increase in incidence of congenital anomalies and cancer after the 1991 Gulf war probably due to use of depleted uranium (Busby et al 2010). The health impact of soil contamination with white phosphorous and Dense Inert Metal Explosive used by the Israeli army in Gaza is still being studied.

Child Social Policy and Unmet Needs for Protection

Challenges to child protection extend beyond economic and political insecurities. Non-conflict humanitarian crises affect children disproportionately. For example, the severe drought in Djibouti in 2009 raised global acute malnutrition among children to 28.8% in the most affected areas (UNICEF 2010a).

Child protection, an international concern since the 1940s, became mandatory in 1990 after the UN Convention on the Rights of the Child came into force. While all Arab countries have ratified the Convention, only Tunisia succeeded to mandate a law against child corporal punishment in both domestic and school settings. In all the other countries, commitment of governments to the decree could not be translated into concrete laws. Only 10 countries, Algeria, Bahrain, Djibouti, Egypt, Jordan, Kuwait, Libya, Oman, UAE, and Yemen, have clear prohibition of corporal punishment in schools (Save the Children 2010). Although 13 of the Arab countries are currently discussing projects of child protection laws or child's rights codes in their constitutional text, there is little hope to see this practice completely eradicated in the region for many reasons. Corporal punishment is still perceived as the best discipline and even when the legislation exists, it needs to overcome the absence of independent bodies to report excesses and specialized courts to take corrective measures to reach implementation.

Even though all countries, except Somalia have ratified the "International Labor Organization Convention on Abolition of Child Labor", at least 13.4 million children (15% of the total child population) still participate in the labor force (ILO 2010), and are exposed to additional abuse and exploitation. The inability of governments to provide families with economic alternatives to child labor is a considerable obstacle to addressing this problem.

Policy fragmentation is a major obstacle to broad-based action on child health. Ministries of health focus on narrowly defined health interventions and do not consider wider goals beyond the health sector while non-health ministries and programs rarely include child health outcomes in their objectives. In countries where international aid has an important influence in public policy, aid programs have generally no mechanisms for intersectoral networking and budgeting. As a result, child health policies and interventions appear to be drifting from one short-term priority to another, undermining sustainability.

Education

One area where policy coherence is urgently needed is child education. While Arab countries have made significant strides in this area, challenges remain. Only nine countries (Jordan, OPT, Algeria, Bahrain, Tunisia, Qatar, Syria, Egypt, and Lebanon) have achieved net primary school enrolment rates exceeding 90% (UNICEF 2009a; Chapter 2). School attrition is connected with the challenge of child poverty and child labor, which raises the need for a multisectoral approach. The focus on universalizing primary education has not been accompanied by efforts to improve the quality of education. Public education often lacks resources to provide children with high quality education that prepares them for the highly competitive labor markets required by modern economies, while private schools attempt to respond to these pressures by overloading curricula with scientific courses. In both sets of schools, cultural, artistic, and sportive education needed for child development is severely lacking.

Child Health Policy

Several Arab countries have undergone health sector reforms, in the context of broader social sector reforms, over the past two decades (see also chapters in Section 6), but these have variable and sometimes conflicting impacts on child health. Reform activities that may adversely impact children include static or shrinking public expenditures on health, much of which goes to secondary and tertiary care, and

increasing privatization of their public health sectors, often in response to World Bank directives (Palma-Solís et al 2009). The result is the increased dependence of families on out-of-pocket health expenditures which remain too high (see Chapter 29), especially as insurance schemes, especially public ones, remain quite limited.

Other reform activities may positively impact children. Many countries have expanded primary health care (PHC) services (Abdullatif 2008). Maternal and child health has traditionally been the cornerstone of PHC in the region. Egypt, Morocco, and Sudan have implemented, with the support of UNICEF, the program of Integrated Management of Childhood Illnesses (IMCI) to improve health workers' skills, health systems, and child health practices by families. The IMCI has been shown to be one of the most successful interventions in countries where it was implemented (UNICEF 2009b).

Starting from the 1980s, school health services became well established in most countries. These are especially effective for achieving the high rate (91%) of immunization (Mackroth et al 2010). However, the quality of school-health programs is far from being perfect; most services are limited to health screening, surveillance, immunization, and hygienic measures, bypassing crucial components of children's development such as psychosocial support and prevention of risk behavior. Lebanon has recently initiated a psychological support system in all public schools but time is needed to evaluate its impact.

There are many reports of quality of child health services but most are not population based. Overall, primary care services appear to be of reasonable quality although many gaps are commonly identified. For example, surveys conducted in a number of Arab countries showed deficiencies in basic procedures happening in primary healthcare settings, such as a weight and temperature taking, assessment of anemia. The hospital care for children suffers from the same impediments encountered by adult patients (see Chapter 31).

While almost all ministries of health have maternal and child health programs commonly headed by pediatricians, our experiences and anecdotal evidence suggest that child public health, as a field of practice, is still not well developed in the region. This is manifested in many ways; for example, the existing child health services are not integrated together to form a true child-friendly health system and equity in such services is not prioritized.

The Way Forward

Given the challenges facing child health and development, a comprehensive approach is needed. We argue that strengthening public health's contribution is a key step. In the area of education and training, high-quality programs on child public health are too few around the region. Public funding and support is needed to develop such programs. In the area of research there are two main gaps that need to be addressed. The social aspects of child health are relatively neglected. One manifestation is the limited attention to vulnerability. For example, Saddik & Nuwayhid (2006) found only nine studies on working children, which is surprising given the gravity of the problem. Another manifestation is the weak adoption of a social-determinants-of-health perspective in research on child health. This challenge is partially related to the problems of available research datasets: data from surveillance systems and disease registries often lack crucial socio-economic information and data from vital registration and demographic census lack health indicators. The Arab League's initiatives on PAPCHILD and PAPFAM and the Demographic and Health Surveys are heading in the right direction toward the production of more comprehensive data.

Health system reforms that secure universal access and reduce financial burden on families, integrate services toward a systems approach, improve public sector performance, and prioritize prevention will positively impact child health in the long term (see example in Box 1). Still, in the short and medium terms much can be done. For example, attending to the current gaps in immunization coverage, specifically in poorer countries and poor and vulnerable groups in all countries, is a priority from an equity perspective. Arab countries have the means today to improve this coverage and eradicate inequities in access to prevention. Improving quality of childcare services, for example through expanding the IMCI program to more countries, is also within the reach of countries. Strengthening the school health programs to become more comprehensive can improve child health outcomes. Gradual integration of positive child development into childcare service is also within reach of the current health system. Last, developing monitoring and evaluating systems can improve the efficacy and efficiency of programs and interventions directed at child health and development.

Box 1. Oral Rehydration Therapy for Diarrhea – A Public Health Success Story in Egypt (Norbert Hirschhorn)

The National Control of Diarrheal Diseases Project (NCDDP) of Egypt began in 1981, became fully operational nation-wide by 1984, and concluded in 1991. The project was designed as a campaign to lower mortality from diarrheal disease in children under 5 by at least 25% within 5 years. The strategies were improving case-management of diarrhea through rehydration and better feeding, ensuring production and distribution of oral rehydration salts, educating families through mass media and health workers through training programs, and creating "rehydration corners" throughout the primary health care and hospital network. The project included a plan for evaluation and research at the start. The NCDDP succeeded in achieving its goals. In local and national mortality surveys, overall infant and childhood mortality fell by at least one-third with the majority proportion in diarrheal deaths. The declines coincided with the peak of NCDDP activities. The case-management improved with plausible sufficiency to account for most of the diarrheal mortality reduction. Changes in other proximate determinants to lowered mortality, such as host resistance or diarrheal incidence, do not plausibly account for the magnitude of the reductions. Improvements in primary care delivery and use of mass media would have been facilitating factors to NCDDP efforts, while deterioration of economic status would have tended to reduce the benefits. This case study shows the potential of simple interventions to have large impact on public health. There is a need to sustain such efforts to improve child health outcomes.

Based on: Miller P & Hirschhorn N (1995) The effect of a national control of diarrheal diseases program on mortality: the case of Egypt. *Social Science and Medicine*, 40(10): S1–S30.

The social policy domain, targeting the social determinants of child health, is another promising field for advocacy. We prioritize two actionable areas. The first is pressures on governments to realize their commitments in international treaties in child protection and rights. A promising trend of recent years has been increasing media attention to child rights and protection. The second is multisectoral policy coherence, especially between health, education, and social affairs ministries, taking into account the influence of aid agencies, where applicable. Advocacy on these two fronts must be broad-based including public health and other social actors including NGOs and civil society whose work has tended to be fragmented. Obviously all parties, including governments, must come together to push the longer term goal of promoting the culture of children's rights to health and protection in all domains, at family, societal, and political levels.

Children are the future adults who will take our society toward peace and security, freedom, equality, and prosperity. We need to provide them with the opportunities to achieve this aspiration. This requires us, in public health, to look at their needs beyond the traditional focus on mortality and morbidity and into all dimensions of child well-being and harmonious development. Matching the strong culture of adoration for children in the region with the culture of child rights provides purpose and direction for public health in its action on child health and its determinants.

References

Abdullah MA (2005) Epidemiology of type I diabetes mellitus among Arab children, *Saudi Medical Journal*, 26(6): 911–917

Abdullatif AA (2008) Aspiring to build health services and systems led by primary health care in the Eastern Mediterranean Region, *Eastern Mediterranean Health Journal*, 14(Sp): 23–41

Achoui M (2003) [Children disciplining within the family context: Reality and attitudes] [in Arabic], *Al Tofoolah Al 'Arabiah*, 16(4): 9–38

Ahmed FA (1990) Gender difference in child mortality, *Egypt Population Family Planning Review*, 24(2): 60–79

Al-Adili N, Shaheen M, Bergstrom S, Johansson A (2008) Survival, family conditions and nutritional status of motherless orphans in the West Bank, Palestine, *Scandinavian Journal of Public Health*, 36: 292–297

Ali AAG (2007) *Child Poverty: Concept and measurement.* Working paper, the Arab Planning Institute – Kuwait

Ali MM, Shah IH (2000) Sanctions and childhood mortality in Iraq, *The Lancet*, 355(9218): 1851–1857

Al-Akour N (2009) Relationship between parental knowledge of fetal gender and newborns' birth-weight among Jordanian families, *International Journal of Nursing Practice*, 15(2): 105–11

Al Hosani H, Salah M, Osman HM, Farag HM, Anvery SM (2005) Incidence of haemoglobinopathies detected through neonatal screening in the United Arab Emirates, *Eastern Mediterranean Health Journal*, 11(3): 300–7

Al-Mazrou YY, Alhamdan NA, Alkotobi AI, Nour OM, Farag MA (2008) Factors affecting child mortality in Saudi Arabia, *Saudi Medical Journal*, 29(1): 102–106

Al-Obaidi AK, Budosan B, Jejrey L (2010) Child and adolescent mental health in Iraq: current situation and scope for promotion of child and adolescent mental health policy, *Intervention*, 8(1): 40–51

Al-Sharbati MM, Al-Hussaini AA, Antony S (2003) Profile of child and adolescent psychiatry in Oman, *Saudi Medical Journal*, 24(4): 391–395

Al-Thamiri D, Al-Kubaisy W, Ali SH (2005) Asthma prevalence and severity among primary-school children in Baghdad, *Eastern Mediterranean Health Journal*, 11(1–2): 79–86

Awqati NA, Ali MM, Al-Ward NJ, Majeed FA, Salman K, Al-Alak M, Al-Gasseer N (2009) Causes and differentials of childhood mortality in Iraq, *British Medical Journal – Pediatrics*, 22(9): 40

Bashour H, Kharouf M (2008) Community-based study of unintentional injuries among preschool children in Damascus, *Eastern Mediterranean Health Journal*, 14(2), 398–405

Bener A, Qahtani RA, Abdelaal I (2006) The prevalence of ADHD among primary school children in an Arabian society, *Journal of Attention Disorders*, 10(1): 77–82

Ben Hamida E, Chaouachi S, Ben Said A, Marrakchi Z (2010) [Determinants of neonatal mortality in a Tunisian population] [in French], *La Tunisie médicale*, 88(1): 41–44

Ben Slama F, Ayari I, Ouzini F, Belhadj O, Achour N (2010) [Exclusive breastfeeding and mixed feeding: knowledge, attitudes and practices of primiparous mothers] [in French], *Eastern Mediterranean Health Journal*, 16(6): 630–5

Betancourt TS, Khan KT (2008) The mental health of children affected by armed conflict: Protective processes and pathways to resilience, *International Review of Psychiatry*, 20(3): 317–328

Black RE, Cousens S, Johnson HL, Lawn JE, Rudan I, Bassani DG, et al, Child Health Epidemiology Reference Group of WHO, UNICEF (2010) Global, regional, and national causes of child mortality in 2008: a systematic analysis. *The Lancet*, 375(9730): 1969–87

Busby C, Hamdan M, Ariabi E (2010) Cancer, infant mortality and birth sex-ratio in Fallujah, Iraq 2005–2009, *International Journal of Environmental Research and Public Health*, 7: 2828–2837

Chaaya M, Jabbour S, El-Roueiheb Z, Chemaitelly H (2004) Knowledge, attitudes, and practices of argileh (water pipe or hubble-bubble) and cigarette smoking among pregnant women in Lebanon. *Addictive Behaviors*, 29(9): 1821–1831

Clark J (2003) Threat of war is affecting mental health of Iraqi children, says report. *British Medical Journal*, 326(7385): 356

Commission on the Social Determinants of Health (CSDH) 2008 *Closing the gap in a generation; Health equity through action on the social determinants of health*. WHO, 2008, Available from: http://www.who.int/social_determinants/thecommission/finalreport/en/index.html [Accessed Jan 2009]

Dashti M, Scott JA, Edwards CA, Al-Sughayer M (2010) Determinants of breastfeeding initiation among mothers in Kuwait. *International Breastfeeding Journal*, 28(5): 7

Dwairy M, Achoui M (2006) Introduction to three cross-regional research studies on parenting styles, individuation, and mental health in Arab societies. *Journal of Cross-Cultural Psychology*, 37(3): 221–229

El Taguri A, Besmar F, Ahmed AM, Betilmal I, Ricour I, Rolland-Cachera MF (2009) Stunting is a major risk factor for overweight: results from national surveys in 5 Arab countries. *Eastern Mediterranean Health Journal*, 15(3):549–562

El-Gilany AH (2007) Determinants and causes of son preference among women delivering in mansoura Egypt. *Eastern Mediterranean Health Journal*, 13(1), 119–128

El-Gilany AH, Amr M (2010) Child and adolescent mental health in the Middle East: an overview. *Middle East Journal of Family medicine*, 8(8): 11–18

El-Mouzan MI, Al-Herbish AS, Al-Salloum AA, Foster PJ, Al-Omar AA, Qurachi MM, Kecojevic T (2010) Regional disparity in prevalence of malnutrition in Saudi children. *Saudi Medical Journal*, 31(5):550–4

El-Sayed SM (2004) *Environmental Security in the Arab World, Paper prepared for presentation at the Meeting of the International Studies Association*. 17–20 March 2004, Montreal, Canada

Emirates news agency (WAM) (2009) *Gaza casualties reach 1, 314*, available from http://www.zawya.com/Story.cfm/sidWAM20090120214000810/Gaza%20casualties%20reach%201,314%20,%20including%20412%20children%20and%20110%20women:%20UNICEF/ [Accessed 28 May 2009]

Fida NM, Al-Aama J, Nichols W, Nichols W, Alqahtani M (2007) A prospective study of congenital malformations among live born neonates at a University Hospital in Western Saudi Arabia. *Saudi Medical Journal*, 28(9): 1367–1373

Gakidou E, Cowling K, Lozano R, Murray C (2010) Increased educational attainment and its effect on child mortality in 175 countries between 1970 and 2009: a systematic analysis. *The Lancet*, 376: 959–74

Galal O (2003) Nutrition-related health patterns in the Middle East. *Asia Pacific Journal of Clinical Nutrition*, 12(3): 337–343

Greiner T (1988) Correlation between birth-weights of infants born in the Yemen Arab Republic and the extent to which mothers said they chewed Qat. *Social Science and Medicine*, 26(7): 769

Gwatkin DR, Rutstein S, Johnson K, Suliman E, Wagstaff A, Amouzou A (2007) *Socio-Economic Differences in Health, Nutrition, and Population, Country reports*. Washington, DC: The World Bank

Hausdorffa WP, Hajjeh R, Al-Mazroud A, Shibld A, Soriano-Gabarroa M (2007) The epidemiology of pneumococcal, meningococcal, and Haemophilus disease in the MENA Region – Current status and needs. *Vaccine*, 25(11): 1935–1944

Higher Relief Commission (HRC) Daily Situation Report: 9/10/2006.

Report No 69, available from, http://www.reliefweb.int/rw/RWFiles2006.nsf/FilesByRWDocUNIDFileName/VBOL-6UEGSR-govlbn-lbn-09oct.pdf/$File/govlbn-lbn-09oct.pdf [Accessed 28 May 2009]

Hong R, Ruiz-Beltran M (2008) Low birth weight as a risk factor for infant mortality in Egypt. *Eastern Mediterranean Health Journal*, 14(5):992–1002

ILO (International Labor Organization) (2010) *International programme on elimination of child labor, Arab states*, available from http://www.ilo.org/ipec/Regionsandcountries/Arabstates/lang – en/index.htm [Accessed 23 December 2010]

Jahan S (2008) Poverty and infant mortality in the Eastern Mediterranean region: a meta-analysis. *Journal of Epidemiology and Community Health*, 62: 745–751

Khader Y, Irshaidat O, Khasawneh M, Amarin Z, Alomari M, Batieha A (2009) Over-weight and obesity among school children in Jordan: prevalence and associated factors. *Maternal and Child Health Journal*, 13(3): 424–431

Khawaja M, Dawns J, Meyerson-Knox S, Yamout R (2008) Disparities in child health in the Arab region during the 1990s. *International Journal for Equity in Health*, 7: 24

Irwin LG, Siddiqi A, Hertzman C (2007) *Early child development: A powerful equalizer*. Final Report for the World Health Organization's Commission on the Social Determinants of Health, 2007, available from http://whqlibdoc.who.int/hq/2007/a91213.pdf [Accessed 15 January 2010]

Mackroth MS, Irwin K, Vandelaer J, Hombach J, Eckert LO (2010) Immunizing school-age children and adolescents: experience from low- and middle-income countries. *Vaccine*, 28(5): 1138–1147

Makhlouf-Obermeyer C (2003) The health consequences of female circumcision: Science, advocacy, and standards of evidence. *Medical Anthropology Quarterly*, 17(3): 394–411

Mirmiran P, Sherafat-Kazemzadeh R, Jalali-Farahani S, Azizi F (2010) Childhood obesity in the Middle East: a review. *Eastern Mediterranean Health Journal*, 16(9)

Myntti C (1993) Social determinants of child health in Yemen. *Social Science & Medicine*, 37(2): 233–240

Nour O (2005) *Child disability in some countries of the MENA region: Magnitude, characteristics, problems and attempts to alleviate consequences of impairments.* Paper Presented at the XXVth IUSSP International Population Conference, Tours, France

Palma-Solís MA, Álvarez-Dardet DC, Franco-Giraldo A, Hernández-Aguado I, Pérez-Hoyos S (2009) State downsizing as a determinant of infant mortality and achievement of Millennium Development Goal 4. *International Journal of Health Services*, 39(2): 389–403

Peden M (2008) World report on child injury prevention appeals to Keep Kids Safe. *Injury Prevention* 14(6): 413–414

Saddik B, Nuwayhid I (2006) Child labour in Arab countries: call for action. *British Medical Journal*, 333(7573): 861–2.

Saggar AK, Bittles AH (2008) Consanguinity and child health. *Paediatrics and child health*. 18(5), 244–249

Salem EM, Abd El-Latif F (2002) Socio-demographic characteristics of street children in Alexandria. *Eastern Mediterranean Health Journal*, 8(1): 64–73

Save the Children – Sweden, the Global Initiative to End All Corporal

Punishment of Children (2010) *Ending legalised violence against children, Global Report 2010.* Nottingham, UK: The Russell Press Limited

Shaheen A, Edwards P (2008) Flying bullets and speeding cars: Analysis of child injury deaths in the Palestinian Territory. *Eastern Mediterranean Health Journal*, 14(2): 406–414

Shaikh U, Ahmed O (2006) Islam and infant feeding. *Breastfeeding Medicine*, 1(3): 164–167

Silink M (2010) The challenge of childhood obesity and diabetes. *The Lancet*, 375: 2211

Tadmouri GO, Nair P, Obeid T, Al Ali MT, Al-Khaja N, Hamamy HA (2009) Consanguinity and reproductive health among Arabs. *Reproductive Health*, 6: 17

Taha D, Ahmed O, bin Sadiq B (2009) The prevalence of metabolic syndrome and cardiovascular risk factors in a group of obese Saudi children and adolescents: A hospital-based study. *Annals of Saudi Medicine*, 29(5): 357–360

Tekce B (1990) Households, resources, and child health in a self-help settlement in Cairo, Egypt. *Social Science and Medicine*, 30(8): 929–940

UNICEF (United Nations International Children's Emergency Fund) (2009a) *The State of the World's Children*, Special edition, UNICEF, November 2009, New York

UNICEF (2009b) *Integrated management of childhood illness*, available from http://www.unicef.org/health/index_imcd.html [Accessed 23 December 2010]

UNICEF (2010a) *News note, New UNICEF report reveals alarming conditions for children in Djibouti,*

14 June 2010, available from http://www.unicef.org/media/media_53968.html [Accessed 23 December 2010]

UNICEF (2010b) *Introduction to immunization*, available from http://www.unicef.org/immunization/index.html [Accessed 23 December 2010]

UNICEF (2010c) *Child protection from violence, exploitation and abuse*, available from http://www.unicef.org/protection/index_genitalmutilation.html [Accessed 23 December 2010]

UNICEF (2010d) *Child Poverty and disparities in Egypt. Building the social infrastructure for Egypt's Future.* UNICEF, Egypt, February 2010

UNRWA (United Nations Relief and Works Agency for Palestine Refugees in the Near East) (2001) *UNRWA Health Report 2001, Department of Health, 2001*, HQs, Amman, Jordan

Watts S, Siddiqi S, Shukrullah A, Karim K, Serag H (2009) *Social determinants in countries in conflict and crisis: The Eastern Mediterranean perspective. Health Policy and Planning Unit, Division of Health System.* Cairo, Egypt: WHO/EMRO

WHO (World Health Organization) (2009) Global Health observatory, available from http://apps.who.int/ghodata/?vid=720 [Accessed 23 December 2010]

WHO (2010) Paediatric HIV, Available from www.who.int/hiv/topics/paediatric/data/en/index1.html [Accessed 23 December 2010]

Yount KM (2001) Excess mortality of girls in the Middle East in the 1970s and 1980s: Patterns, correlates and gaps in research. *Population Studies*, 55(3): 291–308

Chapter

18

The Health of Young People: Challenges and Opportunities

Rima Afifi, Jocelyn DeJong, Krishna Bose, Tanya Salem, Amr A. Awad, and Manal Benkirane

Dramatic events sweeping the Arab region during the winter of 2011 have brought media attention to a long-recognized demographic factor in the region: Arab countries are disproportionately youthful. Indeed, the Arab world now has the largest proportion of youth of its total population of all regions globally (Assaad & Roudi-Fahimi 2007). In 19 Arab countries, around 21% of the total population comprised youth aged 15–24 years old (Assaad & Roudi-Fahimi 2007). Today, the 15 to 29 age-group comprises ≥30% of the population in at least 6 countries and 25–29% in at least 11 others (Brookings Institution 2010). A large proportion of 15- to 24-year-olds is often referred to as the "youth bulge" and is due to the combination of sharp declines in child mortality and belated declines in fertility which has created a significant population momentum (See Assaad and Roudi-Fahimi 2007 and Chapter 3).

The identification of a specific life stage for young people is relatively recent in most of the Arab world. In Morocco, in the 1950s, little boys were welcomed to adulthood right after their circumcision (7–10 years old) and little girls after their menarche (Rachik 2005). Today, the transition to adulthood, in terms of education, marriage, and labor market entry, takes place over a longer period, which calls for a greater policy focus on this group (Assaad & Roudi-Fahimi 2007).

In discussions of young people's issues in the region, education, employment, and risky behaviors get attention – and these concerns have gained increasing attention given recent events – but health is rarely addressed or explicitly considered. This could be a result of health not being seen as a desired outcome but as "a resource for living" (WHO 1984). Health, however, is an essential determinant for achieving the personal and community goals of production and reproduction.

This chapter will present a conceptual framework for analysis of young people's health in the region, and

review the social determinants that influence this. This is followed by a review of the health and selected behavioral and risk factors of young people in the region; and the factors that are protective for this age group. We define young people as those in the age range 10–24 years, following common practices.

Framework for Analysis of Young People's Health

The Ecological Model of Health Promotion (McLeroy et al 1988) suggests that individual behavior is influenced by, and influences, factors at the interpersonal, organizational, community, and policy levels. Attention to such influences is needed to create an environment conducive to young people's health. The literature on young people's health in the region is mostly focused on individual level determinants of health and health behavior. Although necessary, such information is not sufficient to understand, analyze, and intervene to promote young people's health. Social determinants clearly influence young people's health. Socio-economic status, discrimination, and gender relations, for example, can influence a young person's access to information, services, and programs.

Several demographic and social trends affect young people (Chaaban 2009; Chapter 2). The average age at marriage has been rising for both sexes for a number of social and economic reasons (Singerman & Ibrahim 2003), and has resulted in a new phenomenon labeled "waitehood" or "the protracted transition to adulthood that young people … are experiencing as societies move away from traditional production patterns." (Assaad & Ramadan 2008). Greater exposure to global culture often creates rifts between generations, particularly as traditional social networks become more fragmented with greater urbanization and rapid social change. The emerging practice of "electronic" social networks such as FACEBOOK has to be evaluated not only for its clear role in political mobilization during the recent events, but also for its effect on the culture, practices, and expectations of young people. As one young Jordanian woman interviewed during the recent protests stated: "Social media is very important. The worlds of dialogue and information you are exposed to are crucial. They are both enriching and enlightening. Most of all, they allow you to find people all over the world who share the same views and opinions, which effectively demonstrates that no man is an island. This is what galvanized these movements we are witnessing today." (*Guardian* 2011).

The youth bulge augments the working-age population. While this can constitute a great opportunity for economic development, factors such as illiteracy, high youth unemployment, and political instability hinder such development. The Arab region had the highest youth (aged 15 to 24) unemployment rate in the world in 2005 – reaching 26% (Rachik 2005) and is projected to remain the highest (with North Africa) at around 24% in 2010 and 2011 (International Labour Organization 2010). There is a "lack of

harmonization between the outputs of education and training ... and labour market needs" (UNESCWA 2009). We look forward to the time when the changing demographics and social status of young people can be seen as an opportunity to harness vast untapped potential and dynamic energy. As Assaad & Roudi-Fahimi (2007 p.1) note: "The extent to which this large group ... will become healthy and productive members of their societies depends on how well governments and civil societies invest in social, economic, and political institutions that meet the current needs of young people."

If one considers individual determinants as the micro level, and ecological influences and social determinants as the meso-level, there remains a macro level of influences on young people's health which includes international foreign trade and health policy (Fidler & Drager 2006). This includes, for example, promotion and marketing of harmful commodities, especially tobacco, licit and illicit trade of firearms resulting in individual, civil, and inter-country warfare (Moore et al 2006). The framework for analysis of young people's health (Figure 1)

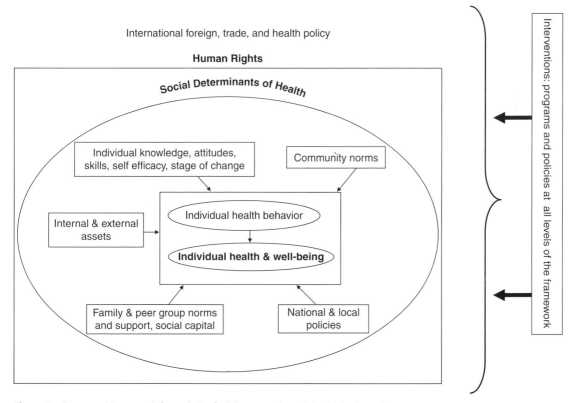

Figure 1. Conceptual Framework for analysis of adolescent and youth health in the region.

suggests that their health and well-being cannot be fully realized without attention to ensuring dignity and the attainment of all human rights, not only the right to health (Atkins et al 2002). Continuous vigilance to advocacy at the outer circles (the macro level) must be within the frame of practice of public health professionals.

Recent literature on young people has shifted from seeing young people as problems and a focus on risk behaviors to considering them as assets, with a focus on protective factors. This paradigm – called positive youth development or an assets approach (Catalano et al 2002) – focuses on all young people, not only those "at risk" and advocates surrounding young persons with an environment that promotes their development, rather than only focusing on preventing risky behaviors. The approach sees young people as contributing to community change by acting as resources and competent citizens in their communities. A focus on positive youth development means that interventions target building life skills and enhancing protective factors.

We understand young people's health as greatly enhanced by involving young people themselves in the assessment and analysis of issues that affect their lives and in the subsequent development, implementation, and evaluation of (promotion) programs. A ladder of young people's participation has been developed (Hart 1992) and suggests levels of possible engagement. We support engagement of young people at the highest levels as a mechanism of enhancing their voice as well as skill building for the positive roles they may take as adults.

The proposed framework is intended to contribute to shaping the dialogue on young people as well as policy, strategy, research, and programs for young people's health in the region.

Social Determinants of Health of Young People

Social determinants are now recognized as the root causes of health status and well-being. They include factors such as income, gender, ethnicity, social class, and education, among others. Although the Arab world is often discussed as one entity, there are many subcultures within it. At the very least, there are three distinct economic strata: the rich oil countries, the middle-income countries of the Levant and North Africa, and the poorest countries such as Yemen.

Selected data on social determinants were recently summarized in a report on youth health in the region (Afifi Soweid & Nehlawi 2007). The percent of persons (not just young people) living below the poverty line ranged from about 7% in Tunisia to 60% in the Comoros Islands. There are vast differences in access to education between countries. Illiteracy for 15–24 year olds ranges from less than 1% in Jordan to 50% in Yemen. The ratio of literacy between women and men aged 15–24 years – an indicator of gender equality, ranges between 0.34 in Yemen to 1.08 in the United Arab Emirates (Afifi Soweid & Nehlawi 2007). The gender gap is still prominent in indicators such as education, employment, and overall status in society (UNICEF 2000).

Inequities in social factors translate into health inequities. Research in the region linking social determinants to health outcomes is still in its infancy, at most disaggregating data by sex and providing regression data on very selected socio-economic status indicators (both rarely). Work on social inequities and their impact on health is increasing (Al-Adili et al 2008; Rezaeian 2007), and needs to be supported.

Although acknowledging the great amount of work yet to be done in individual countries and across the region to advance young people's health and well-being, international politics will continue to limit effectiveness and impact. Violence and conflict fueled by international interests result in displacement, interrupted schooling, disrupted access to basic services, limited opportunities for employment of young people and their families, and disrupted usual livelihoods such as agricultural work (in addition to causing massive death and disability) (SRSG-CAAC et al 2007). Generalized economic sanctions affect children and young people most (see chapters in Section 5). These are social determinants at the global level.

In order to impact young people's health, public health practitioners and researchers need to implement interventions targeted at social determinants and need to play their roles as agents of change (Shuftan 2008), including in prevention of war and conflict.

Health Status, Behaviors and Risk Factors of Young People

While we promote an approach to young people that focuses on healthy development, the data available for the region focuses on health problems – a traditional approach to assessing health for any age group. Youth is generally perceived to be a healthy period. Individuals have passed the threats of childhood infectious diseases and are not yet old enough to acquire chronic diseases. However, a recent study (Patton et al 2009) of young people's (10–24 years) mortality around the world indicated that 2.6 million deaths occurred in this age group in 2004, with 97% occurring in low- to middle-income countries (LMICs). In the Eastern Mediterranean region (EMR), which includes mostly Arab countries, young people had a relative risk of dying of 3.7 as compared to those in high-income countries and the third highest relative risk of LMICs after Africa and South East Asia. Even if one considers mortality to be relatively low in this life stage, it is a critical period in terms of uptake of risky behaviors that influence health and disease later.

A recent review (Afifi Soweid & Nehlawi 2007) found very little information about youth health or health risk behaviors: a total of 83 studies or reports over a 12 year period, translating into about 3.7 studies/reports per country or 0.3 studies/year/country. Several international initiatives have made data about young people's health and risk factor's more available. The partnership between the World Health Organization (WHO) and the US Centers for Disease Control and Prevention (CDC) has resulted in the implementation of the Global Youth Tobacco Survey (GYTS) in Arab countries thus supplying data on smoking for all. Several countries have implemented the more comprehensive Global School-based Student Health Survey (GSHS). Both surveys include young people in grade 7–9.

In this section, we focus on reproductive health, mental health, drug use, tobacco, and obesity. Maternal conditions are the leading cause of mortality for young women and the third largest reason for years lost to disabilities (YLD). Mental health and specifically neuro-psychiatric conditions are a leading cause of YLDs. Drug use influences other risky behaviors and consequences, including injuries, and mental health. Tobacco use and obesity are clear determinants of the epidemic of cardiovascular and other non-communicable diseases. There is a perceived urgency among health professionals in the region, as well as global concern, to tackle these issues. By focusing on these issues for attention we ignore neither other important issues nor the imperative of addressing the needs of young people in their entirety; young people, like people of any other age, do not compartmentalize their lives.

Reproductive Health: In addition to high risk of maternal mortality, adolescent women also have considerable reproductive morbidity (DeJong et al 2005). Only a few of the studies on reproductive morbidity have focused on the special needs of adolescent women. In a pioneering population-based study in Egypt of 508 ever-married women (Khattab et al 1999), 45% of ever-married 14- to 19-year-olds and 55% of 10- to 24-year-olds suffered from reproductive tract infections and 24% of 14- to 19-year-olds and 43% of 20- to 24-year-olds suffered from genital prolapse; yet adolescent married women tended to report serious and non-obstetric complaints much less frequently than older women. The researchers recommended special efforts to reach out to this age group and understand their health-seeking behavior. Young people contribute disproportionately to the HIV epidemic and burden of sexually transmitted infections in the region; yet programs to address sexual and reproductive health education in schools are still under-developed (Abu Raddad et al 2010). The sexual and reproductive health of young people embraces preparation for marriage and reproductive roles as well as addressing the health consequences of sexuality and reproduction in an age-appropriate manner. A focus on sexual and reproductive health *problems* ignores the positive aspects of this age period as identities are formed, relationships beyond the family are fostered, and for many, child-bearing begins.

A comprehensive situation analysis (DeJong & El-Khoury 2006; Shepard & DeJong 2005), found that young people's sexual and reproductive health is under-researched. The limited available information points to considerable unmet need for reproductive health services among young women in particular, both married and unmarried. Provision of such services is still a relatively new concept in a region where the traditional focus has been on maternal health and family planning. There has been political and cultural resistance to addressing the needs of unmarried young people in particular (DeJong & El-Khoury 2006; DeJong et al 2007). While there is emerging literature on young people's reproductive health, studies have focused on topics such as use of family planning services, knowledge about HIV/AIDS (see for example Busulwa et al 2006), and adolescent gender roles (e.g., Jaffer et al 2006) rather than on

Table 1. Legal Minimum Age for Females to Marry in Arab Countries[1] (this table has been updated as of February 2009)

Puberty	Age 9	Age 15	Age 16	Age 17	Age 18	Age 20	Unlegislated
Sudan	Gaza	Kuwait West Bank Yemen	Egypt	Syria[2] Tunisia	Algeria Djibouti[3] Iraq[4] Jordan[5] Lebanon[6] Morocco	Libya	Bahrain Oman Qatar Saudi Arabia UAE

Notes:
[1] All data, unless otherwise noted, has been retrieved from the Women's Learning Partnership for Rights, Development, and Peace (WLP) website at http://www.learningpartnership.org/legislat/family_law.phtml with information compiled from the Emory Islamic Family Law Project, http://www.law.emory.edu/ifl/index2.html, accessed on March 3, 2009
[2] In Syria women can be married at 13 with the permission of a judge
[3] UNFPA report on Djibouti acknowledges that the latest Djibouti Family Code legislates the female age of marriage at 18, see http://www.un.org.dj/UNFPA/CP%202003–2007%20DJIBOUTI.pdf, accessed on January 18, 2009.
[4] Women can get married in Iraq at 15 with parental consent.
[5] A temporary law in Jordan raised the age of marriage for both girls and boys to 18; this remains a temporary law until it is passed and endorsed by parliament.
[6] Lebanon allows marriage at younger ages based on religious affiliation or sect. As described on the Emory Islamic Family Law project, "age of capacity is 18 years for males and 17 for females; scope for judicial discretion on basis of physical maturity and wali's permission from 17 years for males and 9 for females; real puberty or 15/9 with judicial permission for Shi'a; 18/17 or 16/15 with judicial permission for Druze", from http://www.law.emory.edu/IFL/legal/lebanon.htm, accessed January 18, 2009.

the full range of reproductive health conditions young people may experience.

Average age at marriage for women is rising, from between 18 and 21 years in the 1970s, to between 22 and 25 years in the 1990s (Roudi-Fahimi & Kent 2007). This is partly due to the high costs of marriage and securing housing (Rashad et al 2005). In more than a third of countries, the average age at marriage has risen between 4.7 and 7.7 years over a period of 20 years (Abu Raddad et al 2010). However, there are still pockets of early marriage in all countries. As Table 1 illustrates, the legal minimum age at marriage for girls is as low as 15 in Kuwait, the West Bank, and Yemen, and 16 in Egypt. The trend of later age at marriage, combined with a global trend in earlier age of puberty onset, has exposed young people to greater health risks associated with increasing pre-marital sexual activity and rising sexually transmitted infection rates, including HIV (Abu Raddad et al 2010). This risk is heightened by young people's lack of information about their sexual and reproductive health, and lack of access to youth-friendly services. While rigorous studies are few, anecdotal evidence suggests that premarital sexuality is increasing with exposure to global norms through electronic media and networking, increased autonomy of young people and at the same time economic constraints to marriage in many contexts. This raises attendant concerns about lack of health protection given the stigma faced

by unmarried women in accessing contraception. In a study of Lebanese university students, 73.3% of male and 21.8% of female students reported previous sexual relations; among these, 75.6% of females reported never using contraceptives, whereas 86.1% of males had (Barbour & Salameh 2009).

The health implications of changes in the institution of marriage are almost completely unexplored, particularly with the occurrence of nonconventional forms of marriage in countries of the Gulf and Egypt (Rashad et al 2005). For example, *"urfi"* marriage – a practice whereby young people obtain a clandestine marriage certificate to engage in sexual relations but which is unprotected legally or in terms of access to health services – represents a new response of young people to the economic and social impediments to conventional marriage. As Rashad and Osman state, it *"...may represent a coping strategy among youth as a compromise to the economic constraints to marriage and the cultural denial of extra-marital relations"* (Rashad & Osman 2003 p. 9).

For young people with sexual and reproductive health concerns, existing health services do not cater specifically to their needs, and where available, may not always be conveniently located or staffed. There are cultural barriers to young women and men using them. Few government services are equipped to counsel and answer young people's questions pertaining to sexual and reproductive health and there is often little scope for privacy. Confidentiality is not culturally understood to be a right for young people and is not prioritized in health services. This all adds to the known stigma and psychological suffering associated with sexual and reproductive health conditions.

Mental Health: A review of mental health in the EMR identified young people's mental health as an emerging priority (Mohti 2001). The GSHS does not provide a measure of mental health but provides indicators or proxy measures for depression, anxiety, and suicide, such as loneliness, sleep disturbances, and suicide ideation. To date, 11 countries have implemented the GSHS, although not all have selected the same modules. The percent of young persons who reported feeling lonely most or all of the time (asked in seven countries) in the last year ranged from a low of 7.9% in Egypt (2006) to a high of 17.2% in Tunisia (2008). Those who had seriously considered suicide ranged from 12.7% in Morocco (2006) and the UAE (2005) to 19.8% in Tunisia (2008). These figures call for concern.

With respect to mental conditions, most research is focused on countries in conflict, with less focus on adolescents in non-conflict countries or during periods of no conflict. Analysis of patterns of actual suicide among 15–60+ years individuals (Rezaeian 2007) suggested that the peak age for suicide among women was 15–29 years, and that suicide comprised 20% of all deaths due to injuries for women in this age-group. Rates of suicide for both women and men were lowest in high-income countries. Suicide rates in official statistics are likely under-estimates due to social, cultural, and religious taboos on suicide; likewise, mental conditions are under-reported due to stigma attached to such issues (Rezaeian 2007; Jaju et al 2009).

Depressive symptoms seem to be common among young people. Oman implemented a survey in secondary schools as part of the World Mental Health Survey (Jaju et al 2009). Protective factors identified included being male, younger, having good relationships with their social contacts, having a hobby, eating breakfast every day, and sleeping 7–8 hours each night. Risk factors included a high external locus of control and a low internal locus of control score, abuse by parents, a poor relationship with parents, older age, being female, failing a year at school, history of organic illness, and a history of mental illness. Afifi (2006) found that rates of depressive symptoms

are higher in girls than boys and range between 7% and 19%.

Among countries in conflict, exposure to trauma is high for young people in war-affected areas, with boys and older youth generally exposed more than girls and younger youth (Karam et al 2006; Tanios et al 2009; Thabet et al 2008). Exposure to trauma was associated with post-traumatic stress disorder (PTSD) and/or depression and/or anxiety (Giacaman et al 2007a; Karam et al 2006; Tanios et al 2009; Thabet et al 2008). The prevalence of PTSD among young people has ranged from 24% in Lebanon to 69% in Gaza (Elbedour et al 2007; Tanios et al 2009). Prevalence of anxiety disorders also varies: In Lebanon 17.9% reported separation anxiety while 24.9% reported being over-anxious; in Gaza 21.5% exhibited anxiety disorders (Elbedour et al 2007; Tanios et al 2009). As time from trauma passes prevalence of both PTSD and anxiety disorders decrease significantly (Tanios et al 2009). Gender differences in almost every measure of exposure or mental conditions indicate the need to consider gender in both assessment and interventions. Recent research has explored more subtle concepts such as exposure to humiliation and perceived discrimination as indicators of potential mental health problems (Giacaman et al 2007b). The validity of Western biomedical mental illness models to situations of chronic conflict such as that in the Occupied Palestinian Territory has been questioned, suggesting that concepts such as resilience may be a more relevant and valid to context (Rabaia et al 2010). Chapter 15 explores this issue in more detail.

A limited number of interventions in mental health have targeted all young people as opposed to young people with identified clinical disorders. Three interventions with Palestinian youth in Gaza (Thabet et al 2005), Lebanese children and youth in Qana (South Lebanon) (Karam et al 2008), and Palestinian refugees in Beirut (Afifi et al 2010a) did not show an impact despite the presence of a control group in all three. This demonstrates the challenge of promoting mental health in contexts of disadvantage and suggests that "the state of science is still far from determining the effectiveness or specificity of either "social" or "psychological" components of these interventions" (Karam et al 2008 p. 107). Lack of impact also stresses the need for health professionals to enhance their advocacy to prevent exposure to trauma (Thabet et al 2005) and to improve the root causes of ill health such as poverty, unemployment, and discrimination (Rezaeian 2007). Additionally, traditional interventions may not be relevant to context and collective interventions may be more appropriate (Rabaia et al 2010).

Illicit Drug Use: The number of drug users is increasing especially among youth (15–24 years) and women (WHO 2006). Many countries have witnessed rapid social change and emerging or long-term conflict and are vulnerable to health, social, and economic problems related to drug use and dependence (WHO 2006). The region is one of the most important transit areas of the world for illicit drugs. The most common drugs are cannabis, sedatives, opiates, and stimulants (WHO 2006). Among injected drugs, opiates are most commonly used (WHO 2006). Most consumed drugs are locally cultivated: Morocco is the world's leading producer of cannabis resin; Yemen is a prominent producer of khat (*Catha edulis*), and this is legally sold to young people and consumed by these on the streets without restrictions; Iraq is starting to cultivate opium poppy fields.

Considering the size of the problem, there is a dearth of research on prevalence and/or determinants of drug use and abuse among young people. In Egypt, the most abused drugs were alcohol, hashish, stimulants, tranquilizers, hypnotics, and opium. Male university students were more likely to use these substances than females except for tranquilizers and hypnotics where rates of use were similar (Okasha 1999). Secondary school students were most likely to use hashish; the main reason provided for use was entertainment and socializing with friends. Sedatives and hypnotics were the second most used substances to help cope with psychosocial problems or when tired or studying for exams (Okasha 1999). In Bahrain, risk factors for overdose among young people included family problems, relationship problems with the opposite sex, unemployment, and problems of school performance (Al-Ansari et al 2001). In Lebanon, 10% of university students had ever tried tranquilizers, 8% barbiturates, and 4% marijuana; females were more likely to have ever tried the first two, and males the latter (Karam et al 2000). About one-fifth of Bedouin adolescents of the Negev reported use of an illicit drug in the past year. Drug use was more likely among school attendees (rather than drop outs), males, and those stating they were from a secular (rather than devout Muslim) household, those with tolerant attitudes toward use, and who

came from families who were less cohesive and less adaptable (Diamond et al 2008). The GSHS includes a module on alcohol and drugs but only 4 of the 11 Arab countries that have implemented the GSHS chose this module. Prevalence of ever used drugs ranged from 3.4% in Lebanon to 6.9% in Morocco.

Tobacco: There are abundant data to indicate that tobacco use among young people is a public health problem. The GYTS results from Arab countries indicate that among 13- to 15-year-olds, some of the highest ever use of cigarettes is seen in countries of conflict; for examples, 39% of young people in the West Bank, 33% of those in Gaza, and 31.6% of young people in Iraq have ever smoked cigarettes. Even in non-conflict countries rates are high: 34.5% of young people in Saudi Arabia and 32% of young people in Jordan have also ever tried cigarettes. The highest current smoking of cigarettes among young people is in the West Bank (19%). The GYTS also explored attitudes, exposure to advertisement and to free cigarettes, and second-hand smoke. In many countries, more than 50% of young people live in homes where others smoke in their presence. Both knowledge and attitudes (perceived susceptibility) independently protect against cigarette smoking (Yeretzian & Afifi 2009), as do non-smoking behaviors of parents, teachers, and friends (for example, see Afifi et al 2009; El-Tayeb et al 2010; Mandil et al 2007; Maziak et al 2004).

A unique feature of tobacco use is the high rates of use of alternate forms of tobacco such as the *narghile* (waterpipe or hookah). This is evident in current smoking prevalence for any type of tobacco which, in most cases, is greater than that for cigarettes alone. For example, in Lebanon, 61% of students reported currently using a tobacco product, although only 10% currently smoked cigarettes. The GYTS results indicated that in all studied countries, use of tobacco products other than cigarettes (most likely waterpipe) was more common than use of cigarettes. Research has identified the following determinants of *narghile* smoking among middle school, secondary school, or university students: male gender, knowledge of health effects, parental education, parental occupation, crowding index, socio-economic status (private versus public school), parental cigarette and *narghile* smoking, peer use of *narghile*, alcohol use, exercise, seat-belt use, and Internet use (Afifi et al 2009; El-Roueiheb et al 2008; Mandil et al 2007; Maziak et al 2004; Tamim et al 2007).

Obesity: As discussed elsewhere (see Chapters 10, 12 & 13), over-weight and obesity are important public health concerns. Among adolescents, these are perhaps most prevalent in the Gulf countries, and are on the rise. Over-weight rates ranged from 13.4% in Qatar to 32% in Kuwait (Al-Hazzaa 2002; Al-Saeed et al 2003; Al-Sendi et al 2003; Bener & Tewfic 2006). Obesity rates ranged from 1.8% in Qatar to 20% in Saudi Arabia (Al-Hazzaa 2002; Al-Saeed et al 2003; Al-Sendi et al 2003; Bener & Tewfic 2006; Malik & Bakir 2006). Gender differences were evident but differed among countries. The pattern is not so different outside the Gulf. Over-weight rates ranged between 7% (in Egypt) and 37% in Lebanon (Al-Sabbah et al 2008; Blouza-Chabchoub et al 2006; Chakar & Salameh 2006; Hwalla et al 2005; Salazar-Martinez et al 2006). Obesity rates ranged from 3% (in the West Bank) to 12.5% (in Lebanon). Gender differences are again mixed. GSHS results indicate that between 11.8% and 37.6% are over-weight. Prevalence rates for obesity range from 4.4% to 15.6%.

Determinants of over-weight and obesity were varied and included being an expatriate (non-national) in the Gulf, and physical inactivity (Al-Sabbah et al 2008). As for gender and socio-economic status, results are varied (Al-Saeed et al 2003; Hwalla et al 2005). Weight dissatisfaction has been linked to engagement in weight control and other risky behavior (Al-Sabbah et al 2008; Kanaan & Afifi 2009) and therefore may be an important signal for intervention.

Protective Factors in the Lives of Adolescents

Protective factors enhance the likelihood of positive outcomes and lessen the likelihood of engaging in risk behaviors or of adverse outcomes from such behaviors (Jessor et al 1995). In our conceptual framework, these are micro and meso determinants. As adolescents negotiate their way in life, they encounter numerous situations in a world that provides opportunities for progress but also risks to their health and well-being. Early research and intervention focused on assessing and changing risk factors as antecedents for reducing risk behaviors. However, exposure to risk factors alone is not enough to understand the likelihood of engaging in risk behaviors. Some adolescents show remarkable resilience to strong risk exposure. Focusing on the strengths and skills of adolescents has led to a shift toward considering

protective factors that buffer them against risk factors and mitigate their effect. The focus on protective factors (also called developmental assets) recognizes the positive influences within young people themselves and in their social environment that can be supported through programming efforts (WHO 2007). There is now clear evidence that the more protective factors there are in the lives of adolescents the more they are likely to have healthy outcomes (Leffert et al 1998). Both risk and protective factors need to be addressed in order to ensure better outcomes for adolescents (Catalano et al 2002).

Various efforts are under way to assess protective factors or assets among young people. The GSHS, which explores protective factors such as parental monitoring, self-regulation, and others, has been implemented in several countries. The WHO has investigated the relevance and contribution of three protective factors – connection, regulation, and respect for individuality (Barber et al 2005) – that are important in parental roles with adolescents and which in turn influence engagement in specific risk behavior. The latter include alcohol and drug use, interpersonal violence, risky sexual behavior, specific anti-social behavior including truancy and vandalism. These protective factors had a strong and consistent relationship with adolescents' sense of self-efficacy, their social initiative, and reported depression in the absence of such protection.

The Search Institute's 40 developmental assets have been extensively studied, although to date mostly in industrialized countries (see for example, Aspy et al 2004). These assets are grouped into eight categories: four external including support, empowerment, boundaries and expectations, and constructive use of time; and four internal including commitment to learning, positive values, social competencies, and positive identity. Substantial research on these assets has indicated their effectiveness in preventing risky behavior and promoting well-being (see for example, Aspy et al 2004; Scales et al 2000). These protective factors appear to be valid across many cultures (Scales et al 2000), including those in this region as shown in Lebanon (Afifi et al 2010b), and in the OPT (Rabaia et al 2010).

Young People's Voices

As discussed earlier, young people's participation in defining their needs and in the development, implementation, and evaluation of interventions is critical for effective and sustainable improvement in their health. Most research discussed thus far has been quantitative in nature. Qualitative research is also important to provide an in-depth understanding of young people's issues through their own eyes and their perceptions of their reality. Young people's programs across the region are beginning gradually and shyly to involve young people in assessing, developing, implementing, and evaluating programs targeted at them. Such programs are more likely to be relevant to young people's needs and sustainable.

When asked about their lives, young people are articulate, coherent, and eloquent in their descriptions. UNFPA included young people's voices in their State of the World Population report of 2007 through two supplements: Growing Up Urban and Moving Young. UNICEF has sponsored a report entitled: "Will you listen? Young voices from conflict zones." Excerpts from this report indicate that young people can identify the issues that affect their lives.

Young people also engage in programs to impact their communities and change their lives. The Qaderoon mental health promotion project in the Burj El Barajneh Palestinian refugee camp in Beirut, involved young people aged 17–25 as mentors in the implementation of the social skills building program for younger adolescents (fifth and sixth graders). Interviews conducted with youth mentors provided insight into the reasons young people engage in such programs (Makhoul et al 2010).

> "What I liked about the project is that it involves helping the children in the camp. I passed through problems and situations when I was young and I don't want my little brother or cousin or neighbor to commit the same mistakes I did previously. This was one of the major incentives that encouraged me to join this project"
> (p. 1–2 Male #2).

> "I liked the kids more than anything in the project. I liked the kids a lot. I felt that I was benefiting someone. Really for the first time I feel that I am doing something for someone, that is someone in need. I'm doing something that is. I'm doing something good for the camp"
> (p. 4–5 Female #4).

Involving young people is a win-win situation. The paradigm of positive youth development and participatory engagement views young people's involvement as vital to their own development and that of their communities (Hughes & Curnan 2000), and considers young people as "powerful catalysts" in their communities who are capable of working with adults as partners to make these communities safer and more prosperous (Hughes & Curnan 2000). Evidence supports the effectiveness of positive youth development programs (Catalano et al 2002).

Across the region, innovative culturally sensitive programs are addressing young people's health and well-being. They are promoting protective factors and tackling the social determinants of health. Often, they engage young people actively in planning and implementation. Model programs for young people developed in other contexts can be combined with local experiences to provide a rich menu of interventions from which to adapt possible programs for young people. Keeping the framework in mind, young people's policies should ensure that adolescents and young people have access to (i) basic information, (ii) life skills, (iii) comprehensive services, and (iv) safe and supportive environments.

Conclusions and Recommendations

This chapter was written before the events of winter 2011 brought the region and the desire of its citizens for better living conditions, basic rights, and democratic liberties to the focus of world attention. The prominence of young people mutually connected through electronic media networks in the social protests that led to the toppling of successive regimes has been universally noted and emphasized. A clear and welcome shift has implicitly resulted in media coverage of the region from a focus on young people as potentially politically dangerous, to one recognizing their potential and needs. In this way, events have confirmed the thrust of this chapter, which has argued for a paradigm shift in thinking about young people by focusing on their vast potential to influence their own lives and that of their communities. The chapter has also stressed the importance of acknowledging the many determinants at micro, meso, and macro levels that work either to expose young people to potential harm or provide them with opportunities to reach their potential. Although mortality among youth may not be high, the social and economic circumstances of youth and their exposure to risk factors put them in a precarious health position. This ultimately affects their ability to be productive members of society.

The Arab region shares commonalities such as language, the importance of religion, the significance of the family unit (or collective support), and the existence of a large youth population; yet it is also quite diverse in terms of economic conditions, national identities, and history of exposure to the

Global North. Policies and programs to address young people's needs should capitalize on these commonalities while recognizing diversities.

While attention shifts to the needs of young people, it is critically important that their health needs are considered alongside concerns such as education and employment which are more obviously linked to economic development. There is limited research on young people's health, and even less on its social and structural determinants. It is difficult to compare results of research across the region due to differing included age groups, differing definitions, and differing measurement instruments. In keeping with the conceptual framework, research needs to assess the impact of broad determinants of health and health behaviors and be bold enough to tackle the impact of international policy on the health of young people. To do so effectively, and ask the right questions, the research must, by design, be multidisciplinary and multisectoral, and must use multiple methods, including quantitative and qualitative ones.

There are research gaps in important topics, for example, on young people's motor vehicle injuries and fatalities and their determinants, although these are leading causes of young people's death. Because most research has focused on describing problems rather than identifying determinants, it has also typically not been theory-based and this has led to lack of development of theory-based programs. The application of theory at various levels, individual, social network, community, policy, would strengthen the ability of regional research to ask the right questions and provide answers that could be used to develop intervention programs.

A focus on ecologic frameworks and social determinants often suggests problems are larger than life. This chapter has attempted to temper that with a focus on young people as productive active agents of change in their communities and their own lives – with opinions, thoughts, ambitions, energy, and hope. Many innovative programs for young people are under way, but are rarely documented. Data on effectiveness of interventions are critical to ascertain prior to recommending a specific program for replication; therefore, robust evaluation designs using different methods are needed. Partnership among community programs, academic institutions, and national and international development agencies may help improve such designs. Once effectiveness is documented, programs need to be institutionalized within the health, youth, and education systems in the country. Governmental organizations and NGOs need to be engaged early in order to be ready to up-scale effective interventions.

Given the strength of the evidence, programmatic planning should consider a paradigm shift to an emphasis on protective factors – rather than predominantly risk factors as is the case today. Building on the resources and assets of young people, and creating supportive social relationships and communities, is a more cost effective way to promote young people's health.

Finally, expanded indicators of health and well-being – which include an analysis of social determinants and protective factors rather than only risk factors – are needed. This would assist policy makers, government institutions, youth agencies, funders, evaluators, program planners and implementers, researchers, and young people themselves to assess the realities of young people's health, and develop policies and interventions to promote and enhance their well-being.

Young people are windows to the future. The increasing surge of young people in the region creates challenges and opportunities. The opportunities are most easily harnessed through involving young people themselves as resources and assets in diagnosing problems and identifying solutions. The evidence suggests that strong support by adults and institutions in young people's lives is critical to successful navigation of this life phase. An Arabic proverb states: "What is learned in youth is carved in stone" and compels public health professionals in the region to ensure an environment conducive to productive learning for health enhancement leading to productive lives.

Acknowledgment

Krishna Bose is a staff member of the World Health Organization. The author alone is responsible for the views expressed in this publication and they do not necessarily represent the decisions or policies of the World Health Organization.

References

Abu Raddad J, Ayodeji-Akal F, Semini I, Riedner G, Wilson D, Tawil O (2010) *Characterizing the HIV/AIDS epidemic in the Middle East and North Africa: Time for strategic action.* Washington, DC: The World Bank

Afifi M (2006) Depression in adolescents: Gender differences in Oman and Egypt. *Eastern Mediterranean Health Journal,* 12(1–2): 61–71

Afifi RA, Bteddini D, Scales P, Nakkash R (2010b) *Reliability and validity of the Developmental Assets*

Profile in Lebanon. Unpublished manuscript

Afifi RA, Nakkash R, El Hajj T, et al (2010a) Qaderoon youth mental health promotion programme in the Burj El Barajneh Palestinian refugee camp, Beirut, Lebanon: a community-intervention analysis. *The Lancet, peer review abstract posted electronically at: download.thelancet.com/flatcontentassets/pdfs/ . . ./S0140673610608471.pdf* [Accessed: 01 October 2010]

Afifi RA, Yeretzian JS, Rouhana A, Nehlawi MT, Mack A (2009) Neighborhood effects on narghile smoking among youth in Beirut. *European Journal of Public Health,* 20(4): 456–462

Afifi Soweid R, Nehlawi M (2007) *Youth and health issues in the Arab region: The millennium development goals in the Arab region 2007: A youth lens.* Report written for ESCWA, March 2007

Al-Adili N, Shaheen M, Bergstrom S, Johansson A (2008) Deaths among young, single women in 2000–2001 in the West bank, Palestine Occupied Territories. *Reproductive Health Matters,* 16(31): 112–121

Al-Ansari AM, Hamadeh RR, Matar AM, Marhoon H, Buzaboon BY, Raees AG (2001) Risk factors associated with overdose among Bahraini youth. *Suicide & Life Threatening Behavior,* 31(2): 197–206

Al-Hazzaa HM (2002) Physical activity, fitness, and fatness among Saudi children and adolescents, Implications for cardiovascular health. *Saudi Medical Journal,* 23: 144–150

Al-Sabbah H, Vereecken C, Abdeen Z, Coats E, Maes L (2008) Associations of overweight and of weight dissatisfaction among Palestinian schoolchildren (HSBC-WBG2004). *Journal of Human Nutrition and Dietetics,* 22: 40–49

Al-Saeed WY, Al-Dawood KM, Bukhari IA, Bahnassy A (2003) Prevalence and socioeconomic risk factors of obesity among urban female students in Al-Khobar city, Eastern Saudi Arabia. *Obesity Reviews,* 8: 93–99

Al-Sendi AM, Shetty P, Musaiger AO (2003) Prevalence of overweight and obesity among Bahraini adolescents: A comparison between three different sets of criteria. *European Journal of Clinical Nutrition,* 57(3): 471–474

Aspy CB, Oman RF, Vesely SK, McLeroy K, Rodine S, Marshall L (2004) Adolescent violence: The protective effects of youth assets. *Journal of Counseling and Development,* 82: 269–277

Assaad R, Ramadan M (2008) *Did housing policy reforms curb the delay in marriage among young men in Egypt?* Dubai, UAE: Middle East Youth Initiative Policy Outlook

Assaad R, Roudi-Fahimi F (2007) *Youth in the Middle East and North Africa: Demographic opportunity or challenge?* Washington, DC: Population Reference Bureau

Atkins LA, Oman RF, Vesely SK (2002) Adolescent tobacco use: The protective effects of developmental assets. *American Journal of Health Promotion,* 16(4): 198–205

Barber BK, Stolz HE, Olsen JA (2005) Parental support, psychological control, and behavioral control: Assessing relevance across time, method, and culture. *Monographs of the Society for Research in Child Development,* 70(4): 1–137

Barbour B, Salameh P (2009) Knowledge and practice of university students in Lebanon regarding contraception, *Eastern Mediterranean Health Journal,* 15(2): 387–399

Bener A, Tewfic I (2006) Prevalence of overweight, obesity, and associated psychological problems in Qatari's female population, *Obesity Review,* 7(2): 139–145

Blouza-Chabchoub S, Rached-Armouche C, Jamoussi-Kammoun H, Bouchaa N (2006) Frequency and risk factors of obesity in Tunisian adolescent. *Tunisie Medicale,* 84(11):714–6

Brookings Institution (2010) *Understanding the generation in waiting in the Middle East.* Washington, DC: Middle East Youth Initiative at the Brookings Institution. Available from http://www.brookings.edu/~/media/Files/rc/articles/2010/06_middle_east_youth/06_middle_east_youth_map.swf [Accessed 20 February 2011]

Busulwa R, Takiyadddin MY, Azzubeidi AA, et al (2006) Perceptions of the condom as a method of HIV prevention in Yemen. *Eastern Mediterranean Health Journal,* 12(S12): 64–77

Catalano RF, Berglund M, Ryan JAM, Lonczak HS, Hawkins JD (2002) Positive youth development in the United States: Research findings on evaluations of positive youth development programs. *Prevention & Treatment,* 5(15). Available from http://psycnet.apa.org/journals/pre/5/1/15a.pdf [Accessed 13 January 2011]

Chaaban J (2009) Youth and development in the Arab countries: The need for a different approach. *Middle Eastern Studies,* 45(1): 33–55

Chaaya M, El-Roueiheb Z, Chemaitelly H, Azar G, Nasr J, Al-Sahab B (2004) Argileh smoking among university students: A new tobacco epidemic. *Nicotine & Tobacco Research,* 6: 457–463

Chakar H, Salameh PR (2006) Adolescent obesity in Lebanese private schools. *European Journal of Public Health,* 16(6): 648–651

DeJong J, El-Khoury G (2006) Reproductive health of Arab young people. *British Medical Journal,* 333: 849–51

DeJong J, Jawad R, Mortagy I, Shepard B (2005) "The sexual and reproductive health of young people in the Arab countries and Iran". *Reproductive Health Matters,* 13(25): 49–59

DeJong J, Shepard B, Roudi-Fahimi F, Ashford L (2007, April) *Young people's sexual and reproductive health in the Middle East and North Africa Region.* Washington, DC: Population Reference Bureau

Diamond GM, Farhat A, Al-Amor M, Elbedour S, Shelef K, Bar-Hamburger R (2008) Drug and alcohol use among the Bedouin of the Negev: Prevalence and psychosocial correlates. *Addictive Behaviors*, 33(1): 143–151

Elbedour S, Onwuegbuzie AJ, Ghannam J, Whitcome JA, Abu-Hein F (2007) Post-traumatic stress disorder, depression, and anxiety among Gaza strip adolescents in the wake of the second Uprising (intifada). *Child abuse and Neglect*, 31: 719–729

El-Roueiheb Z, Tamim H, Kanj M, Jabbour S, Alayan I, Musharrafieh U (2008) Cigarette and waterpipe smoking among Lebanese adolescents, a cross-sectional study, 2003–2004. *Nicotine & Tobacco Research*, 10(2): 309–314

El-Tayeb S, Nwaru BI, Ginawi I, Pisani P, Hakama M (2010) The role of parents, friends and teachers in adolescents' cigarette smoking and tombak dipping in Sudan. *Tobacco Control*, 20: 94–99

Fidler DP, Drager N (2006) Health and foreign policy. *Bulletin of the World Health Organization*, 84(9): 687

Giacaman R, Abu-Remieh NME, Husseini A, Saab H, Boyce W (2007a) Humiliation: The invisible trauma for Palestinian youth. *The Royal Institute of Public Health*, 121: 563–571

Giacaman R, Shannon HS, Saab H, Arya N, Boyce W (2007b) Individual and collective exposure to political violence: Palestinian adolescents coping with conflict. *European Journal of Public Health*, 17(4): 361–368

Guardian (2011) Young Arabs who can't wait to throw off shackles of tradition (February 14). Available from www.guardian.co.uk/world/ 2011/feb/14/young-arabs-throw-off-shackles-tradition [Accessed 15 February 2011]

Hart RA (1992) *Children's participation: From tokenism to citizenship, Roger Innocenti Essay inness92/6.* Florence, Italy: UNICEF Innocenti Research

Hughes DM, Curnan SP (2000) Community youth development: A framework for action. *Community Youth Development Journal*, 1(1). Available from http://www.cydjournal.org/2000Winter/hughes.html [Accessed 9 April 2010]

Hwalla N, Sibai AM, Adra N (2005) Adolescent obesity and physical activity. *World Review of Nutrition and Dietetics*, 94: 42–50

ILO (International Labour Organization) (2010) *Global employment trends for youth.* Geneva, Switzeralnd: Author

Jaffer YA, Afifi M, Al-Ajmi F, Alouhaishi K (2006) Knowledge, attitudes and practices of secondary-school pupils in Oman: I. Health compromising behaviors. *Eastern Mediterranean Health Journal*, 12(1/2): 35–49

Jaju S, Al-Adawi S, Al-Kharsui H, Morsi M, Al-Riyami A (2009) Prevalence and age-of-onset distributions of DSM IV mental disorders and their severity among school going Omani adolescents and youths: WMH-CIDI findings. *Child and Adolescent Psychiatry and Mental Health*, 29(3): 1–11

Jessor R, Van Den Bos J, Vanderryn J, Costa FM, Turbin MS (1995) Protective factors in adolescent problem behavior: Moderator effects and developmental change. *Developmental Psychology*, 31: 923–933

Kanaan MN, Afifi RA (2009) Gender differences in determinants of weight-control behaviours among adolescents in Beirut. *Public Health Nutrition*, 13(1): 71–81

Karam E, Melhem N, Mansour C, Maalouf W, Saliba S, Chami A (2000) Use and abuse of licit and illicit substances: Prevalence and risk factors among students in Lebanon. *European Addiction Research*, 4: 189–197

Karam EG, Fayyad J, Karam AN, et al (2008) Effectiveness and specificity of a classroom-based group intervention in children and adolescents exposed to war in Lebanon, *World Psychiatry*, 7: 103–109

Karam EG, Mneimneh ZN, Aimee NK, et al (2006) Prevalence and treatment of mental disorders in lebanon: A national epidemiological survey, *The Lancet*, 367: 1000–1006

Khattab H, Younis N, Zurayk H (1999) *Women, reproduction and health in rural Egypt: The Giza Study.* Cairo, Egypt: American University in Cairo Press

Leffert N, Benson PL, Scales PC, Sharma AR, Drake DR, Blyth DA (1998) Developmental assets: Measurement and prediction of risk behaviors among adolescents. *Applied Developmental Science*, 2(4): 209–230

Makhoul J, Alameddine M, Afifi RA (2010) "I felt that I was benefiting someone": Youth as agents of change in a refugee community project, Manuscript submitted for publication

Malik M, Bakir A (2006) Prevalence of overweight and obesity among children in the United Arab Emirates. *Obesity Reviews*, 8: 15–20

Mandil A, Hussein H, Omer G, Turki G, Gaber I (2007) Characteristics and risk factors of tobacco consumption among University of Sharjah students, 2005. *Eastern Mediterranean Health Journal*, 13: 1449–1458

Maziak W, Eissenberg T, Rastam S, et al (2004) Beliefs and attitudes related to narghile (waterpipe) smoking among university students in Syria. *Annals of Epidemiology*, 14: 646–654

McLeroy KR, Bibeau D, Steckler A, Glanz K (1988) An ecological perspective on health promotion programs. *Health Education Quarterly*, 5(4): 351–377

Mohti A (2001) Mental health in the Eastern Mediterranean region of the World Health Organization with a view of the future trends. *Eastern Mediterranean Health Journal*, 5(2): 353–362

Moore S, Teixeira AC, Shiell A (2006) The health of nations in a global context: Trade, global stratification, and infant mortality rates. *Social Science & Medicine*, 63(1): 165–178

Okasha A (1999) Mental health in the Middle East: An Egyptian perspective. *Clinical Psychology Review*, 19(8): 917–933

Patton GC, Coffey C, Sawyer SM, et al (2009) Global patterns of mortality in young people: A systematic analysis of population health data. *The Lancet*, 374: 881–892

Rabaia Y, Giacaman R, Nguyen-Gillham V (2010) Violence and adolescent mental health in the Occupied Palestinian Territory: A contextual approach. *Asia Pacific Journal of Public Health*, 22: 216S

Rachik H (2005) *Jeunesse et changement social*. Morocco: 50 ans de Développement humain et perspectives 2025 (in French)

Rashad H, Osman M (2003) Nuptiality in Arab countries: Changes and implications. *In*: N Hopkins (Ed.) *The new Arab family* (vol. 24, Issues 1–2, p. 20–50). Cairo, Egypt: The American University in Cairo Press

Rashad H, Osman M, Roudi-Fahimi F (2005, December) *Marriage in the Arab world*. Washington, DC: Population Reference Bureau

Rezaeian M (2007) Age and sex suicide rates in the Eastern Mediterranean Region based on global burden of disease estimates for 2000. *Eastern Mediterranean Health Journal*, 13(4): 953–60

Roudi-Fahimi F, Kent MM (2007) Challenges and opportunities – the population of the Middle East and North Africa. *Population Bulletin by Population Reference Bureau*, 62(2).

Available from http://www.prb.org/pdf07/62.2MENA.pdf [Accessed 27 February 2009]

Salazar-Martinez E, Allen B, Fernandez-Ortega C, et al (2006) Overweight and obesity status among adolescents from Mexico and Egypt. *Archives of Medical Research*, 37(4): 535–542

Scales PC, Benson PL, Leffert N, Blyth DA (2000) Contribution of developmental assets to the prediction of thriving among adolescents. *Applied Developmental Science*, 4(1): 27–46

Shepard B, DeJong J (2005) *Breaking the silence and saving lives: Young people's sexual and reproductive health in the Arab States and Iran*. Boston, MA: Harvard University, International Health and Human Rights Program, Francois Xavier Bagnoud Center for Health and Human Rights

Shuftan C (2008) An ethical question: Are health professionals promoters of the status quo or of social change? *Promotion and Education*, 15(3): 30–33

Singerman D, Ibrahim B (2003) The costs of marriage in Egypt: A hidden dimension in the new Arab demography, *In*: N Hopkins (Ed.) *The new Arab family* (vol. 24, Issues 1–2, p. 80–116). Cairo, Egypt: The American University in Cairo Press

SRSG CAAC (Special Representative of the Secretary General for Children and Armed Conflict), GYAN (Global Youth Action Network), UNICEF (United Nations Children's Fund), UNFPA (United Nations Population Fund), UNFPA and Women's Commission for Refugee Women and Children (2007, October) *"Will you listen?" Young voices from conflict zones*

Tamim H, Al-Sahab B, Akkary G, et al (2007) Cigarette and nargileh smoking practices among school students in Beirut, Lebanon. *American Journal of Health Behavior*, 31: 56–63

Tanios CY, Abou-Saleh MT, Karam AN, Salamoun MM, Mneimneh ZN, Karam EG (2009) The epidemiology of anxiety disorders in the Arab world: A review. *Journal of Anxiety Disorders*, 23: 409–419

Thabet AA, Abu-Tawahina A, El-Sarraj E, Vostanis P (2008) Exposure to war trauma and PTSD among parents and children in the Gaza strip. *European Journal of Child and Adolescent Psychiatry*, 17(4): 191–199

Thabet AA, Vostanis P, Karim K (2005) Group crisis intervention for children during ongoing war conflict. *European Child and Adolescent Psychiatry*, 14: 262–269

UNESCWA (United Nations Economic and Social Commission for Western Asia) (2009) *Report of the expert group meeting on reinforcing social equity: Integrating youth into the development process*. Abu Dhabi, 29–31 March 2009

UNICEF (United Nations Children's Fund) (2000) *Talking to tomorrow: Young people in the Middle East and North Africa*. Amman, Jordan: UNICEF Regional Office for the Middle East and North Africa

WHO (World Health Organization) (1984) *Health promotion: A discussion document on the concept and principles*. Copenhagen, Denmark: WHO Regional Office for Europe.

WHO (2006) *Report on the fourth meeting of the regional drug advisory panel on impacts of drug abuse (WHO-EM/MNH/17)*. Cairo, Egypt: WHO Regional office for the Eastern Mediterranean

WHO (2007) *Helping parents in developing countries improve adolescents' health*. Geneva, Switzerland: Author

Yeretzian JS, Afifi RA (2009) 'It won't happen to me': The knowledge attitude nexus in adolescent smoking. *Journal of Public Health*, 31(3): 354–359

Chapter

19

Women's Health: Progress and Unaddressed Issues

Jocelyn DeJong, Hyam Bashour, and Afamia Kaddour

Women's health in the Arab world has received increasing program and research attention since the 1990s. As in other regions, the public health community historically focused on the health of infants and children, with women seen as mothers responsible for children's health. It was not until the 1980s, that adult health attracted real emphasis. The famous Safe Motherhood Conference in Nairobi in 1987 was the first international event emphasizing that maternal mortality, not infant mortality, was the public health indicator that showed the largest discrepancy between developed and developing countries. From the 1960s onward, with the introduction of state-run family planning programs in developing countries, including this region, the main preoccupation of women's health centered around their reproductive role and reducing fertility due to preoccupation with rapid population growth. By the 1990s, growing criticism of targeting fertility in isolation of wider health and well-being, the concept of "reproductive health" –the health consequences of sexuality and reproduction– emerged and was endorsed at the 1994 International Conference on Population and Development (ICPD) in Cairo (Zurayk 1999). Reproductive health was seen in a social, rather than purely a medical, context. While there has been progress in many areas in implementing this approach, gaps prevail and resistance to it has been encountered from political, economic, and administrative perspectives (Langer 2006). Recently, some have criticized "reproductive health," arguing for a broader approach of "women's health" (e.g., Raymond et al 2005).

To understand the relevance of these debates to women's health in this region, we must clarify the origin of the research agendas, public health policies, and social movements which underlie the respective positions on women's health. Conceptually, reproductive health has come to describe an approach which sees women's health and well-being as important in their own right, stressing both the positive and negative aspects of sexuality and reproduction (Cottingham & Myntti 2002). Robust reproductive health implies that every sex act should be free of coercion and infection; every pregnancy intended; and every birth healthy (Tsui et al 1997). Reproductive health includes both women's and men's health but since women bear the heavier health burden associated with reproduction, the focus has been on women. Action on and behalf of reproductive health has galvanized a global advocacy movement. In this region, civil society activism has played a critical role in encouraging more comprehensive policies in this area with action and research beginning well before the ICPD. A network of reproductive health researchers (Box 1) developed a regionally tailored definition of reproductive health as follows: "the ability of women to live through the reproductive years and beyond with reproductive choice, dignity, and successful child-bearing and to be free of gynecological disease and risk."

"Women's health" indicates a prioritization of women's health as distinct from men's and marks a departure from limiting focus to reproductive health and its implicit emphasis on sexuality and reproduction. Some have criticized reproductive health's "bikini approach" and argued that chronic diseases cause a greater burden of ill-health (Raymond et al 2005). Others point to often neglected areas such as mental health, occupational health, or the association between women's multiple roles and their health. In 1994, the National Academy on Women's Health Medical Education adopted the definition of women's health as "...devoted to facilitating the preservation of wellness and prevention of illness in women and includes screening, diagnosis, and management of conditions which are unique to women, are more

Public Health in the Arab World, ed. Samer Jabbour et al. Published by Cambridge University Press. © Samer Jabbour et al., 2012.

Box 1. The Reproductive Health Working Group (RHWG)

The RHWG was established in 1988, from a base at the Population Council in Cairo, in order to study women's health in its broader socio-cultural and policy contexts. A regional group of researchers on reproductive health collectively decided to address three themes: reproductive morbidity, quality of health care, and dignity. These topics reflected their desire to bring to the fore a more explicit attention to women's health care and rights – at a time when international debates were just beginning to question the exclusive focus on fertility reduction in population policies – while resonating with the needs of women in the region. The same process has characterized the development of the group's subsequent research themes, such as conflict and displacement and their impact on reproductive health or quality of life of women with breast cancer, which have emerged simultaneously from their interests and from critical engagement with international debates but which are reflective of regional concerns.

The RHWG does not define a particular research agenda per se; rather, it builds on individual initiatives and consolidates common research topics among its members. Over time, the group has been able to develop, collectively, more appropriate frameworks for conceptualizing health, based on research but also on lived experiences. A central contribution of the RHWG has been the promotion and nurturing of younger scholars in reproductive health who often lack a critical mass of colleagues working on similar topics in their own institutions. This has helped to provide a professional forum within which they can develop and eventually publish their own research while maintaining their institutional base in the region.

From its inception, two elements have characterized the RHWG. The first is inter-disciplinarity – having among its members medical doctors, epidemiologists, biostatisticians, demographers, anthropologists, sociologists, and economists who engage on an equal footing. The second is regionality – making an explicit effort to include researchers from across the region. As a result of these two aspects, the comparative nature of the research is strengthened, with different approaches used to examine a particular issue. Researchers rooted and engaged in specific national contexts learn to appreciate the commonalities and differences in historical and developmental trajectories within the region.

The group has had generous support from the regional office of the Ford Foundation from its inception but has also been successful in attracting funding for particular projects at national level.

Note: for more information on the network see www.rhwg.org

common or more serious in women, or have manifestations, risk factors, or interventions that are different in women."

Precisely because of divisions and debates on terminology and approaches in women's health, this chapter will use a social determinants approach focusing on "reproductive health" but extend the discussion to other health problems. With its focus on women's health, the chapter does not address the vast literature on family planning in the region, which has been well-covered elsewhere. In this volume, chapters on older adults, gender and health, and on adolescent health complement this chapter and together provide a full life-course picture of women's health.

The Determinants of Women's Health and Variations Across the Region

It is impossible to discuss the situation of women's health in the Arab world without reference to the social, cultural, economic, and even political determinants underpinning it. As Glasier & Gulmezoglu (2005) put it: "Perhaps more than any other area of health, sexual, and reproductive health is affected by socio-cultural factors, including gender disparities, taboos, and strongly held behavioral norms." The close connection between women's social status and their health is particularly important in this region whereby the high burden of ill-health faced by women reflects broader gender imbalances whether in the social determinants of health, the social consequences of ill-health, or in the health care system's response to women's health concerns.

The far-ranging demographic changes (see Chapter 3) have clear implications for women's health. For example, the rising average age at marriage, to near 30 for both men and women in parts of North Africa (Fargues 2005), the rising proportion of never-married women in their 30s (Rashad et al 2005) and the increasing numbers female-headed households due to migration and other reasons, all impact women's health. As Rashad et al (2005) have argued, little attention is paid to the health and well-being and health services need of the rising cohort of women who do not marry. Limited evidence from the Occupied Palestinian Territories (OPTs), for instance, found that differences in age and causes of death differ among single women as compared to married women, and the former are more likely to die from medical conditions indicative of barriers in reaching medical care (Al-Adili et al 2008). Throughout the region, unmarried women are not encouraged to seek gynecological screening and care. Overall, women are having fewer children, surviving longer after their reproductive years, and many are not marrying and having children at all. As Saliba & Zurayk (2010) argue, these trends in and of themselves call for a reformulation of women's health priorities.

The region includes some of richest and some of the poorest countries in the world and this is reflected in differentials in women's health and social status (Table 1). Life expectancy, for example, is 20 years higher in Kuwait at 80.1 than in Djibouti at 57.2 and in Yemen at 65.1; similarly, fertility ranges from a high of 5.1 in Yemen and 4.92 in the OPT to below replacement levels in countries such as Lebanon and Tunisia (both 1.84) and UAE (1.9). Maternal mortality ratios are as high as 430 in Yemen and 450 in Sudan and 650 in Djibouti, while being as low as 12 in Qatar and 4 in Kuwait. Chapter 20 provides time-trends in some basic indicators. However, data are lacking for most countries in some areas such as HIV incidence or prevalence among women and risk behaviors for a range of women's health conditions (Table 1).

It is difficult therefore to draw generalizations about women's health across the national income levels. Recent evidence suggests that the burden of mortality and disease, as measured by disability-adjusted life years (DALYs), varies considerably according to income. Deaths and DALYs due to maternal health conditions are lower in high than in low- to middle-income countries while those due to cardiovascular disease and cancer are much higher for high-income countries (Saliba & Zurayk 2010). Disaggregation by national income is not enough; socio-economic differentials within countries must be considered (see Chapter 5). In Egypt, obesity was formerly concentrated among upper-income women but the social gradient has been reversed and obesity now is more common among poorer women (Aitsi 2010). Similarly, health services received vary by socio-economic level. In the 2008 Egyptian Demographic and Health Survey, C-section rates were more than threefold

higher in the highest than in the lowest wealth quintile (44.9% vs. 13.6%) (El- Zanaty & Way 2009). Socio-economic differentials in women's health care utilization are increasingly being analyzed.

Researchers have long recognized a "culture of silence" (Khattab et al 1999) surrounding women's health, manifested in how women are socialized to put their own health after that of family members, and in the sensitivities associated with illnesses that might threaten women's sexuality or reproductive roles. Many women lack autonomy in seeking needed health services. Even when they access health services, they may not be treated with respect or dignity or be given adequate information. Concerned with the need to respect women while receiving health-care services, researchers of the regional Reproductive Health Working Group (RHWG), founded in the late 1980s, incorporated dignity (karama) in their definition of reproductive health (Box 1).

There are limited reviews of women's health in the Arab world (see for example, Obermeyer 1992; Zurayk et al 1997; Aoyama 2001; Roudi-Fahimi 2003; DeJong et al 2005) but all stress the importance of social determinants of women's health. Obermeyer (1992) underscored the role of politicization of religion in influencing women's health and at the same time dispelled stereotypic attempts to draw a one-to-one association between Islam and higher fertility. At the time, women's fertility was high, at an average of six to eight children per woman, and second in the world only to Sub-Saharan Africa, but has since dramatically declined to 3.4 by 2000 (Fargues 2005). Fargues (2005) has pointed to the anomaly that fertility has fallen in a context where patriarchy prevails and female employment remains low. He argues that rising educational levels of women and reforms of personal status legislation are challenging that patriarchal order.

Changes in wider social determinants of health, such as a low but rising female labor force participation of women, have an impact on their own and their family's health. Some countries such as Jordan have made legislative changes that have allowed women who work in the public sector to provide health insurance for their families, an entitlement previously available only to male employees. This is particularly important in a region where public sectors are increasingly becoming feminized (see for example, on Egypt; Assaad & Arntz 2005) as men seek more profitable private sector jobs.

Table 1. Women's Social and Health Indicators

Country	Mortality Life expectancy[xi]	Mortality MM ratio[xii]	Education % Illiterate (>15 years)[xiii]	Current contraceptive use Married 15–49 Any method[xiv]	Current contraceptive use Married 15–49 Modern methods[xv]	Women living with HIV age 15+[i]	Average age at marriage[ii, iii]	Mean age of child-bearing[iv]	Total fertility rate[v]	% Births with skilled attendants[vi]	15–49 Antenatal care, at least once (%)[vii]	% Who smoke any product >15[viii (ix)]	% of women 15+ share of labor force[x]
Algeria	74.1	180	33.6	61	52	6000*	26		2.34	95	58	0.9 (0.3)	31.1
Bahrain	77.7	32	13.6	62	31		25.42	29.7	2.23	99	97	– (2.9)	18.6
Comoros	68.1	400	30.2	26	19	<200	24		3.89	62	74	–	–
Djibouti	57.2	650	n/a	18	17	8700**	n/a		3.79	93	n/a	2.7 –	39.4
Egypt	72.2	130	42.2	60	58	2600***	23.2	28.8	2.82	79	53	– (1.3)	21.8, 15.20[xvi]
Iraq	71.9	300	n/a	50	33		22	30.6	3.96	89	78	– (2.5)	20.4
Jordan	74.9	62	13	57	41		26.3		3.02	99	n/a	– (9.8)	25.5, 11.80[xvii]
Kuwait	80.1	4	6.9	52	39		25	29.6	2.15	100	95	–	25.8
Lebanon	74.4	26	14	58	34	860****	n/a		1.84	98	87	21.4(7.0)	31.1
Libya	77.2	97	21.6	45	26		29		2.64	100	81	–	27.8
Mauritania	59	820	51.7	9	8	2500–8300	28		4.39	61	64	–	–
Morocco	73.9	240	56.8	63	52	5900+	25		2.33	63	42	0.6 (0.3)	26.2+++
OPT	75.3	n/a	9.7	50	39		22		4.92	97	96	–	13.2

Country													
Oman	77.8	64	22.5	24	18		22	30.2	2.98	98	96	– (1.3)	17.4
Qatar	77.2	12	9.6	43	32	24.6	30.4		2.36	100	94	– –	14.0
Saudi Arabia	75.6	18	20.6	24	n/a	22		3.04	96	90	– (3.6)	14.3
Somalia	51.5	1,400	–	15	1	–	–	6.35	33	32	–	–
Sudan	60.1	450	n/a	8	6	23	170,000 ++	4.06	49	75	–	24.9
Syria	76.4	130	23.5	58	43	n/a		3.17	93	51	8 –	30.7
Tunisia	76.4	100	31	60	52	27	1000 +++	1.84	90	79	4.1 (1.9)	28.1
UAE	79.0	37	8.5	28	24	23	30.9	1.9	100	97	– (2.6)	14.6
Yemen	65.1	430	59.5	28	19	21		5.1	36	34	12.8 –	28.2

*3100–12,000; ** 6500–11,000; ***1900–3600; ****<500–2000; + 4100–9100; + + 120,000–250,000; +++ 730–1600; ++++ 21% worked within 12 mo[xviii]. [i, ii, iii, iv, v, x, xi] UNFPA. The State of World Population. Facing a changing world: women, population and climate; [vi] Epidemiological Fact Sheet on HIV and AIDS, 2008; [vii]UN World Fertility Report 2003: http://unstats.un.org/unsd/demographic/products/indwm/ww2005/tab2a.htm. Data years: Algeria (1992), Iran (1996), Kuwait (1996), Libya (1995), Morocco (1994), OPT (1997), Oman (1995), Saudi Arabia (1987), Sudan (1993), Tunisia (1994), UAE (1987), Yemen (1997; [viii] Bulletin on population and Vital statistics in the ESCWA Region. Twelfth issue. Egypt (2008), Jordan (2008), Qatar (2007), Bahrain (2007); [ix] Bulletin on Population and Vital statistics in the ESCWA Region. Twelfth issue. Bahrain (2008), Egypt (2006), Iraq (2000), Kuwait (2007), Oman (2007), Qatar (2007), UAE (2003); [xii] Data from late 1990s – 2001. WHO and UNICEF. Antenatal Care in Developing Countries: Promises Achievements and Missed Opportunities. http://www.childinfo.org/eddb/antenatal/antenatal_full.pdf; [xiii] PAPFAM. Data years: Algeria (2002), Djibouti (2002), Lebanon (2004), Morocco (2003–2004), Syria (2001), Tunisia (2001), Yemen (1997); [xiv] WHO Report on the Global Tobacco Epidemic, 2008. Time of Survey 2005; [xv] UN Statistics Division 2006. Women's Share of Labor Force; [xvi] DHS Egypt 2008-% of currently employed ever married women 15–49; [xvii] DHS Egypt 2008-% of currently employed ever married women 15–49; [xviii] DHS Jordan 2007-% of currently employed ever married women 15–49; [xviii] DHS Morocco 2003–4-% of currently employed ever married women 15–49.

Table 2. Maternity Leave Policies in Arab Countries

Country	Sector (public/ private)	Duration of maternity leave	Report year
Algeria	Public & private sectors	3 months full pay	2010
Bahrain	N/S	60 days (pay N/S)	2010
Djibouti	N/S	14 weeks full/partial pay	2005
Egypt	N/S	90 days full pay	2010
Iraq	Public sector Private sector	6 months 72 days	2010
Jordan	Public sector Private sector	90 days 70 days	2010
Kuwait	Public & private sectors	40 days full pay; 4 months, no pay	2010
Lebanon	Public sector Private sector	60 days full pay 7 weeks full pay	2010
Libya	Public & private sectors	3 months full pay	2010
Morocco	Public & private sectors	12 weeks full pay	2010
OPT	Public & private sectors	10 weeks full/partial pay	2010
Qatar	Public & private sectors	50 days full pay; 60 days, no pay	2010
Saudi Arabia	N/S	10 weeks full/partial pay	2010
Syria	Public & private sectors	120 d for 1st child, 90 for the 2nd, 75 for the 3rd	2010
Tunisia	Public sector Private sector	2 months, full pay 30 days +15 days conditional	2010
Yemen	Public & private sectors	60 days full pay	2010

N/S: Not specified
Sources: The Freedom House Report. Women's Rights in the Middle East and North Africa 2010. Available on http://freedomhouse.org/template. cfm?page=384&key=270&parent=23&report=86

Another important determinant of women's health is the legal situation of women which remains far behind that of other regions. For example, legislated allowances on maternity leave (Table 2) range from a low of 7 weeks in the private sector in Lebanon to 3 months full pay in both public and private sectors in Libya and Algeria, and there is relatively little advocacy on this issue. One major constraint to lengthy maternity leaves in the region is the almost universal reliance on employer liability as a source of funding for maternity leave (ILO 2010). Attempts to revise abortion legislation, in cases, for example, of rape, incest, or congenital malformation, have been few and have remained unsuccessful. Tunisia is the only country where abortion is legal on demand (for a summary of the current status of abortion legislationm, see Hessini 2007). The contribution of unsafe induced abortion to maternal deaths in the region is not known due to the sensitivity of doing abortion research. Clearly, failure to address this public health problem can only result in more maternal health complications or even deaths.

Poverty combined with the lack of priority to women's health within families and communities reduces the chances of health-seeking by women for their own health and raises risks of maternal mortality (Thaddeus & Maine 1994). Lack of financial resources is often cited as a main reason for delays in seeking care. There is limited research on linkages between poverty and women's health or differentials in women's health by social class although there are many studies on women's health in low-income areas (see for example, Kaddour et al 2005). A recent study, using logistic regression analysis of 2005 Demographic and

Health Survey data on Egypt, found that women's lowest wealth quintile was associated with women's relatively low empowerment in household decisions, greater exposure to violence, perception of a lack of healthcare provider, and lack of health insurance as well as predicting the intention to perpetuate female genital cutting on their daughters (Afifi 2009). This connection between poverty and health was also revealed in a study of how women perceive their health in low-income areas of Beirut (Zurayk et al 2007) where women cited physical fatigue and psychological stress of daily life in poverty as direct causes of their ill-health. A promising approach for examining these issues is to analyze the "assets" (see for example, Moser & Dani 2008) which women command (both positive and negative) and how these impact their health (see Chapter 6). There has been surprisingly little research in this area in the region.

Examining women's health and implications of ill-health on their lives through a social determinants of health lens is important for another reason: it may counter arguments that conditions relating to sexuality and reproduction have been over-emphasized in the public health literature and in programs (see Raymond et al 2005). A social justice perspective underscores women's right to experience not only sexuality and reproduction but also to work – whether domestic or paid – and indeed to life in general without undue risk to their health due to gender biases or deficiencies in health services.

Research on Women's Health

Although women's health remains a sensitive issue in Arab countries, pioneering research has been done in this field, which has contributed to international knowledge. For example, as early as the 1970s, Reproductive Age Mortality Surveys (or RAMOS) studies on maternal mortality in Egypt revealed new ways of measuring maternal mortality (Fortney et al 1986). In the 1980s and 1990s, studies on morbidity under the auspices of RHWG (Box 1) in Egypt, Jordan, and Lebanon revealed the heavy and often hidden burden of conditions that women bear. Some of these studies resulted in the development of public health interventions. During the same period, anthropological research on infertility published by Marcia Inhorn on Egypt and later Lebanon represented some of the earliest research on this important health problem in non-Western settings (see Chapter 7). Other important research associated with RHWG was on women's perceptions about the prioritization and severity of health conditions (see for example, Sholkamy & Ghannam 2004), which combines a number of anthropological studies in the region on women's perceptions of their bodies and their health. Giacaman & Odeh (2002) explored women's perceptions of their health in the old city of Nablus; Kaddour et al (2005), Zurayk et al (2007) examined women's understandings of reproductive health in low-income Beirut. More recently, the Choices and Challenges in Changing Childbirth Research Network, which is linked to RHWG with research teams in Egypt, Lebanon, the occupied Palestinian territories, and Syria, has documented the lack of evidence-based practices in childbirth in a region where most births now take place in health care facilities. Recently, this network has begun to explore providers' perspectives on childbirth and the constraints they face in offering quality care (Hassan-Bitar & Wick 2007). The attention to dissemination has made this network of great value in reaching providers, professional associations, as well as women in the communities.

Measurement of Women's Health

Differences in approaches to women's health reflect not only conceptual differences, but also the measurement tools used to assess the burden of ill-health that women bear. Identifying appropriate indicators for measuring the status of, or progress in, women's health in any given context is challenging. Population programs focusing on fertility reduction had the merit of having clear targets and indicators – but reproductive health is much broader in scope and is subject to many difficulties of measurement (Sadana 2000). Similarly, gender-differentiated data on chronic and other diseases are not always available. It is thus difficult to achieve consensus on which indicators to use to evaluate progress in women's health. The omission of reproductive health in its entirety from the Millennium Development Goals (although it was subsequently included in the indicators) at least partly reflects this problem (Crossette 2005).

A number of measurement challenges are of special interest in this region although other regions might have similar challenges. The culture of silence and sensitivity surrounding many women's health issues makes them subject to under-reporting. Because of the relative neglect of many health problems, at least until recently, nationally representative data on the prevalence rates of diverse conditions, such as reproductive morbidity, are often not available. While existing surveys in the region, such as the DHS and PAPFAM, are increasingly providing national data on women's reported morbidity, these do not to correlate well with clinical findings (Sadana 2000; Zurayk et al 1995). The critical issue of maternal mortality is now beginning to receive more public attention, largely thanks to the Millennium Development Goals, but at the same time is very difficult and costly to measure since it is relatively rare, even when the maternal mortality ratio is high, and thus requires large sample sizes.

Bearing in mind these limitations, there nevertheless exists a strong body of mainly descriptive evidence on the heavy burden of ill-health borne by women. We now turn to examine this evidence.

What Health Problems Do Women Suffer From?

Maternal Health Conditions

Maternal health complications cause a large proportion of mortality and disease burden in the Arab region. Using data from the 2008 WHO Global Burden of Disease Report, Saliba & Zurayk (2010) found that, in the Eastern Mediterranean Region, which includes in addition to Arab countries, non-Arab countries with very high mortality rates such as Afghanistan, during women's reproductive age the risk of death from maternal health conditions is higher than the risk from any of the following: cardiovascular disease, cancer, or neuropsychiatric disorders.

A few countries, such as Sudan, Yemen, and Morocco, have much higher maternal mortality ratios than others. Egypt is exceptional because of its recent significant (52%) decline in maternal mortality from 174 to 84 per 100,000 live births (Campbell et al 2005). Throughout the region, access to obstetric care is improving, and the majority of women now deliver with a trained assistant. With greater political attention to maternal mortality, good quality national surveys are becoming available. Egypt, Morocco, Syria, Tunisia, and others have conducted national maternal mortality studies; Egypt conducted two, in 1993 and 2000.

Reproductive Morbidity

In contrast to maternal mortality, few countries have nationally representative data on obstetric complications

Table 3. Prevalence of Reproductive Tract Infection (RTI) and Prolapse From Population-Based Studies in Selected Arab Countries

Country	Sample size and location	RTI (reproductive age)	Genital prolapse (reproductive age)
Egypt	502 (Giza)	51%	56%
Jordan	317 (Ain el Basha)	55%	22%
Lebanon	552 (Beqa'a)	1.2%	49.6%
Oman	1365 (nationally representative)	25%	10%

Sources: Egypt, (Khattab et al 1999); Jordan, (Mawajdeh et al 2003); Lebanon, (Deeb et al 2003); Oman, (Mabry et al 2007).

and morbidities. For example, obstetric fistula is a significant problem in countries such as Sudan and Yemen, but national studies have not been conducted. The few available population-based studies of gynecological or obstetric morbidity date from the early 1990s with the first recognition of the importance of reproductive morbidity in the region and internationally. Evidence indicates a significant burden among ever-married women. In Egypt, an early but innovative and multidisciplinary study, commonly referred to as the Giza study, combined a survey of women in their homes and clinical exams (Khattab et al 1999). A striking 51% of women had reproductive tract infections (RTI) (Table 3) and 56% has genital prolapse (Khattab et al 1999). Few women, however, had brought their conditions to local health services. A number of factors contributed to this observation, but the authors singled out IUD use as well as hygiene-related factors for particular attention. The Giza study was one of the first studies in the region and internationally to point to the relationship between IUD use (and lack of proper screening or monitoring) and reproductive morbidity .

Other studies, mostly small-scale, were conducted in Jordan and Lebanon following the Giza study by a sub-research group on reproductive morbidity as part of RHWG (Table 3). More recently, the first nationally representative study in the region was conducted in Oman. Like the earlier studies, this study combined women's reports and clinical exams (Mabry et al 2007) and found that among ever-married women of reproductive-age, 25% suffered from an RTI and

10% from genital prolapse. More such nationally representative studies are needed.

HIV/AIDS

HIV prevalence among women and the female/male ratio in the region is much lower than in other regions. Women mostly acquire infection through marriage (Abu-Raddad et al 2010), but little is known about HIV risk behaviors among women in general, HIV among female members of at-risk populations in particular, or the female sexual partners of male members of these groups.

Tremendous stigma is attached to sexually transmitted diseases (STDs), and HIV/AIDS specifically, among women in our cultural context; as such this area is relatively under-researched. Internationally, it is known that women are more vulnerable to STDs, including HIV/AIDS, for both biological and social reasons. That women represent a minority of overall reported AIDS cases in this region likely reflects several factors: HIV has not yet spread into the general population in most countries, with the exception of countries such as Sudan; the existing spread of HIV may be confined to male at-risk groups such as injecting drug users and men who have sex with men; or HIV is more stigmatized among women and therefore more likely to be under-reported.

Sensitivity and stigma make it difficult to research women's experiences of living with HIV/AIDS. In a first study in Egypt, Khattab et al (2007) could only interview 12 women, although the study was conducted in partnership with the National AIDS Program. Subjects reported heavy psychological burden and many barriers to health care seeking, particularly for gynecological conditions.

Chronic Diseases

With the epidemiological transition well under way across the region, the burden of chronic diseases is growing for women. Because chronic diseases are discussed elsewhere (see Chapters 12, 13), we focus on three important problems, namely breast cancer, obesity (and low levels of physical activity) and mental health, that are only beginning to receive policy attention.

In their review of WHO Burden of Disease data for 2008, Saliba & Zurayk (2010) found that cancer accounts for approximately 10% of total deaths and 3% of total DALYs among women in the reproductive age (15–44). Breast cancer is the leading tumor for

women and its incidence is increasing. A pattern of early onset of breast cancer is reported in countries such as Egypt and Jordan where between 57% and 68% of all cases were diagnosed before the age of 55, as compared with 35% in the US (Freedman et al 2006). At the same time, there are delays in diagnosing breast cancer that may reflect constraints to accessing care, limited public knowledge as well as deficiency and poor access to screening programs (for research on women's experience of breast cancer in the region, see for example, Doumit et al 2010). In Egypt, for example, although the incidence of breast cancer is lower than in Western countries, the stage at presentation is much more advanced (Corbex 2009).

Obesity is already a major public health issue regionally, particularly in the Gulf countries. The prevalence of obesity is higher in women than men relating to multiparity and higher levels of physical inactivity among women (Musaiger 2004). In the UAE (Sheikh Ismail et al 2009) prevalence of overweight and obesity were 27% and 16% respectively in women aged 20 to 90. Women between 30 and 60 years had the highest prevalence of over-weight (33%) and obesity (24%). High obesity levels among women are not confined to the Gulf region. In urban Syria prevalence of obesity overall was 38.2% but was higher among women at 46.3% in women compared to 28.4% in men (Fouad et al 2006). It was especially high among women with multiparity. In Egypt, 38.4% and 47% of women were over-weight or obese according to the 2008 DHS survey, one of the highest rates of obesity in the world and two times that of the United Kingdom (Aitsi 2009).

Increased urbanization, lack of public spaces as well as appropriate infrastructure for physical activity for women, as well as gender norms limiting women's mobility or discouraging them from being physically active contribute to increasing obesity among women. A qualitative study among female university students in UAE found that women's lack of physical activity was related to perceived gender roles: "Whilst it is generally supported and encouraged among men, women usually abstained from any forms of exercise that might risk the appearance of unfeminine pearls of sweat because girls were meant to look clean." (Berger & Peerson 2009).

Weight problems not only contribute to diabetes, hypertension, and coronary heart disease, but also to musculo-skeletal disorders. In a study of 1266 ever-married women aged 15 to 59 women in poor suburbs of Beirut, Habib et al (2005) found that nearly a fifth suffered from some form of musculo-skeletal disorder; the prevalence of these disorders was related to women's weight and parity.

Mental Health

This is another highly stigmatized health issue in the region and thus subject to under-reporting for both men and women. Nevertheless, Saliba & Zurayk (2010) found that in the Eastern Mediterranean region neuropsychiatric disorders account for almost 3% of deaths and nearly a quarter of total DALYs among women in the reproductive age, reflecting their clear impact on quality of life. As noted in the chapter on gender and health, the mental health of women in the region remains under-researched. In one of a relatively few articles on women's mental health in Muslim/Arab countries, Douki & Nacef (2002) argue that, even in a country such as Tunisia, with its progressive legislation regarding the status of women, women who are mentally ill are not offered the same level of protection as men and suffer from worse clinical and social outcomes. As they note: "The protection of women's mental health is not only a medical challenge, but also a cultural one" in terms of advancing gender equity. Factors such as conflict and economic pressures likely increase the risk of mental health problems among women. Another review, by Eloul et al (2009) concludes that, although rates of depression are significantly higher among women than men, probably related to the burden of postpartum depression, they are comparable to international rates.

The Inter-linkages Between Health Problems and Social Practices and Roles

As in other regions, programs addressing women's health have tended to compartmentalize rather than underscore inter-linkages between health problems. This is clear for physical problems as we discussed in the example of the association of IUD with reproductive morbidity (Khattab et al 1999). Less taken up, however, was research showing that use of oral contraceptive pills can be linked to hypertension (Zurayk et al 1996). Both these findings point to the importance of proper screening of women attending family planning clinics.

Inter-linkages are especially important with regard to mental health. Saliba & Zurayk (2010) show that

DALYs due to neuropsychiatric conditions reach their highest levels among women of reproductive age, meaning that women face multiple disease burdens during this life period. Experiences of violence (Douki et al 2007), gynecological morbidity (Latthe et al 2006), infertility, and even negative obstetric outcomes (Chaaya et al 2002) are associated with depression. Helmy et al (2008) found an association between psychiatric morbidity and hysterectomy in Egypt. Experiences of violence against women (see Chapter 7) have reproductive health implications. In a study in Jordan among 353 women attending reproductive health clinics, 20% said that their husband or another person had tried to interfere with women's effort to avoid pregnancy; this was especially the case for women who reported experiencing violence from their husbands (Clark et al 2008). Efforts to improve women's health in the region must take these inter-linkages into account. We will discuss this again later in relation to health services.

Social Practices or Behaviors With Implications for Women's Health

Such practices include early marriage (see Chapter 18) which, although waning, exists in many pockets. Female genital cutting (FGC) is practiced in four countries – Egypt (latest DHS figures prevalence is over 90%), Sudan (near universal), Yemen (coastal regions, approximate prevalence of 25%), and Djibouti. Action to eliminate FGC started with civil society activism but is increasingly being taken up by governmental bodies. Evidence from the Demographic and Health Survey 2008 in Egypt indicates that control efforts are showing an impact (FGC is further discussed in Chapter 7).

Women's Occupational health

Unlike the literature on inequalities in health status among men which began its focus on links between occupational status and health, that on inequalities in women's health has focused, particularly since the 1980s, on "role analysis" and the often multiple burdens women carry as mothers, spouses, and employees (Khlat et al 2000). Much of that literature, however, has been based in Western European and North American settings where women's formal employment is increasingly the norm. There is little research on the implications of women's varied social roles for their health in this region where female labor-force participation is among the lowest in the world (World Bank 2004).

There is also limited research on occupational exposures on women either in formal work or within domestic labor. Habib et al (2006) report that, in low-income communities in Beirut, the use of certain types of household cleaning products has deleterious effects on women's health. Khawaja & Habib (2007) show that the gendered division of labor may contribute to ill-health; less involvement of husbands in housework was associated with wives' psychological distress, marital dissatisfaction, and overall unhappiness after adjusting for relevant risk factors.

Women's Health Policies and Services

Internationally, momentum for women's health intensified in the 1990s but has faced many setbacks since the late 1990s owing to the change of the US administration, economic problems, and cultural and political resistance to elements of the ICPD agenda. That the comprehensive concept of reproductive health was left out of the Millennium Development Goals (MDGs) and that a population and development conference was not held in 2004, as expected, are cited as evidence of this waning emphasis on reproductive health broadly defined. More recently, there have been arguments that population growth should again be re-emphasized and not just reproductive health (Campbell et al 2007).

It is difficult to make generalizations about the extent to which health policies and services in the Arab region meet women's health needs with the diversity, and changes, in economic and political situations and in health systems. In some countries, the once dominant public sector is eroding with increasing privatization under the pressures of macroeconomic retrenchment, such as in Egypt and Syria, and in others, such as Lebanon, the private sector dominates. One can ask if the emphasis on women's health since the 1994 ICPD has impacted the structure and delivery of health services. There is evidence of institutional changes to better link population programs and women's health. In Egypt and Yemen, the former Population Council was merged with the Ministry of Health to become the Ministry of Health and Population. In the OPT, when the first Palestinian Ministry of Health was created in 1995, it integrated a women's health department. Other countries such as Sudan have renamed departments from Maternal and Child Health to "Reproductive Health." Whether such changes are merely semantic or reflect real changes in the nature of health services would be an important subject of research. Certainly, whereas previously most women's health services focused on pregnancy or avoiding pregnancy with little beyond that scope, there is evidence of a broadening of the scope of services to address such issues as morbidity and infertility.

Trends in service utilization are also positive. Antenatal care use and delivery in hospitals have shown an upward trend across the region. Whereas a generation ago, most women delivered at home, the majority now deliver in health care settings. Except in the poorest countries, it tends not to be the lack of health services for women that is the critical constraint but rather their quality and appropriateness.

Studies conducted by the CCCC research group for example have revealed the limitations in antenatal care in Lebanon and Syria (El-Kak et al 2004; Bashour et al 2005). Research has also documented severe limitations in intrapartum and postpartum care offered in the region. In both Egypt (Campbell et al 2005) and Syria (Bashour et al 2009) quality of care problems by medical professionals were considered a major contributor to maternal mortality.

Studies of childbirth in medical settings in Egypt, the OPT, Syria, Lebanon, and more recently Jordan have documented similar deficiencies. Practices such as episiotomy, routine fetal monitoring, and oxytocin use were found in much higher rates than medically warranted. In research on women's perceptions of their childbirth experience, women express dissatisfaction with their lack of involvement in decisions around childbirth and some hospital routines (such as often not being allowed social support in labor, being restricted in their mobility in labor or choice of position in delivery).

Barriers to health care seeking are many and relate both to the "supply side" of delivery and to obstacles women encounter in seeking services. As the Giza study documented, women may not seek services because local health centers do not provide the full range of health services they need. In other cases, women may distrust health services or feel that they are not dealt with in a respectful manner that respects their dignity. In still other instances, as is the case for breast cancer, for example, women may lack knowledge about the health problem or experience economic barriers in seeking care (Corbex 2009).

Finally, one should not under-estimate political barriers to seeking care in a region which has a strong history of conflicts. In the OPT, for example, a number of pregnant women died at Israeli "checkpoints" as they were not allowed to pass to reach hospitals on time (Giacaman et al 2007). Palestinian health authorities have reported 69 deliveries at checkpoints and 38 newborns and 125 patients have died at these blocks (Abdelwahed 2010). Similar instances of political conflict affecting access to health services occur in other countries such as Iraq and Sudan but have been less documented.

Increasingly a majority of women in the region are accessing services around reproduction, whether for antenatal care and delivery. This presents a valuable opportunity to reach women with prevention and screening for other types of health conditions including chronic problems. It is equally important to reach women not utilizing services, either because of age (older or younger women), marital status (single, divorced, or widows), or financial and other constraints. Innovative examples of reaching such women exist, from mobile clinics offering mammograms in Egypt and services to nomadic populations in Jordan to peer education in university dormitories in Tunisia. Such examples need to be built on to expand coverage and utilization or services. Above all, greater accountability within services to the needs and preferences of women should be a fundamental priority.

Civil Society Activism on Women's Health

Action by civil society on women's health began in the region well before the 1994 ICPD. Organizations, mainly NGOs and women's groups, succeeded in bringing even sensitive issues into the public domain, and in partnership with research organizations, have encouraged government attention to the field. The Palestinian Ministry of Health, for example, established a women's health department on the strength of advocacy and example by pre-existing NGOs such as the women's health program of the Union of Palestinian Medical Relief Committees and the Women's Center for Legal Aid and Counseling. Across North Africa, women's organizations working on violence against women not only established counseling centers ('centres d'écoute') but raised the visibility of the issue and gained the attention of the public and governments.

Civil society activism is not confined to reproductive health. Recent efforts to educate women about the risks of breast cancer and the importance of screening and early detection have proliferated. Egypt has over six such organizations (Araj, SJ, Director Jordan Breast Cancer Program, Personal Communication, July 2009). The Egyptian Breast Cancer Association, for example, aims to inform women from diverse backgrounds by disseminating posters and leaflets and conducting seminars at which specialists are invited to talk about breast cancer and the importance of early detection. The Association also has a support group moderated by breast cancer survivors and provides services/prostheses to women at different cost categories. Jordan has one of the few nationally based efforts, the Jordan Breast Cancer Program (2010) that focuses on public education about early detection, including through a hotline, and national guidelines for screening, prevention, and treatment. Similarly, NGOs in Syria are active in screening for breast cancer. While such success stories are encouraging and NGOs are often very innovative in addressing controversial issues, NGOs are often small in scale and reach a limited number of beneficiaries.

Conclusions and Recommendations

Women's health is integrally linked to the social status of women and is more sensitive to social norms than other areas and this is particularly the case in the Arab world. Partly because of the sensitivity of the topic but also the "culture of silence" surrounding women's health, many health problems remain under-researched and nationally representative data are lacking. However, there is enough evidence for policy action.

We have identified a number of research gaps and the need particularly to look at inter-linkages between different areas of women's health and social practices. Moreover, few governmental or non-governmental women's health programs in the region adopt rigorous approaches to evaluating the impact of their programs. Partnerships with research institutions and universities could strengthen programs to subject them to rigorous evaluation and make them more comprehensive. Other under-researched areas include social, economic, and political determinants of and inequalities in women's health, the health of women post-reproductive age, and the health of adolescent women (married and unmarried) (see Chapter 18). The changing social roles of women, as physicians, health care providers and policy makers, and their impact on health also need more attention. These themes require inter-disciplinary research beyond the collection of data on specific health problems, as is commonly the case today, and into longitudinal and cohort studies that adopt a life course approach to women's health.

As reproductive health services are generally available and utilized widely by women, they represent a main point of access to health services. These services offer a potential channel to address other health issues to which women are increasingly exposed, such as chronic conditions. Effort is needed, however, to reach those not accessing services due to distance, social, and financial barriers, and to address concerns over quality. There is a need for policy debates as to how women's health needs in their entirety and across the life-span of women can be addressed.

Advocacy on behalf of women's health is growing but still weak due to underlying weaknesses of NGOs in the political context of the region and their limited scale of activities, and constraints relating to the status of women and social/cultural resistance to many of the issues involved. From a period of civil society and policy mobilization for reproductive health in the 1990s following the 1994 ICPD, the next decades have seen continued emphasis on women's health internationally and in the region, but also greater awareness of some of the limits to implementation. Governments are increasingly addressing women's health explicitly and collecting relevant gender-disaggregated statistics on which to base programs.

We have argued that health status and health service issues of concern to women should be a starting-point. Women in the region have expressed the need for greater accountability in health service delivery and more information from health care providers about their health. Ultimately only through a combination of increased civil society activism on key women's health issues and critical interdisciplinary research will momentum be created to influence governments to address these problems more comprehensively.

Acknowledgments

The authors gratefully acknowledge the research assistance of Chaza Akik, Silva Kouyoumdjian, and Ghada Saad and the helpful comments of the peer reviewers.

References

Abdelwahed A (2010) Women under siege. Special editorial. *International Journal of Gynecology and Obstetrics*, 108(1): 2–3

Abu-Raddad L, Akala FA, Semini I, Riedner G, Wilson D, Tawil O (2010) *Characterizing the HIV/AIDS epidemic in the Middle East and North Africa: Evidence on levels, distribution and trends, Time for Strategic Action, Middle East and North Africa HIV/AIDS Epidemiology Synthesis Project: World Bank/UNAIDS/WHO*

Afifi M (2009) Wealth index association with gender issues and the reproductive health of Egyptian women. *Nursing and Health Sciences*, 11: 29–36

Aitsi A (2010) What is causing the rapid reversal of the social gradient of obesity among Egyptian women? *Reproductive Health Working Group (RHWG) Annual Meeting*

Al-Adili N, Shaheen M, Bergstrom S, Johansson A (2008) Deaths among young, single women in 2000–2001 in the West bank, Palestine Occupied Territories. *Reproductive Health Matters*, 16(31): 112–121

Aoyama A (2001) *Reproductive Health in the Middle East and North Africa: Well-being for all*. Washington, DC: The World Bank

Assaad R, Arntz M (2005) Constrained geographical mobility and gendered labor market outcomes under structural adjustment: Evidence from Egypt. *World Development*, 33 (3): 431–454

Bashour H, Hafez R, Abdulsalam A (2005) Syrian women's perceptions and experiences of ultrasound screening in pregnancy: Implications for antenatal policy. *Reproductive Health Matters*, 13(25): 147–154

Bashour H, Abdulsalam A, Jabr A, Cheikha S, Tabbaa M, Lahham M, et al (2009) Maternal mortality in Syria: Causes, contributing factors and preventability. *Tropical Medicine and International Health*, 14(10): 1–6

Berger G, Peerson A (2009) Giving young Emirati women a voice: Participatory action research on physical activity. *Health & Place*, 15: 117–124

Campbell M, Cleland J, Ezeh A, Prata N (2007) Return of the population growth factor. *Science*, 315: 1501–1502

Campbell O, Gipson R, Issa AH, Matta N, El Deeb B, El Mohandes A, et al (2005) National maternal mortality ratio in Egypt halved between 1992–93 and 2000. *Bulletin of the World Health Organization*, 83(6): 462–471

Chaaya M, Campbell OM, El-Kak F, Shaar D, Harb H, Kaddour A (2002) Postpartum depression: Prevalence and determinants in Lebanon. *Archives of Women's Mental Health*, 5(2): 65–72

Clark CJ, Silverman J, Khalaf IA, et al (2008) Intimate partner violence and interference with women's efforts to avoid pregnancy in Jordan. *Studies in Family Planning*, 39(2): 123–132

Corbex M (2009) *Situation analysis of breast cancer in Egypt*. Baltimore, MD: USAIDS/John Hopkins University Center for Communication Programs

Cottingham J, Myntti C (2002) Reproductive health: Conceptual mapping and evidence, *In*: G Sen, A George, P Ostlin (Eds.) *Engendering international health: The challenge of equity* (p. 83–109). London, UK: MIT Press

Crossette B (2005) Reproductive health and the Millenium Development Goals: the missing link. *Studies in Family Planning*, 36(1): 71–79

Deeb M, Awwad J, Yeretzian JS, Kaspar HG (2003) Prevalence of reproductive tract infections, genital prolapse, and obesity in a rural community in Lebanon. *Bulletin of the World Health Organization*, 81(9): 639–645

DeJong J, Jawad R, Mortagy I, Shepard B (2005) The sexual and reproductive health of young people in the Arab Countries and Iran. *Reproductive Health Matters*, 13(25): 49–59

Douki S, Nacef F (2002) Women's mental health in Tunisia. *World Psychiatry*, 1(1): 55–56

Douki S, Ben Zineb S, Nacef F, Halbreich U (2007) Women's mental health in the Muslim world: Cultural, religious and social issues. *Journal of Affective Disorders*, 102: 177–189

Doumit M, El Saghir N, Huijer HA, Kelley JH, Nassar N (2010) Living with breast cancer, a Lebanese experience. *European Journal of Oncology Nursing*, 14: 42–48

El- Zanaty F, Way A (2009) *Egypt Demographic and Health Survey 2008*. Ministry of Health, El-Zanaty and Associates, Macro International, Cairo, Egypt

El-Kak F, Chaaya M, Kaddour A, Campbell O (2004) Patterns of ANC in low versus high risk pregnancies in Lebanon. *Eastern Mediterranean Health Journal*, 10(3): 268–276

Eloul L, Ambusaidi A, Al-Adawi S (2009) Silent epidemic of depression in the women in the Middle East and North Africa region: Emerging tribulation or fallacy? *Sultan Qaboos University Medical Journal*, 9(1): 5–15

Fargues P (2005) Women in Arab countries: Challenging the patriarchal system. *Reproductive Health Matters*, 13(25): 43–48

Fortney J, Susanti I, Gadalla S, Saleh S (1986) Reproductive mortality in two developing countries. *American Journal of Public Health*, 76(2): 134–138

Fouad M, Rastam S, Ward K, Maziak W (2006) Prevalence of obesity and its associated factors in Aleppo, Syria. *Prevention and Control*, 2(2): 85–94

Freedman LS, Edwards BK, Ries LAG, Young JL (Eds.) (2006) *Cancer incidence in four member countries (Cyprus, Egypt, Israel, and Jordan) of the Middle East Cancer Consortium (MECC) compared with US SEER*. Bethesda, MD: National Cancer Institute

Giacaman R, Odeh M (2002) *Women's perceptions of health and illness in the context of national struggle in the Old City of Nablus, Palestine*. Cairo, Egypt: Population Council

Giacaman R, Abu-Rmeileh N, Wick L (2007) The limitations on choice: Palestinian women's childbirth location, dissatisfaction with the place of birth and determinants. *European Journal of Public Health*, 17(1): 86–91

Glasier A, Gulmezoglu AM (2005) Sexual and reproductive health: Call for papers. *The Lancet*, 366(9490): 969–970

Habib R, Hamdan M, Nuwayhid I, Odaymat F, Campbell O (2005) Muskuloskeletal disorders among full-time homemakers in poor communities. *Women Health*, 42(2): 1–14

Habib R, El-Masri A, Heath R (2006) Women's strategies for handling household detergents. *Environmental Research*, 101(2): 184–194

Hassan-Bitar S, Wick L (2007) Evoking the Guardian Angel: Childbirth care in a Palestinian hospital. *Reproductive Health Matters*, 15(30): 103–113

Helmy YA, Hassanin IM, Abd El Raheem T, Bedaiwy AA, Peterson RS, Bedaiwy MA (2008) Psychiatric morbidity following hysterectomy in Egypt. *International Journal of Gynaecology & Obstetrics*, 102(1): 60–64

Hessini L (2007) Abortion and Islam: Policies and practice in the Middle East and North Africa. *Reproductive Health Matters*, 15(29): 75–84

ILO (International Labour Office) (2010) *Maternity at work: A review of national legislation/Findings from the ILO database of conditions of work and employment laws*. Geneva, Switzerland: International Labour Organization (ILO)

Jordan Breast Cancer Program (2010) Available from http://www.jbcp.jo [Accessed 15 December 2010]

Kaddour A, Hafez R, Zurayk H (2005) Women's perceptions of reproductive health in three communities around Beirut, Lebanon. *Reproductive Health Matters*, 13(25): 34–42

Khattab H, El Geneidy M, El Nahal N, Shorbagui N (2007) *All alone! The stories of Egyptian Women living with HIV, stigma and isolation*. Cairo, Egypt: Egyptian Society for Population Studies and Reproductive Health

Khattab H, Younis N, Zurayk H (1999) *Women, reproduction, and health in rural Egypt: The Giza Study*. Cairo, Egypt: The American University in Cairo Press

Khawaja M, Habib RR (2007) Husbands' Involvement in housework and women's psychosocial health: Findings from a population-based study in Lebanon, *American Journal of Public Health*, 97: 860–866

Khlat M, Sermet C, Le Pape A (2000) Women's health in relation with their family and work roles: France in the early 1990s. *Social Science & Medicine*, 50: 1807–1825

Langer A (2006) *Cairo after 12 years: successes, setbacks, and challenges.* Lancet, 368: 1552–1555

Latthe P, Mignini L, Gray R, Hills R, Khan K (2006) Factors predisposing women to chronic pelvic pain: systematic review. *British Medical Journal*, 332: 749

Mabry R, Al-Riyami A, Morsi M (2007) The prevalence of and risk factors for reproductive morbidities among women in Oman. *Studies in Family Planning*, 38(2): 121–128

Mawajdeh SM, Al-Qutob R, Schmidt A (2003) Measuring reproductive morbidity: a community-based approach, Jordan. *Health Care for Women International*, 24(7): 635–649

Moser C, Dani AA (eds.) (2008) *New frontiers of social policy. Assets, livelihoods and social policy.* Washington, DC: The World Bank

Musaiger AO (2004) Overweight and obesity in the Eastern Mediterranean Region: Can we control it? *Eastern Mediterranean Health Journal*, 10(6): 789–793

Obermeyer C (1992) Islam, women, and politics: The demography of Arab countries. *Population And Development Review*, 18(1): 33–60

Rashad H, Osman M, Roudi-Fahimi F (2005) *Marriage in the Arab World.* Population Reference Bureau

Raymond SU, Greenberg HM, Leeder SR (2005) Beyond reproduction: women's health in today's developing world. *International Journal of Epidemiology*, 34: 1144–1148

Roudi-Fahimi F (2003) *Women's reproductive health in the Middle East and North Africa.* Population Reference Bureau

Sadana R (2000) Measuring reproductive health: Review of community-based approaches to assessing morbidity. *Bulletin of the World Health Organization*, 78(5): 640–654

Saliba M, Zurayk H (2010) Expanding concern for women's health in developing countries: The case of the Eastern Mediterranean Region. *Women's Health Issues*, 20(3): 171–177

Sheikh Ismail L, Henry CJ, Lightowler HJ, Aldaheri AS, Masuadi E, Al Hourani HM (2009) Prevalence of overweight and obesity among adult females in the United Arab Emirates. *International Journal of Food Sciences and Nutrition*, 60(S3): 26–33

Sholkamy H, Ghannam F (2004) *Health and identity in Egypt: Shifting frontiers.* Cairo, Egypt: American University in Cairo Press

Thaddeus S, Maine D (1994) Too far to walk: maternal mortality in context. *Social Science and Medicine*, 38: 1091–1110

Tsui A, Waserheit JN, Jaaga JG (1997) *Reproductive health in developing countries.* Washington, DC: National Academy Press

World Bank (2004) *Gender and development in the Middle East and North Africa.* World Bank

Zurayk H, Khattab N, Younis N, Kamal O, El Helw M (1995) Comparing women's reports with medical diagnoses of reproductive morbidity conditions in rural Egypt. *Studies in Family Planning*, 26(1): 14–21

Zurayk H, Khattab H, Khalil K, Farag A (1996) A holistic reproductive health approach in development countries: Necessity and feasibility. *Health Transition Review*, 6: 92–94

Zurayk H, Sholkamy H, Younis N, Khattab H (1997) Women's health problems in the Arab world: A holistic policy prospective. *International Journal of Gynecology and Obstetrics*, 58(1): 13–21

Zurayk H (1999) Reproductive health in population policy: A review and look ahead. *In*: A Mundigo (Ed.) *Reproductive health: Programme and policy changes post-Cairo.* Liège, Belgium: International Union for the Scientific Study of Population

Zurayk H, Myntti C, Mylene TS, Kaddour A, El-Kak F, Jabbour S (2007) Beyond reproductive health: Listening to women about their health in disadvantaged Beirut neighborhoods. *Health Care For Women International*, 28(7): 614–637

Chapter

20

The Older Persons: From Veneration to Vulnerability?

Abla Mehio Sibai, Rania A. Tohme, Rouham Yamout,
Kathryn M. Yount, and Nabil M. Kronfol

"It is fitting for the last year of the millennium to be the International Year of Older Persons, with the theme 'towards a society for all ages' – a society that does not caricature older persons as pensioners, but sees them as both agents and beneficiaries of development"
UN Secretary-General Kofi Annan, 1 October 1998

As elsewhere, modernity has brought to the Arab world a great increase in the number of persons living into old age, along with their special needs in health and social welfare (Kinsella & Velkoff 2001). In industrialized countries, the needs of older persons are addressed mainly through governmental retirement schemes and health insurance based either on their contributions during active life or by allocation of tax revenues. In low- and middle-income countries, including the Arab states, it is the family that supplies the main support of its older members (Sokolovsky 1999). When the social and economic equilibrium between providers and recipients of care breaks down or becomes inadequate, inequalities and inequities at both the individual and social levels are aggravated (Bond 1989).

While an ageing population may be considered a human success story, the steady growth of older population in this region poses numerous challenges to a number of resource-scarce countries. The demographic transition in several countries has proceeded rapidly during the past two decades (see Chapter 3), outstripping the nascent systems of health and social welfare, and outpacing the rate of economic growth required to maintain those systems. Although high-income countries are more able than others to adjust to the increased demand of older people for social and health care, the region as a whole is unprepared (UNESCWA 2004). In the absence of social contract, older people become socially vulnerable and their health and well-being are under threat.

This chapter aims to explore the health status and needs of older persons within the particular cultural context of Arab societies. The chapter begins with a brief account of the demographic and socio-political transitions that have altered the situation of older people in the Arab world. It then describes the specific social and economic attributes of older Arabs. Last, the chapter provides an overview of the challenges to healthy ageing, and proposes some public health strategies to meet these challenges.

Definitions

The point at which old age begins is ill-defined, and a question is raised whether there can even be a specific age for "being old" (Tout 1989). Long ago, philosophers defined old age as the time when an individual reached the highest point of physical or spiritual development. According to Hippocrates, this is attained at 56 years; Aristotle proclaimed that point at 35 years for the body and 50 years for the soul (De Beauvoir 1970). Modern social scientists define ageing in terms of social functioning, both in terms of vulnerability and empowerment (Roebuck 1979). To the economist, old age is about eligibility for retirement, related to pension plans and social benefits. The bio-medical definition links old age with limitations in the reserve of the organs and their functions, focusing attention on disability and co-morbidity (Resnick & Dosa 2005).

Old age remains a cultural construct being influenced by the ideals and norms within societies (WHO 2009). In some cultures, the onset of old age in females begins with menopause; in others, men are not regarded as old until they become unable to make a living. In countries where life expectancy at birth does not exceed 60 years, a person is perceived as old much earlier than in countries where life expectancy is more than 80 years. Older people represent

Public Health in the Arab World, ed. Samer Jabbour et al. Published by Cambridge University Press. © Samer Jabbour et al., 2012.

a heterogeneous group; the use of chronological age to define older adults is somewhat arbitrary and not all-embracing. Nevertheless, the classification by chronological age is imperative for comparative purposes across studies and countries. Following the classification used by the United Nations in the context of the International Plan of Action on Ageing (WHO 2009) and based on the cutoff point adopted in most Arab legislations, we consider "60 years and over" to define an older person.

Transitions in the Arab societies
Demographic changes

The ageing of the population has been under way in many Arab countries for the last four decades. Declines in fertility and mortality have changed the age structure of all Arab populations into one characterized by a slow, albeit considerable, increase in the total number and proportion of older persons (Chapter 3). Currently, 5.3% of the Arab population is old, with Lebanon having the highest percentage (10%), followed by Tunisia (9%), Morocco (7.5%), Egypt, and Algeria (7%). Improvements in life expectancy have preceded the decline in fertility; thus the rapid increase in the number of people aged 25–60 years will result in accelerated ageing of the population for the coming decades (UNESCWA 2002). It is estimated that, by the year 2050, the percentage of older persons will exceed 15% in over 13 out of the 22 countries of the region (United Nations 2007; Table 1).

Socio-economic Changes

The transition of Arab economies from being based on agriculture to domination of service industry, coupled with globalization, has transformed older adult care in three ways. Rapid urbanization has favored the nuclear family, shattering traditional family life, and exposing people to Western ideas that promote individualistic social ideals at the expense of kin-based culture (Faour 1989). Economic globalization has imposed free trade, increasing the gap between the rich and the poor across and within countries. Recurrent economic crises in middle- and low-income Arab countries, with increased rates of unemployment, have depleted already scarce financial resources and have worsened the living standards of families (see Chapter 2). These countries have also

witnessed out-migration of youth seeking work, along with increased entry of women in the labor market to fulfill the increasing needs of their families (Yount 2003). The latter factors undermine current patterns of family-based old-age care, leading to further marginalization of the aged.

Policy Changes and Political Conflicts

A myriad of internal and external factors, including weak states, corruption, and pressure from international organizations for "structural adjustment," drove some Arab countries to privatize public social and health services. Privatization of the health sector deprived wide segments of the older population of affordable quality health care. Furthermore, a number of countries (Occupied Palestinian Territory [OPT], Lebanon, Iraq, Sudan, and Somalia) are caught in permanent war or occupation, and some others are affected periodically by violent conflicts or political tensions, which exacerbate social and economic vulnerabilities.

The Ageing Experience in Arab Societies

While the living conditions of older persons and opportunities available to them vary from one Arab country to another, older people in the region share common features that have important implications for their health care. These include strong family norms mandating care for seniors by juniors, but also low levels of educational attainment, weak pension systems, and, for women, high rates of widowhood and solitary living.

Cultural Attributes

Overall, socio-cultural norms and religious values in Arab societies demand respect toward the aged and emphasize family relations as a key resource for older adults (Barakat 1993). Older people are considered a resource to their families and their communities; they are praised for their life experiences and quality of advice (Ajrouch et al 2008). To symbolize this attitude, in the spoken and formal Arabic language, words used to describe an older person clearly connote respect and veneration. For example, "al sheikh" (الشيخ) is commonly used to designate either an older person or the chief of a tribe. The terms "hajj" (الحاج) or "hajjah" (الحاجة), originally used to show deference to those who have accomplished the highest religious duty of pilgrimage, is commonly addressed to an

Table 1. Demographic Changes in Arab Countries

	GDP/capita (US$)[1]	TFR		U5 Mr		LEB-2005			LE60-2005		% 60 & over[2]		
		1970–1975	2000–2005	1970	2005	Total	Males	Females	Males	Females	2005	2025	2050
Algeria	7,062	7.4	2.5	220	39	71.7	70.4	73	17	20	7	11	24
Bahrain	21,482	5.9	2.5	82	11	75.2	73.9	77	18	20	4	10	24
Comoros	1,993	7.1	4.9	215	71	64.1	62	66.3	15	17	5	7	14
Djibouti	2,178	7.2	4.5	–	133	53.9	52.6	55.2	15	16	5	7	13
Egypt	4,337	5.9	3.2	235	33	70.7	68.5	73	16	18	7	10	19
Iraq	–	7.2	4.9	127	125	57.7	55.7	59.9	15	16	5	6	13
Jordan	5,530	7.8	3.5	107	26	71.9	70.3	73.8	17	19	5	8	19
KSA	15,711	7.3	3.8	185	26	72.2	70.3	74.6	17	19	4	9	19
Kuwait	26,321	6.9	2.3	59	11	77.3	75.7	79.6	17	22	3	10.5	25
Lebanon	5,584	4.8	2.3	54	30	71.5	69.4	73.7	17	19	10	15	26
Libya	10,335	7.6	3	160	19	73.4	71.1	76.3	17	21	6	10	23
Mauritania	2,234	6.6	4.8	250	125	63.2	61.5	65	15	16	4	6	12
Morocco	4,555	6.9	2.5	184	40	70.4	68.3	72.7	17	19	7.5	13	23
Oman	15,602	7.2	3.7	200	12	75	73.6	76.7	18	20	4	9	21
OPT	–	7.7	5.6	–	23	72.9	71.3	74.4	17	19	–	–	–
Qatar	27,664	6.8	2.9	65	21	75	74.6	75.8	18	20	2	4.5	20
Somalia	–	7.3	6.4	–	225	47.1	45.9	48.2	14	15	4	5	7
Sudan	2,083	6.6	4.8	172	90	57.4	56	58.9	16	17	5	7	13
Syria	3,808	7.5	3.5	123	15	73.6	71.8	75.5	17	19	5	8	19
Tunisia	8,371	6.2	2	201	24	73.5	71.5	75.6	17	20	9	15	28
UAE	25,514	6.4	2.5	84	9	78.3	76.8	81	20	23	2	5	18
Yemen	930	8.7	6	303	102	61.5	60	63.1	15	17	4	5	10

TFR = total fertility rate; U5Mr = under-5 mortality rate per 1000 live birth; LEB = life expectancy at birth; LE60 = life expectancy at age 60.
Sources: 1- UNDP (2008); 2- Population Division of the Department of Economic and Social Affairs of the United Nations Secretariat (2009).

Table 2. Illiteracy, Labor Force Participation, and Solitary Living of Older Adults (Age 60 Years and Over) in Arab Countries

Country	Illiteracy		Labor force participation		Living alone	
	Men	Women	Men	Women	Men	Women
Algeria	76.6	94.6	27.1	6.2	0.8[b]	2.9[b]
Bahrain	–	–	38.3	0.6	0.6	0.9
Comoros	–	–	83.8	24.4	1.1	1.8
Djibouti	82.7[b]	95.0[b]	61.9	21.2	2.1[b]	14.4[b]
Egypt	27.8	76.2	17.5	2.8	3.9	13.1
Iraq	69	93.2	46.8	1.7		
Jordan	36.7	82.5	27.9	4	3.3	10.7
KSA	68.1	94.5	32.6	1	–	–
Kuwait	30.7	69	15.5	0.6	0.3[a]	1.9[a]
Lebanon	46.0[b]	63.2[b]	41.1	4.4	6.2[b]	17.3[b]
Libya	–	–	42.5	4.2	–	–
Mauritania	–	–	63.4	22.9	–	–
Morocco	75	96.6	38.9	4.7	2.3	9.2
Oman	75.4	93.3	30.2	3.6	–	–
OPT	–	–	18	2.3	1.8	9.4
Qatar	46.3	80.4	51.3	3.7	–	–
Somalia	–	–	87.2	24.1	–	–
Sudan	61.3	91.8	61	16.3	5.6	15.4
Syria	54.1	77	52.4	16.2	1.9	6.8
Tunisia	66.6	94.3	35.8	2.9	1.9	3.7
UAE	–	–	31.8	1.3	–	–
Yemen	66.4[b]	98.0[b]	27.1	6.8	2.3	6

–: missing data.
All data obtained from: United Nations. (2007) except: a. Shah et al 2002; b. League of Arab States (2008).

older person regardless of whether he/she has been pilgrims. The nature and the structure of the patrilineal family bolster power and authority in old age, especially to women and those married and with sons (Olmsted 2005).

Educational Attainment and Economic Security

Educational attainment has a direct influence on people's health. Historical trends in ever-schooling in all Arab countries show that men gained access to education earlier and completed a higher number of grades than did women. Currently, rates of illiteracy among older women exceed 90% in the majority of Arab countries, including Yemen, Morocco, Algeria, Saudi Arabia, Djibouti, Iraq, Oman, and Sudan (League of Arab States 2008). Among men the rates range between 28% in Egypt and 82% in Djibouti (United Nations 2007) (Table 2). Recent data indicate that gender gaps in educational attainment will, in the coming generations of older adults, diminish and even reverse because of faster gains in schooling among young women (Yount & Sibai 2009).

Comprehensive old-age pension schemes in the Arab region are rather scarce and inconsistent across countries extending to less than 25% of the Arab population in general (UNESCWA 2004). These schemes are limited to those who have worked in the formal sector (Overbye 2005). While the old-age benefit may be as high as 65% of the insured person's prior average monthly earnings in Kuwait, the basic benefit does not exceed 2.5% of the insured person's average monthly earnings in Libya (US Social Security Administration 2006). As a consequence, a substantial share of older men in these settings continue to work often well beyond the legal age of retirement (Yount & Sibai 2009). This phenomenon is in marked contrast to countries with developed social protection where withdrawal from the labor force is common practice at older age. The percentage of older men who continue to work is highest in poorer Arab countries, reaching up to 87% in Somalia, 84% in Comoros, and 61% in Sudan (Table 2) (United Nations 2007). Research is needed to explore whether this phenomenon of extended periods of work reflects personal preferences of older people to remain active, or responses to absence of public safety nets in the Arab states.

Women's participation in the labor force is low (Table 2). The 2008 data from the International Labor Organization (ILO) report show that participation rates are actually the lowest in the world. Adult female employment-to-population ratio is 24.7% for the Middle East (including Iran) and 27% for North Africa versus 53.1% world average, and 50.4% in developed economies and the European Union. In comparison, male employment-to-population ratios are 81.7% for the Middle East and North Africa, and 80.3% for the world average (ILO 2009). The poorer countries, specifically Comoros, Djibouti, and Somalia, have higher rates of female employment, up to 60% (ILO 2009). These estimates may not reflect the full picture of women's employment since a substantial proportion of women who work do so irregularly to meet their family responsibility, or limit their involvement to the informal sector, mainly in service and agriculture. Consequently, women are more vulnerable than men to financial dependency in their old age.

Living Arrangements and Family Support

Co-residence is one of the means by which Arab families fulfill the support due to their older relatives (Khadr 1997; Shah et al 2002; Yount & Khadr 2008). Historically, the main investment during one's active

life is to raise children who will then protect their aged parents from isolation and deprivation. A large family, especially with several sons, has long been considered as old age "social security" (Prothro & Diab 1973) and this probably remains true today in many settings (Yount 2005). However, co-residence of three generations or more has begun to disappear from some Arab societies. For instance, Prothro & Diab (1973) showed that the majority of women in the Arab Middle East who were married in the 1960s has never lived with their in-laws. Yet, the intensity of family ties has not weakened. It is observed in several countries that married children and their parents aspire to live in the same neighborhoods, sometimes on different floors of the same building (Khadr 1997; Yount 2003). Grandparents, especially grandmothers, are often involved in the organization of family life and education and babysitting of grandchildren, thus providing themselves and their children with a feeling of usefulness.

As elsewhere, men in Arab countries tend to marry women of a younger age (Carr & Bodnar-Deren 2009). Given the longer life expectancy of women, older women are more likely to lose the support of a spouse in their later years. This situation may lead to increased dependency on male relatives (Yount 2003). Across countries, the percentage of older women living alone is much higher than that of older men, up to 17.3% in Lebanon, 15.4% in Sudan, and 14.4% in Djibouti (United Nations 2007; League of Arab States 2008) (Table 2). Recent studies conducted in the region highlight the heterogeneity in circumstances urging intergenerational co-residence of older Arabs (Khadr 1997; Shah et al 2002). Whereas wealth and higher standards of living increase the likelihood of co-residence with adult children in Egypt and Kuwait, the reverse is true in Lebanon where solitary living is a marker of greater independence and the financial means to purchase privacy, thus challenging long held assumptions about family relations in the country (Tohme et al 2011).

The prevalent culture in the region commonly allots a special place for seniors in the family hierarchy and obligates the offspring to serve and provide care and financial support to parents and grandparents (Yount et al 2009). The intensity of financial exchanges across generations of the same family modifies the attributes of old-age vulnerability. Indeed, financial deprivation leading to marginalization is less likely to affect older persons, when these enjoy the right to support inside their families. The situation may be expectedly different if the family itself is suffering grave social exclusion. Therefore, the well-being of an older adult is linked with the availability of offspring to protect him/her from loneliness, unworthiness, insecurity and indigence, as much as it is determined by the combination of income, savings, and social benefits, as suggests a study demonstrating the intensity of intergenerational exchange in Egypt (Yount et al 2009). Consequently, infertility or a social path that had led a person to become childless, carries potentially substantial social cost in older age (Inhorn & Van Balen 2002), especially in women, in light of the increased need of women to be supported (Yount et al 2009). This is all the more true considering the weak formal social safety nets for older people. It is important to address this determinant of health in a region witnessing in some of its areas an increase in numbers of never married women and to a lesser extent, men (see Chapter 3) who will become childless older persons.

Challenges in Health and Health Care Systems for Older Adults

Health Profile of Older People

Along with population ageing, the health profile in the region has changed considerably over the last three decades. Non-communicable diseases (NCDs), notably cardiovascular diseases, cancer, diabetes and musculoskeletal disorders, are looming as the most important causes of morbidity and mortality, imposing far greater demands on health care systems already constrained by scarce resources. In a survey in nine Arab countries, the percentage of older adults reporting at least one chronic disease ranged between 13.1% in Djibouti and 63.8% in Lebanon; the majority of the countries having rates above 45% (League of Arab States 2008) (Table 3). Differences in prevalence rates are likely to be partly attributed to reporting biases and undiagnosed diseases.

Ill health in old age is often influenced by factors that operate well before the onset of old age, including early life and occupation. The circumstances of childhood (Buxton et al 2005) and the socio-economic (Grundy & Sloggett 2003), demographic and geographic context of early life pre-define health in old age (Grundy & Holt 2000). As elsewhere in the world, substantial differences in the health profile of women

Table 3. Selected Health Characteristics of Older Adults (Age 60 Years and Over) in Arab Countries

Country	Suffering from at least one chronic disease	Prevalence of disability	Current cigarette smokers
Algeria	55.2	7.5	20.9
Djibouti	13.1	17.2	6.0
Lebanon	63.8	15.3	24.7
Morocco	45.8	5.1	6.1
Syria	43.2	9.9	22.5
Tunisia	54.1	15.5	50.3
Yemen	40.0	15.2	24.6
Libya	55.1	10.1	12.0
Palestine	33.3	7.5	15.5

Source: League of Arab States (2008).

and men also exist, with rates of cardiovascular diseases higher in men, and rates of diabetes, obesity, musculoskeletal disorders, osteoporosis, and depression higher in women (Yount & Sibai 2009). High prevalence rates of functional disability are noted in Djibouti (17.2%), Tunisia (15.5%), Lebanon (15.3%), and Yemen (15.2%) (Table 3) (League of Arab States 2008). These levels are expected to rise along with the growing number and percentage of older persons.

Of significance are the alarming levels of obesity (around 40%), most notably among older women in the oil-rich countries such as Kuwait, Bahrain, the United Arab Emirates (UAE), and in Tunisia (Harzallah et al 2005; Jackson et al 2001; Musaiger & Al-Mannal 2001). Obesity by itself increases the risk of mortality (Adams et al 2006) but also increases cardiovascular risk through associated co-morbidity with hypertension, unfavorable blood lipid profiles, and diabetes (Miller et al 2005). The online Diabetes Atlas of the International Diabetes Foundation lists five Arab countries among the "Top Ten" in world prevalence of diabetes among 20–79 year olds with UAE, Saudi Arabia, and Bahrain ranking second, third, and fifth, respectively. Lifestyle changes and ongoing nutrition transition, characterized by a consistent rise in per capita calorie supply and increased consumption of fat and refined carbohydrates, have been reported as important factors affecting levels of obesity among populations in high-income Arab countries (Sibai et al 2010). Arab culture traditionally values "plumpness" as an attractive physique for women, and as a sign of health and affluence; this has been suggested as an additional cause for the prevalence rates of obesity among women (Kandela 1999). With old age, women acquire exceptional power within a family, equaling or surpassing that of men, and hence, may start to delegate household responsibilities to their grown-up daughters or their daughters-in-law (Yount 2003). The exemption from domestic chores adds to restricted physical activity, leading to weight gain.

Behavioral risk factors play an important role in the epidemiological transition. When risk factors are not dealt with earlier in life, the incidence and prevalence of age-related NCDs and complications become more likely. Wide variations have been reported in the rates of cigarette smoking across Arab countries. While older men in Bahrain, Egypt, Jordan, Lebanon, Morocco, and Tunisia appear to show relatively high rates of smoking, ranging between 30% and 50% (Tazi et al 2003; Musaiger 2004; CDC 2006; Chaaya et al 2006), contemporary rates in Oman and the UAE are much lower (7–15%) (Al-Riyami & Afifi 2004; Ministry of Health UAE 2003). Except for a few countries such as Bahrain (24.8%) and Lebanon (17.3%), the prevalence of smoking among older women does not exceed 5% (Musaiger 2004; Chaaya et al 2006). This is likely to change in the coming generations of older adults because of more rapid uptake of smoking among girls compared to boys. Waterpipe smoking is also on the increase among younger and older adults alike (Maziak et al 2004), with available data suggesting a prevalence rate of around 11% among older adults (Chaaya et al 2006; Table 3).

Health Systems and Health and Social Care Resources

Resources devoted to the health sector, and the coverage and benefits provided by health care systems to older persons vary considerably amongst and within Arab countries. While public health services are widely provided in oil-rich GCC countries, Syria and Jordan, out-of-pocket health expenditures represent often the most important source of financing care. It is not surprising that the poorer the country, the larger the share of out-of-pocket expenses (Yount & Sibai 2009). Furthermore, available services for the older persons are generally welfare-based and, except

for a few countries (Oman, Jordan, and Syria), health interventions are largely specialized and curative in nature. The burden of health care delivery to the older population has been shouldered mostly by the public sector in its roles of stewardship. An ageing population challenges the health care system in most countries and raises the importance of health reforms.

Since co-residence or quasi-co-residence is a common feature between parents and adult children (Yount et al 2009), many older adults live at home and receive care from their children, spouses, or other close relatives. With a decline in the number of children and increasing involvement of women in the labor market, families are less able to meet the needs of their older relatives (Yount & Khadr 2008). In some countries, privileged families have opted for in-home long-term care given by full-time, paid, foreign domestic workers. This new form of home care is not only an alternative, but a valuable solution in the absence of family members. Specialized home care is generally unavailable (Youssef 2005), and there is limited social and economic support for caregivers (Atallah et al 2005).

Nursing homes and old-age institutions are considered as the last resource when families cannot afford to care for their frail, severely ill, or disabled older members at home (Margolis & Reed 2001; Sinunu et al 2009). While accurate numbers are not available, the proportion of institutionalized older adults remains low in most Arab countries (Boggatz & Dassen 2005). In Tunisia, for instance, the estimated prevalence of institutionalization among persons aged 65 years and older does not exceed two per thousand (Radhouane 2004). In the UAE and Lebanon, this ranges between seven and 14 per thousand, which is still six times lower than those in the United States (Margolis & Reed 2001). Cultural norms toward older care, the stigma associated with placing older relatives in nursing homes, and the dependence on local or foreign house-helpers among the richer societal categories, may explain the low rates of institutionalization.

A number of countries have made important strides over the past several years, enabling the older person to "age in place." Qatar and Jordan have introduced the Family Welfare Programme to reach older persons in their homes, providing health-related services *in situ*. Tunisia supports families through a special program entitled National Program to Assist the Elderly within Their Families and facilitates the hosting of an older person by volunteer families. In Egypt, home services operate through specialized units within the Ministry of Social Solidarity. Bahrain, Oman, Qatar, Tunisia, and Saudi Arabia, have established mobile units providing medical and other services to reach older people within their families (Sibai & Kronfol 2008). Qatar, Saudi Arabia, Oman, Lebanon, and Syria have convened meetings and conferences and published brochures to raise awareness of health problems of older people. These activities seldom involve "lay" older persons, or emphasize the "life course perspective" in healthy ageing.

Toward the Implementation of Sustainable Ageing Policies

The exigencies of new social and economic realities and the emerging burden of NCDs threaten the well-being of older Arabs in two ways. First, the social norms and duties toward the old have been altered by urbanization and modernization of lifestyles and values. A decline in fertility rate, an increasing percentage of women entering the workforce, and a region afflicted by decades of migration, wars, and political violence, have over the years distorted family cohesion and the role of children in caring for their old parents. Second, with the rise in inflation and unemployment, and the expense of living in cities, families in most Arab countries are getting poorer. Thus, a retired dependent parent often depletes family savings because of chronic disease or catastrophic illness (Boggatz & Dassen 2005; Seoud et al 2007). While richer families can provide older members with dignified living, aged members of poorer families are more likely to be in a situation of deprivation. The limited family resources and the need to "ration" family expenses may lead to clashes between generations, which undermines cultural traditions and may threaten the health and well-being of older adults. Government and non-governmental old-age care systems fail to secure minimal health and social needs of seniors (Myers & Nathanson 1982).

There is an urgent need for policy makers to focus on improving the quality of life of older citizens, to provide health care and social security in old age, and to develop a support system, leaning on the family-based care that still functions (UNESCWA 2004). These ambitious goals can be reached solely by inter-sectoral work directed toward securing diverse aspects of supportive and dignified environments for

older persons. We propose four broad strategies to promote and maintain healthy ageing.

Promoting Health and Well-Being in Old Age: A Life-Course Perspective

Risk for chronic illnesses, such as diabetes and heart disease, originates in early childhood (Bibbins-Domingo et al 2007). Although genetic predispositions and individual variations exist, health in old age reflects the living circumstances and actions during the whole life span. While it is "never too early and never too late" to change behaviors, adopting healthier lifestyles in early ages and adapting to age-associated changes thereafter present opportunities to influence how people age (Oxley 2009). To decrease out of pocket health care costs, governments and organizations need to provide free or low cost relevant prevention programs for older people. Health education materials that teach "self-care" and "active ageing" are additional means to advance lifelong health promotion. Social responsibility for health is one of the main priorities identified in the Jakarta Declaration on Health Promotion into the twenty-first century (Madi & Hussain 2008). Hence, younger relatives and family members should learn the principles of active ageing, and be more involved in promoting healthy habits and provision of care to their older relatives.

Integrated Health Systems

The continuum of care for older people ranges from primary care to specialized and palliative care in hospitals and nursing homes, buttressed throughout by informal care of family and relatives. The challenge is to develop an integrated health and social system in which various caregivers play their role in complementary channels to cover the needs of older persons. Integrated systems will include health insurance, services, family-centered care, and information.

Health Insurance

Older people have a greater need for services due to increased morbidity and disability, but lesser resources due to their withdrawal from the labor force. Without insurance coverage or free services, they and their families have to rely on out-of-pocket purchase of health services including medicines, eyeglasses, hearing aids, and other assistive devices. Catastrophic illnesses involving surgery, diagnostic scanning, and chronic treatment for cancer are known to absorb large amounts of family budgets and drive older persons and their families to unexpected poverty. Many older persons in Arab countries lack even minimal health insurance benefits, and cannot afford paid health services. Illustratively, in Lebanon, subscribers to the National Social Security Fund lose their health insurance upon retirement, at the very time when it is most needed (Abyad 2001).

Health Services

The increasing burden of degenerative chronic diseases and proportion of older persons with disabilities will require an integrated net of health care, along with new skills required of health care professionals and workers. A key feature of a comprehensive model of care for older people is a "geriatric philosophy" with commitment to a "holistic approach to care, including the central role for the primary care physician" (MacAdam 2008). Currently, different providers attend to co-morbidities among older persons within a fragmented vertical disease-centered health care system. Most Arab countries lack physicians, nurses, community workers, and social welfare personnel trained in gerontology. Units catering to long-term and palliative care to alleviate the burden on family members are not adequately provided even in countries with a developed public health sector. Integrated, patient-centered primary health care with comprehensive multidisciplinary assessment of medical, functional, psychological, and social needs ameliorates poor health outcomes and reduces health costs (Oxley 2009).

Family-Centered Care

Societal changes in family structures and roles have created a shortage in available family members who can give care. Full-time immigrant caregivers, when afforded, resolve only part of the problem. These play the roles of a house-maid, a companion, or a guard who also provides long-term care to older adults dependent on help in daily living (Margolis & Reed 2001). However, these workers have no formal qualifications and cannot replace nurses or nursing assistants. Long-term care, whether provided by family members or paid-caregivers, is a physically and mentally taxing responsibility, and it is not unusual for caretakers to incur health problems themselves (Seoud et al 2007).

Informational Support

Using various channels of communication, governments and non-governmental organizations can promote community awareness and understanding of existing health facilities and resources tailored to the needs of older people. Older people-friendly directories of services provided by the government, various nursing homes, and NGOs are still insufficient. Older persons and their caregivers often lack access to information about available assistance, when it exists. This undermines sound decisions on the choice of needed health services or on utilization of existing resources.

Promoting Social and Health Research of Old Age

In most Arab countries, research data on older adults is scarce. Policies for developing health programs need to be based on understanding the reality of life experiences, on epidemiological trends, and on the utilization rates of health and social care services. Population databases are needed to track the rapid socio-economic and demographic changes that affect older adults. A standard set of survey instruments, harmonized definitions and measurements, and comparable social, economic, and health indicators will be essential to map equity and inequity, and geographic disparities within and between Arab countries. In-depth, social research is also crucial to capture changes in the social, cultural, and family norms in relation to older adults. There is also a need to promote, support and fund research on older adults within the region.

Old Age Care in the Development Agenda

Older persons are valuable social and human capital. The Arab culture that draws from the wisdom of older persons is weakening in face of the emerging economic and social realities endured by most modern Arab societies. Organized community groups and civil associations that advocate and lobby for the rights of older persons, similar to those found for other vulnerable population groups, are scarce if not totally lacking in the region. Government programs continue to be geared toward other segments of the population perceived to be more vital for the nation, such as children and women of reproductive age.

So far, public participation and legislative representation of older persons in Arab countries appear to be related more to the position of the older persons in the society, associated with economic and political power, than to institutionalized policy structures and processes. The right of older people to health and social protection is not a luxury; it is an essential component of social equity and a must in the development agenda. For older adults to reach real social and economic independence, it is imperative to implement multi-sectional policies, and mainstream the issues of older people into economic, social, and health development projects. This involves active participation of the older people themselves in strategy development, where they can voice their preferences and ideals (Heywood et al 2002). Special attention to vulnerable older people, in particular those who are childless, lonely, disabled, poor, or caught in war and violence, is part of equitable access to resources for all age groups.

Conclusions

Although quite diverse in their resources and policies, Arab countries share the potential of being age-friendly societies owing to the particular family-based culture. However, with ageing of the population over the coming decades coupled with the changing cultural, social, and economic conditions of modern families, maintaining health autonomy and social integration in old age will become increasingly challenging. Improving health and social welfare of older people can be realized with a combination of enhanced preventive health services, increased health literacy, coordinated health care systems, reinforced family role, and policy integration across a number of governmental and non-governmental agencies.

References

Abyad A (2001) Health care for older persons: A country profile – Lebanon. *Journal of the American Geriatrics Society*, 49: 1366–1370

Adams KF, Schatzkin A, Harris TB, et al (2006) Overweight, obesity, and mortality in a large prospective cohort of persons 50 to 71 years old. *New England Journal of Medicine*, 355(8): 763–778

Ajrouch KJ, Antonucci TC, Akiyama H, Abdulrahim S (2008) *Older men and family relations in Lebanon: An exploratory study. Presented at Global Trends and Challenges Facing the Arab Family.* Lebanese American University-Byblos Campus, June 20–21, 2008

Al-Riyami AA, Afifi M (2004) Smoking in Oman: Prevalence and characteristics of smokers. *Eastern Mediterranean Health Journal*, 10(4/5): 600–609

Atallah R, Nehme C, Seoud J, Yeretzian J, Zablit C, Levesque L, et al (2005) Caregivers of elderly people with loss of autonomy in Lebanon: What is the context of their health care? *Recherches des Soins infirmiers*, 81: 122–138

Barakat H (1993) The Arab family and the challenge of change. *In: The Arab world, society, culture and state* (p. 97–118). Los Angeles, CA: University of California Press

Bibbins-Domingo K, Coxson P, Pletcher MJ, Lightwood J, Goldman L (2007) Adolescent overweight and future adult coronary heart disease. *New England Journal of Medicine*, 357(23): 2371–2379

Boggatz T, Dassen T (2005) Ageing, care dependency, and care for older people in Egypt: A review of the literature. *International Journal of Older People Nursing* in association with *Journal of Clinical Nursing*, 14(8b): 56–63

Bond J (1989) Political economy as a perspective in the analysis of old age. *In*: C Phillipson, M Bernard, P Strang (Eds.) *Dependency and interdependency in old age* (p. 48–53). UK: British Society of Gerontology

Buxton J, Clarke L, Grundy E, Marshall CE (2005) The long shadow of childhood: Associations between parental social class and own social class, educational attainment and timing of first birth; results from the ONS Longitudinal Study. *Population Trends*, 121: 17–26

Carr D, Bodnar-Deren S (2009) Gender, aging and widowhood. *In*: P Uhlenberg (Ed.) *International handbook of population aging* (p. 705–728). Netherlands: Springer

CDC (Centers for Disease Control and Prevention) (2006) Assessing risk factors for chronic disease – Jordan, 2004. *Morbidity and Mortality Weekly Report*, 55(23): 653–655

Chaaya M, Sibai AM, El-Chemaly S (2006) Smoking patterns and predictors of smoking cessation in elderly populations in Lebanon. *International Journal of Tuberculosis and Lung Disease*, 10(8): 917–923

De Beauvoir S (1970) *La vieillesse [The coming age]*. Paris, France: Gallimard (in French)

Faour M (1989) Fertility policy and family planning in the Arab countries. *Studies in Family Planning*, 20(5): 254–263

Grundy E, Holt G (2000) Adult life experiences and health in early old age in Great Britain. *Social Science and Medicine*, 51(7): 1061–1074

Grundy E, Sloggett A (2003) Health inequalities in the older population: The role of personal capital, social resources and socio-economic circumstances. *Social Science and Medicine*, 56(5): 935–947

Harzallah F, Alberti H, Ben Khalifa F (2005) The metabolic syndrome in an Arab population: A first look at the new international diabetes federation criteria. *Diabetic Medicine*, 23: 441–444

Heywood F, Oldman C, Means R (2002) *Housing and home in later life*. Buckingham, UK: Open University Press

ILO (International Labour Organization) (2009) *Global employment trends for women*. Geneva, Switzerland: ILO

Inhorn M, Van Balen F (2002) *Infertility around the globe: New thinking on childlessness, Gender, and reproductive technologies*. Berkeley, CA: University of California Press

Jackson RT, Al Mousa Z, Al-Raqua M, Prakash P, Muhanna A (2001) Prevalence of coronary risk factors in healthy adult Kuwaitis. *International Journal of Food Sciences and Nutrition*, 52: 301–311

Kandela P (1999) The Kuwaiti passion for food cannot be shaken. *The Lancet*, 353: 1249–1250

Khadr ZA (1997) *Living arrangements and social support systems of the older population in Egypt, Unpublished doctoral dissertation*. Ann Arbor, MI: University of Michigan

Kinsella K, Velkoff V (2001) *An aging world*. Washington, DC: Government Printing Office

League of Arab States (2008) *Pan Arab project on Family health (PAPFAM) survey- comparative report*

MacAdam M (2008) *Frameworks of integrated care for the elderly: A systematic review, CPRN research report*. Available from http://www.cprn.org/documents/49813_EN.pdf [Accessed April 2009]

Madi HH, Hussain SJ (2008) Health protection and promotion. *Eastern Mediterranean Health Journal*, 14(1): 15–22

Margolis SA, Reed RL (2001) Institutionalizing older adults in a health district in the United Arab Emirates: Health status and utilization rate. *Gerontology*, 47(3): 161–167

Maziak W, Ward KD, Afifi Soweid RA, Eissenberg T (2004) Tobacco smoking using a waterpipe: A re-emerging strain in a global epidemic, *Tobacco Control*, 13: 327–333

Miller WM, Nori-Janosz KE, Lillystone M, Yanez J, Peter A, McCullough PA (2005) Obesity and lipids. *Current Cardiology Reports*, 7: 465–470

Ministry of Health-UAE (United Arab Emirates) (2003) *National family health study*. United Arab Emirates: Ministry of Health

Musaiger AO (2004) Health status, lifestyle and nutrient intake of home resident elderly in Bahrain. *Nutrition and Health*, 17(4): 285–295

Musaiger AO, Al-Mannal MA (2001) Weight, height, body mass index and prevalence of obesity among the adult population in Bahrain. *Annals of Human Biology*, 28(3): 346–350

Myers G, Nathanson C (1982) Aging and the family. *World Health Statistics Quarterly*, 35: 225–238

Olmsted JC (2005) Gender, ageing and the evolving patriarchal contract. *Feminist Economics*, 11: 53–78

Overbye E (2005) Extending social security in developing countries: A review of three main strategies. *International Journal of Social Welfare*, 14: 305–314

Oxley H (2009) *Policies for healthy ageing: An overview*. OECD Health Working paper no. 42. Available from http://www.olis.oecd.org/olis/2009doc.nsf/LinkTo/NT00000BDE/$FILE/JT03259727.PDF [Accessed 15 April 2009]

Population Division of the Department of Economic and Social Affairs of the United Nations Secretariat (2008) *World Population Prospects: The 2008 Revision*. Available from http://www.esa.un.org/unpp [Accessed 2 October 2009]

Prothro ET, Diab LN (1973) *Changing family patterns in the Middle East*. Beirut, Lebanon: Librairie du Liban

Radhouane G (2004) *The elderly in Tunisia*. Available from http://www.inia.org.mt/data/images/bold/Bold0204.pdf#page=17 [Accessed 15 September 2009]

Resnick NM, Dosa D (2005) Geriatric medicine. *In*: AS Fauci, et al, (Eds.) *Harrison's principles of internal medicine* (16th edition). US: McGraw Hill Medical

Roebuck J (1979) When does old age begin? The evolution of the English definition. *Journal of Social History*, 12(3): 416–428

Seoud J, Nehme C, Atallaha R, et al (2007) The health of family caregivers of older impaired persons in Lebanon: An interview survey. *International Journal of Nursing Studies*, 44: 259–272

Shah N, Yount KM, Shah MA, Menon I (2002) Living arrangements of older women and men in Kuwait. *Journal of Cross-Cultural Gerontology*, 17: 37–55

Sibai AM, Kronfol N (2008) *Situation analysis of population ageing in the Arab countries: The way forward towards implementation of MIPAA*, ESCWA, Technical Paper 2. Available from http://www.escwa.un.org/information/publications/edit/upload/sdd-08-tp2-e.pdf [Accessed 15 November 2008]

Sibai AM, Nasreddine L, Mokdad A, Adra N, Tabet M, Hwalla N (2010) Nutrition transition and cardiovascular disease risk factors in the MENA countries: Reviewing the evidence. *Annals of Nutrition and Metabolism Journal*, 57: 193–203

Sokolovsky J (1999) *Living arrangements of older persons and family support in less developed countries, UN Population Division, technical meeting on population ageing and living arrangements of older persons*. New York, NY, 8–10 February 2000

Tazi MA, Khalil SA, Chaouki N, Chergaoui S, Lahmouz F, Srairi JE, et al (2003) Prevalence of the main cardiovascular risk factors in Morocco: Results of a national survey, 2000. *Journal of Hypertension*, 21: 897–903

Tohme RA, Yount KM, Yassine S, Shideed S, Sibai AM (2011) Socioeconomic resources and living arrangements of older adults in Lebanon: Who chooses to live alone? *Ageing and Society*, 31: 1–17

Tout K (1989) What is ageing? *In*: K Tout (Ed.) *Ageing in developing countries* (p. 5–16). UK: Oxford University Press for Help Age International

United Nations (2007) *World population ageing 2007*. New York, NY: United Nations

UNDP (United Nations Development Programme) (2008) Human development index. *Human Development Report* 2007/2008

UNESCWA (United Nations Economic and Social Commission for Western Asia) (2002) *The Arab plan of action on ageing to the year 2012*. Available from http://www.escwa.un.org/information/publications/edit/upload/sd-02-01.pdf [Accessed 15 December 2010]

UNESCWA (2004) *Ageing in the Arab Countries: Regional variations, policies and programmes*. Available from http://www.monitoringris.

org/documents/strat_reg/unescwa1.pdf [Accessed 15 December 2010]

US Social Security Administration (2006) *Social security programs throughout the world*. Available from http://www.ssa.gov/policy/docs/progdesc/ssptw/index.html [Accessed 15 December 2010]

WHO (World Health Organization) (2009) *Definition of an older or elderly person: Proposed working definition of an older person in Africa for the MDS project*. Available from http://www.who.int/healthinfo/survey/ageingdefnolder/en/index.html [Accessed 1 April 2009]

Yount KM (2003) Ageing in the Arab States, *In*: S Joseph (Ed.) *Encyclopedia of women and Islamic cultures: Family, body, sexuality and health* (vol. 3). Leiden, Netherlands: Brill

Yount KM (2005) Resources, family organization, and violence against married women in Minya, Egypt. *Journal of Marriage and Family*, 67(3): 579–596

Yount KM, Cunningham S, Agree EM, Engelman M (2009) Gender, generation, and economic transfers in Ismailia, Egypt. *In*: *Family support networks and population ageing* (p. 39–47). Doha, Qatar: Doha International Institute for Family Studies and Development and UNFPA

Yount KM, Khadr Z (2008) Gender, social change and living arrangements among older Egyptians during the 1990's. *Population Research and Policy Review*, 27: 201–225

Yount KM, Sibai AM (2009) The demography of aging in Arab countries. *In*: P Uhlenberg (Ed.) *International handbook on the demography of aging* (p. 277–331). Netherlands Springer

Youssef RM (2005) Comprehensive health assessment of senior citizens in Al-Karak governorate, Jordan. *Eastern Mediterranean Health Journal*, 11(3): 334–348

The Well-Being of Migrant Women: Between Agency and Restraint

Sawsan Abdulrahim and Ynesse Abdul Malak

The past decades of the twentieth century have witnessed a "feminization of labor migration," and a rampant increase in the number of women crossing international borders in search of economic opportunities (Hondagneu-Sotelo 1999; Ehrenreich & Russell Hochschild 2002). A large proportion of female migrants work in domestic service, an economic niche that has historically providing employment for poor women in different social and national contexts (Pedraza 1991; Hill Collins 2000). The profession is highly gendered, provides low-wages and high risk for exploitation. It has increasingly become "racialized," in that the overwhelming majority of domestic workers in any setting are either foreigners or belong to the most disadvantaged social groups (Anderson 2000).

Migrant women from countries of the global South are highly visible in the Arab world and constitute a significant proportion of low-wage labor migration. In 1996, the proportion of women in the total migratory flows from the three top Asian sending countries – Indonesia, Sri Lanka, and the Philippines – to the Middle East was between 25–30% (Gamburd 2000). In the Gulf Cooperative Council, the majority of the general female migrants and 90% of Sri Lankan female migrants work specifically in the domestic service sector (Massey et al 1998; Gamburd 2000). An estimated 130,000 to 200,000 migrant domestic workers live and work in Lebanon (ILO 2008). On average, 300 applications are processed each day for housemaids in the United Arab Emirates (UAE) (Sabban 2002). The presence of domestic workers is not limited to middle- or high-income countries in the region; it is estimated that 6000 to 8000 Ethiopian housemaids live and work in Yemen (de Regt 2007).

The International Labor Organization (ILO) identifies domestic workers as the largest group of unprotected workers in the Arab region. A combination of factors – such as lack of protective government policies, unregulated private employment agencies, and the nature of domestic labor as work performed in the privacy of homes and away from public scrutiny – amplify the vulnerability of this group whose well-being is determined by the intersection of gender, class, and migrant status. Migrant women generally have less access to resources compared to men and are affected by the accumulated disadvantage of their gender, low socio-economic status, and inability to access resources that are limited to citizens. Given the large number of migrant domestic workers in Arab countries and the social determinants that increase their vulnerability to poor health outcomes, focusing on the health of this group is an important component of examining health in the region.

In this chapter, we review the literature on the health of migrant domestic workers. We were not surprised by the dearth of scholarly research on this particular topic. We were, however, amazed by the flurry of writings, reports by international organizations, and media projects describing the plight of this social group in Arab countries. Whereas women are generally less visible in migration research (Pessar & Mahler 2003), women migrant domestic workers have recently dominated the writings on migration in this region. Their living conditions have been the subject of numerous scholarly writings (Shah et al 1991; Haddad 1999; Silvey 2004; Moukarbel 2009, Jarallah 2009) and reports prepared by international organizations (Jureidini 2002; Sabban 2002; Esim & Smith 2004; Workshop Report 2005). These conditions have been emphatically described as "slavery" or "slave-like" (Abu Habib 1998; Jureidini & Moukarbel 2004; Haddad 1999). The plight of migrant domestic workers has stimulated media projects such as

Public Health in the Arab World, ed. Samer Jabbour et al. Published by Cambridge University Press. © Samer Jabbour et al., 2012.

documentary films and "blogspots" that chronicle stark cases of abuse and suicides (Ethiopian suicides 2011).

Relying on a wealth of resources, of which very little addresses health specifically, this chapter discusses how current policies and social conditions put migrant women at risk for negative health outcomes. It focuses on three levels of determinants – government policies, private "middleman" agencies, and individual employers. Employing a nuanced and gendered analysis throughout the chapter, we do stop at describing this group of migrants as passive victims but as individuals who strive to promote their own health through proactive strategies. We highlight some of these strategies and the resources women draw upon to reduce the harmful health effects of structural constraints and daily mistreatment. The chapter ends with a section in which we outline priorities for action and future research areas. Throughout, we strive to build a case for acknowledging the rights of migrant women in this region and for beginning to examine the long-term consequences of migration on their health and well-being. In an effort to contextualize the flow of migration of women to Arab countries, we first present a concise theoretical review on the economic sociology of migration.

Migration: A Theoretical Framework

The definition of migration, or what constitutes a migrant, is loose and changing. Some definitions use citizenship status, length of residence in the host country, or reason for migration (Schramm 2006; Fargues 2005). This chapter focuses on women who leave their countries of origin to go to the Arab region voluntarily for economic reasons. We refer to these women as migrants, not expatriates or temporary workers. While there is a fine line between what constitutes voluntary versus forced migration in cases where poverty, racism, and social exclusion force people to cross national boundaries for economic survival. This chapter does not purport to address the complex issues and gross human rights violations that negatively affect the well-being of refugee or trafficked women.

A number of theoretical frameworks have been developed to explain migration both at the micro- and macro-structural levels. Economic explanations fall within micro-level human capital theories and suggest that individuals migrate in order to maximize

the economic return on their education and experience (Borjas 1989). This view has been criticized as utilitarian and male-centric by scholars who have documented the high proportion of women in migration flows and called for bringing gender into the study of migration (Pedraza 1991; Donato et al 2006). Whereas many women migrate to improve their economic position, their migration is an outcome of family or community decisions and takes shape through a socio-cultural process mediated by gendered ideologies (Salazar Parreñas 2001; Mahler & Pessar 2006). Migration can either reaffirm or reconfigure gender ideologies depending on factors at the level of the state, the family, or the individual (Pessar & Mahler 2003).

Conversely, a macro-structural perspective on migration focuses on understanding the global, political, and economic factors that shape population mobility. Pedraza (1991) and Sassen (1999) have argued that migration flows are very selective and take structured forms that reflect large-scale economic transformations in both sending and receiving countries. With globalization, unequal structural links between poor and rich countries have increased the flow of low-wage female service workers from some African and Asian countries to Western Europe and the United States (Salazar Parreñas 2001). Structural adjustment programs and policy changes pushed by the World Bank and the International Monetary Fund to promote privatization and free markets in developing countries, have rendered poor women extremely vulnerable and with no option but to migrate to the global North to work for very low wages (Chang 2000). These programs lead to government withdrawal of funding from public services such as health and education, social disinvestments that disproportionately affect women in developing countries.

In addition to the micro- and macro-level explanations, social and cultural capital theories constitute important frameworks to explaining why certain migration flows persist despite restrictive policies. Although structural factors initiate migration flows initially, it is social networks and institutions that maintain them in the long term (Portes 1987). Migration flows, which are originally propelled by external structural factors, develop an internal dynamic determined by social networks that lower the cost and risks to future migrants (Pedraza 1991; Massey et al 1998). Further, cultural norms explain why female migration takes place from some sending countries but not others. Cultural norms that support female participation in the labor force in the Philippines, for example, encourage migration whereas the exclusion of women from household decision making and the social stigma attached to female mobility in Bangladesh have discouraged it (Oishi 2002). The migration of women from Bangladesh to work in domestic service in Arab countries has increased in recent years.

Writings on migrant domestic workers in the Arab region corroborate the theoretical frameworks. A study by Silvey (2004) described how the migration flow of Indonesian women to Saudi Arabia was sustained by macro-level economic arrangements. While Indonesia benefited from remittances, Saudi Arabia's economy also benefited from having access to a low cost and compliant labor force. In Indonesian society, women have historically taken on both reproductive and productive responsibilities, a factor which contributed to the success of the Indonesian state efforts to promote female migration, as these efforts did not sever cultural norms (Silvey 2004). The presence and quality of migrant social networks in the receiving country constitute important factors in directing and maintaining migration flows into the Arab region (Schramm 2006). Specifically, social capital theory is compatible with observed trends of Asian and African women migrants usually moving into Arab countries where they have relatives and friends (Oishi 2002).

The Social Determinants of Domestic Workers' Health

In the Arab region, inadequate data constrain an examination of the health of migrants in general let alone migrant domestic workers. The majority of Arab countries do not collect data on non-citizens and only a few of the sending countries collect statistics on their expatriate population (Schramm 2006). No publicly available data on immigrants exist in major receiving countries, such as the Gulf Cooperative Council countries and Libya. Credible socioeconomic and health data are very limited in others (Fargues 2005). The outcome of this limitation is predictable: our literature review revealed that practically no studies on the health of migrant domestic workers in the Arab region exist; specifically, almost nothing has been published on the long-term health consequences of migration. Further, while the subject of the rights of migrant domestic workers continues

to be highlighted, the link between policies, social conditions, and health is yet to receive attention.

Given the paucity of evidence, we chose to direct our attention to presenting in broad strokes how existing policies and social conditions negatively influence the health of women migrants in the region. Drawing on the available writings, we focused on the following inter-related and mutually enforcing constellation of factors: (1) state policies designed to extract labor from migrants at the lowest cost while at the same time limiting their integration in host societies; (2) exploitative and un-monitored practices on the part of private "middleman agencies" such as employment and health insurance companies; and (3) the private setting in which domestic service is performed which further increases women's vulnerability to exploitation. In addition to these factors, we found that existing literature and writings have neglected to explore two important areas. First, the prevalent view that migration in Arab countries is a temporary phenomenon prevents serious exploration into the long-term health effects of migration on women. Second, the focus in the media on extreme cases of abuse, some of which lead to suicide, while intended to draw attention to the violence some women experience, unfortunately distracts from discussions on women's daily experiences with stress and discrimination. Examining how poor working conditions and day-to-day experiences with discrimination and social exclusion grind away at the health of the majority of domestic workers is both timely and warranted.

Writings on gender and migration have implicated state policies in both sending and receiving countries in increasing the vulnerability of female migrants (Pessar & Mahler 2003). Sending countries treat poor women as a "safety valve, " promoting their migration to reduce the effects of unemployment and to increase the country's foreign exchange through remittances. In many instances, state and private institutions actively recruit women to migrate abroad to work in domestic service (Mahler & Pessar 2006). In Sri Lanka and Indonesia, women's out-migration is initiated, managed, and controlled with the active involvement of state actors (Gamburd 2000; Silvey 2004). A number of receiving countries in the region have historically instituted policies to recruit massive numbers of migrants (Massey et al 1998). These workers are allocated to different levels in the hierarchy based on nationality, with Asian women, most of whom work as housemaids, occupying the bottom rank. Massey and colleagues (1998) compared migration in the Gulf Cooperative Council system to old guest worker programs in the United States and Germany that were designed to extract labor from migrants while preventing their social and political integration. To illustrate, none of the Gulf countries allows migrants to obtain residency without having a job, none recognizes the right to family reunification (e.g., allowing the domestic worker to bring her children with her), and none guarantees social and health benefits that are available to citizens.

A policy most responsible for the exclusion of migrants in general, and female domestic workers specifically, is the sponsorship or *kafala* system, whereby the employee is under the "protection" of the employer and not international labor standards. *Kafala* is engrained in most state policies in the Arab region; it allows the employer to bind a domestic worker into a 1- to 3-year contract and to withhold her passport and other legal documents to prevent her from escaping (Sabban 2002). Binding a worker to a contract in this manner is akin to what has historically been termed "indentured servitude" (Galenson 1984); it is still commonly practiced and legally protected in countries such as Lebanon, Saudi Arabia, and UAE. *Kafala* provides employers with heightened power and limits domestic workers' ability to freely remove themselves from exploitative or abusive working conditions. Domestic workers who run away from their employer without their own identifying documents become "illegal" from the perspective of the state, a factor that further increases their vulnerability.

Because *kafala* operates through 1- to 3-year contracts, the system gives the impression that migration in the Arab region is a short-term phenomenon. Evidence, however, highlights that domestic workers extend their stay in the host country for years past the expiration of their initial contract, whether to remain separated from an abusive husband back home or because they have not saved enough money to enhance their social status upon return to their country of origin (Gamburd 2000; Pessar & Mahler 2003). Recent studies in Yemen and Jordan have shown that migrant women do not necessarily return home at the termination of their initial contracts, and some live in the host country for up to 20 years (de Regt 2007; Frantz 2008). Research conducted by the authors of this chapter revealed that some migrant women from West African countries have been living and working in Lebanon for over 17 years. Those who continue to work as freelancers after their contract with their original sponsor ends fall into undocumented status, a situation that invariably increases their vulnerability to economic exploitation by employers and in public spaces.

In addition to state actors, private middleman industries have proliferated to recruit domestic workers and to match them with potential employers in Arab countries. Anecdotal evidence abounds on the deceptive practices of some recruitment agencies, both in the sending and receiving countries, many of which operate without regulation by any professional body. The majority of these agencies are unregistered in the country's Ministry of Labor. Ethnographic studies on migrant women who worked in the Arab region have narrated blatant cases of fraud and corruption on the part of recruitment agents (Gamburd 2000), and international organizations have called for states to monitor the practices of agencies. One of the private institutions that benefits from the transnational migration of women but that has received little attention is the health insurance industry. In most Arab countries, employers are required to purchase a health insurance plan for their migrant domestic worker as part of her residency and work permit package. There is limited information on the nature of these insurance plans; anecdotal evidence suggests that migrant women do not benefit from them when the need arises.

A study on the adequacy of health care for Filipina domestic workers in Lebanon argued that the health insurance mandated by the Lebanese Ministry of Labor as part of migrant women's employment is designed to protect the employer but provides very little protection to domestic workers themselves (Abi Chaker et al 2008). The study revealed that health insurance coverage reimburses the employer for a maximum of $7500 in the case his/her domestic worker was hospitalized for a severe illness before returning her (or her body remains) to the country of origin. The insurance does not cover medical bills for preventive tests, outpatient visits, medications, antenatal care or delivery in the case of pregnancy. Abi Chaker et al conclude by highlighting the inadequacy of mandatory health insurance for migrant women but leaves many questions unanswered: (1) what is the justification for not including preventive or maternity services in a health insurance plan?; (2) who profits from these health insurance plans and why do employers (and employees) continue to pay for them?; and (3) where do migrant women seek health services when needed? The Lebanese Ministry of Labor increased the cap for mandatory insurance coverage in 2008 from $7,500 to $23,000 but the gaps in health coverage have remained.

We conducted in-depth interviews with 50 migrant domestic workers from African countries in Lebanon to explore a number of questions, one of which relates to the choices women make when they need health care. Even though most women interviewed reported that they have health insurance, only a few indicated that they ever used it or intend to use it if the need arises. Our findings revealed that health insurance offered very little if any protection to women when they needed health care. Women who lived in their employer's home, a very common arrangement in Lebanon, had to rely on the personal values and good will of the employer to cover medical bills. Often, domestic workers distinguished between a "nice Madame, " who helped them pay for a doctor's visit and allowed them to take time off when ill, and a "not so nice Madame, " who told them to take a pill to get rid of the pain or fever and get back to work. In quite a few cases, a domestic worker who fell ill during her years of work in Lebanon invested a disproportionately high amount of her wages on medical care. While migrant women incur medical costs first and foremost, the migrant community sometimes provides a buffer in the case that a member experiences unforeseen circumstances. Only women who are well integrated into their ethnic community can access this form of instrumental support. Social integration requires time and freedom to attend community events, which is often not afforded to live-in domestic workers who may or may not be allowed to leave the home of the employer on their own.

The nature of domestic labor as work performed in the privacy of homes places migrant women at an increased risk for exploitation and abuse. The vulnerability to sexual harassment has been amply addressed in feminist writings on domestic service (Hill Collins 2000; Hondagneu-Sotelo 1999; Salazar Parreñas 2001). Silvey (2004) further argued that cultural norms which promote strict segregation between the sexes in some Arab countries further increase migrant women's vulnerability to sexual abuse. Even in the majority of cases where physical and sexual abuse does not take place, what distinguishes domestic labor from other economic spheres is that a number of

work-related conditions that have direct bearing on women's well-being are privately negotiated between the employer and employee. The employer holds more power in these negotiations and she can set the number of hours a domestic worker works and the wages she earns. For a salary between $150 and $300 – depending on the host country and the national background of the domestic worker – employers often expect domestic workers to perform a variety of tasks such as cleaning, cooking, and providing care to children and often to an elderly person in the household. The domestic worker may or may not get one day off a week, may or may not have a private sleeping space, and may or may not be given the freedom to prepare her own food. All these basic needs and health-promoting conditions cannot be taken for granted but are negotiated in private and within the confines of an unequal relationship. A study conducted by Grete Brochmann in the early 1990s among housemaids returning from the Middle East to Sri Lanka reported that 49% worked more than 16 hours a day and 72% did not receive any weekends off during their contract period (cited in Gamburd 2000).

Even if conditions related to work hours and days off have drastically improved since Brochmann's study, migration remains a stressful process of uprooting. Migrants experience loneliness, marginalization, and discrimination that invariably affect their mental health. Studies suggest that social networks and social support serve to buffer the damaging effects of stress on physical and mental health of migrants (Kuo & Tsai 1986; Murphy & Mahalingam 2004). Inability to integrate into social networks in the host country or to maintain transnational relations can have detrimental effects on the psychological well-being of migrant women. In a qualitative study that sought to explore how Sri Lankan women cope post-migration, women described how staying in touch with family members eased their worries while having limited contact with family negatively affected their mental health (Faraj 2006). A participant in the study was quoted as saying: "When I receive a letter from Sri Lanka, I feel good, no problem. When I don't receive letters or a phone call, my head begins to wonder, I don't feel good." The findings of a clinical study conducted in Kuwait provided compelling evidence if the consequences of poor social integration on migrant women (Zahid et al 2004). The authors showed that the most important stressor reported by domestic workers admitted to a psychiatric hospital was having little or no contact with family members back home and limited access to ethnic social networks in the host country.

Migrant Women Reclaiming Agency

Most writings on domestic workers in the Arab region have primarily focused on glaring human rights violations and paid scant attention to women's day-to-day interactions with stressful and health-demoting conditions both in the homes of employers and in public spaces. In the media, and even in some academic writings, domestic workers are generally presented as victims of severe abuse. The 2005 movie *Maid in Lebanon* (Director Carol Mansour, Beirut: Forward Film Production), for example, presents a dichotomy between good employer and bad employer, while at the same time stereotyping migrant women as passive victims or extremely dedicated employees that are happy to serve their employers without protesting the inequality they experience daily. The study we conducted with African domestic workers in Lebanon presented a different reality. Statements made by these workers revealed that they not only saw their social conditions as an outcome of structural inequality but that they refused to accept it as a normal state of affairs. We do not deny that physical, sexual, or psychological abuse of migrant workers take place or that migrant women are offered very little self protection. We however highlight women's capacity to actively improve their living conditions and avoid victimization.

A number of scholarly writings have emphasized the importance of acknowledging women's agency and their ability to take action to reduce their vulnerability and enhance their social location (Pessar & Mahler 2003; Hondagneu-Sotelo 2001). Gamburd's (2000) book on Sri Lankan women who worked in the Middle East falls within this genre of feminist writings. She reported that, despite strenuous past working conditions, all participants in her ethnographic study presented themselves as active agents and none as helpless victims. In *Agency: Women's Work Experiences Abroad*, Gamburd (2000) narrated numerous stories of how women exercised agency and drew upon all available resources to increase their income and savings, to extricate themselves from compromised working conditions, and even to escape war and arrive home safely. de Regt's

(2007) work on Ethiopian women in Yemen similarly presented a case for the "importance of giving attention to women's agency" (p. 3) and the varied mechanisms they employ in order to enhance their working conditions. She argued that examining the different migration trajectories of Ethiopian women allows observing the different types of decisions and proactive steps women make to exert more control over their own lives.

Reviewing a few studies from the region and reflecting on some of our own data, we argue that many domestic workers exercise agency to improve both their living and working conditions, and in turn their mental health, through two mutually reinforcing mechanisms. First, because social isolation can have detrimental effects on mental health, migrant women actively invest in building and maintaining social networks with members of their ethnic community in the host country. Based on interviews and observations in one household shared by Ethiopian and Eritrean migrant domestic workers in Lebanon, Beyene (2005) argued that women make considerable investments to maintain social networks with compatriots as a way to improve their living conditions in the host country and to enhance their well-being. The author discussed how the household, maintained mostly by freelancers, served as the epicenter in which emotional and instrumental support were exchanged.

A second mechanism employed by female migrants in some contexts, albeit not possible in all Arab countries, is maintaining distance from the employer by leaving a live-in arrangement and working as freelancers. Removing themselves from being bound by one sponsor, although technically "illegal" in many countries in the region, is an important strategy migrant women employ to improve their working conditions. Freelancing provides domestic workers with numerous benefits, the most important being higher wages and less vulnerability to exploitation. Freelancing women have more time during evenings and weekends to network with other women from their country of origin. Data from our study revealed that many migrants view the first two-years of work in Lebanon as a "right-of-passage, " a difficult period of time during which women endure long hours of work, low pay, and social isolation, until their live-in contract expires and they move into freelancing. This move comes with uncertainty and a high investment of financial and emotional resources. In most cases, however, women spoke about the economic payback of freelancing, which allowed them to save more money and send their families more remittances. Moreover, women we interviewed spoke about other health-promoting benefits to freelancing that went beyond economic returns to reveal women's capacity to act not only to survive but to live in dignity. One woman we interviewed stated: "You go to your home, they [employers] give you respect. When you stay with them [work in a live-in arrangement], there is no respect."

Recommendations for Future Action and Research

Paid domestic labor is becoming increasingly concentrated among women who are disadvantaged due to their social location before migration and who become doubly excluded in the host country due to their gender and non-citizen status. One of the most important factors that negatively affect the well-being of migrant workers in the Arab region in general and domestic workers specifically is inadequate protection through policies and laws. Some Arab countries have taken positive steps in recent years, ratifying labor laws to improve the conditions of migrant workers and offer them better protection. Jordan, for example, was the first to issue a new law that covers work contracts which ensure the basic rights of migrant workers (Baldwin-Edwards 2005). This law indirectly covers migrant domestic workers and stipulates the employer's obligation to provide the residency permit, pay the worker's wages in a timely manner, and provide her with one day of rest. The employer is not allowed to retain or confiscate the migrant worker's passport or other personal documents. Recently, the Lebanese Ministry of Labor, along with the United Nation's High Commissioner of Human Rights and the ILO, signed a unified labor contract that guarantees domestic workers one day of rest a week and limits the number of work hours to 10 per day. In a more drastic step in 2009, Bahrain began discussing amending its labor law in order to end the *kafala* system, whereby migrant workers would be sponsored by the country's labor authority and not by individual employers. The amended law, unfortunately, excludes domestic workers.

Despite promising developments, without establishing mechanisms to ensure enforcement and to monitor employers and recruitment agencies, policies on paper remain only a first step toward instituting real change in the region. Even with better protection to migrant workers, there remains a dilemma between policies designed to maintain migration in the Arab region as a short-term phenomenon and the reality that many female migrants extend their stay long after their initial contracts expire. Long-term migration necessitates the development of strategies to reduce the emotional, social, and economic costs of migration, a burden that will solely fall on the shoulders of migrant women as long as state policies refuse to acknowledge migration as anything but short term. Mobilization for change in this area promises to be a major feat as migrants are excluded from the political process in virtually all Arab states (Fargues 2005). Without allowing immigrants themselves to organize and demand an overhaul of existing policies, change promises to be slow in coming.

Despite the wealth of writings on the plight of migrant workers in the Arab region, our review revealed gaps in social scientific research on the well-being of this social group. There is a dearth of information and writings on how policies and social conditions influence the health of domestic workers and how women interact with these policies and take action to enhance their living conditions and social status. Based on our synthesis of the international literature on migration and gender and our reading of the literature in the Arab region, we propose that three areas of action research deserve concerted exploration. First, given that migration in general comes with separation from established social networks and in many cases with severe emotional stress, the mental health of female migrants constitutes one critical area of research and action. Studying the mental well-being of migrants has received significant attention in the international public health literature (McKay et al 2003). With the exception of one clinical study by Zahid and colleagues (2004), we could not locate any research that specifically addressed the mental well-being of women migrants. As severing contact with family members back home is inevitable, enabling domestic workers to embed in social networks in host countries becomes critical to enhancing their mental well-being.

Second, in line with the evidence that low-wage labor migration is not as short-term as policies intend for it to be, the long-term health of migrant women as they live for decades in the host country is an important area of investigation. As we have explicated in this chapter, many migrant women opt to renew their contracts and extend their stay in the host country, oftentimes entering middle and even old age away from home. A proportion of migrant women begin to experience chronic illnesses such as hypertension and diabetes in the host country, but have little or no access to social or health benefits. Whereas the international literature on migration and health focuses on chronic illnesses (McKay et al 2003), most of the attention on health and migrant domestic workers in Arab countries has focused on screening them for sexually transmitted and other infectious diseases. Investigating the effects of migration on the premature development of chronic conditions such as diabetes or hypertension will open the door to exploring crucial policy questions such as: Who is responsible for the health of female migrants as they age – their country of origin that has benefited from their remittances or the host country that has extracted their labor at the lowest cost?

Finally, a gendered view on migration and health necessitates serious attention to the sexual and reproductive health of migrant women, an area that is virtually untouched in the writings on domestic workers in the Arab region. Migrant women's sexual and reproductive health should not be limited to screening them for HIV and other sexually transmitted infections but should extend to the rights of women to exercise sexual and reproductive rights. Currently, state policies, not to mention the preferences of employers, virtually prevent migrant women from making decisions about sexuality, reproduction, or mothering. Domestic workers are often hired to provide childcare to the employer while at the same time forced to leave their own children behind. Some sociological writings have explored the concept of "transnational mothering," whereby migrant women continue to mother their children across national boundaries (Hondagneu-Sotelo 1997). With the exception of Gamburd's (2000) work on Sri Lankan women and a qualitative study conducted in Lebanon (Faraj 2006), the subjective experiences of migrant women who are denied the right to motherhood by the state and the employer have not been fully explored. This is an important area of research and the reproductive rights of migrant women ought to be integrated into the reproductive health agenda in the Arab region. In cultural contexts where the ability to bear children has direct bearing on social status and is an important determinant of overall well-being, valuing only the productive capacities of female migrants and denying them their reproductive rights highlights glaring contradictions.

In conclusion, despite the emotional and physical costs of migration, many women from poor countries of the "Global South" will continue to migrate in search of economic opportunities. In this chapter, we examined the health of female migrants in the region as an outcome of a constellation of social conditions that operate at the levels of state policies, private agencies, and individual employers. Our aim was to explicate how factors that operate at the structural and individual level interact and reinforce the vulnerability of domestic workers. We also highlighted how migrant women themselves resist and take proactive steps to reduce their vulnerability and to improve their living and working conditions, and in turn their well-being. In proposing areas for action and future research, we argued that host countries in the Arab region, which benefit from the low-wage labor of migrants, share responsibility for the long-term health consequences of migration. Finally, we suggested that a comprehensive approach to the health of migrant domestic workers necessitates acknowledging the rights of migrants in general to organize and to participate in the political process.

References

Abi Chaker S, Abou Ghannam G, El Chakhtoura N, Hani A, Harb N (2008) *Health care of Filipino domestic workers in Lebanon: Is it adequate? Social and preventive medicine, IV report.* Faculty of Health Sciences, American University of Beirut

Abu Habib L (1998) The use and abuse of female domestic workers from Sri Lanka in Lebanon. *Gender & Development*, 6(1): 52–56

Anderson B (2000) *Doing the dirty work? The global politics of domestic labour.* London, UK: Zed Books

Baldwin-Edwards M (2005) *Migration in the Middle East and Mediterranean. A regional study prepared for the Global Commission on International Migration, Mediterranean Migration Observatory, University Research Institute for Urban Environment and Human Resources.* Greece: Panteion University

Beyene J (2005) *Women, migration and housing: A case study of three households of Ethiopian and Eritrean female migrant workers in Beirut and Naba'a.* Masters' Thesis, American University of Beirut

Borjas GJ (1989) Economic theory and international migration. *International Migration Review*, 23(3): 457–485

Chang G (2000) *Disposable domestics: Immigrant women workers in the global economy.* Cambridge, MA: South End Press

de Regt M (2007) *Ethiopian women in the Middle East: The case of migrant domestic workers in Yemen. Paper prepared for the African Studies Seminar* (February 15, 2007). Leiden, the Netherlands: Africa Studies Centre

Donato KM, Gabaccia D, Holdaway J, Manalansan M, Pessar PR (2006) A glass half full? Gender in migration studies. *International Migration Review*, 40(1): 3–26

Ehrenreich B, Russell Hochschild A (2002) *Global woman: Nannies, maids and sex workers in the new economy.* London, UK: Granta Books

Esim S, Smith M (2004) *Gender and migration in Arab States: The case of domestic workers, international labour organization: Regional Office for Arab States, Beirut Ethiopian suicides. . . and Nepalese and Eritrean and Bengali and Sri Lankan and Filipino and Malagasy who work as domestic workers in Lebanese homes* (2011) Blog. Available from http://www. ethiopiansuicides.blogspot.com/ [Accessed 10 November 2011]

Faraj L (2006) *"Me no pain, me too happy": The voice of migrant Sri Lankan domestic workers in Lebanon.* Research report submitted in fulfillment of the MPH degree at the Faculty of Health Sciences at the American University of Beirut.

Fargues P (2005) *Mediterranean migration – 2005 Report. Cooperation project on the social integration of immigrants, migration and the movement of persons.* Florence, Italy: EUI-RSCAS CARIM Consortium

Frantz E (2008) Of maids and madams: Sri Lankan domestic workers and their employers in Jordan. *Critical Asian Studies*, 40(4): 609–638

Galenson DW (1984) The rise and fall of indentured servitude in the Americas: An economic analysis. *The Journal of Economic History*, 44(1): 1–26

Gamburd MR (2000) *The kitchen spoon's handle: Transnationalism and Sri Lanka's migrant housemaids.* Ithaca, NY: Cornell University Press

Haddad R (1999) A modern-day "slave trade" Sri Lankan workers in Lebanon. *Middle East Report*, 211: 39–41

Hill Collins P (2000) *Black feminist thought: Knowledge, consciousness, and the politics of empowerment.* New York, NY: Routledge

Hondagneu-Sotelo P (1997) "I am here, but I am there": The meaning of Latino transnational motherhood. *Gender and Society*, 11(5): 548–571

Hondagneu-Sotelo P (1999) *Gender and U.S. immigration: Contemporary trends.* Berkeley, CA: University of California Press

Hondagneu-Sotelo P (2001) *Doméstica: Immigrant workers cleaning and caring in the shadows of affluence.* Berkeley, CA: University of California Press

ILO (International Labor Organization) (2008) *Promoting the rights of women migrant domestic workers in Arab States: The case of Lebanon, Issue Brief 1.* International Labour Organization, Regional Office for Arab States

Jarallah Y (2009) Domestic labor in the Gulf countries. *Journal of Immigrant and Refugee Studies*, 73: 3–15

Jureidini R (2002) *Women migrant domestic workers in Lebanon.* Geneva, Switzerland: International Migration Programme

Jureidini R, Moukarbel N (2004) Female Sri Lankan domestic workers in Lebanon: A case of 'contract slavery'? *Journal of Ethnic & Migration Studies*, 30(4): 581–607

Kuo WH, Tsai YM (1986) Social networking, hardiness, and immigrant's mental health. *Journal of Health and Social Behavior*, 27: 133–149

Mahler SJ, Pessar PR (2006) Gender matters: Ethnographers bring gender from the periphery toward the core of migration studies. *International Migration Review*, 40(1): 27–63

Massey DS, Arango J, Hugo G, Kouaouci A, Pellegrino A, Taylor JE (1998) *Worlds in motion: Understanding international migration at the end of the millennium.* Oxford, UK: Oxford University Press

Moukarbel N (2009) *Sri Lankan housemaids in Lebanon: A case of symbolic violence and everyday forms of resistance.* Amsterdam, the Netherlands: Amsterdam University Press

McKay L, Macyntire S, Ellaway A (2003) Migration and health: A review of the international literature. *MRC Social & Public Health Sciences Unit, Occasional Paper No 12*

Murphy EJ, Mahalingam R (2004) Transnational ties and mental health of Caribbean immigrants. *Journal of Immigrant Health*, 6(4): 167–178

Oishi N (2002) *Gender and migration: An integrative approach, The Center for Comparative Immigration Studies.* Working Paper, 49. La Jolla, California

Pedraza S (1991) Women and migration: The social consequences of gender. *Annual Review of Sociology*, 17: 303–325

Pessar PR, Mahler SJ (2003) Transnational migration: Bringing gender. *International Migration Review*, 37(3): 812–846

Portes A (1987) The social origins of the Cuban enclave economy in Miami. *Sociological Perspectives*, 30(4): 340–372

Sabban R (2002) *United Arab Emirates: Migrant women in the United Arab Emirates, the case of female domestic workers, GENPROM Working Paper no. 10, Series on Women and Migration, Gender Promotion Programme.* Geneva, Switzerland: International Labour Office

Salazar Parreñas R (2001) *Servants of globalization: Women, migration, and domestic work.* Stanford, CA: Stanford University Press

Sassen S (1999) *Guests and aliens.* New York, NY: The New Press

Schramm C (2006) *What do we know about international migration from the Middle East and North Africa?, A migration literature review.* Florence Summer School on Euro-Mediterranean Migration and Development

Shah N, Al-Qudsi S, Shah M (1991) Asian women workers in Kuwait. *International Migration Review,* 25(3): 464–486

Silvey R (2004) Transnational domestication: State power and Indonesian migrant women in Saudi Arabia. *Political Geography,* 23(3): 245–264

Workshop Report (2005) *Report of the awareness raising workshop on the situation of women migrant domestic workers in Lebanon, Beirut.* 28–30 November 2005, ILO

Zahid MA, Fido AA, Razik MA, Mohsen MA, El-Sayed AA (2004) Psychiatric morbidity among housemaids in Kuwait, a prevalence of psychiatric disorders in the hospitalized group of housemaids. *Medical Principles and Practice: International Journal of the Kuwait University, Health Science Centre,* 13(5): 249–254

Chapter

22

Workers' Health: A Social Framework Beyond Workplace Hazards

Rima R. Habib, Fadi A. Fathallah, and Iman Nuwayhid

I roam the streets of Beirut very early in the morning looking for a job on a construction site. I accept any available job regardless of hazards. Pay is decided by the site supervisor at the end of the first week. There is no room for negotiation. It is take it or leave it.
Migrant construction worker, Beirut, Lebanon

Workers' health is an issue that is relevant to all people in Arab countries, as it is in the rest of the world. Workers engage in both paid and unpaid work in an effort to support themselves and their families but also their communities. Workers' health is a human rights issue that has clear social and economic benefits to populations. The paraphrased statement above reflects several of the prominent issues impacting workers in Arab countries – financial insecurity, exploitation, hazardous work environments, and migration, to mention a few. These issues are at the heart of the social justice agenda and, if not resolved, will impede true changes in the lives of the working population. Accomplishing this goal, however, requires a new paradigm of thought, one that acknowledges that workers' health is determined both by the physical and psychosocial conditions of the workplace and also by the interaction of working conditions with environmental, social, economic, and political factors *beyond* the work environment (Krieger, 2010). In this sense, this chapter departs from the narrow "hazard" focus of occupational health usually found in the literature, to encompass a broader view, which incorporates social change and social justice as necessary components for the improvement of workers' health.

People spend most of their waking hours working or thinking about work. For some, work represents a main source of livelihood, as well as an opportunity for personal growth, expression of ideas and talent,

and social interaction. But for many, work is also fundamental to basic survival and can be a daily source of anxiety, sacrifice, and hazard. Consequently, the health of workers is partly dependent on guarantees of a safe work environment – preventing injury and illness – which also provides an environment where dignity is respected and aspirations are nurtured. On the other hand, it is important to recognize that workers do not live in isolation. Their lives do not strictly revolve around work, but extend beyond the workplace to include interactions with outside social networks and communities, which are instrumental in determining work and life opportunities.

Many factors affecting workers' health are established a priori to employment. Education, ethnicity, gender, age, economic status, home circumstances, past work, and health experiences determine work opportunities and partly define work disparities. For example, in some contexts women are prohibited by law or social restrictions from certain jobs, children are driven to work at an early age by poverty, family obligation, or structural violence, and migrant workers accept menial and hazardous jobs at minimal pay with meaningless or no social protections and/or health insurance. In these circumstances, people's expectations for opportunity or vertical mobility are likely regulated by powerful determinants such as economic position, social status, and evolving economic and social conditions that affect them (CSDH 2008).

Improving working conditions is also crucial for the safety, health, and security of any working population. Optimal work environments require commitment and social and political policies that value the health of workers over the economic benefits reaped by business and industry. This conflict often determines the establishment and enforcement of occupational health and safety regulations in most countries. Although specific to country context, workers' health is usually negotiated through a tripartite system of workers, employers, and government institutions. However, this system is rarely balanced or fair, as governments tend to typically cooperate with employers who are more represented in the government structure. In neoliberal economies, this government path has often been justified by a fallacy that protecting employers' interests will generate more financial profits that trickle down into better revenues to the local economy.

Knowledge of workers' health in the Arab world is still relatively thin, as research has been constrained by financial, expertise, and institutional limitations. Furthermore, the literature focuses on the hazards of work environments and lacks an expansive articulation of workers' health issues in the region. This chapter aims to draw out some of the major issues affecting workers' health in the Arab world, with a particular emphasis on vulnerable working populations. It explores economic and employment concepts, such as globalization, social exclusion, psychosocial workplace hazards, and government intervention, which have had varied effects on worker populations. Later the chapter identifies gaps in occupational health research in the Arab world and concludes by discussing the importance of adopting a social justice perspective for occupational health in the region and its implication for local and regional decision makers.

The Workforce in the Arab World

The World Bank (2009) estimates that the labor force in the Arab world is more than 100 million, representing one third of the region's population. However, this figure is likely an underestimate, as it excludes people working in informal occupations and women who work from their home or in support of small to medium size family enterprises. As in much of the rest of the world, most employed people in Arab countries work in the service sector. This sector represents 35–82% of the workforce depending on the country (Table 1). In contrast, the percentage of workers in the agricultural sector in most Arab countries ranges, at the bottom end, from 0% to 26%. Yemen (54%), Morocco (43%), and Egypt (31%) are notable exceptions, as many people are still employed in the agricultural sector. The industrial sector has a relatively limited capacity in most countries (11%–28%). The Kingdom of Saudi Arabia (KSA), Libya, Qatar, Tunisia, and the UAE are the exceptions, with more

than 30% employed in industrial jobs. The government/public sector remains a sizeable employer in most Arab countries, reflecting the limited economic development and rampant underemployment in the region. Unemployment in the region varies by country, with lower rates in oil producing nations (2%–6%), but higher rates elsewhere (8%–33%) (World Bank 2009). It is worth noting that unemployment statistics from the region are not very reliable, as epidemiological studies often cast doubts on official figures provided by governments.

Two demographic trends differentiate Arab countries from other parts of the world. The first, which is women's relative exclusion from the workforce, is a result of social norms that define gender roles and expectations. Participation of women in the workforce is low (averaging 32%) in the Arab world compared to the global average of 55% (ILO 2007). Women's participation is below 25% in nine Arab countries – Egypt, Iraq, Jordan, Lebanon, Morocco, Palestine, Saudi Arabia, Syria, and Yemen, while it exceeds 50% in Comoros, Djibouti, Mauritania, and Somalia. The second labor force trend is the widespread employment of migrants. This has played a substantial role in regional economic and employment developments. Economic migration from Arab and non-Arab countries has acutely impacted the Gulf countries, as expatriates represent a sizeable proportion of the working population in the UAE (91%), Qatar (85%), Kuwait (83%), and Oman (78%) (ITUC 2007). The figure for KSA, which is 82%, represents only those insured under the umbrella of the General Organization for Social Insurance (GOSI 2009). Expatriates employed in government institutions are not covered by GOSI. Migrant workers are mostly employed as vendors, service, construction, and agriculture workers, and as domestic helpers (CSDH 2008).

Workers' Health in the Region
Work Conditions

The health and safety of workers' in the Arab world has been all but neglected by public and private sector decision makers. To be modest, workers' health has not been a priority of governments, while the Western model of workplace-oriented intervention and regulation promoted by international organizations has been relatively ineffective. Most Arab governments have not signed onto the bulk of international labor treaties, and among regional signatory countries poor

Table 1. Population and Labor Force Distribution by Sector Characteristics in Countries in the Arab World[*]

Country	Population (million)	Labor force (in millions)	Labor force by sector (%)		
			Agriculture	Industry	Services
Algeria	37	14	20.7	26	53
Bahrain	0.8	0.4	1.5	28	67.8
Comoros	0.6	0.3	–	–	–
Djibouti	0.8	0.3	–	–	–
Egypt	75	24	31.2	22	46.6
Iraq	27	7	17	17.8	65.1
Jordan	6	1.5	3.6	21.8	74.5
Kuwait	3	1.4	0	18.3	81.7
Lebanon	4	1.5			
Libya	6	2.3	19.7	30	50.2
Mauritania	3	1.3			
Morocco	31	11	43.3	20.3	36.3
Oman	3	1.0	6.4	11.2	82.1
Palestine	4	0.8	15.6	23.8	59.5
Qatar	0.9	0.5	3	41.6	55.2
Saudi Arabia	24	9	4.7	19.8	75.2
Somalia	9	3.4	–	–	–
Sudan	39	12	–	–	–
Syria	20	6.4	27	25.6	47.3
Tunisia	10	3.7	25.8	33.6	39.1
UAE	4	2.7	4.9	39.8	54.4
Yemen	22	5.4	54.1	11.1	34.7

[*]Adapted from: (ILO 2007) & (World Bank 2009).

implementation and enforcement is endemic. Occupational health researchers are partly complicit in this development, as they have reinforced the research and policy paradigms which isolate occupational exposures as a focal point of workers' health while neglecting more salient issues affecting workers in the region. Specifically, occupational health research has failed to capture how social determinants of health *synergize* with occupational exposures, leading to more complex health problems among workers and their communities.

Workplace hazards, be they chemical, biological, safety, ergonomic, or physical, are the primary source of morbidity and mortality among the exposed workers. Similarly, psychosocial hazards, such as poor management styles, stressful work environments, lack of democratization at work, and workplace discrimination – may lead to specific psychosocial problems or indirectly cause illness or death. All of these workplace hazards may collectively interact with outside environmental, social, economic, and political factors that determine health. As an example, people living in poorer countries typically suffer greater rates of malnutrition and communicable diseases, which may be caused by conflict, drought, and inadequate government policies (World Bank 2009). Although not traditionally occupational health issues, they are inescapable realities that bear serious consequences for workers and the workplace.

Poor workplace safety and health is a serious problem facing Arab and migrant workers in the Arab countries. Several publications have documented occupational health and safety risks in a variety of work settings across the region. Studies have discussed the effects of environmental pollution on fishermen in Egypt (Osfor et al 1998), dermatological problems among Egyptian porcelain craftsmen (Gabal et al 1994), slaughterhouse-workers (Gabal & el Geweily 1990), ammonia-exposed employees in the fertilizer industry (Ballal et al 1998), and noise-induced hearing loss in the manufacturing industry (Ahmed et al 2004), to mention a few. Several other studies have been published on health care settings and have studied a number of infectious diseases, illnesses, and injuries among various health care workers, including physicians, nurses, laboratory technicians, and dentists in KSA (see for example Abbas et al 2007; Abou-Atme et al 2007; Al-Haj & Lagarde 2002; Al-Haj et al 2003). Surveys of workplaces, especially small industrial workshops (less than 10 workers), in Lebanon and most other Arab countries revealed inadequate ventilation, illumination, sanitation, and housekeeping conditions that might contribute to poor health outcomes as well as general lack of safety measures and emergency plans and absence of basic personal protective equipment to workers (authors' observations 2000–2010; Taha 2000).

Occupational health and safety conditions nonetheless may differ in enterprises that observe international industry-specific standards such as in the large oil companies in oil-producing countries, e.g., ARAMCO in Saudi Arabia or Qatar Petroleum in Qatar. These enterprises adopt standards that are much stricter than most regional standards.

Work-Related Injuries and Diseases

Table 2 reports on some recent statistics from the Arab world. Agriculture is the leading sector in the number of fatal accidents in almost all countries in the region. This is consistent with the experience of other countries in the world. The number of work-related accidents causing three or more days of absenteeism varies widely among countries in the Arab world; more than 15% of the workforce are affected in certain countries (namely Djibouti, Somalia, and

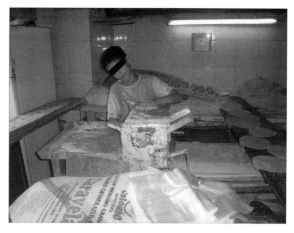

Figure 1. An 11-year-old child worker in a bakery – handling dough with hand inside a sharp flattener, Tripoli, Lebanon. RR Habib, 2009: Health and Safety in Lebanese Bakeries: From Policy to Practice. Photograph taken by Hind Farah.

Sudan) as compared to less than 5% in a few others (Algeria, Bahrain, and Oman). In comparison, the number of accidents as a percentage of the workforce in Sweden is less than 1%, in Malaysia about 3%, and in the United States is about 8% (ILO 2007; World Bank 2009). The work-related mortality rate is especially high in several Arab countries, most notably Egypt, Sudan, and Algeria. It is prudent, however, to note that differences might also be due to varied reporting systems, poor surveillance systems, or inconsistent case definitions. The ILO estimates the global cost of work-related fatalities, injuries, and disabilities at 4 percent of the gross domestic product (GDP) (ILO 2003b). Only a few published studies from Arab countries reported on the cost of work-related health outcomes; however, selective measures of cost were used falling short of a comprehensive measure of the national burden of work-related illnesses and injuries. For example in Lebanon, a national survey using insurance payouts estimated the cost of work-related injuries in insured workplaces at more than $13 million a year (Fayad et al 2003). No other national figures exist on the cost of work-related injuries and illnesses in Lebanon.

Political, Legal, and Economic Determinants of Workers' Health

This section addresses the social determinants of workers' health focusing on regulation, social exclusion, and global economy.

Table 2. Work-Related Illnesses and Accidents in the Arab World[*]

Country	Number of work-related fatal accidents by sector			Accidents >3 days absence		Work-related disease		Work-related mortality		Deaths by dangerous substance	
	Agriculture	Industry	Services	N (1000)	%**	N (1000)	%	N (1000)	%	N (1000)	%
Algeria	229	130	472	634.5	4.53	8.0	0.06	8.8	0.06	1.9	0.01
Bahrain	1	10	10	16.5	4.11	0.2	0.05	0.2	0.06	0.0	0.01
Comoros	41	2	5	36.4	12.13	0.2	0.06	0.2	0.08	0.1	0.02
Djibouti	59	5	10	57.0	19.01	0.3	0.10	0.4	0.12	0.1	0.03
Egypt	1,339	734	869	2245.1	9.35	22.4	0.09	25.4	0.11	5.5	0.02
Iraq	205	99	525	632.8	9.04	4.7	0.07	5.5	0.08	1.2	0.02
Jordan	18	34	113	125.2	8.35	1.0	0.07	1.1	0.08	0.2	0.02
Kuwait	3	21	113	105.0	7.50	1.6	0.11	1.7	0.12	0.4	0.03
Lebanon	50	70	80	152.5	10.17	1.0	0.07	1.2	0.08	0.3	0.02
Libya	67	83	82	176.7	7.68	1.1	0.05	1.3	0.06	0.3	0.01
Mauritania	175	16	50	183.8	14.14	0.9	0.07	1.2	0.09	0.3	0.02
Morocco	1,227	266	330	1390.9	12.64	11.9	0.11	13.7	0.12	3.0	0.03
Oman	9	3	2	10.9	1.09	0.1	0.01	0.1	0.01	0.0	0.00
Palestine	–	–	–	–	–	–	–	–	–	–	–
Qatar	2	15	20	28.0	5.59	0.2	0.04	0.2	0.05	0.1	0.01
Saudi Arabia	183	276	370	632.5	7.03	7.4	0.08	8.2	0.09	1.8	0.02
Somalia	578	43	109	556.8	16.38	2.8	0.08	3.6	0.10	0.8	0.02
Sudan	1,560	70	729	1800.7	15.01	9.2	0.08	11.6	0.10	2.5	0.02
Syria	510	184	196	678.7	10.61	6.2	0.10	7.1	0.11	1.5	0.02
Tunisia	157	118	150	324.3	8.77	3.5	0.09	3.9	0.10	0.8	0.02
UAE	33	51	140	170.6	6.32	2.3	0.08	2.5	0.09	0.5	0.02
Yemen	381	83	176	487.8	9.03	4.6	0.09	5.3	0.10	1.1	0.02

[*]Adapted from Takala (2005); **Percentage of total labor force.

Occupational Health and Safety Regulations

Several labor regulations in the Arab countries address issues of work such as hiring, firing, organization and representation, number of working hours and days, benefits, maternity and sick leaves, vacations, and compensation among others. In spite of its centrality, health is not explicitly considered in these regulations. These issues are typically regulated and monitored by the ministries of labor with minimal contribution of public health authorities or professionals. The latter group tends to focus on work hazards and their impact on health and safety and what is "traditionally" referred to as occupational health and safety regulations. However, regulations to protect workers from work hazards and promote their health have been deficient. An ILO sponsored study carried out by Habib (2007; 2009) assessed the main obstacles to promoting workers' health and safety in 18 Arab countries. The study found that the overall attention given to Occupational Health and Safety (OHS) in the Arab world is generally inadequate, and the political commitment to effectively handle OHS issues on par with international standards is still lacking. Many governments in the region have refrained from ratifying OHS ILO conventions, partly because of disagreements with aspects of the treaties or as a result of administrative, financial, and human resource limitations (Habib 2007; 2009). Yet by failing to adopt, implement, and enforce these conventions or, more importantly, develop contextually relevant standards, Arab governments have left their working populations vulnerable to workplace hazards and other work-related health problems.

The study depicts a heterogeneous picture of OHS regulations across the Arab world, which appears less than ideal under close scrutiny (Habib 2007; 2009). Enforcement of OHS regulations, especially what relates to hazard control, safety measures, and prevention, often goes by the wayside in most Arab countries. OHS inspectors, if available, are small in number, under-equipped, improperly trained, and often disempowered to take actions against violations in most Arab countries. In a few countries, such as the KSA, the labor inspectors are trained before taking their jobs, have the power to access firms without prior notice, and are empowered to take action to ensure compliance with the provisions pertaining to workers' health and safety (The Saudi Network 2007).

Compensation for work-related injuries might be covered through accident insurance or the legal system, but the vast majority of work-related illnesses and health outcomes remain undetected or absent from legal coverage (Habib 2007; 2009). Within individual Arab countries, disparities exist between different worker groups. Workers in specific industries might benefit from relatively more established health and safety regulations, as is the case with the oil and large construction companies that adhere to international guidelines. Meanwhile, the majority of workers in other sectors lack the same protections afforded by these industries.

Social Exclusions

The term "social exclusion" is defined differently by different social scientists and policy bodies (Atkinson & Hills 1998). In this chapter, it will be used to include people and communities that are discriminated against or excluded from the work sphere because of health reasons or disability, their nationality, gender, and social class. The intention of this section is to apply the concept and alert the reader to its criticality to occupational health since it addresses work and consequently opportunities in life.

Nationality/Place of Origin

Place of origin plays an important role in determining workers' positions in Arab societies. Immigrant

workers come from diverse backgrounds and cultures, have varied skill-sets, educational backgrounds, and access to social capital (CSDH 2008). Workers from the developing world immigrate to the region in search of steady employment and sources of familial remittance (Reinert 2007). Many of those work in unsafe environments, their economic situation leading them to accept difficult jobs characterized by hazardous conditions (Al-Neaimi et al 2001).

Economic migrants from South East Asia and Africa face difficult integration into Arab societies. Institutional and non-institutional racism impacts immigrant workers in a variety of ways. Both skilled and unskilled workers face subjugation and alienation at the workplace (Gamburd 2004; Vora 2008), while government policy and poor enforcement allow employers leeway in determining salaries and working conditions (Nuwayhid 2004; Shaham 2008). This relationship has unskilled workers competing over minimal salaries that fail to accommodate local living standards (Shaham 2008). Ethnic discrimination in the workplace is also perceived as a problem in skilled and professional occupations, as Westerners and Arabs are paid higher salaries and have better job status than people from other parts of the world (Gulfnews.com 2009).

Gender

In the Arab world, gender equality is another complex issue to engage. Governments and communities need to negotiate important cultural traditions against mounting pressures to reinterpret women's role in society. In the extreme, several governments in the region dictate the social and economic activities of women at the workplace and in the social sphere (*The Economist* 2008). Other Arab governments interfere less in the lives of women, yet custom and tradition play an important role in defining women's working and living conditions (Khatib 2008). Accordingly, working women receive fewer job-related benefits, lower salaries, and fewer opportunities in the job market (CSDH 2008). Women working in the same or equivalent jobs often receive lower salaries than male counterparts and have fewer chances for advancement (Jamali et al 2008), while female immigrants working in the service and domestic industries experience an intensified disadvantage, as they face the triple burden of poverty, sexism, and cultural estrangement (Gamburd 2004).

Informal Sector

It may be argued that those employed in the informal sector are not socially excluded but depend on a different network of connections, support, and communication. This is partly true but in general the informal sector describes work that is not formally incorporated into economic institutions and an only option for those who either cannot join the formal sector for lack of economic or education skills or who fall out of the formal sector. Jobs in the informal sector include day-labor, street vending, garbage recycling, garment making from home, and temporary or casual jobs. Work in the informal sector is typically marked by poverty, which leads to powerlessness, exclusion, and vulnerability (ILO 2002). Informal work is also often excluded from many of the regulatory frameworks that govern labor relations and contracts. Many workers in this sector often do not pay taxes (and are often too poor to contribute), and, therefore, lack adequate access to public services and benefits. Informal workers are also vulnerable to harassment, corruption, bribery, and other forms of abuse. The informal sector presents a challenge to many governmental authorities that must devise ways of incorporating informal workers into legislative frameworks that protect their rights as workers and ensure their health. Gauging the size of the informal sector in Arab countries is difficult, as most governments do not provide statistics on this group of workers; yet several governments reached out to these workers with various forms of assistance (Isaia 2005; Loewe 2004).

Unemployment

Unemployment is a social and economic phenomenon that is a key element of social exclusion especially if associated with poverty or limited economic alternatives. It affects many people globally and is associated with both physical and psychological health outcomes that have measurable impacts on quality of life (WHO 2008). Employment even in less desirable jobs and workplaces as compared to unemployment is linked with a variety of health benefits ranging from better mental health to improved access to health resources (CSDH 2008; Dooley et al 1996). Individuals cope with unemployment by utilizing varied resources at their disposal, from those provided by government and private organizations, as well as social networks. However, if it lasts, unemployment becomes a critical public health

concern, as it contributes to health inequalities and social injustice within communities and countries and between nations.

National unemployment rates are reported at an average of 13.4% for the Arab world, and range from 1.7% (Kuwait) to 44% (Djibouti) (World Bank 2009); however, rates may vary dramatically among regions of the same country. Of relevance to the Arab world is the lack of adequate social protection programs in some countries, such as unemployment benefits and social security; hence, "unemployed workers" tend to slip further into poverty and insecurity.

Poor Health and Disabilities

Poor health, specific diseases, and physical and mental disabilities are also grounds for social exclusion and job discrimination. Foreign workers in most Arab Gulf countries testing positive for HIV and selected communicable diseases will be dismissed from their work and immediately deported. These phobias from "stigmatized" diseases are rampant in most Arab countries. The ILO and many civil society groups are active in promulgating more inclusive policies. Similarly, and in spite of national acts and participation in international conventions on disability in most Arab countries (United Nations 2006), workers with compromised health or disability are not easily employed. This is more prominent in times of high unemployment and prevalence of cheap foreign labor. No studies on these issues have been published in the scientific literature.

Global Economy

Uneven economic growth worldwide has put developing countries in the Arab world under more pressure to capitulate to international economic pressures. This has led to unplanned and unregulated growth that has had serious consequences for workers, resulting in high rates of work-related fatalities, injuries, and illnesses. Workers' health and safety has been generally overlooked due to overwhelming economic challenges (Christiani et al 1990; Nuwayhid 2004; O'Neill 2000). On the other hand, despite the prosperity of oil-rich Gulf countries, migrant workers still face harsh working conditions and limited rights and protections (ITUC 2007). A case in point is the construction boom in Dubai, where pressure to keep up with unprecedented building demands had serious consequences on migrant construction worker populations. Construction workers, 90% of whom were migrants, experienced high accident rates due to unsafe working conditions that were compounded by unfavorable employment and legal stipulations (ITUC 2007). In the KSA, for example, 50.2% of the 86,211 work-related accidents reported in 2009 were among the construction workers. More than 90% of them were non-Saudis (GOSI 2009).

National regulations are further restricted by trade agreements or the urge to attract foreign businesses and investors. Global economic forces pressure governments to forego occupational health and safety regulations in order to undercut foreign competition, reduce the cost of production, and gain a competitive edge. International regulations (such as those promulgated by the ILO) are meant to ensure international minimum standards of practice; yet this is not always achieved or enforced by local agents. Occasionally, employers and unions in one country might cooperate in favor of national economic or employment interests at the expense of other countries which follow international conventions. This pattern is encouraged by free-market economic principles that pit the consumer-driven demands of leading industrial nations against the resource scarce, investment-starved desperation of many developing countries.

In addition, the liberalization and integration of global markets in the past two decades has seriously influenced employment and working conditions in some Arab countries. The relocation of labor-intensive manufacturing from technically advanced countries to countries with a low-wage base and few regulations (CSDH 2008; Fröbel et al 1980) has recently spread to Arab countries. The textile industry in Jordan's Export Processing Zones (EPZs), which employ mostly migrant workers from Asia, is a striking example of this phenomenon. Migrant workers in textile factories in Jordan have been reported to work up to 16 hours a day in poor working conditions with abusive employment contracts (ITUC 2007).

Selected Working Groups

This section reviews published research on agricultural workers, working children, and women homemakers in Arab countries. These worker groups were selected partly because of the availability of information, but also because of their relative exclusion from workers' health discourses in the region and around the world.

Agricultural Workers

When I grow up, I wish for my kids a better future than mine.
... I like to go back to school.

A child in a family of migrant agricultural workers in the Bekaa valley in Lebanon

Agricultural work is one of the most dangerous occupations to engage in and has one of the highest morbidity and mortality rates of any occupation globally (ILO 2003a). Agricultural workers are typically exposed to chemical, biological, physical (such as heat, noise, etc.), mechanical (i.e., falls, abrasions, tool injuries), and psychological hazards that have harmful health effects. The social contexts surrounding agricultural work – migration, discrimination, poverty, low social status, and limited social protections – also likely have an interactive effect with occupational hazards impacting this worker group.

Chemical hazards such as pesticides can lead to acute illnesses, poisonings, reproductive problems, and possibly cancer (ITUC 2007). Agricultural workers in the Arab world have been reported to suffer from deleterious health outcomes due to pesticide exposures, including cardiac complications (Saadeh et al 1997), respiratory diseases and symptoms (Salameh et al 2006), cancer (Safi et al 2002), and psychiatric disorders (Amr et al 1997). In most Arab countries, however, oversight institutions and agencies have not been able to ensure that workers receive appropriate protective equipment for handling chemicals and that bans on illegal chemicals are enforced.

Physical injuries related to falling from high places (ladders, trees, or terraces) and tool use (i.e., abrasions, musculoskeletal pain) are another major source of morbidity in agricultural work (Frank et al 2004). Although epidemiological studies have yet to capture reliable statistics on physical injuries in farm workers in Arab countries, it is likely that injuries are common and go undertreated as many farms are isolated from health services and most farm workers lack access to basic health provisions. Heat-related illnesses are also likely to affect this working group (Schulte & Chun 2009), especially since most Arab countries have very hot and humid climatic conditions.

Several studies from around the world discuss the psychosocial problems affecting agricultural workers. A qualitative study found that Lebanese farm workers typically live in low quality housing with leaks, poor

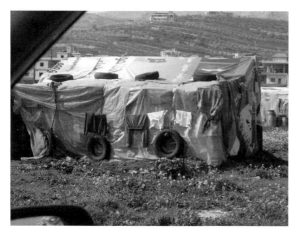

Figure 2. The home of migrant agricultural workers in the Bekaa Valley, Lebanon. RR Habib, 2010b: Migrant Agricultural Workers in Lebanon: Our Harvest of Shame. Photo taken by Lubna Haidar.

ventilation, and overcrowded conditions (Habib 2010b, 2010c). Agricultural workers reported workplace exploitation, precarious work and housing conditions, and problematic workplace power dynamics. Migration also affects this worker group as many farm workers in the Arab region are migrants. Cultural or linguistic barriers and social practices leave migrant workers vulnerable to exploitation, abuse, discrimination, and legal persecution (Ahonen et al 2007). Migrant workers often lack basic access to health care services and other social resources protective of their health (Habib & Fathallah 2009; Habib 2010a, 2010b).

Working children

I have been working with my uncle in his mechanics shop for the last 3 years. I open the shop at 8 am and leave work not before 8 pm. I usually take half an hour for lunch but most of the times I prefer to take a stroll to enjoy a breath of fresh air.

12 year-old Lebanese boy, Tripoli, Lebanon

Child labor is a persistent issue affecting youth in Arab countries. People under the age of 18 in poor and developing countries join the labor force primarily for economic reasons or following drop outs from school systems that offer limited opportunities (Saddik & Nuwayhid 2006). Alternatively, working at an early age may benefit many of these children, allowing them to contribute to family incomes and build a career for later life (Hartung et al 2005). The magnitude of child labor in the Arab world is not well

documented but it is reportedly more prevalent in poorer Arab countries – in rural, agricultural areas and in poor neighborhoods of urban centers such as Cairo in Egypt and Casablanca in Morocco.

Capturing the health effects on child labor poses several difficulties for research. It is difficult for studies to identify health outcomes that only appear many years after initial exposure. Moreover, children who are healthier and more able typically handle the most labor- or mentally intensive jobs, presenting potential selection biases and nuanced exposure profiles that limit the generalizability in most cross-sectional and case-control study designs. The studies that are available from the region typically utilize simpler study designs because of their relative ease and the limited resources available for research projects (Saddik & Nuwayhid 2006).

Child entrance into the labor force has troubling impacts on school attendance and basic education. Young Egyptian girls enlisted into family domestic tasks were found to have lower rates of school attendance (Assaad et al 2010). In Yemen at least 20% of the children aged 14 years or younger entered the labor force, resulting in low school attendance (Dyer 2007). Overwhelming poverty and poor educational systems have led many children to forego an education for early work opportunities, limiting the possibilities for economic advancements. Dyer (2007) advocates for an educational policy that permits individuals and families to remain financially afloat, while governments provide contextually appropriate quality educational services that meet the needs of working children.

Given the link between education and health, ensuring that child laborers are provided with the necessary life skills should be a focus of interventions targeting younger workers. Occupational health policies should also acknowledge that younger workers are at risk for age specific health problems, such as stunted growth or neurological development-related disorders. These issues must be addressed, while taking into consideration families' and communities' reliance on child labor for economic solvency. Solutions must accommodate the contextual realities of child labor, while minimizing the impact of work on child workers' health and well-being.

Women and Housework

My day starts at 5:30 am and ends around 10 pm. I take care of my children's food, hygiene, school, and studies;

of my hemiplegic mother-in-law; and of my husband who owns a shop near home. I usually replace my husband in the shop for 2 hours a day to allow him time to have lunch, take an afternoon nap, and shop for merchandise. I do not mind the long hours of work, but I miss a warm thank you from my husband when he returns home in the evening.

A 38 year old mother of two boys in
Nabaa, suburb of Beirut, Lebanon

The reported low labor force participation of women in Arab countries is somewhat misleading, as many women still work in the informal sector and almost all women are in charge of domestic work at home. These activities, important as they are, are not accounted for by most employment models. Specifically, women's involvement in domestic labor has substantial economic value, as housework and child rearing facilitate family functioning, enabling children's education and assisting the work activities of economically active family members. Unfortunately, homemaking is also overlooked by a majority of the occupational health literature, despite its occupational relevance to most women around the world.

Housework is traditionally performed by women and involves regular tasks, such as cleaning, cooking, purchasing, etc., in addition to family care duties like child rearing and care giving (Coltrane 2000). Research comparing housework to paid work has found that many household tasks are more energy intensive than some types of paid work (Brooks et al 2004). More to that, housework is a potential source of hazard, which is comparable to other occupational settings that share its biomechanical and psychosocial characteristics (Habib et al 2006b, 2010; Messing 1998; Yip et al 2004).

Relatively few studies from the region have explored the health hazards related to homemaking. A study by Smith (1998) in Egypt reports that women commonly suffer burns from household activities or as a result of domestic abuse. Their social status as homemakers has also made treatment of these burns particularly difficult. Alternately, studies in Lebanon have found that women engage in heavy paid and unpaid workloads and engage in much more housework than men (Habib et al 2006b, 2010, 2011). Homemakers in these communities may also spend many unnecessary hours cleaning because of social pressures from family members, neighbors, and acquaintances (Habib et al 2006a). Lebanese homemakers reported high 12 month prevalence of

musculoskeletal symptoms (77%) (Habib et al 2005, 2009, 2011) and may also be at risk of exposure to hazardous cleaning products due to improper handling and overuse (Habib et al 2006a).

Challenges and Opportunities
Research on Workers' Health

Research on workers' health in the Arab world is neither comprehensive nor coordinated. A majority of studies are of cross-sectional design and generally focus on assessment of specific hazards with occasional links to health outcomes. A PubMed search revealed a rather small number of publications. Much of the published research is in report form or in national journals not cited by PubMed. Studies of working women, migrant workers, and working children are few in number, as are studies examining social issues and the impact of globalization, financial fluctuations, and discriminatory policies on the health of workers.

Similar to other fields of research in the Arab world, research on workers' health is conducted mostly in academic institutions or in response to requests typically from governmental and regional agencies (e.g., Arab Science and Technology Foundation, and the Qatar Foundation). However, research funding for projects related to workers' health has been rather limited compared to other fields. Most reported studies have been conducted in some countries targeting a limited number of occupations and worker populations, especially in larger countries such as Egypt and Saudi Arabia. These studies focused on specific themes including pesticide exposure among agricultural workers, injuries and diseases among health care workers, respiratory diseases, musculoskeletal disorders and ergonomic exposures among industrial and office workers, in addition to limited studies on various exposures among other Arab worker populations.

Three striking observations characterize research on workers' health in the Arab world. First, it is hazard and workplace focused with almost total absence of a framework on the social determinants of health. Second, it lacks governmental or agency funds since these are directed to what is perceived as higher priority health problems. Third, in contrast to the model adopted by many industrialized countries, there are no national agencies dedicated to the development, coordination, and implementation of national research agendas on occupational health and safety, such as the National Institute for Occupational Safety and Health (NIOSH) in the US. At the regional level, however, the Institute of Occupational Health and Safety (IOHS) under the Arab Labour Organization (ALO) aims to oversee health and safety issues in the Arab world. The IOHS acts as a link between the ILO and the Arab countries and has recently been designated by the ILO as a regional International Occupational Safety and Health Information Center. To our knowledge, the IOHS so far neither has the necessary mandate nor adequate funding to make a significant impact on workers' health in Arab countries. Given the significance of workers' health in terms of both human and economic costs, there is an urgent need for national, regional, and international agencies in funding research, education, and training related to workers' health issues in the Arab world. The funding approach should be comprehensive, encompassing not only the traditional physical aspects of the risks and hazards, but also the social and economic dimensions related to workers' health.

Workers' Health as a Social Agenda

Prominent arguments supporting workers' rights often address two divergent sets of interests: humanitarian appeals and economic effects. Most recent ILO documents refer to "decent work" as a basic human right and, in the same breath, as an opportunity to improve businesses' "productivity and profitability... [Decent work] makes good business sense" (Takala 2005 p. 3). Unifying economic and social interests into one appeal might strengthen the persuasiveness of the argument to support workers' health. However, this appeal allows room for business interests to forego worker protection out of economic convenience. What happens to OHS when protecting workers does not make "good business sense" to the employer? In addition, many workers are willing to sacrifice benefits and safe working conditions in order to support their families. Such circumstances leave many workers having to choose between two unnecessary evils: unemployment and abject poverty or marginal employment and difficult or harmful working conditions. "Workers would rather die of disease than go hungry," as stated by a Lebanese worker in the recently shut down asbestos-cement industry (personal communication 2005).

Given the complex processes and factors affecting workers in the region and recognizing that workers'

health is not perceived as a priority in the Arab world, how can this issue move forward?

Foremost, health professionals and policy makers should engage in the fundamentals of the debate and try to shift the conversation on workers' health away from economic justifications to arguments based on basic human rights. Such an unconditional commitment to workers' health and safety might be rather difficult to achieve in most countries and especially in Arab countries. After all, providing "decent work" should be an all-inclusive effort that seeks increased social commitments, structural and political change, and the wider inclusion of workers and their communities in decision making. Workers and their communities should be the focal point of this comprehensive effort. Unlike their counterparts in developed countries, most workers in the Arab world lack knowledge of OHS needs. Awareness and training campaigns should be launched to inform and educate workers on how to embrace occupational health and safety in their daily life. In other words, we should seek to make "workers' health and safety" a household term and concept in the Arab world.

Equally important is the role of labor unions and syndicates. Unionization, which has not been a priority in the Arab world, has proved important in securing healthy and safe environments in many technically advanced countries. Ensuring legal protection and support for disempowered workers might improve their economic and social standing within the region. Organizing these workers poses a unique challenge for advocates of workers' rights, as in many cases, their cultural background, lower social and economic position, and vulnerability hinders their participation in efforts to improve their working and life conditions. Currently, labor unions in Arab countries are either weak, constitute a subset of the ruling political system, or are totally focused on wages and compensation issues. Workers' health is perceived within the context of hazards, diseases, and injuries that require facility intervention rather than national regulations.

At the macro level, OHS should be mainstreamed as an integral component of public and environmental health, and placed into a broader political, social, and cultural framework. With the recent call for a revival of primary health care in the region, workers' health may have an opportunity to be integrated in a comprehensive system of health care. Governments, employers, and communities that fail to protect minorities and vulnerable segments of society invite inequality, social instability, and conflict (CSDH, 2008). Evidence is badly needed to support such arguments and advance a social agenda. This requires comprehensive OHS national and regional surveillance systems and databases as an essential step in identifying research and intervention priorities, which clearly calls for well trained and socially committed professionals in occupational health.

References

Abbas MF, Atwa M, Emara, A (2007) Seroprevalence of measles, mumps, rubella and varicella among staff of a hospital in Riyadh, Saudi Arabia. *Journal of the Egyptian Public Health Association*, 82(3–4): 283–297

Abou-Atme YS, Melis M, Zawawi KH, Cottogno L (2007) Five-year follow-up of temporomandibular disorders and other musculoskeletal symptoms in dental students. *Minerva Stomatol*, 56(11–12): 603–609

Ahmed HO, Dennis JH, Ballal SG (2004) The accuracy of self-reported high noise exposure level and hearing loss in a working population in Eastern Saudi Arabia. *International Journal of Hygiene and Environmental Health*, 207(3): 227–234

Ahonen EQ, Benavides FG, Benach J (2007) Immigrant populations, work and health – a systematic literature review. *Scandinavian Journal of Work, Environment & Health*, 33(2): 96–104

Al-Haj AN, Lagarde CS (2002) Statistical analysis of historical occupational dose records at a large medical center. *Health Physics*, 83(6): 854–860

Al-Haj AN, Lobriguito AM, Lagarde CS (2003) Occupational doses during the injection of contrast media in paediatric CT procedures. *Radiation Protection Dosimetry*, 103(2): 169–172

Al-Neaimi YI, Gomes J, Lloyd OL (2001) Respiratory illnesses and ventilatory function among workers at a cement factory in a rapidly developing country. *Occupational Medicine (Lond)*, 51(6): 367–373

Amr MM, Halim ZS, Moussa SS (1997) Psychiatric disorders among Egyptian pesticide applicators and formulators. *Environmental Research*, 73(1–2): 193–199

Assaad R, Levison D, Zibani N (2010) The effect of domestic work on girls' schooling: Evidence from Egypt. *Feminist Economics*, 16: 79–128

Atkinson AB, Hills J (Eds.) (1998) *Exclusion, employment and opportunity*. London: Centre for Analysis of Social Exclusion, London School of Economics

Ballal SG, Ali BA, Albar AA, Ahmed HO, al-Hasan AY (1998) Bronchial asthma in two chemical fertilizer producing factories in eastern Saudi Arabia. *The International Journal of Tuberculosis and Lung Disease*, 2(4): 330–335

Brooks AG, Withers RT, Gore CJ, Vogler AJ, Plummer J, Cormack J (2004) Measurement and prediction of METs during household activities in 35- to 45-year-old females. *European Journal of Applied Physiology*, 91(5–6): 638–648

Christiani DC, Durvasula R, Myers J (1990) Occupational health in developing countries: Review of research needs. *American Journal of Industrial Medicine*, 17(3): 393–401

Coltrane S (2000) Research on household labor: Modeling and measuring the social embeddedness of routine family work. *Journal of Marriage and the Family*, 62: 1208–1233

Commission on Social Determinants of Health (CSDH) (2008). *Closing the gap in a generation: Health equity through action on the social determinants of health*. Geneva: Commission on Social Determinants of Health (CSDH)

Dooley D, Fielding J, Levi L (1996) Health and unemployment. *Annual Review of Public Health*, 17: 449–465

Dyer C (2007) Working children and educational inclusion in Yemen. *International Journal of Educational Development*, 27: 512–524

Fayad R, Nuwayhid I, Tamim H, Kassak K, Khogali M (2003) Cost of work-related injuries in insured workplaces in Lebanon. *Bulletin of World Health Organization*, 81(7): 509–516

Frank AL, McKnight R, Kirkhorn SR, Gunderson P (2004) Issues of agricultural safety and health. *Annual Review of Public Health*, 25: 225–245

Fröbel F, Heinrichs J, Kreye O (1980) *The new international division of labour*. Cambridge: Cambridge University Press

Gabal MS, el Geweily M (1990) Dermatologic hazards among slaughterhouse workers. *Journal of the Egyptian Public Health Association*, 65(1–2): 191–206

Gabal MS, Helmy GA, Faris R (1994) Occupational dermatoses among workers in a porcelain manufacturing factory. *Journal of the Egyptian Public Health Association*, 69(5–6): 425–438

Gamburd MR (2004) Money that burns like oil: A Sri Lankan cultural logic of morality and agency. *Ethnology*, 43(2): 167–184

The Economist (2008). Gender gulf: Women in the Gulf seek to prise open the male-dominated world of banking. *The Economist*, 387: 86. Available from http://www.economist.com/node/11024384

General Organization for Social Insurance (GOSI) (2009) *Annual statistical report: 1430*. Riyadh: General Organization for Social Insurance (GOSI)

Gulfnews.com (2009) Discrimination 'a big issue'. *Gulfnews.com*. Available from http://gulfnews.com/news/gulf/uae/employment/discrimination-a-big-issue-1.238803 [Accessed 4 February 2011]

Habib RR, Hamdan M, Nuwayhid I, Odaymat F, Campbell OM (2005) Musculoskeletal disorders among full-time homemakers in poor communities. *Women Health*, 42(2): 1–14

Habib RR, El-Masri A, Heath RL (2006a) Women's strategies for handling household detergents. *Environmental Research*, 101(2): 184–194

Habib RR, Nuwayhid IA, Yeretzian JS (2006b) Paid work and domestic labor in disadvantaged communities on the outskirts of Beirut, Lebanon. *Sex Roles*, 55(5–6): 321–329

Habib RR (2007) *Overview of the occupational safety and health situation in the Arab region*. Damascus: International Labour Office

Habib RR (2009) *Occupational Health and Safety in the Arab World*. Presented in a Special Session on 'Occupational Health and Safety in Asia'. In the Proceedings of the 29th International Congress on Occupational Health. Cape Town, South Africa, 22–27 March 2009

Habib RR, Fathallah FA (2009) *Migrant women agricultural workers in Lebanon – A health perspective*. Paper presented at the Migration and Urbanization Workshop

Habib RR, Fathallah FA, Hamdan M (2009) *Women's paid and unpaid work in a disadvantaged community*. Paper presented at the International Ergonomics Association 17th World Congress on Ergonomics, Beijing, China

Habib RR (2010a) Farm workers: Double marginalization. *Al-Akhbar*, 1 January 2010

Habib RR (2010b) *Migrant agricultural workers in Lebanon: Our harvest of shame*. Paper presented at the

American Public Health Annual Meeting. Denver, Colorado, 6–10 November 2010

Habib RR (2010c) *Migrant agricultural workers in Lebanon: An understudied population*. Paper presented at the 21st International Symposium on Epidemiology in Occupational Health: Occupational Health under Globalization and New Technology. Taipei, Taiwan, 21–25 April 2010

Habib RR, Fathallah FA, Messing K (2010) Full-time homemakers: Workers who cannot "go home and relax". *International Journal of Occupational Safety and Ergonomics*, 16(1): 113–128

Habib RR, El Zein K, Hojeij S (2011). Hard work at home: Musculoskeletal pain among female homemakers. *Ergonomics (In press)*

Hartung PJ, Porfeli EJ, Vondracek FW (2005) Child vocational development: A review and reconsideration. *Journal of Vocational Behavior*, 66: 385–419

International Labour Organization (ILO) (2002) *Resolution concerning decent work and the informal economy*. Paper presented at The General Conference of the International Labour Organization, 90th Session

International Labour Organization (ILO) (2003a) *Facts on agriculture*. Available from http://www.ilo.org/ [Accessed 7 January 2011]

International Labour Organization (ILO) (2003b) *Safety in numbers: Pointers for global safety culture at work*. Geneva, Switzerland: International Labour Office (ILO)

International Labour Organization (ILO) (2007) *ILO Key Indicators of the Labour Market (KILM), Fifth Edition (Version W010) [Computer Program]*. Geneva: International Labour Organization

Isaia E (2005) Microfund for women: A case history of microcredit in Jordan. *Savings and Development*, 29: 441–468

International Trade Union Confederation (ITUC) (2007) *Migrant workers in the Middle East*, (No. Union View #7). Brussels: International Trade Union Confederation

Jamali D, Sidani Y, Kobeissi A (2008) The gender pay gap revisited: Insights from a developing country context. *Gender in Management*, 23: 230–246

Khatib L (2008) Gender, citizenship and political agency in Lebanon. *British Journal of Middle Eastern Studies*, 35(3), 437–451

Krieger N (2010) Workers are people too: Societal aspects of occupational health disparities – an ecosocial perspective. *American Journal of Industrial Medicine*, 53(2): 104–115

Loewe M (2004) New avenues to be opened for social protection in the Arab world: The case of Egypt. *International Journal of Social Welfare*, 13: 3–14

Messing K (1998) Hospital trash: Cleaners speak of their role in disease prevention. *Medical Anthropology Quarterly*, 12: 168–187

Nuwayhid IA (2004) Occupational health research in developing countries: a partner for social justice. *American Journal of Public Health*, 94(11): 1916–1921

O'Neill DH (2000) Ergonomics in industrially developing countries: Does its application differ from that in industrially advanced countries? *Applied Ergonomics*, 31(6): 631–640

Osfor MM, Abd el Wahab AM, el Dessouki SA (1998) Occurrence of pesticides in fish tissues, water and soil sediment from Manzala Lake and River Nile. *Nahrung*, 42(1): 39–41

Reinert KA (2007) Ethiopia in the world economy: Trade, private capital flows, and migration. *Africa Today*, 53(3): 65–89

Saadeh AM, Farsakh NA, al-Ali MK (1997) Cardiac manifestations of acute carbamate and organophosphate poisoning. *Heart*, 77(5): 461–464

Saddik B, Nuwayhid I (2006) Child labour in Arab countries: Call for action. *BMJ*, 333: 861–862

Safi JM, Abou-Foul NS, el-Nahhal YZ, el-Sebae AH (2002) Monitoring of pesticide residues on cucumber, tomatoes and strawberries in Gaza Governorates, Palestine. *Nahrung*, 46(1): 34–39

Salameh PR, Waked M, Baldi I, Brochard P, Saleh BA (2006) Chronic bronchitis and pesticide exposure: A case-control study in Lebanon. *European Journal of Epidemiology*, 21(9): 681–688

Schulte PA, Chun, H (2009). Climate change and occupational safety and health: Establishing a preliminary framework. *Journal of Occupational and Environmental Hygiene*, 6(9): 542–554

Shaham D (2008) Foreign labor in the Arab Gulf: Challenges to nationalization. *al Nakhlah*, 1–14

Smith S (1998). Treating burns as if gender mattered. *Links*, March (3)

Taha AZ (2000) Knowledge and practice of preventive measures in small industries in Al-Khobar. *Saudi Medical Journal*, 21(8): 740–745

Takala J (2005) *Introductory report: Decent work – safe work*. Geneva: Safe Work- International Labour Office

The Saudi Network (2007) *Saudi labor and workmen law, English Translation*. Available from http://www.the-saudi.net/business-center/labor_law.htm [Accessed 14 January 2011]

United Nations (UN) (2006) Convention on the rights of persons with disabilities. Available from http://treaties.un.org [Accessed 7 January 2011]

Vora N (2008) Producing diasporas and globalization: Indian middle-class migrants in Dubai. *Anthropological Quarterly*, 81(2): 377–406

World Health Organization (WHO) (2008) *The World Health Report 2008: Primary health care now, more than ever*. Geneva: WHO

World Bank (2009) *2009 World development report*. Washington, DC: Development Data Group

Yip YB, Ho SC, Chan SG (2004) Identifying risk factors for low back pain (LBP) in Chinese middle-aged women: A case-control study. *Health Care for Women International*, 25(4): 358–369

23

Conflict and Health: Meeting Challenges to Insecurity

Hani Mowafi and Rayana Bou-Haka

Large-scale humanitarian emergencies are growing globally and are common in the Arab world. Fifteen of the 22 Arab countries, with 85% of the region's population, have been in protracted conflict situations over the past two decades (Musani & Shaikh 2008). The following chapters in this section illustrate various aspects of public health in three conflict situations (Iraq, Lebanon, and the Occupied Palestinian Territory [OPT]). They highlight how communities have actually responded to conflicts, and identify ways to increase their capacity to respond to such crises in the future. This chapter aims to build toward and supplement the discussions in these chapters through reviewing key concepts common to various forms of humanitarian emergencies and, more specifically, through examining the effects of conflict on health in the region. Based on our review, we propose a research agenda to build a knowledge base that enables stronger action on conflict-related health challenges.

> **What is the duration of a "crisis" or an "emergency?"**
>
> Conflicts in the Arab world defy notions of "crises" and "emergencies" as discrete events in time. Rather, they are characterized by a prolonged nature with periods of increased intensity and without well-defined conclusions. Darfur has been considered a humanitarian "emergency" since 2003; Somalia has been in "crisis" since the early 1990s; and the Occupied Palestinian Territories has seen decades of low-level conflict with severe indirect impacts on public health (e.g., food insecurity) punctuated by periods of intense conflict with spikes in direct impact from violence.

Characteristics of Humanitarian Emergencies

Humanitarian emergencies, which include natural disasters, technological disasters, and those resulting from war or other conflicts, are often multi-faceted and complex. A widely used definition of emergencies is that of the United Nations Inter-Agency Standing Committee: "humanitarian crisis in a country, region or society where there is total or considerable breakdown of authority resulting from internal or external conflict and which requires an international response that goes beyond the mandate or capacity of any single agency and/or the ongoing United Nations country program" (UN-OCHA, 1999). Emergencies commonly represent an exacerbation of lower-level crises, increased recognition of previously under-appreciated human suffering from long-standing events, or a combination. Acute-on-chronic crises exacerbate underlying societal problems; exploit long-standing vulnerabilities; and strain communities already beyond capacity in their ability to deliver services.

The vast majority of crises are predictable. Many are preventable or can be significantly mitigated through hazard reduction and preventive efforts. Whether through surveillance of natural phenomenon as in drought, early warning systems or through monitoring systems of political and social tensions that herald impending conflict, early recognition of the potential for a crisis is essential for early mobilization of resources to prevent or mitigate crises.

Humanitarian crises disproportionately affect vulnerable populations or vulnerable members of a population. That opportunities are repeatedly missed to reduce the impact of crises on vulnerable populations indicates that policy makers have at best a fundamental misunderstanding of vulnerability, or worse, willfully neglect certain populations in order to exacerbate vulnerability.

Regardless of their causes, humanitarian emergencies have direct and indirect public health effects. Conflict-related direct consequences – physical or mental trauma, for example – are followed by indirect consequences like increases in preventable diseases, food insecurity, and lack of access to basic services.

Conflict, Displacement, and Health

A hallmark of humanitarian emergencies is large-scale population displacement. Perhaps, nowhere is this more evident than in the Arab world. There are over 7 million refugees in the Middle East and North Africa (MENA) (UNHCR 2009; UNRWA 2009). Millions more are internally displaced persons (IDPs) and/or stateless persons. Musani & Shaikh (2008) note that "The world's highest proportion of [IDPs] still lives in the Eastern Mediterranean Region".

Major displacements have included the repeated displacement of Southern Lebanese communities due to war with, and occupation by, Israel; massive internal and refugee displacement of Iraqis after the 2003 war; internal and cross-border displacement in Sudan and Somalia throughout the past 15 years; and the decades-long displacement of Palestinians. The IDPs suffer from degrading health services, poorer living conditions, decreased access to clean water and sanitation, and social suffering through loss of ties to land, livelihood, and social support (Marx 1992; ICRC 1999; Batniji et al 2009). Large-scale displacements also threaten economic, social and environmental stability and political security (Adelman 2001). There is a paucity of policies and institutions to deal with these phenomena in the region (Fargues & Bensaad, 2007; Grabska, 2006).

Displacement in the region is urban where services and economic opportunities attract the displaced. Whether living among local populations as do Iraqis in Jordan and Syria; in urban refugee camps as do Palestinians around the region; or in shantytowns on the outskirts of large capitals like Cairo and Khartoum; addressing the needs of displaced populations is a challenge to already strained local governmental social services. Urbanization of displacement is important in light of evidence of already alarming health inequalities in urban centers.

Many displaced people hide, fearing being designated as illegal immigrants in host countries rather than as asylum seekers or refugees – a common situation as many Arab countries are not signatories to the Refugee Convention (Mowafi & Spiegel 2008).

Civilians flee to escape threats to personal security but this option is not always available. In the winter 2008–09 Israeli attack on the Gaza Strip, Palestinian civilians were literally trapped with nowhere to flee. By preventing civilian flight through controlling borders, Israeli and Egyptian authorities deprived Palestinian civilians of a primary means of initial response – flight to safety.

There is limited research on the health effects of displacement in the region. Most studies focus on the direct health effects of active conflict and are conducted primarily by and for the relief agencies (Shami 1993). Research is needed to relate the health effects of the acute phase to pre-existing conditions that contribute to vulnerability and to the health impacts during the often-prolonged phase of post-conflict displacement.

The Challenge of Services for Displaced Populations

Frequently, the displaced have no legal rights to access public services. Current UN agency mandates and international covenants do not give clear guidance on what constitutes an appropriate set of services for displaced populations. A policy framework is needed to allow displaced people to access basic health services, shelter, and livelihoods. Existing guiding UN principles are frequently not adhered to necessitating assistance from international organizations. In Jordan and Syria, the cost of providing health services to Iraqi refugees is UNHCR's costliest health program per beneficiary (Spiegel et al 2010). The diffusion of the displaced into the local populace makes identifying them and providing them services more difficult. The provision of special services for the displaced strains local infrastructures and can create friction with the poor of the host population. Work is needed with mid-level community health officials from host countries to gauge their understanding of health risks posed by uncovered populations in their midst and to promote actions to mitigate risks.

Social Disruption

Conflict, war, and displacement disrupt infrastructure, trade, transportation, and other norms of daily life causing "social transformation" (Castles 2003). Social exchange, communication, and transaction are interrupted. Only the strongest pre-existing social relationships remain. Early on during displacement, family and cultural ties can form the foundation of a new stripped-down social order (Marx 1990, 1992). Understanding how this social capital functions can help develop interventions to empower populations to be their own first resource during crisis. Social capital is increasingly understood as a determinant of health and well-being (see Chapter 6). This is no less true in conflict.

Communities in the Arab world have highly developed social networks which become critical during crisis and form the basis for communal resilience in the face of adversity as highlighted in the example of the Lebanese Shiite community during the 2006 war with Israel (Chapter 26). These communities had strong civilian, religious, and social networks developed over 30 years of various conflicts. A religiously infused notion of "resistance" and the experience of reliance on communal resources created a shared sense of struggle and worthiness that resulted in a surprising degree of noted resilience.

Conflict and war "not only create miseries among individuals ... they destroy a society where people lead stable daily lives" (Shinoda 2004). This destruction manifests itself as a decline in overall *human security* where people's relationships to home, family, and sense of place in society are made tenuous by sudden dislocations. Ethnicity, social position, economic class, and other social characteristics can be the fault lines along which conflicts occur. However, such shared characteristics, along with individuals' personal relationships, also form the bases for social capital. Such networks represent the first and most immediate line of support. For example, functional social networks alleviated the negative health effects among long-term displaced populations in Lebanon (Choueiry & Khawaja 2006). Assessing the degree of "intactness" of social networks among populations in crisis, through qualitative and quantitative approaches, helps focus on the needs of the displaced and provides more robust information regarding a community's coping capacity.

Health Patterns in Conflict

The Arab world has diverse economies (see Chapter 2). On average, development indicators parallel those of low- and middle-income countries. However, averages mask important disparities between groups (see Chapter 5). It follows that the epidemiology of

conflict will also reflect, and may exacerbate, these disparities. Subgroup analysis is essential for research looking to document and analyze this impact.

Besides direct impacts of wars and violent conflicts, including violent death, injury, disability, psychological trauma, and sexual violence, indirect impacts occur due to displacement, inadequate shelter, destruction of infrastructure, failure of social networks, and collapse of public health systems (Brennan & Nandy 2001). Like people, systems use coping strategies to mitigate the effects of crisis. Flexible health systems that can rapidly reorganize to meet new challenges are more resilient. Rationing of medicines and supplies; changing procedures and health protocols to optimize use of resources; the shifting of less complicated clinical tasks to nonclinical personnel are strategies that may be employed. Grave health conditions, such as massive malnutrition and epidemics, can arise when the system's capacity to cope is overwhelmed.

Infectious Diseases

A disproportionate number of outbreaks of international health importance occur in countries affected by complex emergencies (Salama et al 2004; Spiegel 2005). If the integrity of the public health and medical systems is crippled, threats arise as happened in Iraq, where outbreaks of cholera and meningitis occurred in the aftermath of both Gulf wars (ICRC 1999). A large measles outbreak in 2009 was traced to lack of access to health services and the breakdown of the immunization program. Immunization rates plummeted to 35% following the 2003 invasion (Geoghegan 2007). Member of unvaccinated families fleeing to neighboring countries represented a public health concern because of reduced herd immunity in host populations (Mowafi 2007).

While overall prevalence of HIV/AIDS in the Arab world is low (DeJong et al 2005; Obermeyer 2006), the risk of HIV transmission increases during conflict and displacement, especially with increasing high risk behaviors including injection drug use and commercial sex practiced by individuals impoverished by conflict. Additionally, displaced populations have dis-incentives for seeking diagnosis and treatment due to the "enormous stigma and rights issues surrounding HIV" (DeJong et al 2005 p. 161; Obermeyer 2006).

Children in war

– While Iraq's under-5 mortality ranks in the middle range when compared with other developing countries, it has worsened faster than any other country. In 1990, the infant mortality rate (IMR) was 50 per 1000 live births. By 2007 IMR had climbed to 125 (Geoghegan, 2007).

– In both Sudan and Yemen over 40% of children under-5 have moderate or severe malnutrition (Save the Children, 2008).

– Somalia has perhaps the worst health indicators in the Arab world; material mortality rates are among the highest globally with 1 in 12 women dying from a pregnancy-related cause. Coverage with life-saving interventions is abysmal with only 5% of children fully immunized against diphtheria, pertussis, and tetanus and of those with diarrhea only 5% receive oral rehydration therapy (ORT) (Save the Children 2008).

The Hidden Violence of Conflict: Mental Health and Trauma

Researchers have documented the links between exposure to conflict and mental health problems (see Chapters 14 & 15). In a nationally representative study of nearly 3000 Lebanese adults, war trauma correlated with mental disorders (Karam et al 2006). Being a refugee for part of the war (displacement) was associated with the highest prevalence (37.7%) as compared with witnessing a dead body, seeing someone killed or severely injured (18%), losing a loved one (10.2%) or personally sustaining a life-threatening injury (3.1%). Although this survey was conducted more than a decade after the end of the Lebanese civil war, it demonstrates the lasting mental health effects of displacement. The Iraq Mental Health Survey (IMHS) in 2006/7, the first and only nationwide mental health survey there, showed that nearly 17% of the 4332 adult respondents had a mental disorder in their lifetime with a large percentage of documented cases related to the period starting with the 2003 war (WHO 2009). The 30-day and 1-year prevalence of disorders were similarly high.

Many countries do not have enough resources to provide mental health services to the general population let alone to victims of violence and displacement (Chynoweth & McKenna 2007). The result is that such services are often neglected, incomplete, or provided based on models developed in Western, non-

conflict settings that may not be appropriate or acceptable to those affected by conflict (Okasha 2003; Bader et al 2009).

In many Arab societies, mental illness remains stigmatized and commonly under-diagnosed. Therefore, perhaps the most vulnerable of displaced people are those with severe mental illness prior to displacement. This is especially so for those previously untreated (Jones et al 2009). Even those with well-controlled conditions can decompensate when facing the loss of support networks, familiar surroundings, and livelihoods. Many sufferers of mental health problems do not seek care or do so through medical centers and report physical rather than psychosocial complaints. "Somatisation" is well described among populations displaced in the region and among those resettled in Western countries (Jamil et al 2002; Okasha 2003; Choueiry & Khawaja 2006). Addressing this problem requires incorporating mental health screening and treatment at the primary care level. Services are also needed for displaced populations coping with the stress of isolation and social dislocation, substance abuse, and emotional or mood disturbances.

Emergency mental health programs in the region need to focus on several tracks simultaneously – assisting displaced people to establish social networks and social capital; training primary care practitioners to recognize and treat basic mental health ailments; establishing referral paths for victims of severe physical and sexual trauma; and contextualizing psychosocial programs to fit social attitudes and culture. The mental health programs for Iraqi refugees in Syria and Jordan are steps in the right direction. The WHO, in collaboration with host governments, has established multi-disciplinary mental health teams incorporating psychosocial counselors, physical and occupational therapists and medical practitioners. The teams have been models of mental health care and have trained similar teams from around the region. These efforts look to be sustainable through development of masters-level training programs at the national universities in each country. The Jordanian ministry of health plans to incorporate these teams into permanent staff in its facilities (Mowafi 2010).

Women's Health and Gender-Based Violence

With displacement and social dislocation women and girls can experience a loss of gender equity gains

(Kholy 2008). In addition to violence experienced prior to or during the flight from home, displaced women and girls also suffer exploitation in places of refuge. Without legal status many engage in sex work to support their families (Chynoweth & McKenna 2007; Zoepf 2007). Others are kidnapped and trafficked to other countries for prostitution (USAID 2004). In such an environment, a comprehensive set of health services is needed including emergency contraception, prevention of sexually transmitted illnesses, and counseling and forensic medicine services to assist victims of sexual crimes. These services are lacking or inadequate in many of the region's health systems to meet the needs of large, displaced populations.

Healthcare services for the displaced and those affected by war are variable (McGinn 2000; Plumper & Neumayer 2006). Conservative norms and attitudes in Jordan, Syria, the Gulf countries, and Iraq make it harder for displaced women to access services including basic contraception (Ladek 2007). It is reported that displaced Iraqi women and girls were uncomfortable with the conservative customs in their places of displacement. Health workers, agencies and the displaced themselves reported more unattended births and miscarriages.

Violence against women has risen dramatically in Iraq. Internally displaced women fear venturing out alone in public due to a rise in kidnapping and rape by armed groups (Chynoweth & McKenna 2007). The social stigma attached to crimes of sexual violence discourages women from accessing treatments for injuries, wounds, and sexually transmitted illnesses. Reporting sexual assaults and rapes can also lead to serious social and cultural consequences, such as rejection or violence for having caused shame to the family (Foran 2008). Women displaced both inside and outside Iraq find non-governmental organization (NGO) and local health clinics ill-prepared to address sexual violence (Chynoweth 2008).

Environmental Degradation and Health in Conflict

War and conflict cause environmental degradation through destruction of resources such as clean water supplies and agricultural fields increasing risk of illness and food insecurity. The Arab world is especially vulnerable because of its limited resources (see Chapter 4). The region has the lowest per capita availability of water in the world with half of the region living under water stress. The combined scarcity of water and desertification limits agricultural and grazing lands and brings farming and pastoralist communities into conflict over resources. In Sudan, Jordan, and Syria, drought has contributed to humanitarian crises. In Iraq, the destruction of water and sanitation systems due to the accumulating effects of neglect, sanctions, and war has resulted in outbreaks of cholera and other water-related illnesses (MOH-Iraq & WHO-Iraq 2008).

The use of environmental contaminants as weapons of war has potential serious long-term effects. Examples are white phosphorous in the Israeli attack on the Gaza Strip (Batniji et al 2009; McGirk 2009), depleted uranium (DU) in shells dropped on Iraq in the 1991 Gulf War, and Saddam Hussein's use of chemical weapons in Kurdish areas. While there is disagreement over the long-term health effects of DU (McDiarmid 2001; Bem & Bou-Rabee 2004), its presence in the environment is a major concern to affected populations.

Detritus of war such as unexploded ordinance, landmines, and cluster bombs maim and kill civilians for decades and isolate nearby communities from one another. "It is estimated that 18 countries in the [Eastern Mediterranean] region have dormant and active landmines" (WHO EMRO 2002). Landmines are serious issues in Lebanon, Iraq, Yemen, Egypt, Libya, and the Western Sahara; some estimate that one-third of the countries' land mass are contaminated (Leaning 2000). In addition to injury and death to livestock, landmines degrade the environment (Leaning 2000). Fearful populations abandon abundant natural resources and arable land and are forced to move into marginal and fragile environments which speeds depletion of biological diversity. Additionally, landmine explosions disrupt essential soil and water processes.

Finally, some combatants despoil the environment as a strategy of war or retreat as in the first Gulf War when the Iraqi military released 10 million barrels of Kuwaiti oil into Gulf waters and set fire to 732 oil wells causing destruction of marine ecosystems and severely polluting the atmosphere of surrounding countries (Leaning 2000).

Measuring Impact of Conflict

Assessing the impact of conflict in a diverse setting such as the Arab world is difficult. We need new ways

305

to conceptualize and measure such impact. This is especially true in the domain of health as there are acute and long-term consequences. An expansive concept should focus on health and not simply its absence – on function rather than dysfunction. New qualitative measures of community functioning are required to assess the health impact of conflicts on heterogeneous communities beyond simply documenting the self-articulated concerns of affected populations. To be useful for analysis across crises and to generalize conclusions for policy making these measures need to examine the relationships between conflict and behaviors of populations – both to help predict impending crises as well as plan for their effects. Such measures must also capture the costs of conflicts that have tangible if unmeasured impacts on human health and livelihoods. Instruments should capture longer-term impacts and the aggregate suffering accumulated across repeated crises.

Examining societal response to crises can provide useful insights. We need to understand not only how well societies rebuild after destruction but also what choices are made to build back better. The destruction of existing order produces short-term dysfunction, but also the opportunity to re-imagine how things could be done differently. The choices made will reflect societies' needs, powerful interests, and the degree to which people are empowered to act in what they see as their best interest. Empowerment (or lack thereof) may contribute significantly to a sense of human security (insecurity) that impacts personal well-being in times of crisis (see Chapter 36).

Working with health data in wartime faces the problem of a few frames of reference to which one can compare findings. Conflicts occur in resource-constrained countries with inadequate surveillance and civil registration systems. As such, baseline data are often either unavailable or inaccurate (Brennan & Nandy 2001; Guha-Sapir et al 2005). Using data to mitigate the health impact of conflict therefore requires a surveillance system that provides early warning of food insecurity, public health concerns, and population movements. It is not yet clear what indicators would be the best predictors of impending crises. New indicators are needed to measure peoples' attitudes and behaviors and their current health. Just as drought and famine early warning systems use certain coping behaviors in times of water scarcity as markers of impending drought, so too, may war and civil conflict cause similar changes in pre-emergency behavioral or health indicators that can provide an alert to decision makers that the conditions may be ripening for an impending crisis. Pilot programs in East Africa and Afghanistan have attempted to integrate such pre-emergency health indicators into early warning systems. An early warning system for infectious disease has been implemented in Somalia, Sudan, Afghanistan, and the OPT with the assistance of WHO and is currently being evaluated.

The revolution in digital communications is changing the way Arab societies communicate with one another and with the world. Coverage of mobile communications networks is near complete and even some remote parts have Internet access. Until robust, well-resourced health surveillance systems are routinely available one solution may be to turn to bottom-up solutions. New surveillance paradigms should be developed that take advantage of "crowdsourcing" where a large number of users can provide information in a de-centralized fashion. This can rapidly generate health information in times of conflict by harnessing the power of the region's greatest untapped resource – its people.

> **Box 1. Ushahidi**
>
> This is a simple example of how a network can be used in times of emergency to predict impending crisis. *Ushahidi*, meaning "testimony" in Swahili, is a crisis information system originally developed by programmers in East Africa. It gathers real-time data through SMS, email, and Internet from a large number of public users – hence called *crowdsourcing*. It then rapidly analyzes the data to produce useable information that is sent back to field users to inform them of potential risks. The original network was used by human rights activists in Kenya to inform people of incidents of violence around the country. Ordinary citizens accessed the network through their mobile phones to report human rights abuses and to seek out safe havens away from violent attacks. In a subsequent iteration, an Ushahidi network was established for the Arab news network Al Jazeera during its "War on the Gaza Strip" coverage. The network used a "trusted network" of journalists on the ground who sent reports of locations of artillery and air-strikes around the Gaza Strip. This network proved to be one of the fastest and most robust documentations of events on the ground and was entirely generated by people inside the Gaza Strip itself at a time when outsiders were barred access to the besieged territory (Ushahidi.com, 2009).

Emergency Preparedness and Response

Parts of the Arab world display many characteristics of unstable environments, making these areas fertile ground for conflicts and complicating the response to even minor humanitarian crises. These characteristics include: (a) contested government legitimacy; (b) limited ability to govern (impaired ability to identify needs, determine priorities, mobilize and allocate resources); (c) weak political and social institutions; (d) dispersed and dispossessed communities; (e) and disarticulated civil societies (Zwi 1999). When violence occurs, military and security forces dominate the response as they are highly funded (Shinoda 2004). Therefore, they can mobilize the most resources (human, material, and logistical), have more professionalization than civil service branches and bring command structures with defined roles that can be useful in the chaos after a humanitarian emergency (Beeril 2008). In theory, when they are effective and properly directed, security forces can monopolize the use of force to limit civil disorder and secondary violence as well as to facilitate orderly distribution of assistance to victims.

In reality, reliance on security forces for response in humanitarian emergencies has potential perils. Militaries are not trained in large-scale response – especially caring for large civilian populations. With civil or political unrest, security forces can become partisans or can target sectors of the civilian population thought to support the opposition. The main problem, however, is that their humanitarian role will always be secondary to their national security mission (Beeril 2008). In these cases, Arab governments rely on para-statal organizations such as Red Crescent Societies. These are commonly semi-official NGOs, not independent agencies that function as an arm of the executive power as in Syria, or under a royal charter as in Jordan which places them in parallel to the main health system under the ministry of health.

Evidence suggests that neither militaries nor para-statal NGOs engage in serious efforts to prepare and protect populations in advance of impending disasters (Leaning 2008). Over-reliance on these organizations locks Arab governments into a reactionary mode with too few professionals available to plan for protecting civilians. There are currently no degrees in civil disaster response or emergency preparedness in the region. The challenge remains to increase the numbers of trained emergency response health professionals and to integrate these into a coordinated emergency health plan.

Aid Workers at Risk

Ten of the 60 "hotspots" worldwide with smoldering crises or deteriorating political and social situations that could lead to crisis (Beeril 2008) and 25% of the countries with active armed conflict on their territory (Leonard & Melanie 2010) are in MENA. When the need for assistance overwhelms the capacity of local governments, societies frequently turn to humanitarian international NGOs for assistance. But use of aid agencies is complicated as "humanitarian space – physical locations that are safe from attack in a conflict, respect for core humanitarian principles of independence, impartiality, and neutrality, and the ability of aid agencies to access and help civilians affected by conflict – has shrunk substantially because of political polarization and a perception by combatants that humanitarian assistance is merely an instrument of interference by foreign powers" (Spiegel et al 2010). Humanitarian workers are increasingly the targets of hostile action in conflict. The most common cause of death of these workers has shifted from road traffic injuries in the 1970s–80s, to violent trauma now as workers are themselves the targets of belligerence (Brennan & Nandy 2001). The number of attacks against aid workers has risen steadily recently; in 2008, the fatality rate of aid workers exceeded that of UN peacekeepers (Stoddard et al 2009). Attacks in Sudan and Somalia made up more than 60% of attacks (Stoddard et al 2009). Most aid workers are targeted for political or economic reasons rather than being random victims of violence (Haver 2007).

While injuries and deaths of foreign, especially Western, aid workers receive considerable media attention, most aid workers are not foreigners but members of local communities. National staff represent 90% of field workers and 79% of all victims of violence perpetrated against humanitarian workers (Haver 2007). The absolute numbers of incidents against them and the disturbing trend in relative rates of violence demonstrate their vulnerability. In 2005, for the first time, the reported rate of incidents against national staff (7/1000) surpassed that of international staff (6/1000) (Haver 2007). While national staff of aid agencies in the region sometimes enjoy greater community acceptance than foreign workers, they may be at risk for being members of ethnic or religious groups that are party to a conflict.

Politics of Humanitarian Emergencies

A key difference between man-made and natural disasters is in their implications on developing political will for action (Spiegel 2005). Building political support for intervention after natural disasters is often easier than for conflict. Victims of natural disasters are seen as "blameless." There is no concern for stirring the ire of an opposing party when intervening on their behalf. They are easier to fundraise for and organizations are more willing to dedicate resources to serving in natural emergencies. In contrast, interventions in conflicts bring political risks. (Note the silence of Arab States and lack of operational presence by Arab forces and NGOs in the conflict in Darfur, Sudan.) Conflicts with layered political entanglements, commercial interests, and geostrategic importance cannot easily be resolved without the action and agreement of a large number of actors.

Politics also influence public attitude and attention towards suffering. Witness the world's outrage when flights bearing humanitarian aid were delayed for even a few days after the massive earthquake that destroyed Haiti in January 2010. Contrast this with the relative silence as humanitarian aid is denied entry by the Israeli and Egyptian forces to the Gaza Strip for months on end. In both cases, large civilian populations living in high-density conditions of urban poverty were affected, destruction of infrastructure resulted in tremendous direct and indirect morbidity and mortality, and suffering of civilians was highly publicized in media. However, the presence of partisan forces in the Gaza Strip and conflict with neighboring Israel lead to siege as a security strategy. Initial widespread international condemnation eventually yielded to quiescence as Israel, with complicity from the Egyptian regime, simply waited out the world's brief attention span. The suffering continues.

Several factors are fundamental to understanding why interventions to stop conflict-related humanitarian emergencies are prevented, limited, or delayed. These include ongoing conflict, insecurity and tensions, lack of capacity, lack of infrastructure in remote regions, the structure of international organizations like the United Nations and the bases for international law. While serving to build consensus for many international actions, the United Nations itself is at times hamstrung by its very architecture and the limits placed on it by international law and respect for sovereignty (Burkle 2005). Many interventions are thwarted through the use of Security Council vetoes (274 vetoes between 1945 and 1992) with many more examples of threatened vetoes that halt discussion well before any formal vote.

Regional and world powers also have competing interests (strategic, economic, financial, and cultural) that lead them to prevent outside interventions and mitigate the effect of sanctions or political isolation against their allies. Recent examples include Chinese protection of Sudan from international censure over violence against civilians in Darfur and repeated United States protection of Israel from international censure over its policies in the OPT and Lebanon. China sees Sudan as a strategic ally to meet its growing demand for oil. The United States has strong political ties to Israel. Many conflicts in the region continue due, in part, to such geopolitical stalemates.

Steps Forward: Supporting Community Capacity

Where civil society plays an important role in humanitarian assistance rapid and flexible responses to crises are possible. Such is the case in Lebanon and the OPT where weak central government control leaves more room for non-governmental action. The ensuing chapters highlight community action during recent conflicts in these two settings. Social organizations affiliated with political and religious groups were highly instrumental in dissemination of information, communal action during emergency, as well as in the post-emergency phase. The experiences gained by relief and health practitioners under prolonged conflict in Lebanon and OPT contribute to this flexibility and resilience. These experiences build individual and institutional memory and ability to cope with new emergencies.

One of the great challenges of humanitarian work in the coming decades will be to democratize hazard mitigation and response to humanitarian emergencies (Alexander 2003). The purpose is to encourage and empower "people to take responsibility for their own ... safety, to achieve a more participatory approach to disasters, to improve equity ... to share decision-making" in the aftermath of humanitarian crises. An outstanding example is a study of a training intervention for rural pre-hospital providers in Northern Iraq (Husum et al 2003). Training local laypersons in basic first aid led to a dramatic drop in mortality (from 40% to 14.9%) from trauma, largely from landmines. Such a move requires changing attitudes and political culture and organization (Alexander 2002). Good emergency preparedness requires institutions with strong leadership that are responsive to their stakeholders – the public. This is difficult since many governments in the region remain either unwilling or unable to identify, mitigate, and respond adequately to humanitarian emergencies that threaten their most vulnerable citizens.

A Research Agenda to Inform Future Action

The Arab world provides many case studies illustrating the impact of conflict on health that provide interested researchers precious learning opportunities. Lamentably, the body of research and lessons learned from crises are not commensurate with the region's experience. Such research is critical to moving the agenda for action forward. We identify four strategic directions for research.

First, the wide range of conflict types, duration, affected populations, and impact provide the opportunity for comparative analysis to better identify the impacts of conflict on health in the region.

Second, the number and recurrence of conflicts in the region create the imperative for developing tools that are contextualized to local needs. Part of developing a region-specific set of tools will be challenging and empowering different groups – academic, scientific, humanitarian – to define the parameters for this research agenda. For example, we know that conflicts and humanitarian emergencies do not affect all communities equally. As Chapter 26 discusses, examples of community resilience are a fertile ground for research, which can inform us about the capacity of affected communities to respond to future crises. There are few measures today to assess such capacity.

Third, with regard to large scale and long-term displacement, research needs to document the health and social cost of displacement, and identify disparities in health among displaced and other marginalized populations. Currently, weak surveillance systems in Arab countries must be advanced to capture disaggregated data on displaced people within host country populations. The challenges of service provision, health surveillance, and demands on highly strained local resources need also to be studied. Action-oriented research can inform efforts to relieve the observed tensions between displaced populations and host communities. Another focus for policy research is how to identify and provide services to displaced populations in the context of unmet needs for the poor citizens of host countries.

A final research imperative is identifying determinants of human security during prolonged conflicts. New instruments to measure human security – including the social capital on which people draw under crisis – and track threats must be developed and validated. Chapter 36 examines health and human security in more details.

Conclusion

This chapter and the following ones in this section illustrate aspects of public health in conditions of conflict and political crisis and highlight the challenges faced by populations, humanitarian actors, and decision makers. Now is the time to not only synthesize what is known about the impacts of conflict on health but also to sharpen our tools for analysis and research. The agenda for action also requires challenging communities to increase their degree of civic engagement – despite the discouragement of dominating governments. Practitioners need to draw on the strengths of local populations – strong family and communal ties, recent and persistent practical experience with conflict, and national or communal "narratives" of resilience – to help communities mitigate the impact of violence and conflict on health and human security.

Acknowledgment

Rayana Bou-Haka is a staff member of the World Health Organization. The author alone is responsible for the views expressed in this publication and they do not necessarily represent the decisions or policies of the World Health Organization.

References

Adelman H (2001) From refugees to forced migration: The UNHCR and human security. *International Migration Review*, 35(1): 7–32

Alexander D (2002) From civil defence to civil protection – and back again. *Disaster Prevention and Management*, 11(3): 5

Alexander D (2003) *A feckless world: Warfare, disasters and democracy.* Shrivenham, UK: Cranfield University, Royal Military College of Science

Bader F, Sinha R, Leigh J, et al (2009) Psychosocial health in displaced Iraqi care-seekers in non-governmental organization clinics in Amman, Jordan: an unmet need. *Prehospital & Disaster Medicine*, 24(4): 312–320

Batniji R, Rabaia Y, Nguyen-Gillham V, et al (2009) Health as human security in the occupied Palestinian territory. *The Lancet*, 373(9669): 1133–1143

Beeril C (2008) *Strengthening of the coordination of emergency humanitarian assistance of the United Nations, General Assembly, 63rd Session, General Plenary Meeting.* New York, NY: International Committee of Red Cross

Bem H, Bou-Rabee F (2004) Environmental and health consequences of depleted uranium use in the 1991 Gulf War. *Environment International*, 30(1): 123–134

Brennan RJ, Nandy R (2001) Complex humanitarian emergencies: A major global health challenge. *Emergency Medicine*, 13(2): 147–156

Burkle FM Jr (2005) Integrating international responses to complex emergencies, unconventional war, and terrorism. *Critical Care Medicine*, 33(1): S7–S12

Castles S (2003) Towards a sociology of forced migration and social transformation. *Sociology*, 37(1): 13–34

Choueiry N, Khawaja M (2006) Displacement and health status in low-income women: Findings from a population-based study in Greater Beirut. *Journal of Migration and Refugee Issues*, 3(1): 1–13

Chynoweth S, McKenna M (2007) *Iraqi refugee women and youth in Jordan: Reproductive health findings, a snapshot from the field.* New York, NY: Women's Commission for Refugee Women and Children

Chynoweth S (2008) The need for priority reproductive health services for displaced Iraqi women and girls. *Reproductive Health Matters*, 16(31): 10

DeJong J, Jawad R, Mortagy I, Shepard B (2005) The sexual and reproductive health of young people in the Arab countries and Iran. *Reproductive Health Matters*, 13(25): 49–59

Fargues P, Bensaad A (2007) *Senders turned into receivers: Transit migration in the Middle East and North Africa 8th Mediterranean Research Meeting* (Workshop 16). European University Institute-Robert Schuman Centre for Advanced Studies, Florence.

Foran S (2008) *Access to quality health care in Iraq: A gender and life-cycle perspective* (p. 28). Amman, Jordan: UNOCHA

Geoghegan T (2007) *State of the world's mothers 2007* (p. 70). Westport, CT: Save the Children Foundation

Grabska, K (2006) *Who asked them anyway? Rights, policies and wellbeing of refugees in Egypt.* Cairo: American University in Cairo, Center for Forced Migration and Refugee Studies.

Guha-Sapir D, van Panhuis WG, Degomme O, Teran V (2005) Civil conflicts in four African countries: A five-year review of trends in nutrition and mortality. *Epidemiologic Review*, 27(1): 67–77

Haver K (2007) Duty of care? Local staff and aid worker security. *Forced Migration Review*, 28: 10–11

Husum H, Gilbert M, Wisborg T, Van Heng Y, Murad M (2003) Rural prehospital trauma systems improve trauma outcome in low-income countries: A prospective study from North Iraq and Cambodia. *Journal of Trauma*, 54(6): 1188–1196

ICRC (International Committee of the Red Cross) (1999) *Iraq: 1989–1999, a decade of sanctions.* Available from http://www.icrc.org/eng/resources/documents/misc/57jqap.htm [Accessed 15 December 2010]

Jamil H, Hakim-Larson J, Farrag M, Kafaji T, Duqum I, Jamil LH (2002) A retrospective study of Arab American mental health clients: trauma and the Iraqi refugees. *American Journal of Orthopsychiatry*, 72(3): 355–361

Jones L, Asare JB, El Masri M, Mohanraj A, Sherief H, van Ommeren M (2009) Severe mental disorders in complex emergencies. *The Lancet*, 374(9690): 654–661

Karam EG, Mneimneh ZN, Karam AN, Fayyad JA, Nasser SC, Chatterji S, Kessler RC (2006) Prevalence and treatment of mental disorders in Lebanon: a national epidemiological survey. *The Lancet*, 367(9515): 1000–6.

Kholy AME (2008) *Cost of conflict for women in the Arab world.* Alexandria, Egypt: Institute for Peace Studies

Ladek DG (2007) *Iraq displacement year in review.* Amman, Jordan: International Organization for Migration

Leaning J (2000) Environment and health: Impact of war. *The Canadian Medical Association Journal*, 163(9): 1157–1161

Leaning J (2008) Disasters and emergency planning. *In*: *International Encyclopedia of Public Health* (p. 4614): Academic Press.

Leonard SR, Melanie DB (2010) Responsibility for protection of medical workers and facilities in armed conflict. *The Lancet*, 375 (9711): 329–340

Marx, E (1990) The social world of refugees: A conceptual framework. *Journal of Refugee Studies*, 3(3): 189–203

Marx E (1992) Palestinian refugee camps in the West Bank and the Gaza Strip. *Middle Eastern Studies*, 28(2): 281–294

McDiarmid MA (2001) Depleted uranium and public health. *British Medical Journal*, 322(7279): 123–124

McGinn T (2000) Reproductive health of war-affected populations: What do we know? *International Family Planning Perspectives*, 26(4): 174–180

McGirk J (2009) Gaza's health and humanitarian situation remains fragile. *The Lancet*, 373(9663): 531–531

MOH-Iraq (Iraq Ministry of Health) & WHO (World Health Organization) Iraq (2008) *Situation report on diarrhea and cholera in Iraq.* Amman, Jordan: WHO

Mowafi H (2007, July 2007) [Conversation with Dr. Hisham al Moussad, WHO Country Director, Amman, Jordan]

Mowafi H (2010, May) [Conversation with Dr. Hisham al Moussad, WHO Country Director, Amman Jordan]

Mowafi H, Spiegel P (2008) The Iraqi refugee crisis: Familiar problems and new challenges. Journal of the American Medical Association, 299(14): 1713–1715

Musani A, Shaikh IA (2008) The humanitarian consequences and actions in the Eastern Mediterranean Region over the last 60 years – a health perspective. Eastern Mediterranean Health Journal, 14: S150–S156

Obermeyer CM (2006) HIV in the Middle East. British Medical Journal, 333(7573): 851–854

Okasha A (2003) Mental health services in the Arab world. Arab Studies Quarterly, 25(4): 14

Plumper T, Neumayer E (2006) The unequal burden of war: The effect of armed conflict on the gender gap in life expectancy. International Organization, 60(3): 723–754

Salama P, Spiegel P, Talley L, Waldman R (2004) Lessons learned from complex emergencies over past decade. The Lancet, 364(9447): 1801–1813

Save the Children (2008) State of the world's mothers. Westport, CT: Save the Children

Shami S (1993) The social implications of population displacement and resettlement: an overview with a focus on the Arab Middle East. International Migration Review, 27 (101): 4–33

Shinoda H (2004) Operational phases of human security measures in and after armed conflict: The link between humanitarian aid and peace-building. Paper presented at the Annual meeting, International Studies Association, Montreal, Quebec, Canada, Available from http://www.allacademic.com/meta/p74186_index.html [Accessed 15 July 2010]

Spiegel PB (2005) Differences in world responses to natural disasters and complex emergencies. Journal of the American Medical Association, 293(15): 1915–1918

Spiegel PB, Checchi F, Colombo S, Paik E (2010) Health-care needs of people affected by conflict: future trends and changing frameworks. The Lancet, 375(9711): 341–345

Stoddard A, Harimer A, DiDomenico V (2009) Trends in violence against aid workers and the operational response Humanitarian Practice Group (vol. HPG Policy Brief 34). London, UK: Overseas Development Institute

UNHCR (2009) UNHCR Statistical online population database. Available from http://www.unhcr.org/statistics/populationdatabase [Accessed 19 October 2010]

UNRWA (2009) UNRWA in figures: As of 30 June 2009. Geneva, Switzerland: UNRWA

USAID (2004) Literature review and analysis related to human trafficking in post-conflict situations. Washington, DC: USAID

Ushahidi.com (2009) Ushahidi: Crowdsourcing crisis information (FOSS). Available from http://www.ushahidi.com/ [Accessed 30 April, 2009]

WHO EMRO (World Health Organization – Regional Office for the Eastern Mediterranean (2009) Iraq Mental Health Survey 2006/7 (p. 107). Baghdad, Iraq: WHO.

WHO EMRO (Eastern Mediterranean Regional Office) (2002) Health under difficult circumstances: The impact of war, disasters and sanctions on the health of populations. Cairo, Egypt: WHO EMRO

Zoepf K (2007, May 29) Desperate Iraqi refugees turn to sex trade in Syria. New York Times. Available from http://www.nytimes.com/2007/05/29/world/middleeast/29syria.html [Accessed 15 January 2011]

Zwi A (1999) Community and institutional preparedness and resilience of health systems technical guidelines – Emergency management essentials. London, UK: WHO

Chapter

24

Health Status and Health Services in the Occupied Palestinian Territory

Rita Giacaman, Rana Khatib, Luay Shabaneh, Asad Ramlawi, Belgacem Sabri, Guido Sabatinelli, Marwan Khawaja, and Tony Laurance

Editors' note: This chapter is an article that appeared in the *Lancet* series on Health in the Occupied Palestinian Territory launched in March 2009. It is reproduced with permission from the Lancet with minor formatting changes. All articles and commentaries in the series are accessible from the *Lancet* Web site at: http://www.thelancet.com/series/health-in-the-occupied-palestinian-territory

We describe the demographic characteristics, health status, and health services of the Palestinian population living in Israeli-occupied Palestinian territory, and the way they have been modified by 60 years of continuing war conditions and 40 years of Israeli military occupation. Although health, literacy, and education currently have a higher standard in the Israeli-occupied Palestinian territory than they have in several Arab countries, 52% of families (40% in the West Bank and 74% in the Gaza Strip) were living below the poverty line of US$3·15 per person per day in 2007. To describe health status, we use not only conventional indicators, such as infant mortality and stunting in children, but also subjective measures, which are based on people's experiences and perceptions of their health status and life quality. We review the disjointed and inadequate public-health and health-service response to health problems. Finally, we consider the implications of our findings for the protection and promotion of health of the Palestinian population, and the relevance of our indicators and analytical framework for the assessment of health in other populations living in continuous war conditions.

Introduction

"The conditions in which people live and work can help to create or destroy their health."

Commission on Social Determinants of Health (CSDH 2006).

WHO's Commission on Social Determinants of Health (Jong-wook, 2005) has drawn attention to the effects on health of low income, inadequate housing, unsafe workplaces, and lack of access to health facilities. Conflict is an additional hazard to health, not only because it causes injury, death, and disability, but also because it increases physical displacement, discrimination, and marginalization, and prevents access to health services. Constant exposure to life-threatening situations in a conflict setting is an additional, specific social determinant of health, which can lead to disease (WHO 2008c; Stewart-Brown, 1998).

This is the first of five reports about the health status and health services in the Israeli-occupied Palestinian territory – the West Bank (including Palestinian Arab East Jerusalem) and the Gaza Strip. We emphasize the complexity of factors that contribute to Palestinian health and health-system problems: ongoing colonization – i.e., continued land confiscation and the building of Israeli settlements on Palestinian land; fragmentation of communities and land; acute and constant insecurities; routine violations of human rights; poor governance and mismanagement in the Palestinian National Authority; and dependence on international aid for resources. These and other factors have distorted and fragmented the Palestinian health system and adversely affected population health.

Here, we describe the demographic characteristics and the health status of the Palestinian population living in the occupied Palestinian territory. We have used not only conventional indicators, such as infant mortality, but also subjective measures based on people's experiences and perceptions of their health status and quality of life. We draw on the human-security framework to analyze and understand the effects on health and well-being of the socio-political conditions in the occupied Palestinian territory.

Public Health in the Arab World, ed. Samer Jabbour et al. Published by Cambridge University Press. © Samer Jabbour et al., 2012.

First developed by the UN development program (UNDP) for the 1994 human development report, the human-security framework is used to explore multiple threats and new causes of insecurity (Jolly & Basu Ray, 2006; King and Murray, 2001). This framework focuses on people and their protection from social, psychological, political, and economic threats that undermine their well-being (Leaning 2004). Also, it emphasizes the capability of people to manage daily life, and the importance of social functioning and health. The framework has important implications for health and human development (Chen & Narasimhan 2004) because health is a vital core of human security and is susceptible to various threats and insecurities, such as destruction of infrastructure, lack of access to health services, food shortage, job insecurity, and poor quality of health care (Caballero-Anthony 2004), all in addition to the toll of death, morbidity, and disability caused by war.

We also briefly look at public-health and health-services responses to prevailing health problems, which will be dealt with in detail in the last report of this Series (Mataria et al 2004). We conclude by considering the implications of our findings for protection and promotion of health of the Palestinian population, and the relevance of the indicators and analytical framework we have adopted for the assessment of health in other situations of constant conflict.

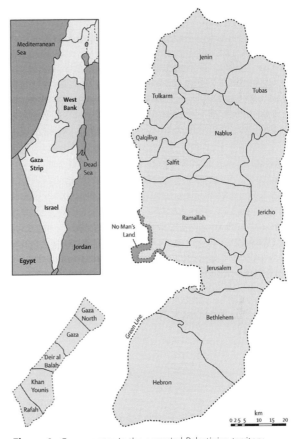

Figure 1. Governorates in the occupied Palestinian territory.

Historical Overview

The term Palestinians refers to the people who lived in British Mandate Palestine before 1948, when the state of Israel was established, and their descendants. As documented by several Israeli historians (Rogan & Shlaim 2001), more than three-quarters of the Palestinian population were forcibly dispossessed and expelled between 1947 and 1949, becoming refugees in neighboring Arab states (Kimmerling 1992). This traumatic situation – called the *nakba* (or catastrophe) by Palestinians – is engrained in the collective memory, and is still felt by third-generation refugees, especially those living in refugee camps (Baker & Shalhoub-Kevorkian 1999). Since then, Palestinian identity has been reinforced through resistance to dispossession and extinction (Said, 1974).

Palestinians identify themselves as Arabs because of the common language and culture with other Arab nationalities, but maintain their distinctive identity as Palestinians (Khalidi 1991). Most Palestinians are Muslim (94%), about 6% are Christian, and only a few are Jewish (Usher 2004). At present, about 4·5 million Palestinians are refugees from the 1948 Arab–Israeli war and their descendants are registered by the UN Relief and Works Agency for Palestine Refugees in the Near East. Almost a third of Palestinian refugees still live in camps inside and outside the occupied Palestinian territory (UNRWA 2009a), although these camps are now urban settlements, not tents.

The occupied Palestinian territory is the term used by the UN for those parts of Palestine occupied by Israel after the Arab–Israeli war of 1967 (UN, 2008). It consists of the West Bank, including East Jerusalem (Figure 1), and the Gaza Strip, and has a population of 3·77 million, 1·8 million of whom are registered refugees.

In 1991, a peace conference on the Middle East was convened in Madrid between Israel and Palestinians and Arab states. Several subsequent negotiations led to mutual recognition between Israel and the Palestine Liberation

Panel

A brief history of the occupied Palestinian territory

1917

The Balfour Declaration stated that the British Government favors the establishment of a home for the Jewish people in Palestine, emphasizing that nothing should be done to undermine the civil and religious rights of non-Jewish communities in Palestine.

1920–48

British Mandate of Palestine.

1948

First Arab–Israeli war. Creation of Israel on most of British Mandate of Palestine, with two-thirds of Palestinians forcibly dispossessed and dispersed, and made into refugees in neighboring Arab countries.

1950–67

West Bank annexed by the Hashemite Kingdom of Jordan. Gaza Strip came under Egyptian military administration.

1967

Arab–Israeli war. Israel occupied the rest of Palestine (the West Bank, including Palestinian Arab East Jerusalem, and the Gaza Strip) and parts of Syria.

1987

First Palestinian popular uprising (intifada) against Israeli military occupation.

1993

The signing of the Declaration of Principles on Interim Self-Government Arrangements (the Oslo Accords), and handing over of selected spheres of administration, including health care, to an interim Palestinian National Authority. This authority was intended to govern parts of the West Bank and Gaza Strip during a transitional period when negotiations of a final peace treaty would be completed.

2000

Interim political solution exploded with the second Palestinian uprising, fueled by widespread discontent with the failure of the Oslo Accords to address accelerating Israeli confiscation and colonization of Palestinian lands in defiance of international law, and by the shortcomings of the Palestinian National Authority.

2002

Israel's military incursions of the West Bank, and the ransacking of several Palestinian ministries and institutions, including the Palestinian Central Bureau of Statistics, the Palestinian Ministry of Education and Higher Education, various other research and cultural institutions, and radio and television stations.

2005

Israel withdrew its settlements from the Gaza Strip in August, 2005, but continued to retain control over access to the Gaza Strip by land, sea, and air.

2006–08

Democratic election of Islamic Hamas to majority in the Palestinian National Authority. Israel and key Western states responded by boycotting its administration.

Diplomatic ties and international donor funding were cut, and Israel withheld Palestinian tax revenues, which together form about 75% of the budget of the Palestinian National Authority.

Israeli military closure policies intensified, and fragmentation continued to be reinforced. By February, 2008, and after the Annapolis summit, the closure system was tightened even further and included over 600 checkpoints and barriers erected by the Israeli military on roads to restrict Palestinian movement, compared with about 518 such barriers to movement in 2006.

November 2008 to January 2009

The truce with Hamas is broken (Nov 4, 2008). Israel invades Gaza Strip (Dec 27, 2008). Destruction of infrastructure and buildings, including homes, universities, schools, clinics, mosques, and welfare organizations. Hundreds of civilians are killed and thousands injured, intensifying Gaza's humanitarian crisis.

Organization and, in 1993, the Declaration of Principles on Interim Self-Government Arrangements (Question of Palestine 2008), otherwise known as the Oslo Accords.

The Oslo Accords aimed to achieve a resolution to the conflict and established the Palestinian National Authority for a transitional period, during which negotiation of a final peace treaty would be completed (UN 2009). On the basis of these accords, the authority assumed control over some, but not all, areas of the West Bank and Gaza Strip. The agreement divided the occupied Palestinian territory into three zones. The Palestinian National Authority assumed control of all civilian administration, including health, and became responsible for security in zone A, which includes the main urban areas of the West Bank, but only about 3% of the land. The Palestinian National Authority has civilian authority, but shares security responsibility with Israel in zone B, which includes about 450 Palestinian towns and villages, and covers about 27% of the West Bank. The authority has no control over the remaining 70% of the occupied Palestinian territory, zone C, which includes agricultural land, the Jordan valley, natural reserves and areas with low population density, and Israeli settlements and military areas (UNCTAD 2008). Fundamental issues, such as the status of East Jerusalem, refugees and the right of return or compensation, Israeli settlements, security arrangements, and borders were left for later negotiations (IMFA 2008).

The Palestinian National Authority did not have, and still does not have, sovereignty over borders, movement of people and goods, and control over land and water (Giacaman 1998). Over time, the authority became troubled by other shortcomings, including corruption, absence of collective decision making and integrated planning, and the appointment of excessive numbers of civil servants as reward for the so called revolutionary heroism, political support, or both, causing a major drain on the national budget (Shu'aybi & Shikaki 2000). By September, 2000, the Palestinian National Authority collapsed with the second Palestinian uprising (*intifada*). The uprising was fuelled by widespread discontent, on the one hand for the shortcomings of the authority, and on the other for the acceleration of Israeli confiscation and colonization of Palestinian lands in defiance of international laws (Hammami & Hilal 2001). These developments undermined an already fragile system of public services, including health services.

Since 2000, life for Palestinians has become much harder, more dangerous, and less secure. Under the justification of protecting Israelis from Palestinian violence, a massive wall is being constructed between Israel and the West Bank, incorporating areas of the West Bank into Israel, and hundreds of Israeli military checkpoints have been established accompanied by curfews, invasions, detentions, the use of lethal force against civilians, land confiscations, and house demolitions, all of which have made ordinary life almost impossible. These events entail the systematic collective punishment of the Palestinian population living in the occupied Palestinian territory. According to the Israeli human-rights organization B'tselem, almost 5000 Palestinians – mainly civilians, including more than 900 children – have been killed by Israeli military action between September, 2000, and June, 2008, and over 1000 Israeli civilians and military personnel have been killed by Palestinians (B'tselem 2008), mainly in suicide attacks. Many people were seriously wounded and disabled (Palestinian Central Bureau of Statistics 2008a; Baker & Kanan 2003). During the preparation of this report, almost 1400 Palestinians living in the Gaza Strip were killed, and thousands injured, with many civilians among the casualties. The high burden of injury and trauma on

individuals, health services, and society is discussed more fully by Batniji and colleagues (Batniji et al 2009) in this Series.

Evidence exists of severe damage to infrastructure and institutions, homes, schools, private businesses, cultural heritage sites, and the Palestinian National Authority ministry buildings, equipment, and data-storage facilities, especially during the Israeli invasions of West Bank towns in 2002. The UN, the World Bank, and the Government of Norway have estimated the loss, due to infrastructural and physical damage during the March to April Israeli military invasions of 2002, at about US$361 million (UN 2009). Israeli invasions have also caused widespread food and cash shortages, psychological distress, and serious interruption of basic services, including crucial health services (Giacaman et al 2004).

Since 2002, the construction of the separation wall has continued, in defiance of the international commission of jurists' decision that the wall constitutes a serious violation of international human-rights law and international humanitarian law (International Commission of Jurists 2008). The Israeli high court of justice has repeatedly ruled that the route of the wall should be dictated by security considerations and not by Israeli settlement expansion plans (Harel, 2008). The construction of this wall has meant the confiscation of thousands of hectares of fertile Palestinian agricultural land, restrictions on freedom of movement, division of communities, and worsening economic conditions. In 2006, although still not defining the state's borders, Israel announced that the route of the separation wall followed official aspirations for a new border (Myre, 2006). This means that Israel will have annexed approximately 10% of the West Bank, including Palestinian farmland and key water sources, and incorporated most Israeli settlements. Israeli military closures and their effects on the movement of goods and people have become increasingly severe in the occupied Palestinian territory, causing an economic crisis (with the gross domestic product per person in 2007 falling to 60% of its value in 1999) (The World Bank 2008): rising unemployment and a serious decline in living standards (FAO 2007), all of which are associated with negative health outcomes (EMRO 2008d; Benach et al 2007). The Israeli military closures restrict Palestinian access to basic services, such as health and education, and separate communities from their land and places of work. In the West Bank, the physical separation has been tightened even further; by June, 2008, over 600 checkpoints and barriers to movement had been erected by the Israeli military on roads to restrict Palestinian movement, compared with an average of 518 in 2006 (UNICEF 2009).

The failure to reach a permanent peace agreement and the continuing expropriation of land for settlements and roads, which has continued unabated since 1967, the failure to establish an independent Palestinian state, and the disillusionment of the population with the Palestinian National Authority could explain the unexpected majority of parliament seats achieved by Hamas (the Islamic resistance movement) in elections for the Palestinian legislative council in January, 2006. Despite the overwhelming electoral support for Hamas, Israel and key Western countries responded by boycotting and isolating the newly elected administration because of Hamas' refusal to meet three criteria: recognition of Israel's right to exist, renunciation of violence, and adherence to interim peace agreements with Israel (Reuters 2008). Diplomatic ties and international donor funding were cut, and Israel withheld Palestinian tax revenues, which together form about 75% of the budget of the Palestinian National Authority (Human Rights Watch 2007).

The withholding of taxes and international aid created a severe political and financial crisis, with the Palestinian National Authority unable to pay the salaries of 165,000 civil servants. This situation led to intermittent strikes by civil servants, including health personnel; worsening service provision; severe shortages of medication and equipment; and a health-system crisis (WHO 2006). Poverty and dependence on food aid increased. The World Food Program indicated sharply reduced access to food, with evidence that a third of Palestinian households were food insecure and highly dependent on assistance (FAO 2009). The consequences of this situation were institutional decline, degraded governance, economic crisis, breakdown of social networks, and growing internal violence.

In February, 2007, a national unity government was formed with representatives from the two main Palestinian parties: Fatah (the Palestinian national liberation movement) and Hamas (US Department of State 2007). But the national unity government was not accepted by Israel, most European countries, and North America, and soon collapsed (Sayigh 2007). An emergency government was established, and Israel and the international community finally ended the boycott of the Palestinian Authority.

However, factional clashes continued and in June, 2007, Hamas took control of the Gaza Strip (BBC News 2007). Israel had withdrawn its settlements from the Gaza Strip in August, 2005, but retained control over access to the Gaza Strip by land, sea, and air. A separation wall or fence surrounds Gaza and, since the takeover by Hamas, Israel has maintained a strict siege, with people and goods allowed in or out only for essential humanitarian purposes (Human Rights Watch 2007; Sayigh 2007). Incursions by the Israeli military continued until a limited truce was agreed in June, 2008. The truce was broken on Nov 4, 2008.

The effects of the siege on economic and social conditions in Gaza have been devastating. There is a great shortage of fuel and cooking gas, and power cuts are frequent. Economic activity has almost completely ceased. Unemployment was around 33% of the active workforce in 2007, and rose to 37% in 2008. The percentage of Gazans who live in deep poverty has been steadily increasing, rising from nearly 22% in 1998 to nearly 35% in 2006. With the continued economic decline and the implementation of even stricter closures on Gaza, the poverty rate in 2008 is expected to be higher than it was in 2006. Food insecurity has continued to rise reaching 56% in 2008. In addition, 60% of households regard emergency assistance as a secondary source of income, with increased numbers of families relying on assistance, making present coverage by main assistance providers insufficient (The World Bank 2008; WFP/UNRWA/FAO 2008). The Israeli military invasions in December, 2008, to January, 2009, of the Gaza Strip severely intensified this pre-existing humanitarian crisis.

Health of Palestinians in the Occupied Palestinian Territory

Table 1 shows data for the 3.77 million Palestinians living in the occupied Palestinian territory, including comparisons with neighboring countries. A total of 46% of the population is younger than 15 years of age, an indication of the high fertility rate and falling infant mortality. The fertility rate was very high during the 1960s until the early 1990s, and then declined. Since 2000, fertility has remained stable at about five children per woman (Figure 2). Infant mortality rates fell until the mid-1990s (Figure 3), contributing to the high proportion of children in the population

Table 1. Demographic and Socio-ecomomic Characteristics of the Population Living in the Occupied Palestinian Territory and Neighboring Countries

Total population	OPT	Jordan	Lebanon	Syria	Egypt	Israel
	3,770,606	5,700,000	3,900,000	19,900,000	73,400,000	7,300,000
Number of registered Palestinian refugees	1,765,499	1,880,740	411,005	446,925	"	"
Number of Palestinian refugees living in camps	669,096	330,468	217,441	120,383	"	"
Number of Palestinians living in Israel	"	"	"	"	"	1184466
Palestinians aged <15 years	45.7%	37.0%	27.00%	37.0%	33.0%	28.00%
Palestinians aged ≥65 years	3.0%	3%	8%	3%	5%	10%
Male average life expectancy at birth (years)	71.7	71.0	69.0	71.0	68.0	78.0
Female average life expectancy at birth (years)	73.2	72.0	73.0	75.0	73.0	82.0
Infant mortality rate (per 1000)	25.3	24.0	17.0	19.0	33.0	3.9
Average number of children per woman	4.6	3.5	2.3	3.5	3.1	2.8
Adult literacy rate (aged ≥ 15 years)	93.9%	91.1%	88.0%	81.0%	61.0%	97.1%
Combined primary, secondary, and tertiary gross enrolment ratio	82.4%	78.1%	84.6%	64.8%	76.9%	89.6%
Average unemployment in individuals aged ≥15 years	21.5%	15.0%	10.0%	12.0%	10.0%	8.5%

Sources: Palestinian Central Bureau of Statistics 2008b; UNRWA 2007a; Palestinian Central Bureau of Statistics 2007a, 2006; UNDP 2008a; Population Reference Bureau Data finder 2008a; UNDP, 2008b; WHO 2008b; Population Reference Bureau Data finder 2008b; EMRO 2008a; UNDP 2008c; Population Reference Bureau Data finder 2008c; EMRO 2008b; UNDP 2008d; Population Reference Bureau Data finder 2008d; EMRO 2008c; UNDP 2008e; Population Reference Bureau Data finder 2008f; UNDP 2008f.

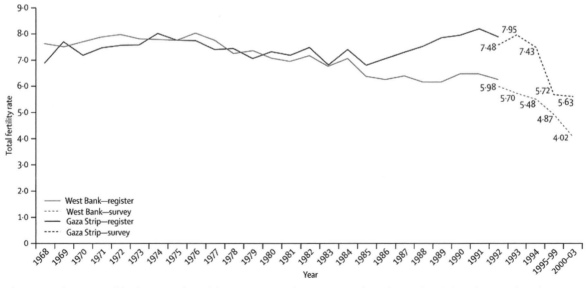

Figure 2. Palestinian total fertility rate and trends between 1968 and 2003. Data are from Khawaja (2000), the Palestinian Central Bureau of Statistics (2007a, 2006, 1995) and other sources.

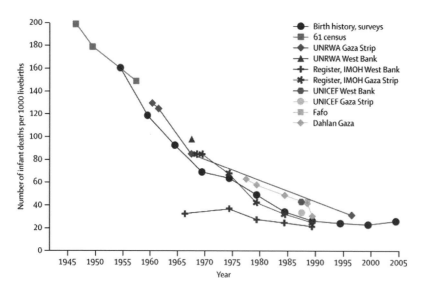

Figure 3. Number of infant deaths per 1000 livebirths between 1945 and 2005. Sources: Palestinian Central Bureau of Statistics 2007c, 2006, 1995; Dahlan; Abu Libdeh Hovensen & Brunborg 1993; Hill 1983; Israel Ministry of Health 1994; Abu Libdeh et al 1992; UNRWA 2003) IMOH=Israeli Ministry of Health. UNRWA=UN Relief and Works Agency.

(Abdul Rahim et al 2009). Health of children, and data quality, are discussed in more detail by Abdul Rahim and colleagues (2009) in this Series.

Palestinians are undergoing a rapid epidemiological transition (Husseini et al 2009). Non-communicable diseases, such as cardiovascular diseases, hypertension, diabetes, and cancer, have overtaken communicable diseases as the main causes of morbidity and mortality. The prevalence of HIV/AIDS is very low, and the population is deemed free of poliomyelitis, as judged by WHO criteria. Communicable diseases of childhood have already been mostly controlled with effective immunization program (Palestinian National Authority 2010).

Standards of health, literacy, and education are generally higher in the occupied Palestinian territory than in several Arab countries, but substantially lower than in Israel (Table 1). By contrast with the decline between 1967 and 1987, infant mortality stalled at around 27 per 1000 during 2000–06, the same as that reported in the 1990s (Figure 3), which suggests a slowdown of health improvements, a possible increase in health disparities (Tang et al 2008), or an indication of deteriorating conditions (Gould 1998).

The rate of stunting in children younger than 5 years (defined as height for age >2 SDs below the median of the US National Center for Health Statistics and WHO Child Growth Standards (2008a) has risen from 7.2% in 1996 (Palestinian National Authority 2006) to 10.2% in 2006. Stunting during childhood is an indicator of chronic malnutrition, and is associated with increased disease burden and death (Palestinian Central Bureau of Statistics 2007b), including compromised cognitive development and educational performance (Mendez & Adair 1999; Walker et al 2005; Black et al 2008) and obesity and chronic diseases in adulthood (Sawaya et al 2003).

The incidence of pulmonary tuberculosis increased in the Gaza Strip from 0.83 per 100,000 in 1999 to 1.31 per 100,000 in 2003. The incidence of meningococcal meningitis also rose in the West Bank and Gaza Strip from 3.0 per 100,000 in 1999 to 4.6 per 100,000 in 2003, and that of mental disorders rose by about a third, from 32.0 per 100,000 in 2000 to 42.6 per 100,000 in 2003 (Abu Mourad et al 2008). Data for mental disorders are obtained from yearly health reports, which consistently indicate increases in the frequency of most diseases (WHO 2006). However, whether these data show real changes, including those due to the violence and social damage of Israeli occupation, or due to better information-gathering methods and coverage, is unclear. Furthermore, such data do not distinguish between mild and severe disorders.

To assess the quality of life in Palestinians living in the occupied Palestinian territory, the WHO quality of life-Bref (WHO 2008d) was used in a 2005 survey, containing a representative sample of adults from the general population, after addition of some questions relevant to the Palestinian context (Mataria et al 2009a). Life quality in the occupied Palestinian territory proved lower than that in almost all other

Table 2. Quality of Life Scores in the Occupied Palestinian Territory and Selected Other Countries

	Physical domain	Psychological domain	Social domain	Environmental domain
	Mean (St Dev)	Mean (St Dev)	Mean (St Dev)	Mean (St Dev)
OPT[*]	14.2 (3.2)	13.3 (2.5)	14.8 (3.1)	11.2 (2.3)
All countries	16.2 (2.9)	15.0 (2.8)	14.3 (3.2)	13.5 (2.6)
Argentina[†]	12.1 (2.2)	10.6 (2.9)	10.8 (3.5)	10.7 (2.3)
Israel	15.5 (3.0)	14.2 (3.0)	13.0 (3.8)	12.6 (2.6)
Netherlands[‡]	18.3 (3.0)	16.6 (2.8)	15.8 (3.3)	15.9 (2.8)

Domain means are estimated on a range from 4 (low quality of life) to 20 (high quality of life).
The sample of occupied Palestinian territory was derived through a three-stage random sampling procedure, selecting 1008 responders who were ≥18 years old from all governorates and localities in the West Bank and Gaza Strip. The WHO field trials included adult participants recruited from outpatient facilities and the general population. OPT = occupied Palestinian territory.
[*]The difference between the mean for the occupied Palestinian territory and overall mean from all countries surveyed by WHO was significant (p<0·05) for all domains.
[†]Lowest score.
[‡]Highest score.

countries included in the WHO study (Table 2). Furthermore, the study showed that most responders had high levels of fear; threats to personal safety, safety of their families, and their ability to support their families; loss of incomes, homes, and land; and fear about their future and the future of their families (Table 3).

Feelings in the population include *hamm* – a local Arabic term that combines different feelings, such as the heaviness of worry, anxiety, grief, sorrow, and distress – frustration, incapacitation, and anger. Feelings of deprivation and suffering were also high. Most people reported being negatively affected by constant conflict and military occupation, closures and siege (including the separation wall), and inter-Palestinian violence.

In a study based on 3415 adolescents of the Ramallah district (Giacaman et al 2007a), Palestinian students reported the lowest life-satisfaction scores compared with 35 other countries (Figure 4). Collective exposure to violence was associated with negative mental health. After adjustment for sex, residence, and other measures of exposure to violent events, exposure to humiliation was also significantly associated with increased subjective health complaints. Such subjective data should be interpreted with caution because subjective measures can be complicated by people understanding and responding to questions in different ways (Salomon et al 2004). However, self-rating of health measures offer "something more – and something less – than objective medical ratings" (Quesnel-Vallee

2007), especially because of the incomplete understanding of what true health is.

In May, 2002, in a survey of a representative sample of households in the five West Bank towns invaded by the Israeli military during March and April, 2002 (Giacaman et al 2004), responders reported high psychological distress at home, including sleeplessness, uncontrollable fear and shaking episodes, fatigue, depression, and hopelessness, and enuresis and uncontrolled crying episodes in children. Distress was highest in Ramallah (93%), Tulkarm (91%), Jenin (89%), Bethlehem (87%), and Nablus (71%). It was also associated with the imposition of curfews, bombing and shooting, loss of home, displacement, degradation of quality of housing, including interruption of utilities such as electricity and water, and the consequent destruction of food supplies, shortages of food and cash, and no access to medical services.

According to the UN, studies done in the Gaza Strip in 2008 also showed high distress and fears, especially in children (UN 2008). Children were highly exposed to traumatic events, such as witnessing a relative being killed, seeing mutilated bodies, and having homes damaged. These studies also reported several psychosocial problems, including behavioral problems, fears, speech difficulties, anxiety, anger, sleeping difficulties, lack of concentration at school, and difficulties in completing homework.

Palestinians are people who were never safe (Das 2006), even before the 1967 Israeli occupation of the West Bank and Gaza Strip. The trauma of the 1948

Table 3. Insecurities and Threats in a Random Sample of the Population of the Occupied Palestinian Territory

Question	Sample (n)	Not at all	A little	Moderate amount or more	Very much or extremely
To what extent do you fear for yourself in your daily life?	1008	19% (1.24)	24% (1.35)	27% (1.40)	30% (1.44)
To what extent do you fear for your family in your daily life?	1004	5% (0.69)	9% (0.90)	19% (1.24)	67% (1.48)
To what extent do you fear for the safety of your family?	1004	5% (0.69)	12% (1.03)	19% (1.24)	64% (1.51)
To what extent does your family fear for your safety?	1007	4% (0.62)	9% (0.90)	17% (1.18)	70% (1.44)
To what extent do you currently feel threatened by not being able to provide for your family?	994	7% (0.81)	16% (1.16)	24% (1.35)	53% (1.58)
To what extent do you currently feel threatened by losing your family income?	980	8% (0.87)	15% (1.14)	19% (1.25)	58% (1.58)
To what extent do you currently feel threatened by losing your home?	999	23% (1.33)	19% (1.24)	12% (1.03)	46% (1.58)
To what extent do you currently feel threatened by losing your land?	633	21% (1.62)	18% (1.53)	14% (1.38)	47% (1.98)
To what extent do you currently feel threatened by displacement or uprooting?	1000	24% (1.35)	16% (1.16)	16% (1.16)	44% (1.57)
To what extent do you feel worried over your future and the future of your family?	1008	3% (0.54)	11% (0.99)	18% (1.21)	68% (1.47)

Note: Data are percentage (SE)
Source: The Palestinian Quality of Life Study, December, 2005. Data were calculated by the authors using the Palestinian life quality dataset.

nakba – the dispossession and dispersion of Palestinians – is imprinted in the collective consciousness to this day. Moreover, Palestinians' quality of life is very low, and their daily lives are constantly under threat. People live in alarm and pain because of current life events, but also because of the history of mass trauma that is part of their collective consciousness. Their sense of future is shaped by past and present violations. Their experiences of violations inform their future, and expectation of danger and threats prepares them ceaselessly for how to respond (Kleinman et al 1996), and to undertake daily life.

Palestinians have been enduring social suffering (Kleinman et al 1996) associated with war – a notion that includes socio-cultural aspects of the experience of pain, and entails new ways of treatment and management that go beyond biomedical conceptualizations. Social suffering seeks to explain people's realities in ways that cannot be explained by objective measurements (Wilkinson 2006). Personal psychological or medical problems are regarded as inseparable from societal issues (Darby 2006).

The idea of social suffering combines into a single space conditions that are usually separated into sectors (such as health, welfare, and judicial) because these conditions originate in the overpowering injustices that social forces inflict on human experience (Das 2006). Social suffering removes the artificial division between health and social

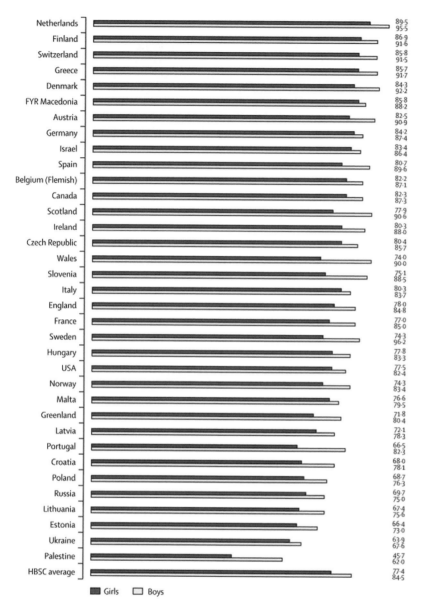

	Girls	Boys
Netherlands	89·5	95·5
Finland	86·9	91·6
Switzerland	85·8	91·5
Greece	85·7	91·7
Denmark	84·3	92·2
FYR Macedonia	85·8	88·2
Austria	82·5	90·9
Germany	84·2	87·4
Israel	83·4	86·4
Spain	80·7	89·6
Belgium (Flemish)	82·2	87·1
Canada	82·3	87·3
Scotland	77·9	90·6
Ireland	80·3	88·0
Czech Republic	80·4	85·7
Wales	74·0	90·0
Slovenia	75·1	88·5
Italy	80·3	83·7
England	78·0	84·8
France	77·0	85·0
Sweden	74·3	96·2
Hungary	77·8	83·3
USA	77·5	82·4
Norway	74·3	83·4
Malta	76·6	79·5
Greenland	71·8	80·4
Latvia	72·1	78·3
Portugal	66·5	82·3
Croatia	68·0	78·1
Poland	68·7	76·3
Russia	69·7	75·0
Lithuania	67·4	75·6
Estonia	66·4	73·0
Ukraine	63·9	67·6
Palestine	45·7	62·0
HBSC average	77·4	84·5

Figure 4. Life-satisfaction scores of 15-year-old students in 35 selected countries. Source: HBSC=health behavior in school-aged children.

issues in ways that promote an understanding of how both individual and collective suffering pose threats to health. In the Palestinian context, the shared experience of violence and trauma has implications for a shared sense of need for community security.

Humiliation is a central tactic of war, often cited by the Israeli and international press as one of the daily experiences that Palestinians must withstand (Haaretz 2003) and as a form of Israeli control over Palestinian lives. In the occupied Palestinian territory,

violence includes chronic exposure to humiliation, which is associated with negative mental health (Giacaman et al 2007b). Humiliation is a form of violation, identified as a component of the suffering of victims of war in need of acknowledgment and restoration of dignity (Leaning 2004). The strong sense of family and community in Palestinians of the occupied Palestinian territory has helped them to sustain high community cohesion and communal survival (Barber 2001), despite the realities described above, including constant humiliation.

321

Health System

The current Palestinian health system is made up of fragmented services that grew and developed over generations and across different regimes. During the nineteenth century, Christian missionaries from the Western countries established some hospitals that are still operating in East Jerusalem. During the early part of the 20th century, the British Mandate expanded these services (Ben-Arieh 1995).

The 1948 nakba led the UN General Assembly to establish the UN Relief and Works Agency in 1949 (UNRWA 2009b). Since then, the UN Relief and Works Agency has been delivering various key services to registered Palestinian refugees, including food aid, housing, education, and health services, not only in the occupied Palestinian territory, but also in Jordan, Lebanon, and Syria.

From 1950 to 1967, the West Bank was annexed by the Hashemite Kingdom of Jordan, and the Gaza Strip came under Egyptian military administration. Although Egyptian and Jordanian state services for education and health expanded, rural areas in the West Bank, where most people lived, remained mainly untouched by these developments (Graham-Brown 1984). Palestinians responded by building a network of charitable health services. During this period, private Palestinian medical services also grew and developed (Barghouthi & Giacaman 1990).

Between 1967 and 1993, health services for Palestinians in the occupied Palestinian territory were neglected and starved of funds by the Israeli military administration, with shortages of staff, hospital beds, medications, and essential and specialized services, forcing Palestinians to depend on health services in Israel (Giacaman 1994). For example, in 1975 the West Bank health budget was substantially lower than that of one Israeli hospital for the same year (Katbeh 1977). The Palestinian response was to create independent Palestinian services through health, women's, agricultural, and student social-action groups, all promoting community steadfastness on the land (*sumud*). This response also led to the development of a Palestinian health and medical care infrastructure, independent of the Israeli military that still helps to meet the health needs of the population, especially during emergencies.

The Palestinian Ministry of Health was established after the Oslo accords in 1994, and inherited, from the Israeli military government, health services that had been neglected. Supported by massive funding from international donors (Schoenbaum et al 2005), the ministry has since upgraded and expanded the health-system infrastructure by institution building and human-resource development (Hamdan & Defever 2003). The number of hospitals, hospital beds, and primary health care centers in the country increased, a public-health laboratory was established, and a health-information system and a planning unit were set up. Planning for the development of the health sector began during this period, and entailed some coordination with the UN Relief and Works Agency, local non-governmental organizations, and the private medical sector in developing policies and protocols (Giacaman et al 2003).

By 2006, the number of hospital beds managed by the Palestinian Ministry of Health had increased by 53% compared with that of 1994, with a similar increase in the number of available hospital beds in non-governmental organizations and private sectors (Palestinian National Authority 2010). The Palestinian Ministry of Health currently operates 24 of 78 hospitals, which have 57% of all hospital beds in the West Bank and Gaza Strip (Table 4). Also, the number of primary health care facilities increased between 2000 and 2005 (Table 5), with 416 of 654 centres managed by the Palestinian Ministry of Health. 170 facilities opened in less than 13 years. Similarly, the UN Relief and Works Agency facilities have increased in number, but not those of non-governmental organizations.

By 2006, about 40,000 people were employed in different sectors of the health system, with 33% employed by the Palestinian Ministry of Health (Table 6). Health-related human resources in Palestinian institutions of higher learning also grew. Although a shortage of health personnel exists in many specialties (especially in family medicine, surgery, internal medicine, neurology, dermatology, psychiatry, pathology, anesthesiology, nephrology, nursing, and midwifery), there is an excess in others (such as dentistry, pharmacy, laboratory technology, and radiology technology) (Palestinian National Authority 2010), suggesting the need for rationalization of the educational programs of Palestinian institutions of higher learning.

At present, all four main health-service providers (the Palestinian Ministry of Health, the UN Relief and Work Agency, non-governmental organizations, and the private medical sector) contribute to all areas of health care. However, because of various factors, including little health-service development under the Israeli military administration between 1967 and

Table 4. Distribution of Hospital Beds by Health Care Provider

	West Bank (population: 2,350,000)			Gaza Strip (population: 1,420,000)			OPT (population: 3,770,000)		
	Number of hospitals	Number of beds (1.2*)	Percentage of beds	Number of hospitals	Number of beds (1.4*)	Percentage of beds	Number of hospitals	Number of beds (1.3*)	Percentage of beds
PMoH	12	1316	44.4%	12	1548	75.4%	24	2864	57.1%
UNRWA	1	63	2.1%	0	0	0.0%	1	63	1.3%
NGOs	20	1183	40.0%	8	399	19.4%	28	1582	31.6%
Private	21	399	13.5%	2	34	1.7%	23	433	8.6%
PMS	0	0	0.0%	2	72	3.5%	2	72	1.4%
Total	*54*	*2961*	..	*24*	*2053*	..	*78*	*5014*	*100%*

*Hospital beds per 1000 people.
Pop=population. UNRWA=UN Relief and Works Agency. PMoH=Palestinian Ministry of Health. PMS=Police medical services.
NGOs=non-governmental organizations.
Source: The Palestinian National Authority.

Table 5. Distribution of the Primary Health Care Facilities by Health Care Provider in 2000 and 2005

	2000			2005			Increase in PHC facilities %
	West Bank	Gaza Strip	Total	West Bank	Gaza Strip	Total	
Population	2,011,930	1,138,126	3,150,056	2,372,216	389,789	3,762,005	–
PMoH PHC facilities	316	43	359	360	56	416	16%
NGO PHC facilities	145	40	185	130	55	185	0%
UNRWA PHC facilities	34	17	51	35	18	53	4%
Total PHC facilities	495	100	595	525	129	654	10%
Number of people PHC facilities	4065	11381	5294	4519	10774	5752	–

UNRWA = UN Relief and Works Agency; PHC = primary health care; PMoH = Palestinian Ministry of Health; NGO = non-governmental organization.
Source: Palestinian National Authority.

1993, and poor governance and mismanagement of the Palestinian Authority, current services have been unable to provide adequately for people's needs, especially in tertiary health care. Therefore, the Palestinian Ministry of Health continues to refer patients elsewhere (Israel, Egypt, and Jordan), leading to a substantial drain of health resources.

Conventional indicators of health-system function, focusing on the number of patients who use services, the number of hospitals, hospital beds, and primary health care facilities, and the number of personnel, mask an underlying issue of low quality of care. Several types of health services fail to meet consistent standards for training, equipment, and overall quality. This low quality of care is partly due to restricted mobility inhibiting effective health-system function, management, and accountability; the presence of under-qualified health care providers; and weak institutional capacity for monitoring and assessment (Schoenbaum et al 2005; Wick et al 2005). This issue will be addressed more fully in the other reports of this Series.

The Palestinian Ministry of Health recognizes its weak role in the organization, regulation, and

Table 6. Health Employees

	Number			Ratio per 1000 people							
	OPT			OPT			Other countries				
	WB	GS	Total	WB	GS	Total	Jordan	Egypt	Israel	UK	Canada
Physicians	4337	3711	8048	1.8	2.6	2.1	2.0	0.50	3.8	2.3	2.10
Dentists	1355	680	2035	0.6	0.5	0.5	1.3	0.10	1.2	1.1	0.60
Pharmacists	2242	1600	3842	1.0	1.1	1	3.1	0.10	0.7	4.5	0.70
Nurses	2452	4200	6652	1.0	2.9	1.7	3.0	2.00	6.3	12.2	10.00
Midwives	..	..	449	..	..	0.1	0.3	<0.1	0.2	0.6	..
Paramedics	7421	3100	10521	3.0	2.2	2.7	1.2	0.10	..	2.8	..
Administrative	4263	3257	7520	1.7	2.3	1.9	3.2	0.10	..	21.2	..

OPT = Occupied Palestinian Territory; GS = Gaza Strip; WB = West Bank.
Source: Palestinian National Authority.

supervision of the health sector, and in the coordination of policy making and planning among health care providers, especially those of the private sector. Several factors, some internal and some external to the health and political systems, account for the inability of the ministry of health to assume the stewardship role needed to build a health system.

First, despite substantial funding and efforts made by the Palestinian Ministry of Health to build a Palestinian health system, the obstacles to planned development have proved too great. Restrictions placed by Israel since 1993 on the free movement of Palestinian goods and labor across borders between the West Bank and Gaza, and within the West Bank, have had damaging effects not only on the economy and society (Roy 1999), but also on the attempts of the Palestinian National Authority at system building. The physical separation (USAID 2007) and complicated system of permits required to go from the Gaza Strip to the West Bank resulted in the emergence of two Palestinian Authority ministries of health, one in the Gaza Strip and the other in the West Bank. Since 2007, this separation has been further compounded by the political divide between Fatah and Hamas.

Second, the absence of any control by the Palestinian National Authority over water, land, the environment, and movement within the occupied Palestinian territory has made a public-health approach to health-system development difficult, if not impossible. These issues have been exacerbated by the dysfunctional political and institutional systems of the authority;

the damaging effects on ministries of using the authority resources for patronage to secure loyalty; marginalization of the Palestinian Legislative Council; and corruption and cronyism (Sayigh 2007), all of which led to a rapid increase in the number of health-service employees of the Palestinian National Authority without evident improvement in the quality of health services (Giacaman et al 2003). These factors have adversely affected an already fragile health service.

Third, the multiplicity of donors with different agendas and the dependence of the Palestinian National Authority on donor financial assistance have also caused program fragmentation. Most occupied Palestinian territory health budget is financed by donor agencies. The Palestinian Authority is estimated to have received US$840.5 million in aid between 1994 and 2000 (Sayigh 2007). Donors have an influential role in determining the policy of the authority (Hamdan et al 2003). The American Rand Corporation has indicated that donors prefer to support infrastructural – mostly equipment and construction – over the operating expenses of the Palestinian National Authority health sector (Schoenbaum et al 2009), which have increased as a result of expanded infrastructure and the introduction of modern equipment. The consequences of this substantial but uncoordinated investment will be considered in more detail by Mataria and colleagues (2009b) in this Series.

All these interacting factors have contributed to undermine the ability of Palestinians to build a health system from existing health services. In addition to the need for control over resources for health care, building an effective health system requires sovereignty, self-determination, authority, and control over land, water, the environment, and movement of people and goods, all of which are relevant for the protection and promotion of health. The international community has not appreciated the degree to which the Palestinian National Authority is "less than a state, yet expected to act like a state" (Sayigh 2007).

Discussion

We have shown that, after a period of improvement in Palestinian health in the occupied Palestinian territory, socio-economic conditions have deteriorated since the mid-1990s, with a humanitarian crisis emerging in the Gaza Strip and intensifying as a result of the Israeli military invasion in December, 2008, and January, 2009, and because of destruction of homes and infrastructure, the death and injury of civilians, and shortages of food, fuel, medicines, and other essentials, all requiring urgent world concern. We have also described the severe constraints imposed on the Palestinian National Authority in its attempts to build the Palestinian health care and other systems in response to threats to the health of the population. Ironically, the year when the UN announced its Millennium Development Goals was also the year when the occupied Palestinian territory fell into a phase of political and economic crisis, with widespread poverty and a high prevalence of extreme poverty.

Our analysis of Palestinian health in the occupied Palestinian territory has used not only conventional indicators of health, such as infant mortality and stunting in children, but also survey data for subjective measures of people's experiences, life quality, and ratings of health status. The human security framework prompted us to consider and analyze health more comprehensively, and has shown some of the indicators that need to be measured beyond body counts and traditional measures of morbidity. Indicators of human insecurity and social suffering seem essential in the study of the consequences for health and well-being of war and conflict. We hope that our analysis of the Palestinian experience will assist in extending and informing the debate on the notion of health, and on the way that it is monitored and assessed, especially during conflict. Data summarized

here indicate that conventional explanations of poor health need to move to grounds that are often ignored, including the consequences for health of social, economic, and political exclusion, and the lack of basic freedoms, disempowerment, fear, and distress (Marmot 2006).

Because of the current political and contextual constraints, no comprehensive agenda for improving health and services in the occupied Palestinian territory can be outlined with any confidence. Recommendations for improving Palestinian health-service performance and the quality of care will be outlined in the other reports in this Series, in addition to recommendations to assist international donors to develop policies that are appropriate to the extraordinary contextual needs of the population. Policies must take into account the need to protect Palestinians from the severe insecurities of continuous colonization and war-like conditions, where the home front is the battlefront (Jolly & Basu Ray 2006; Leaning et al 2004a). Neither the Palestinian National Authority nor the international community have succeeded in protecting Palestinian civilians either from Israeli aggression or from the consequences of recent inter-Palestinian violence.

Our account of Palestinian health under Israeli military occupation – the longest occupation in modern history – also calls for the protection of the basic human rights of Palestinians, in compliance with the Geneva Conventions, including the right to justice and to health. This demand for rights and justice is at the center of plans to improve Palestinian health. However, it cannot be met by medical and humanitarian interventions alone, because such interventions leave the causes of ill health in the occupied Palestinian territory untouched. We concur with the judgment of the World Bank that economic growth cannot be achieved and donor assistance will not produce durable results without serious improvements in security, dismantling Israeli restrictions on the movement of people and goods, and achieving progress on Palestinian reform and institution building (The World Bank 2007).

Finally, we return to where we started – the WHO Commission on Social Determinants of Health – and the evidence that it has assembled on the factors that affect health and identifying what can be done to improve health (CSDH 2008). Our analysis shows that, although substantial aid can alleviate some of the short-term effects of a socio-economic crisis, it does not tackle the root causes of ill health. Hope for improving the health and quality of life of Palestinians will exist only once people recognize that the structural and political conditions that they endure in the occupied Palestinian territory are the key determinants of population health.

Acknowledgments

We thank the *Lancet* Palestine Steering Group (Iain Chalmers, Jennifer Leaning, Harry Shannon, and Huda Zurayk) for reading, discussing, and commenting on several drafts of this report; Graham Watt, Andrea Becker, Margaret Lock, and Karl Sabbagh for their valuable comments and support, and Will Boyce for the provision of the life satisfaction figure contained in this report; Medical Aid for Palestinians UK, University of Oslo, Institute of General Practice and Community Medicine, and the Norwegian Programme for Development, Research, and Education for their financial contributions that made the workshops related to this Series possible; and the anonymous reviewers of this report, whose comments improved this final draft substantially.

References

Abdul-Rahim HF, Wick L, Halileh S, et al (2009) Maternal and child health in the occupied Palestinian territory. *Lancet*, 373(9667): 967–977

Abu Libdeh Hovensen G, Brunborg H (1993) Population characteristics and trends. *In*: M Heiberg, G Ovensen (Eds.) *Palestinian society in Gaza, West Bank and Arab Jerusalem. A survey of living conditions* (p. 35–38). Oslo, Norway: FAFO

Abu Libdeh H, Smith C, Nabris K, Shahin M (1992) *Survey of infant and child mortality in the West Bank and Gaza Strip*. Jerusalem, OPT: UNICEF and the Jerusalem Family Planning and Protection Association

Abu Mourad T, Radi S, Shashaa S, Lionis C, Philatithis A (2008) Palestinian primary health care in light of the National Strategic Health Plan 1999–2003. *Public Health*, 122: 125–139.

Baker A, Kanan H (2003) Psychological impact of military violence on children as a function of distance from traumatic events: The Palestinian case. *Intervention*, 1: 13–21

Baker A, Shalhoub-Kevorkian N (1999) Effects of political and military trauma on children: The Palestinian case. *Clinical Psychological Review*, 19: 935–950

Barber BK (2001) Political violence, social integration, and youth functioning: Palestinian youth from the Intifada. *Journal of Community Psychology*, 29: 259–280

Barghouthi M, Giacaman R (1990) The emergence of an infrastructure of resistance: The case of health. *In*: JR Nassar, R Heacock (Eds.) *Intifada, Palestine at the crossroads* (p. 73–87). New York, NY: Praeger

Batniji R, Rabaia Y, Nguyen-Gillham V, et al (2009) Health as human security in the occupied Palestinian territory. *Lancet*, 373(9669): 1133–1143

Benach J, Muntaner C, Santana V (Chairs) (2007) *Employment conditions and health inequalities. Final report to the WHO. Employment conditions knowledge network (EMCONET), Commission on Social Determinants of Health (CSDH)*. September 20, 2007

Ben-Arieh Y (1975) The growth of Jerusalem in the nineteenth century. *Annals of the Association of American Geographers*, 65: 263–264

Black RE, Allen LH, Bhutta ZA, et al (2008) Maternal and child undernutrition 1. Maternal and child undernutrition: Global and regional exposures and health consequences. *Lancet*, 371(9608): 243–260

B'tselem (2008) Statistics, fatalities. Available from http://www.btselem.org/english/statistics/Casualties.asp [Accessed 13 August 2008]

Caballero-Anthony M (2004) Human security and primary health care in Asia: Realities and challenges. *In*: L Chen (Ed.) *Global health challenges for human security* (p. 234–255). Boston, MA: Harvard University Press

Chen L, Narasimhan V (2004) Global health and human security. *In*: L Chen (Ed.) *Global health challenges for human security* (p. 183–189). Boston, MA: Harvard University Press

Commission on Social Determinants of health (CSDH) (2006) *Closing the gap in a generation: Health equity through action on the social determinants of health, Final report of the Commission on Social Determinants of Health*. Available from http://whqlibdoc.who.int/publications/2008/9789241563703_eng.pdf [Accessed 29 Nov 2008]

Commission on Social Determinants of Health (CSDH), The World Health Organization (2006) WHO/WIP/EQH/OI/2006. Available from http://www.who.int/social_determinants/resources/csdh_brochure.pdf [Accessed 30 November 2008]

Dahlan A (2006) *Levels and trends of infant and child mortality in the Gaza Strip: A fieldwork survey.*

Darby P (2006) Security, spatiality and social suffering. *Alternatives*, 31: 453–473

Declaration of principles on interim self-government arrangements. Available from http://www.mfa.gov.il/MFA/Peace%20Process/Guide%20to%20the%20Peace%20Process/Declaration%20of%20Principles [Accessed 25 March 2008]

Giacaman G (1998) In the throes of Oslo: Palestinian society, civil society, and the future, In: Giacaman G, Lonning D (Eds.) *After Oslo: New realities, old problems* (p. 1–51). London, UK: Pluto Press

Giacaman R (1994) *Health conditions and services in the West Bank and Gaza Strip.* United Nations Conference on Trade and Development, UNCTAD/ECDC/SEU/3. September 28

Giacaman R, Abdul-Rahim HF, Wick L (2003) Health sector reform in the occupied Palestinian Territory (OPT): Targeting the forest or the tree? *Health Policy Planning,* 18: 59–67

Giacaman R, Abu-Rmeileh NME, Husseini A, Saab H, Boyce W (2007b) Humiliation: The invisible trauma of war for Palestinian youth. *Public Health,* 121: 563–571

Giacaman R, Husseini A, Gordon NH, Awartani F (2004) Imprints on the consciousness. *European Journal of Public Health,* 14: 286–290

Giacaman R, Shannon H, Saab H, Arya N, Boyce W (2007a) Individual and collective exposure to political violence: Palestinian adolescents coping with conflict. *European Journal of Public Health,* 17: 361–368

Gould WT (1998) African mortality and the new 'urban penalty'. *Health Place,* 4: 171–181

Graham-Brown S (1984) Impact on the social structure of Palestinian society. In: N Aruri (Ed.) *Occupation, Israel over Palestine* (p. 223–254). UK: Zed Books Limited

Hamdan M, Defever M, Abdeen Z (2003) Organizing health care within political turmoil: The Palestinian case. *International Journal of Health Planning and Management,* 18: 63–87

Hamdan M, Defever M (2003) Human resources for health in Palestine: A policy analysis. Part I: Current

situation and recent developments. *Health Policy,* 64: 243–259

Hammami R, Hilal J (2001) An uprising at the crossroads. *Middle East Report,* 219: 2–7

Harel A (2008) *IDF to dismantle 2·5 kilometers of separation fence at cost of NIS 50m.* Available from http://www.haaretz.com/hasen/spages/1006195.html [Accessed 29 July 2008]

Hill A (1983) The Palestinian population of the Middle East. *Population and Development Review,* 9: 293–316

Human Rights Watch (2007) *World report.* Available from http://hrw.org/englishwr2k7/docs/2007/01/11/isrlpa14707.htm [Accessed 30 November 2007]

Humiliation at the Checkpoints (2008) *Haaretz.* Available from http://www.haaretz.com/hasen/pages/ShArt.jhtml?itemNo=315603&contrassID=2&subContrassID=3&sbSubContrassID=0&listSrc=Y [Accessed 8 August 2008]

Husseini A, Abu-Rmeileh NM, Mikki N, et al (2009) Cardiovascular diseases, diabetes mellitus, and cancer in the occupied Palestinian territory. *Lancet,* 373(9668): 1041–1049

International Commission of Jurists in Israel (2008) *Israel's separation barrier: Challenges to the rule of law and human rights: Part III and IV.* Available from http://www.icj.org/news.php3?id_article=3411&lang=en [Accessed 20 March 2008]

Israel Ministry of Health (1994) *Health in Judea/Samaria and Gaza 1967–1994.* Jerusalem, Israel: State of Israel and Ministry of Health

Jolly R, Basu Ray D (2006) The human security framework and national human development reports. Human Development Report Office. National Human Development Report Series, NHDR occasional paper 5. *May 2006*

Jong-wook L (2005) Public health is a social issue. *Lancet,* 365: 1005

Katbeh S (1977) The status of health services in the West Bank. Jordan Medical Council 1977, (in Arabic)

Khalidi R (1991) Arab nationalism: Historical problems in the literature. *American Historical Review,* 96: 1363–1373

Khawaja M (2000) The recent rise in Palestinian fertility: Permanent or transient? *Population Studies,* 54: 331–346

Kimmerling B (1992) Sociology, ideology, and nation-building: The Palestinians and their meaning in Israeli sociology. *American Sociological Review,* 57: 446–460

King G, Murray CJL (2001) Rethinking human security. *Political Sciences,* 116: 585–610

Kleinman A, Das V, Lock M (1996) Introduction. *Daedalus,* 125: XI–XX

Leaning J, Arie S, Holleufer G, Bruderlein C (2004a) Human security and conflict: A comprehensive approach. In: L Chen (Ed.) *Global health challenges for human security* (p. 13–30). Boston, MA: Harvard University Press

Leaning J, Arie S, Stites E (2004b) Human security in crisis and transition. *Praxis,* XIX: 9–10

Marmot MG (2006) Status syndrome: A challenge to medicine. *Journal of the American Medical Association,* 295: 1304–1307

Mataria A, Giacaman R, Stefanini A, Naidoo N, Kowal P, Chatterji S (2009a) The quality of life of Palestinians living in chronic conflict: Assessment and determinants. *European Journal of Health Economics,* 10: 93–101

Mataria A, Khatib A, Donaldson C, et al (2009) The health-care system: An assessment and reform agenda. *Lancet,* 373(9670): 1207–1217

Mendez MA, Adair LS (1999) Severity and timing of stunting in the first two years of life affect performance on cognitive tests in late childhood. *Journal of Nutrition,* 129: 1555–1562

Myre G (2008) *Olmert outlines plans for Israel's borders, The New York Times*. Available from http://www.nytimes.com/2006/03/10/international/middleeast/10mideast.html [Accessed 7 August 2008]

New Palestinian Cabinet Sworn. *In*: BBC News. Available from http://news.bbc.co.uk/2/hi/middle_east/6760975.stm [Accessed 26 November 2008]

Palestinian Central Bureau of Statistics (1996) *Demographic survey 1995*.

Palestinian Central Bureau of Statistics (2006) *Demographic and health survey 2004, Final report* 2004, February, 2006

Palestinian Central Bureau of Statistics & League of Arab States (2007a) *Palestinians Family Health Survey*, Preliminary Report, April, 2007

Palestinian Central Bureau of Statistics (2007b) *Palestinian family health survey, 2006: Preliminary report, 2007*, Ramallah-Palestine: 20

Palestinian Central Bureau of Statistics (2007c) Palestinians in numbers 2007, *May*, 2008

Palestinian National Authority, Ministry of Health (2010) *Health Planning Unit, National Strategic Health Plan, Medium Term Development Plan 2008–2010*. Draft: 14

Palestinian National Authority & Palestinian Central Bureau of Statistics (2006) *Demographic and health survey – 2004, Final report*. February, 2006. Ramallah-Palestine: 150

Palestinian National Authority & Palestinian Central Bureau of Statistics (2008a) *Injured Palestinians in Al-Aqsa Uprising (Intifada), by year and tool of injury*. Available from http://www.pcbs.gov.ps/Portals/_pcbs/intifada/98dd344c-21be-4672-a252-c6890e201d58.htm [Accessed Aug 13, 2008]

Population Reference Bureau Datafinder (2008a)Available from http://www.prb.org/Datafinder.aspx [Accessed 23 July 2008]

Population Reference Bureau Datafinder (2008b) Available from http://www.prb.org/Datafinder/Geography/Summary.aspx?region=123&region_type=2 [Accessed 23 July 2008]; http://www.prb.org/Datafinder/Geography/Summary.aspx?region=126&region_type=2 [Accessed 23 July 2008]

Population Reference Bureau Datafinder (2008c) Available from http://www.prb.org/Datafinder/Geography/Summary.aspx?region=130&region_type=2 [Accessed July 23, 2008].

Population Reference Bureau Datafinder (2008d) Available from http://www.prb.org/Datafinder/Geography/Summary.aspx?region=9&region_type=2 [Accessed 23 July 2008]

Programme of Assistance to the Palestinian People (2008) *Palestinian economy. Country: Land, people and government*, UNCTAD. Available from http://r0.unctad.org/palestine/economy1.htm [Accessed 25 March 2008]

Quesnel-Vallee A (2007) Self-rated health: Caught in the crossfire of the question for 'true' health? *International Journal of Epidemiology*, 36: 1161–1164

Question of Palestine (2008) *History*. Available from http://www.un.org/Depts/dpa/ngo/history.html [Accessed 20 March 2008]

Reuters (2008) *Britain's Hamas boycott counterproductive – lawmakers*. Available from. http://www.reuters.com/article/middleeastCrisis/idUSL10906661 [Accessed 13 August 2008]

Rogan EL, Shlaim An (2001) *The war for Palestine. Rewriting the History of 1948*. Cambridge, MA: Cambridge University Press

Roy S (1999) De-development revisited: Palestinian economy and society since Oslo. *Journal of Palestine Studies*, 28: 64–82

Said EW (1974) Arabs and Jews. *Journal of Palestinian Studies*, 3: 3–14

Salomon J, Tandon A, Murray CJL (2004) Comparability of self rated health: Cross sectional multi-country survey using anchoring vignettes. *British Medical Journal*, 328: 258–264

Sawaya AL, Martins P, Hoffman D, Roberts SB (2003) The link between childhood undernutrition and risk of chronic diseases in adulthood: A case study of Brazil. *Nutrition Review*, 61: 168–175

Sayigh Y (2007) Inducing a failed state in Palestine. *Survival*, 49: 7–40

Schoenbaum M, Afifi AK, Deckelbaum RJ (2005) Strengthening the Palestinian health system. *Rand Corporation*, 2005

Shu'aybi A, Shikaki K (2000) A window on the workings of the PA: An inside view. *Journal of Palestine Studies*, 117: 90

Skevington SM, Lotfy M, O'Connell KA (2004) The World Health Organization's WHOQOL-BREF quality of life assessment: Psychometric properties and results of the international field trial, A report from the WHOQOL Group. *Quality of Life Research*, 13: 299–310

Stewart-Brown S (1998) Emotional wellbeing and its relation to health. Physical disease may well result from emotional distress. *British Medical Journal*, 17: 1608–1609

Tang S, Meng Q, Chen L, Bekedam H, Evans T, Whitehead M (2008) Tackling the challenges to health equity in China. *Lancet*, 372: 1493–1501

The United Nations (2008a) *Question of Palestine*. Available from http://www.un.org/depts/dpa/ngo/history.html [Accessed 16 August 2008)

The United Nations (2008b) *Socio-economic achievements of the Palestinian people, 1993 – present. Building a public administration under the Palestinian Authority.*

Available from http://www.un.org/
Depts/dpi/palestine/ch9.pdf
[Accessed 14 January 2009]

The World Bank (2007a) *Two years
after London: Restarting Palestinian
economic recovery. Economic
monitoring report to the
Ad Hoc Laison Committee.*
2 September 2007

The World Bank (2007b) *Implementing
the Palestinian reform and
development agenda. Economic
monitoring report to the Ad Hoc
Laison Committee.* Available from
http://siteresources.worldbank.org/
INTWESTBANKGAZA/
Resources/WorldBank
AHLCMay2,08.pdf [Accessed
1 December 2008]

The World Health Organization
(2008a)*Health status statistics:
Morbidity, children under five
years of age.* Available from
http://www.who.int/healthinfo/
statistics/indchildren
stunted/en/index.html [Accessed 21
June 2008].

UNDP. Human Development Reports
(2008a) *Egypt.* Available from
http://hdrstats.undp.org/
countries/country_fact_sheets/
cty_fs_EGY.html [Accessed 23 July
2008].

UNDP. Human Development Reports
(2008b) *Israel.* Available from
http://hdrstats.undp.org/
countries/country_fact_sheets/
cty_fs_ISR.html [Accessed 23 July
2008]

UNDP. Human Development Reports
(2008c) *Jordan.* Available
fromhttp://hdrstats.undp.org/
countries/country_fact_sheets/
cty_fs_JOR.html [Accessed July 2008]

UNDP. Human Development Reports
(2008d) *Lebanon.* Available from
http://hdrstats.undp.org/
countries/country_fact_sheets/
cty_fs_LBN.html [Accessed July
2008]

UNDP. Human Development Reports
(2008e) *Occupied Palestinian
Territories.* Available from http://
hdrstats.undp.org/countries/

country_fact_sheets/cty_fs_PSE.
html [Accessed July 2008]

UNDP. Human Development Reports
(2008f) *Syrian Arab Republic.*
Available from http://hdrstats.undp.
org/countries/country_fact_sheets/
cty_fs_SYR.html [Accessed July
2008]

UNICEF (2009)*UNICEF humanitarian
action update. Occupied Palestinian
territory.* Available from http://
www.reliefweb.int/rw/rwb.nsf/
db900SID/EGUA-7MLPG6?
OpenDocument [Accessed 14
January 2009]

United Nations, The World Bank,
Government of Norway (2009)
*Press release: Damage to civilian
infrastructure and institutions in
the West Bank estimated at 361
Million.* Jerusalem. Available from
http://www.reliefweb.int/rw/
rwb.nsf/db900sid/OCHA-
64CRTW?OpenDocument&
RSS20&RSS20=FS&Click=
[Accessed 13 January 2009]

United Nations (2008) *Gaza Strip inter-
agency humanitarian fact sheet.*
Available from http://domino.un.
org/pdfs/GSHFSMar08.pdf
[Accessed 2 August 2008]

UNRWA (2007) *Headquarters.*
Available from http://www.un.org/
unrwa/publications/pdf/uif-june07.
pdf [Accessed 24 December 2007]

UNRWA (2007) *Health Annual
Reports,* 1964–2003

UNRWA (2009a)*Establishment of
UNRWA.* Available from http://
www.un.org/unrwa/overview/
index.html [Accessed 13 January
2009]

UNRWA (2009b) *Statistics.* Available
from http://www.un.org/unrwa/
publications/index.html [Accessed
14 January 2009]

US Department of State (2007) *Quartet
statement on the agreement to form
a national unity government,*
Washington, DC: Office of the
Spokesman. Available from http://
www.state.gov/r/pa/prs/ps/2007/
february/80368.htm [Accessed 26
November 2008]

USAID (2007) *West Bank/Gaza
overview.* Available from http://
www.usaid.gov/pubs/bj2001/ane/
wbg/ [Accessed 30 November 2007]

Usher G (2004) Who are the
Palestinians? *New Statesman,* July
12, 2004: 18–20

Walker SP, Chang SM, Powell CA,
Granthan-McGregor SM (2005)
Effects of early childhood
psychosocial stimulation and
nutritional supplementation on
cognition and education in growth-
stunted Jamaican children:
Prospective cohort study. *Lancet,*
366: 1804–1807

WFP/UNRWA/FAO (2008) *Joint rapid
food security survey in the occupied
Palestinian territory.* Available from
http://documents.wfp.org/
stellent/groups/public/documents/
ena/wfp181837.pdf [Accessed 2
December 2008]

WHO Country Office in Jordan (2008)
Available from http://www.emro.
who.int/jordan/HealthIndicators.
htm [Accessed 23 July 2008]

WHO (2006) 8th issue, Health sector
surveillance indicators, monitoring
health and health sector in the OPT,
Jerusalem. *World Health
Organization,* 8 November 2006

Wick L, Mikki N, Giacaman R,
Abdul-Rahim H (2005) Childbirth
in Palestine. *International Journal
of Gynaecology and Obstetrics,*
89: 174–178

Wilkinson I (2006) Health, risk and
'social suffering'. *Health Risk
Society,* 8: 1

World Food Program, FAO (2009)
*West Bank and Gaza Strip.
Comprehensive food security and
vulnerability analysis (CFSVA).*
Available from http://home.wfp.
org/stellent/groups/public/
documents/vam/wfp191001.pdf
[Accessed 13 January 2009]

World Health Organization Regional
Office for the Eastern
Mediterranean (WHO/EMRO)
(2008b) *Country profiles.* Available
from http://www.emro.who.int/

329

emrinfo/index.asp?Ctry=egy [Accessed 23 July 2008]

WHO/EMRO (2008c) *Country profiles.* Available from http://www.emro. who.int/emrinfo/index.asp? Ctry=leb [Accessed 23 July 2008]

WHO/EMRO (2008d) *Country profiles.* Available from http://www.emro. who.int/emrinfo/index.asp? Ctry=syr [Accessed 23 July 2008]

WHO/EMRO, West Bank and Gaza Office (2008e) *Occupied Palestinian Territory. WHO in the occupied Palestinian territory.* Available from http://www.emro.who.int/Palestine/ index.asp?page=inpalestine [Accessed 23 July 2008]

World Health Organization/ West Bank and Gaza Office (2006) *Community mental health development in the occupied Palestinian territory: A work in progress with WHO.* WHO West Bank and Gaza Office. September 2006

World Health Organization (2008c) *Social determinants of health in countries in conflict: A perspective from the Eastern Mediterranean Region.* WHO/EMRO, Cairo, Egypt, 2008

World Health Organization (2008) *WHO quality of life-bref (WHOQOL BREF.* Available from http://www. who.int/substance_abuse/ research_tools/whoqolbref/en/ [Accessed 23 July 2008]

Chapter

25

Public Health in Crisis: Iraq

Salman Rawaf and David Rawaf

Iraq is a resource-rich country with three main sources of fortune: water, abundant reserves of oil and gas, and an educated populace. Long known to the world as *Mesopotamia*, Iraq's history goes back to the origins of civilization. Here, the first urban literate civilization was born; writing was invented by the Sumerians; mathematics, astronomy, and law by the Babylonians; and literacy and arts by the Assyrians. Kofa, 70 miles from Baghdad, and later Baghdad became the center of the Muslim world. The Ottoman Empire took control in the sixteenth century, followed by the British colonization at the end of the First World War. Iraq became an independent kingdom in 1921. In 1958, a republic was proclaimed but a series of military dictators have ruled the country since, the latest being Saddam Hussein, overthrown by the US-led invasion in 2003. This invasion, and subsequent occupation, was only a chapter in a series of tragic events that have devastated Iraq since 1980. This chapter describes the profound public health impacts of repeated wars and their consequences, critically examines efforts since 2003 to rebuild the health system, and proposes concrete steps to strengthen public health.

Population Health and Health Services Prior to the First Gulf War (Until 1980)

Iraq was a high- to middle-income country with a modern social infrastructure (Acheson 1992; UN & World Bank 2003). Abundant in natural resources, the Gross National Production (GNP) per capita in 1987 was $3508. Access to free comprehensive health services was nearly universal. Medical facilities and the public health system were well developed, probably the best in the region at the time, with a good capacity to respond to major public health issues.

Health indicators were better than neighboring countries. Health services were provided through well-staffed facilities including 185 (currently 220) public hospitals (a proportion of which offered specialist services) and at least 1600 (currently 2170) primary care health centers. Additionally, there were many private and military health establishments. Medical education was well-developed with 12 medical schools (currently 20). International agencies described the health infrastructure during this period as "a first class range of medical facilities including well-established public health services, hospitals, primary care facilities and ample production and supply of medicine and medical equipment" (UN & World Bank 2003).

Population Health and Health Services Under Recurrent Wars and Sanctions (1980–2003)

The public health impact of wars, sanctions, civil unrest and economic deterioration can be seen through examining three periods: the Iraq–Iran War (1980–1988); the period starting with the invasion of Kuwait, the US-led war to drive Iraqi forces out, the uprisings, and their brutal crushing, in the North and South, repeated attacks on Iraq and UN Sanctions (1990–2003); and the aftermaths of the 2003 US-led invasion.

1980–1988

The first few years of the Iraq–Iran war had limited impact on public health: it was business as usual in terms of development and capacity building, thanks to Iraq's large foreign reserves of more than $35 billion and support of Arab Gulf States. Nevertheless,

Public Health in the Arab World, ed. Samer Jabbour et al. Published by Cambridge University Press. © Samer Jabbour et al., 2012.

some health professionals lost their lives in the war and many left Iraq. From 1982 to 1987, the war was deadlocked and in 1984 the "war of cities" started with heavy tolls on civilian populations of both countries. In August 1988, Iran accepted a ceasefire, and Iraq declared a "victory." But what type of victory could this be, and at what cost, considering the more than 750,000 dead, the many more injured, the ravaged economy and enormous foreign debts of $85–$100 billion with the total cost of the war exceeding $500 billion? (Bennis & Moushabeck 1992)?

While Iraqis were relieved with the end of the war, several sinister movements were developing. Iraqi Kurds took advantage of Saddam's pre-occupation with war efforts and seized control of part of northern Iraq. Immediately after the declaration of the ceasefire with Iran, the central government launched the *Anfal* campaign (February to September 1988) where hundreds of villages were destroyed; thousands of people were killed or injured with large numbers fleeing to Turkey and Iran.

During most of the war years, health services remained functioning and up-to-date despite the population demands. However, gradually the health system, as other public services, started to deteriorate and incur huge debts. Damaged infrastructure continued to deteriorate. Internal and external migration of health professionals intensified. The government focused on a few national priorities, which did not include health and education. Re-construction of damaged towns and cities was slow due to limited financial resources.

1990–2003

Another catastrophe for Iraq and the Arab region unfolded in August 1990 with the invasion of Kuwait. Immediately afterward, the UN imposed on Iraq one of the harshest punitive sanctions in its history, the impact of which was immediately noted on Iraq's war-devastated economy. Under UN Resolution 678, a loose US-led coalition of 34 countries launched Operation Desert Storm on 17 January 1991 to "expel Iraqi troops from Kuwait." The 43-day campaign included an intensive air campaign followed by ground invasion of southern Iraq. The public health impact of yet another war proved devastating, resulting in a large loss of human life in addition to a complete breakdown of the civilian infrastructure, or more precisely, of what was left from the previous war. A UN

Under-Secretary General characterized the situation as "*nothing that we had seen or read had quite prepared us for the particular form of devastation which has now befallen the country. The recent conflict has wrought near-apocalyptic results upon the economic infrastructure of what had been, until January 1991, a rather highly urbanized and mechanized society. Now, most means of modern life support have been destroyed or rendered tenuous. Iraq has, for some time to come, been relegated to a pre-industrial age, but with all the disabilities of post-industrial dependency on an intensive use of energy and technology*" (Ahtissari 1991).

International mainstream media glorified the 1991 war, promoting the use of so-called "smart bombs" that achieve a "surgical precision" with minimal "collateral damage." In reality, the precision-guided bombs accounted for only 8.8% of the 84,200 tons of munitions dropped on Iraqis. Most of the bombs (91.2%) were unguided "dumb bombs" with an estimated accuracy of only 25% (Middle East Watch 1991). Depleted uranium was heavily used. Many highlighted that US-led forces violated international laws in not avoiding civilian casualities, in targeting civilians' infrastructures, and in using illegal weapons (Middle East Watch 1991; Clark 1992a, 1992b; Smith 1992). In 1991, uprisings in the North by Kurds and in the South by Shiites against Saddam's regime were brutally crushed leaving at least 30,000 dead, hundreds of villages destroyed, and large numbers of refugees and displaced. The public health impacts are summarized in Table 1.

The socio-economic impact of the wars and sanctions was heavy. Immediately after the 1991 war, with tightening of sanctions, inflation and poverty levels rose dramatically. In 1995, with an estimated gross domestic product (GDP) of US$715 and unemployment levels greater than 50%, almost half of families did not earn enough money to meet basic needs and lived below the poverty line. By January 2003, nearly 60% of Iraqis (approximately 14 million) depended entirely on government food subsidies that, by international standards, represented the minimum for human sustenance. Depleted resources forced many families to sell whatever they could. Local currency depreciated considerably. In 1989, one Iraqi dinar equaled US$3.30. In 2003, 2500 dinars equaled US $1. An average doctor earned around $7–10 a month and a school teacher $3–5 a month.

A grave humanitarian tragedy was unfolding as a vast majority of Iraqis were struggling to survive.

Table 1. The Public Health Impact of 1991 Gulf War and Its Aftermath

Area of impact	Magnitude/comments
Military casualties	100,000–200,000 Iraqi soldiers, mainly conscripts (many under "turkey's shooting" policy)*
Civilian casualties	–50,000 to 150,000 as a direct consequence of air bombing (3000 sorties a day), ground invasion and lack of humane living conditions (Middle East Watch 1991; Clark 1992a,b) –500,000 excess deaths among children under the age of 5 (Ali et al 2003) (Figure 2)
Civilian infrastructures	– Total devastation of what was a modern and growing civilian infrastructure –11 oil refineries, five oil pipelines, production facilities, and many oil tankers were hit (Clark 1991).
The environment	The massive air bombardment and land invasions left extensive damage to the environment and habitability of vast areas (Clark 1991)
Damage to health facilities	– 28 hospitals, 52 centers, and all military medical facilities were destroyed – Many hospitals were rendered dysfunctional – Surgical capacity was reduced to less than 10% (MOH-Iraq 2004; UNICEF-WHO 2003)
Civil uprising	– 30,000 killed by the brutal crushing of the uprisings in the North and South – Hundreds of villages were destroyed in Northern Iraq and in some cases chemical weapons were used (Johns 1999; Saletan 2003; Dybvik 1991) – >2,000,000 people fled for their lives – The march Arabs were relocated following the draining of the marshlands
Human rights abuses	Large scale terror and abuses started during the Iraq-Iran war era intensified the 1991 war and the uprisings. Many mass graves were later uncovered (Burns 2006; Johns 1999; Al-Shawaf & Rawaf 1995)
Dividing Iraq	– A security zone was created in the North (April 1991) and a no-fly zone in the South (May 1991). The UN declared these zones as "illegal" (Pilger 2000)
Tightening UN punitive sanctions	– Tightening of the UN punitive sanctions. They have had deleterious effects on all aspects of Iraqi life, and in particular people's health (Kandela 1998)
Impacts on health and services	– Infant mortality: rose from 47 per 1000 live births during 1984–89 to 108 per 1000 in 1994–1999 – Under 5 mortality: rose from 56 to 131 per 1000 live births (Eastman-Abaya 2000; Wakai 2000) – Health care fell below acceptable standards; large scale shortage of drugs; surgical practices were severely affected by the lack of sutures, anesthesia, medications, cauterizing devices, surgical gloves, and many other essential materials (Barnouti, 1996) – Human resource training declined substantially under the intellectual embargo and the complete international isolation (Al-Shawaf & Rawaf 1995; Richards & Wall 2000; Sansom 2004)
Severe restrictions on Iraqis' movements	Iraqi's movements were severely restricted within Iraq and internationally. This has had tremendous impacts on the medical education and training, especially as Iraqi professionals and institutions had many international links

In 1996, the situation was described as "18.8 million people in a refugee camp, one third of them are children, of whom at least 100,000 are now dead: not from war, but from hunger" (Table 1) (Simons 1996 quoting Salman Rawaf, p. 109). Hospital wards filled with malnourished children and much of the population maintained only a marginal nutritional status. Large numbers had a food intake lower than that of disaster-stricken populations in Africa. While various reports described the UN sanctions as leading to persistent deprivation, chronic hunger, endemic malnutrition, massive unemployment and widespread human suffering, Madeleine Albright, the US State Secretary, asserted in 1996 on *60 Minutes*

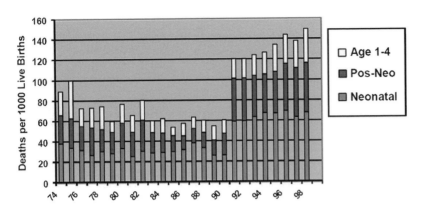

Figure 1. Infant mortality.

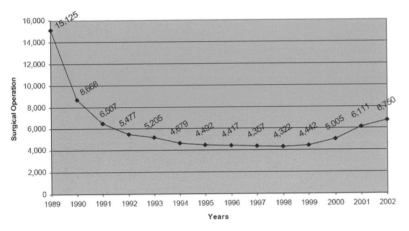

Figure 2. Surgical practices affected.

that US policy objectives were worth the deaths of thousands of Iraqi children. Eventually an estimated half a million Iraqi children would be sacrificed to the sanctions. Despite many warning reports by international agencies, including those of the UN such as the Food and Agriculture Programme, the UN continued the punitive sanctions. In 1996, Iraq was bankrupt. On its knees, it accepted the UN Security Resolution 986 (1995) and its "Oil-for-Food Programme" (OFFP 2004), allowing Iraq to export $1 billion worth of oil, 5% of which was paid to Kuwait as war compensation and $130 million allocated to the North where the majority of Iraqi Kurds were protected by the no-fly zone. Despite the OFFP, 12 million Iraqis lacked secure access to food and depended on the monthly food rations.

During this period, Iraq was subjected to frequent military attacks, the worst being a massive air raid in 1998 authorized by President Clinton under the pretext of lack of cooperation with inspectors searching for weapons of mass destruction (WMDs). The entire country fell to the mercy of many international organizations and non-governmental organizations (NGOs) providing poor quality services, in an unplanned and uncoordinated manner. Inspectors captured the media with confrontations with the Iraqi authority blamed for hiding WMDs. Meanwhile, ordinary people were subjected to the real WMDs: the increased brutality of the regime, UN punitive sanctions, and frequent military attacks on their economic and social infrastructures. Eastman-Abaya (2000) argued, "The UN, acting for the geopolitical interests of USA and Britain, is deliberately bringing about the destruction of Iraqi society."

During this period, population health dramatically deteriorated. Infant mortality soared to 108 per 1000, under-5 mortality 131 per 1000, and maternal mortality over 117 per 100,000 live births (Figure 1). Many senior physicians fled to neighboring countries and Europe. Health care fell below acceptable standards. Large scale shortage of drugs was reported. Surgical practices were severely affected due to lack of essential equipment (Figure 2) (Barnouti 1996). Human resource training declined substantially under the intellectual embargo and the complete international isolation.

Population Health and Health Services Following the US-Led Invasion in 2003

On the pretext of fabricated threats to the West from Saddam's WMDs, the US/British allied forces launched *"Operation Iraqi Liberation"* on March 20, 2003, without a UN mandate and despite vast international and popular protests. Once again military action brought more devastation to the economic, social, and health infrastructures in addition to the large numbers of deaths and injuries. During the 42 days of war, allied forces targeted a large number of public buildings, utilities, and communication networks. Some public hospitals and primary care centers were directly targeted: around 7% of hospitals were damaged and more than 12% were looted (Garfield 2003). Civil chaos was a main characteristic of the early weeks of the post-war period with widespread lootings, destruction of public buildings and private businesses, and total paralysis of civilian lives. This chaos emerged following the immediate abolition by the allied forces of the Iraqi army, its security forces, and civil servants. Coalition forces failed to protect public buildings and offices – except for the Ministry of Oil – despite international warnings. While the war was won, there was no clear post-war plan to win the peace (Frankish 2003; de Ceukelaire et al 2003).

As invasion turned into occupation, and occupation triggered an out-of-control insurgency and sectarian bloodshed from 2003 to 2008, much of the blame was allotted to Lieutenant-General Jay Garner and US Administrator to Iraq Paul Bremer, and the successive civil administrators and their Coalition Provisional Authority (CPA). Bremer took catastrophic decisions, first disbanding the army and the entire governmental civil structure and then ordering a blanket "de-Baathification" of the country. Many people with much needed expertise were either killed, imprisoned, or fled the country. Bremer fomented the insurgency, advised by new elites from outside Iraq, and did not understand the country he was to run (Rawaf 2005). Many Iraqis were angry at the way the CPA handled public service funds. Out of $20bn raised in oil revenues during the US-led rule, $8.8bn went unaccounted for. The sudden departure of Bremer in June 2004, without explanations for the missing billions, raised questions about the failure to prevent widespread fraud (BBC 2005).

While the majority of Iraqi people welcomed the removal of Hussein's regime and his three decades of tyranny and dictatorship, the post-war management failed to provide the promised security, freedom, and prosperity. Basic living commodities, such as safety, electricity, water, and petrol, were not available and promised rehabilitation and development efforts were halted. Between 2003 and 2008 many Iraqis found themselves again struggling to survive with almost 60% still solely dependent on monthly government food subsidies.

For the first time in Iraq's history, a clear and destructive ethnic and sectarian divide emerged. This division remained until June 28, 2004, when limited Iraqi sovereignty, under Prime Minister Ayad Allawi, was restored. Sectarian rivalries led to many revenge killings, displacements, and serious damage to businesses and properties and divided many areas as no-go zones to the opposite religious sects and amounted in many places to "ethnic cleansing." Such a division was a fertile ground for insurgency and organized crime. The continued occupation remains a source of embitterment among Iraqis.

The security situation was grave. More than 4 million people, mainly graduates, left the country, including 18,000 out of 34,000 physicians by 2006 (UN 2006). Some estimated that universities and hospitals had a loss of up to 80% of their professional staff. Approximately 2.8 million people were displaced internally (Zarocostas 2006). More than 200,000 people were killed by insurgencies, coalition forces, and criminals including an estimated 2,000 doctors by 2006. In October 2006, Jan Egeland, UN Under Secretary General indicated that "1,000 Iraqis are fleeing their homes every day, 365,000 people have been displaced in the last eight months, with 1.5 million displaced people throughout Iraq, revenge killings are totally out of control, 100 people are killed every day" (UN 2006). Many of those fleeing were highly educated people including doctors. Classified Pentagon documents leaked in October 2010 showed that there were more than 109,000 violent deaths instigated or committed by government forces and their agents between 2004 and the end of 2009 (BBC 2010).These included 66,081 civilians, 23,984 people classed as "enemy", and 15,196 members of the Iraqi security forces. These figures contradict earlier claims that the US coalition forces did not keep records of civilians killed. Many people were kidnapped including more than 250 doctors by 2006 (Zarocostas 2006; Ismael 2008). It is estimated that operations by the occupying forces and Iraqi police have killed twice as many Iraqis, most of them civilians, as attacks by "insurgents" (Youssef 2004).

Since 2008, parts of Iraq have witnessed considerable improvements in security. However, violence, corruption, mis-governance, unemployment, and lack of real investment in reconstruction remain real features of Iraq today. Table 2 summarizes the main impact of the 2003 invasion and subsequent mis-governance.

In a survey of Iraqi public opinion in December 2004 (IRI 2004) unemployment and health care were the two most important issues of concern to Iraqis (43% and 32%, respectively) despite ongoing violence. Furthermore, 14.2% cited access to health care as their first priority and 28.4% as their second. We will examine a limited number of health system issues that have proved crucial since 2003.

The health system. The level of devastation and neglect of the civil infrastructure in Iraq was somewhat of a surprise to the American administrators who took over the management of the health system. While they were keen to rebuild the Iraqi health system they were certainly lacking the experience of health systems outside the United States, were unfamiliar with critical aspects of assessment, always imposing an American model of health services, were reluctant to work with local and international organizations and unwilling to listen to other views. All these were contributing factors for achieving so little (Rawaf et al 2004; Burkle & Noji 2004). In a meeting of WHO Iraq and CPA Health Team in preparation for the Joint Workshop on Health Priorities in August 2003, one CPA member stated that the best thing for Iraqis is to privatize all the 198 large public hospitals and keep public only the 1700 primary care centers and public health functions. With this attitude, the experienced WHO team was thereafter mainly absorbed in "damage limitation" exercises rather than providing badly needed technical support.

Lack of security is one of the main negative influences on health in Iraq (*Lancet* 2003). Despite improved security since 2008, "insurgents" and criminals continue to threaten the life of doctors on a daily basis. Health professionals live and work in the most difficult working circumstances, under a hostile environment of violence, human right abuses, the

Table 2. Public Health Impact of the 2003 US-Led Invasion and Subsequent Occupation

Area of impact	Magnitude/comments
Military casualties	> 20,000
Civilian casualties	98,000 – 200,000 (Roberts et al. 2004; Horton, 2004)
Health professional casualties	> 2,000 Doctors; >1,500 other health professionals
Civilian infrastructures	All ministries (except Ministry of Oil), were looted. Destruction to civilian infrastructures including hospitals and clinics
The environment	No real assessment has been conducted but evidence accumulating of pollution and contamination (cluster bombs)
Food security	60% of population is still solely dependent on food distributed by the government each month; 1/3 of children are chronically malnourished
Damage to health facilities	– 7% of hospitals were damaged; 12% were looted
Human rights abuses	Committed by all parties including the coalition forces (e.g. Abu Ghraib Prison), government and para-government forces, resistance movements, insurgents, ethnic and sectarian militias (e.g. Al-Mahdi Army, Kurdish Militias, others), criminals
Impacts on health and services	Limited health sector capacity but gradual and steady improvements; 18,000 doctors left the country, but some started to return; Improvement in all health indicators; Fluctuations in supply of medicine

Note: Many violent deaths either by the coalition forces or "insurgents" and others were not reported (Al-Rubeyi, 2004). This does not include the losses of allied forces.

risk of raids on hospitals, and blocking of ambulances and lack specialists in many areas (Labonte 2005; Al Sheibani et al 2006; Al-Khalisi 2010). Not surprisingly, an estimated of 8000 doctors have left Iraq since 2003.

Table 3. Iraqi Military and Civilian War-Related Casualties 1980–2008

Health status	Iraq-Iran War	Gulf War 1991	Gulf War 2003	Post-War Iraq 1 May 03–31 Dec 08
Dead (plus reported civilians)	250,000 – 500,000	63,000 – 100,000 (2,300)	Over 4,000	98,502 (IBC) Up to 2004 -100,000 (excluding Fallujah)
Wounded (plus reported civilians)	300,000	40,000 – 78,000 (6,000)	N/A (5,163)	No data
Missing in action	N/A	N/A	5,500	
Prisoners of war	65,000 (59,830 returned to Iraq)		8,622 (nearly 8,000 released)	
Conflict casualties (in Northern Iraq, between Barazani & Talabani Parties 1991–2003)			35,000 – 37,000	
Dead (internally displaced people) – North and South		14,000 + 6,000		No data but 2m were displaced internally
Uprising vengeance/insurgents attacks		3,500 (in 2 months after war)	No accurate figures are available but estimate around 100,000 – 150,000 (maybe more)	
Unexploded ordinance (UXO) related deaths/injuries	N/A		70,000+ limb injuries	

Policy and governance. The lack of a national health policy and, for many years, weak command and control due to limited management capacity at the Ministry of Health (Alwan 2004) have undermined public health. The centralized system provides little delegated power to the 20 health directorates in each of the 18 Governorates (the capital Baghdad has three directorates), despite the Local Governments Act of 2008. The health information system is weak with severely limited information technology and poor analytical skills.

Health care provision. Early comparative data of pre- and post-2003 war indicates that health system performance has improved but this does not equal the significant effort put forward by the Iraqi government. Hospital admissions have increased, yet efficiency is very low (bed occupancy on average is 47%). Lack of medications and poor quality of care in the public sector are major concerns and the reason for the shift to the private sector. This has increased the share of private providers in the health economy. Lack of control and regulation of providers has allowed many small private hospitals and small diagnostic clinics to operate in the larger cities. Additionally, no system exists to regulate professional practice and prices or monitor the quality of care. Indeed,

many of the non-governmental organizations, under the pretext of bridging the gaps in services due to deteriorating public services, operate services of questionable quality.

The Situation Today

Since 1980, wars, sanctions, insurgency, and other forms of violence have caused unspeakable loss of human life and suffering (Table 3): over two and a half million people have died, more have been displaced, and many have been left with permanent disabilities due to war injuries. Iraq lost an estimated $5–10 trillion in damages through lost production, possible lost income from investment, wasted expenditures on weapons, penalties and compensation, and interest paid on loans (Strategic Foresight Group 2009). Despite two free elections in 2005 and 2010, Iraq today is still technically under occupation, mandated under the restriction of Chapter 7 of the UN Security Council, services debt despite its level of suffering, and is incapable of ensuring security to its citizens. The overall economic situation has improved, with GDP per capita increasing from $450 prior to 2003 to $2000 in 2009. However, more than 50% still live on less than $1 per day and around 60% receive monthly basic food rations of rice, flour, and cooking oil.

Population Profile

With a population estimate of over 30 million (Figure 1), Iraq is a youthful country with a median age of 19 and 41% of the population under the age of 15 years (WHO 2010). With a population growth rate of 3.4% annually and depleted health and social resources, meeting the challenges of public health is difficult. Since 1927, national censuses have been undertaken but information is not collected on ethnicity or religious sects. Estimates show that Arabs constitute more than 80%, with the rest being Kurds (13%), Turks, and other minorities. Muslims comprise 95% and Christians approximately 4%. These statistics must be cautiously approached as inter-ethnic and religious marriages are very common (Rawaf et al 2004). Table 1 summarizes the most recent and main health and social indicators.

Population Health and Health of Vulnerable Groups

Public health has improved compared with 2003 when the entire health system had collapsed, but the picture remains very challenging. In 2010, the health budget was around $5 billion, about 3.1% of government expenditure, as compared with $16 million in 2002. However, out-of-pocket health care expenditures exceeded 50%. Most of the health infrastructure has not been fully rehabilitated. Shortages of doctor and health professionals remain widespread despite improvements in their salaries, which are now equivalent to neighboring countries. Under-5 mortality rate is 30/1000 live births, down from 131/1000 in 2002. However, these achievements, significant and commendable, are short of both expectations and populations needs. Public health is still at its worst compared to the baseline of 1980. Life expectancy remains low, mainly due to terrorism-linked fatalities and a relatively high infant and child mortality.

Despite data limitations, it is known that Iraq currently experiences a dual burden of disease. Non-communicable diseases, such as cardiovascular disease and cancer, are leading causes of death (in line with other countries in the Gulf region), but infectious diseases, especially gastroenteritis remain the major causes of morbidity (Table 5) (Alwan 2004;

Table 4. Iraq – Selected Demographic, Socio-economic, and Health Indicators

Indicator	Year	Value or unit
Demographic		
Total population	2008	30,000,000 E
	2009	32,326,011 E*
Population growth rate	2008	3.0 – 3.4
Average household size	2008	7.7
Total fertility rate/1,000	2008	5.0
Crude birth rate/1,000	2007	37.0
Crude death rate/1,000	2007	8.0
% Population over the age of 65	2007	2.8
Socio-economics		
Adult literacy rate	2010 (E)	67% estimate
Per capita GDP ($US)	2002	450
	2006	1,457
	2009	2,000
Health		
Life expectancy at birth		
Males	1997–2010**	58 (1997); 59.2 (2001); 68.6 (2010)
Females	1997–2010**	59 (1997); 62.3 (2001); 71.4 (2010)
Infant mortality rate/1,000	2008 (E)	44.0 (107 in 2003)
Child mortality rate < 5/1,000	2008 (E)	41.0
Maternal mortality rate	2008	84/100,000 live birth (117 in 1999)
Hospital admission rate	2003	71.1/1,000 pop***
Physician/population	2008	0,6/1,000 pop (total 16,721)
Nurse/population	2008	1.2/1,000 (32,304) mostly male
Hospital beds public/private	2009	13.3/10,000 [36.850/2.220]
Public/private hospitals	2009	220/100***

+ No explanation is available for such a large difference.
* OFFP implantation was started in 1997.
** Bed occupancy is around 47.5%, which reflects the inefficiency of the system.
*** The private hospitals are small, not regulated and concentrated in Baghdad, the capital.
Source: MOH-Iraq (2008, 2009).

Table 5. Iraq: Burden of Disease 2008

Rank	Cause of mortality	Cause of morbidity
1	Cardiovascular diseases	Gastroenteritis
2	Accidents	Accidents
3	Tumors	Bronchitis
4	Senility	Abortion
5	Septicemia	Pneumonia
6	Renal failure	Cardiovascular diseases
7	Cerebrovascular strokes	Malignant neoplasms
8	Hypertension	Inguinal hernia
9	Diabetes mellitus	Urinary tract infections
10	Acquired asthma	Diabetes mellitus

Source: MOH-Iraq 2008.

MOH-Iraq 2004, 2008, 2009; Rawaf et al 2004). This is not surprising as only 72% of the population have access to clean water and 20% to proper sewage disposal. Waste disposal is still a major public health problem. Accidents are the second major cause of both mortality and morbidity. The data do not provide detailed explanation but we assume this high figure could be attributed to the high level of violent deaths and injuries, domestic accidents as well as RTA.

Women pay the heavy tolls of wars. As husbands and sons were drafted, more than one million women are estimated to have lost their husbands in the various wars since 1980. Many women became the "bread winners" in very difficult circumstances. Approximately a third of women give birth without skilled health attendants and another 15–20% faced high risks to health and are in need of advanced medical support. This may explain the high maternal mortality (Table 4). Current data on the nutritional status of pregnant women are not available. In 2000, 24.3% of registered newborns had low birth weight (less than 2.5 kg) as compared with 4.5% in 1990.

Children have suffered immensely from war, sanctions, and violence. Today more than 4.5 million children are orphans, mostly due to war and violence, and this is a major concern in Iraq. Compared to other countries in the region, child health indicators were reasonably good in the 1970s and 1980s, but dramatically declined following the 1991 Gulf War. UN agencies estimate that one out of eight children die before the age of 5 years, one-third are malnourished, and one quarter do not have access to safe water. The three major killers accounting for 70% of under-5 mortality, namely diarrheal diseases, acute lower respiratory infections, and measles, are preventable. Childhood cancers are very high in comparison with other countries (8% of all cancers in Iraq compared with 0.5–1% across Europe) (MOH-Iraq 2000). The most common cancers are leukemia, lymphomas, and brain tumors. This high prevalence of cancer is localized in the southern governorates and many Iraqis attribute these high rates to the use of depleted uranium used during the 1991 Gulf War.

The more than two million internally displaced people pose a major public health challenge. Most live in camps with poor sanitation, lack adequate water and other living facilities, and are at high risk of both physical and mental problems. The majority have poor access to health services.

The Health System

In the 1980s and 1990s, the health system was founded on a philosophy of health for all and free care at the point of delivery. It was mainly publicly funded with a small proportion of out-of-pocket contributions. It was based on primary care as the first point of contact, with secondary and tertiary care provided through 185 public hospitals. One can say that both medical education and health service delivery were shaped on the British undergraduate medical education model and the National Health Service. However, from the mid-1980s the vast majority of the national wealth was directed to war efforts and other projects and diverted away from public services. Such an under-investment and severe UN sanctions meant that the health system could not respond to people's basic health care needs.

In the mid-1990s, the health system was operating at 10% of its capacity, mainly due to lack of medicine and medical supplies. Lacking resources, the health system became more centralized thus gravitating delivery towards a hospital-based service. This was mainly due to the nature of imported goods and medical supplies under the Oil-for-Food Program, which ignored primary care. The health system was further weakened by lack of investment in salaries, training, and recurring maintenance expenses. The government introduced two measures to soften the financial pressure: it facilitated the growth of the private sector by removing regulations in 1994 and in 1998, allowed public hospitals to charge recovery fees, mainly to support doctors' salaries and minimize "brain-drain."

During and immediately after the US-led invasion of 2003, the Ministry of Health and some key health facilities were damaged. About 7% of hospitals were damaged and 12% were looted. More than 30% of primary care facilities were destroyed as were the two major public health laboratories in Baghdad and Basra. Health departments, hospitals, and primary health centers lost vital equipment, refrigerators, furniture, and air conditioners.

Between 2004 and 2008, health services improved through rehabilitation of existing facilities, construction of new ones (mainly primary care centers), and development of training programs inside and outside Iraq. The progress was below expectation due to insecurity, exodus of medical staff, lack of expertise in planning, epidemiology and analysis, lack of experienced health leadership, lack of stability in the MOH, and distorted central and governorate health priorities. Since 2008 health service delivery has substantially improved with improved security and stability of leadership in the MOH.

Many challenges burden the health system today. Being highly politicized, it has fallen victim to political and sectarian rivalries since 2003. Eight ministers and many rapid changes within senior and middle management, based on sectarian alliances, have left the system with little or no clear direction. There is a clear lack of leadership to steer the complex political and operational agenda of reconstruction after years of neglect and destruction. Many of the current leaders have little experience to handle the complex and multi-dimensional issues of health system development. Expenditure on health remains low (currently 3.1% of government expenditure) in relation to population health needs (Alwan 2008). Resource allocation is based on historical arrangements and not linked to need, performance, or development.

The health system is highly centralized and bureaucratic with little delegated powers at Governorate, hospitals, and health clinics levels. This slows decision making and undermines innovation and ability to respond to local health challenges. The counter argument against decentralization at this stage of Iraq's political and civil development is the lack of trust due to the very high level of corruption at all levels of government and society.

Hospital care dominates the health system although a recent effort was launched in 2010 to strengthen primary care. Only one third of primary care needs today are met by primary care centers with the rest met by hospital services and the private sector. Despite a high level of mental health problems as the result of conflict and daily living problems (Fleck 2004), mental health resources are severely limited. Primary care centers are overcrowded with some recently opened clinics operating at nearly triple their capacity (Dorell 2007) and coping with a daily load exceeding 120 patients per doctor. Deteriorating infrastructures, shortage of medical equipment, poor documentation and lack of integrated IT systems, lack of guidelines, the absence of referral systems, uneven geographical distribution of doctors along with security concerns have all led to the poor performance of primary care centers. The poor physical conditions of public facilities contribute to increased use of private facilities and consequently higher out-of-pocket payments. The private sector of small hospitals and disconnected networks of clinics, however, remains largely unregulated.

Human resources for health are a major challenge. The exodus of large numbers of health professionals, who are unlikely to return in the near future (Wilson 2006; Dorell 2007) and the shift of many others to the private sector create a difficult situation. Almost all doctors in primary care centers are not family medicine board certified. While Iraq enjoys the benefit of both the Arab Board for Higher Medical Specializations and its National Iraqi Board, the needs by far exceed available training opportunities. The system is loaded with civil servants with no clear role or job description. Governments understandably use public employment to reduce high rates of poverty and unemployment but there must be more effective use of available employees. Recent unpublished figures indicate that employees of these centers do not adhere to the official working hours and many give less than 20 hours a week. There is a lack of sufficiently trained doctors and a poor distribution of the limited number of doctors available with the system.

There has been little improvement in quality of services. Lack of maintenance, shortage of drugs, inadequately trained staff, lack of practice guidelines and lack of accountability and measures of effectiveness all contribute. Most, if not all, services are not people-centered. Barely able to cope with demands on limited resources, most of the population believes that primary health clinics cannot provide services of quality similar to those in hospitals. In addressing this issue, the WHO in 2009 proposed a "Basic Health Service Package" to "ensure delivery of equitable and accessible health services through four layers of health facilities starting from the community health house up to the district hospital level" (WHO 2009). However, such packages are designed for low-income countries and not to resourced countries like Iraq.

From a public health perspective, two crucial issues need to be addressed. The mal-distribution of services, especially primary care, of health professionals and of power for decision making to meet local need, leads to inequitable access to services. Lack of emphasis on effective public health interventions is mainly due to the orientation, organization, and structure of the health system, which is disease-focused rather than population health-oriented.

With UN support, the health system is currently undergoing major reform as part of broader public service reform (UN 2010). The impact is unclear given the current environment of political immaturity, insecurity, and pervasive corruption.

The Future of Public Health

Addressing the many challenges facing public health requires a systematic approach. Such an approach should be based on addressing the wider determinants of health. Iraq has high levels of unemployment (currently estimated to be around 20%, including 28% of those aged 15–29); poor housing with many displaced families; damaged electricity, water, and sanitation systems; neglected education; and a devastated environment. It is difficult to improve health without addressing these determinants.

The type of health system Iraq needs is determined by Iraq's particularities. The current health system, established in the 1920s, is limited by strong centralization and bureaucracy. An opportunity was missed in 2003 to develop a modern adaptive health system (Rawaf 2005; Rowson 2005) as occupation failed to identify the urgent population needs. With the second largest oil reserves in the world, Iraq is resource-rich. Spending on equitable universal

health coverage of the highest quality is the best method of wealth distribution in such a context. Therefore, a state-funded national health system is the best approach for Iraq. This model should include free services at delivery point with co-payments restricted to a small contribution such as for dental and prescription costs; be primary care and public health-led; and have strong monitoring and performance management to eradicate corruption and misuse of power.

Policy development. Medium and long-term health and health care policies must address the physical and psychological health burden that Iraqis have endured since 1980. Both national and local (Governorate) evidence-based policies should address significant geographical and socio-economic disparities. The technical limitations at the Ministry of Health, Kurdistan Regional Government, and Governorate levels should be addressed. Policies should not only address standards but also how to improve outcomes of service delivery, motivate health workers, improve efficiency, eliminate waste and corruption, and base services according to assessed population health needs (WHO 2010).

Health system financing. Since 2003 there has been no consensus in Iraq on establishing a single payer as the best option given the country's circumstances, its resources, and past experiences. Various financing methods have been proposed (Alwan 2008) but none will tackle the inequitable distribution of power, money, and resources. Iraqi constitutions since 1958 have stipulated that all citizens are comprehensively entitled to free health service. Furthermore, Iraqis rate health as one of their highest priorities despite the security problem. In choosing a financing model key principles should be considered: critically assessing needed services; achieving universal coverage; securing social protection from financial consequences of ill-health; optimizing use of human and financial resources through good governance and eliminating waste and corruption; investing in technology; motivating the health workforce; and strictly regulating the private sector.

We strongly believe that Iraq can offer to spend more than 9% of its GDP on health; this will allow it to achieve the proposed health system model. Additional resources could be raised through taxes imposed on cigarettes, alcohol, air travel, use of large cars as well as business corporate taxation, among many examples (WHO 2010).

Increasing the government's contribution to the health economy from the current 78% to at least 85% can achieve health system stability and sustainability. Low incomes among many Iraqis (54% live on less than $1 a day) must also be considered. A cyclical three-year spending review that includes appropriate annual percent increases (2.65% to meet the needs of annual population growth, 2% for medical technology, plus annual inflation) is needed. With an annual population growth of 3.4%, by the year 2025 the population will increase by 65% of its current size. Raising sufficient resources for health alone will not guarantee universal access. The right health system and the trained workforce need to be in place.

Service provision and delivery. To establish, out of the wreckage of Iraq, a functioning health system would be a daunting task considering the limited experiences available in Iraq. We argue for four priority needs. First, is the *full reconstruction and rehabilitation* of damaged infrastructures and services. This requires proper needs assessment, planning, financial modeling and projections, efficiency strategy, and above all the workforce and expertise to deliver. Reconstruction started in 2003 but has been marred by poor planning and massive corruption.

Second, a *strategy for human resources for health* is needed. Rebuilding the once-renowned and highly skilled workforce is a long-term process that requires planning, considerable investment, and leadership. Third, the new Iraq health system model should be *primary care-led based on family medicine.* The whole population should be registered with primary care as the gatekeeper for the entire health system. Primary care is very effective in terms of costs, prevention, and clinical services (Starfield et al 2005; Rawaf et al 2008). Again, the challenge is significant, especially in terms of the workforce: At least 15,000 to 18,000 fully trained

family physicians are needed. The MOH needs a triangulated strategy for workforce development: Increase training slots in all specialties including public health and family medicine; create a program of on-the-job training particularly in family medicine; and recruit international doctors and nurses to bridge the acute gaps in the workforce.

Lastly, there is a need for *focus on efficiency, effectiveness, and safety* through good management, high level training, continuous professional development, monitoring, and above all regulations.

Health regulations and laws. With rapid changes in health, population expectations, medical knowledge, and complexity of services, the regulation of health professionals, institutions, and service delivery is vital to protect the public, health professionals, and managers. In the twenty-first century, it is unacceptable for the MOH to combine the functions of policy development, delivery and regulation, or for trade unions to combine the conflicting roles of professional regulations and licensing, serving the interest of their paid members rather than the public. Independent regulatory bodies, with the public serving on it as lay members and supported by strong laws to ensure impartiality and full protection of public interests, are needed. Since 1991 the enforcement of already-weak regulations was softened due to the pressure of sanctions. The extensive private sector flourished. Many practitioners had neither the qualifications nor the experience to practice independently and set up practice without proper license, monitoring, and control.

Organizational fitness and development. Currently, the health system works below capacity due to the inter-related factors of low numbers of health professionals, the lack of high-level training, and poor organization and management of the health economy. In Figure 3, we propose a direction for health system planning and development based on at least four

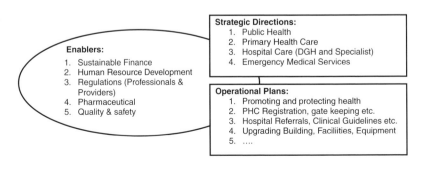

Figure 3. Developing the Iraqi health system.

strategic directions, as many as 10 operational plans, and at least six enablers.

Conclusion

The story of public health in Iraq is a tragic one but is only a fraction of the calamities that Iraq has faced since 1980. Dictatorship and misgovernment have brought devastating consequences, not only for Iraq but for the entire region. It will take Iraq many years, if not decades, to recover. We have described in this chapter a process of dismantling a country and destroying the whole population by default and design. However, the Iraqi people across their long history have proved to be very resilient. With the trilogy of tyranny and misgovernment, UN sanctions, and the unfounded WMDs behind us, Iraq is on the path to full freedom, and will be able to recover and achieve its aspirations. The people of Iraq should never have to suffer again, as long as leaders maintain vision and keep the interest of people at heart and in mind.

References

Acheson ED (1992) Health problems in Iraq. *British Medical Journal*, 304: 455–456

Ahtissari M (1991) *Report on humanitarian needs in Iraq in the immediate post-crisis environment by a mission to the area led by the Under-Secretary-General for Administration and Management*, 10–17 March 1991. S/22366. New York: UN, 20 March 1991. Available from www.casi.org.uk/info/undocs/s22366.html [Accessed 10 December 2010]

Ali MM, Shah IH (2000) Sanctions and childhood mortality in Iraq. *The Lancet*, 355: 1851–1857

Ali MM, Blacker J, Jones G (2003) *Annual mortality rates and excess deaths of children under five in Iraq, 1991–98*. Geneva, Switzerland: World Health Organization

Al-Khalisi N (2010) The perils of being a doctor in Baghdad. *British Medical Journal*, 341: 253

Al-Rubeyi BI (2004) Mortality before and after the invasion of Iraq in 2003. *The Lancet*, 364: 1834

Al-Shawaf T, Rawaf S (1995) Human rights in Iraq. *British Medical Journal*, 310: 130

Al Sheibani BIM, Hadi NR, Hasson T (2006) Iraq lacks facilities and expertise in emergency medicine. *British Medical Journal*, 333: 847

Alwan A (2004) *Health in Iraq*. Baghdad, Iraq: Ministry of Health

Alwan A (2008) Health-sector funding: Options for funding healthcare in Iraq. *Eastern Mediterranean Health Journal*, 14: 1372–1379

Barnouti HN (1996) Letter from Iraq. Effect of sanctions on surgical practice. *British Medical Journal*, 313: 1474–1475

BBC (2005) Iraq reconstruction funds missing. Available from http://news.bbc.co.uk/1/hi/programmes/file_on_4/4216853.stm [Accessed 10 December 2010]

BBC (2010) Wikileaks: Iraq war logs 'reveal truth about conflict'. Available from http://www.bbc.co.uk/news/world-middle-east-11612731 [Accessed 23 October 2010]

Bennis P Moushabeck M (Eds.) (1992) *In: Beyond the storm*. Edinburgh, UK: Canongate

Burkle FM, Noji EK (2004) Health and politics in the 2003 war with Iraq: lessons learned. *The Lancet*, 364: 1371–1375

Burns JF (2006) *Uncovering Iraq's horrors in desert graves*. New York Times. 5 June 2006. Available from http://www.nytimes.com/2006/06/05/world/middleast/05grave.html?_r1 [Accessed 10 December 2010]

Clark R (1991) Carbon release in the Persian Gulf. *Earth Island Journal*, Summer 1991

Clark R (1992a) *War crimes: A report on United States war crimes against Iraq*. Washington, DC: Maisonneuve Press

Clark R (1992b) *The fire this time. US war crimes in the Gulf*. New York, NY: Thunder's Mouth Press

de Ceukelaire W, Jabbour S, Stephens C (2003) The people of Iraq face a grim future with or without a war. *The Lancet*, 362: 1938

Dorell O (2007) Medical exodus worsens Iraq's ills, *US Today* 17 August 2007. Available from http://www.usatoday.com/news/world/iraq/2007–08–17-medical-exodus_N.htm [Accessed 18 January 2009]

Dybvik R (1991) *Situation 'fluid' in southeast Iraq and Kurdish north: Government establishing some control*. Public Diplomacy Query 6 March 1991. Available from http://www.fas.org/news/iraq/1991/910306–175102.htm [Accessed 18 January 2009]

Eastman-Abaya R (2000) Life after sanctions: The fate of Iraq. *The Lancet*, 356: 685

Fleck F (2004) Mental health a major priority in reconstruction of Iraq's health system. *Bulletin of World Health Organization*, 82: 555

Frankish H (2003) Health of the Iraqi people hangs in the balance. *The Lancet*, 361: 623–625

Garfield R (2003) Challenges to health service development in Iraq. *The Lancet*, 362: 1324

Horton R (2004) The war in Iraq: Civilian causalities, political responsibilities. *The Lancet*, 364: 1831

IRI (International Republican Institute) (2004) *Survey of Iraqi public opinion*. Washington: IRI, December 2004. Available from www.iri.org [Accessed 27 February 2005]

Ismael ST (2008) *The impacts of physicians' migration on provision* of health care in Iraq after the 2003 US led invasion. Master Degree Thesis, London, UK: LSHTM, University of London

Johns D (1999) *The crimes of Saddam Hussein: Suppression of the 1991 uprising.* Frontline world. Available from http://www.pbs.org/frontlineworld/stories/iraq501/events_uprising.html [Accessed 12 January 2009]

Kandela P (1998) Shortages distort the social fabric of Iraq. *The Lancet,* 351: 9117

Labonte R (2005) Iraq doctor tells of health crimes. *British Medical Journal,* 331: 2529

Lancet Editorial (2003) Act now to secure Iraq's health. *The Lancet,* 362: 1249

Middle East Watch (1991) *Needless deaths in the Gulf War: Civilian casualities during the air campaign and violations of the laws of war.* US: Human Rights Watch

MOH-Iraq (Ministry of Health – Iraq) (2000) *Iraq cancer registry.* Baghdad, Iraq: MoH

MOH-Iraq (2004) *Statistical manual, 5th Issue.* Baghdad, Iraq: MoH, Department of Health and Vital Statistics

MOH-Iraq (2008) *Health compass.* Baghdad, Iraq: MoH, Department of Health and Vital Statistics)

MOH-Iraq (2009) *A basic health service package in Iraq.* Iraq: Ministry of Health

Pilger J (2000) *Labour claims its actions are lawful while it bombs Iraq, its people and sells arms to corrupt states.* 7 August 2000. Available from http://www.johnpilger.com/page.asp?partid=308 [Accessed 17 January 2009]

Rawaf S, Bahri S, Alsheikh G, Mahgoub A (2004) Public health in Iraq. *Public Health Medicine,* 5: 75–79

Rawaf S (2005) The health crisis in Iraq. *Critical Public Health,* 15: 181–188

Rawaf S, De Maeseneer J, Starfield B (2008) From Alma-Ata to Almaty: A new start for primary health care. *The Lancet,* 372: 1365–1367

Richards LJ, Wall SN (2000) Iraq medical education under intellectual embargo. *The Lancet,* 35: 1093–1094

Roberts L, Lafta R, Garfield R, et al (2004) Mortality before and after 2003 invasion of Iraq: Cluster sample survey. *The Lancet,* 364: 1857–1864

Rowson M (2005) Commentary on Rawaf: The health crisis in Iraq. *Critical Public Health,* 15: 189–190

Saletan W (2003) *Shia Folly, Slate.* Available from http://www.slate.com/id/2080606/ [Accessed 12 January 2009]

Sansom C (2004) The ghost of Saddam and UN sanctions. *The Lancet Oncology,* 5: 143–145

Simons G (1996) *The scourging of Iraq. Sanctions, law and natural justice.* London, UK: MacMillan Press

Smith JE (1992) *George Bush's war.* New York, NY: Henry Holt

Starfield B, Shi L, Macinko J (2005) Contribution of primary care to health systems and health. *Milbank Q,* 83: 457–502

Strategic Foresight Group (2009) *Cost of conflict in the Middle East,* Mumbai, India: Strategic Foresight Group

UN (United Nations) (2006) *Jan Egeland, UN Under-secretary General: UN Press Conference on Iraq* New York: United Nations

UN (United Nations) (2010) *Iraq Public Service Modernization Programme.* Iraq: UNDP – Iraq Office

UNICEF/WHO (2003) *Iraq: Social sectors watching briefs: Health and nutrition.* Prepared by Dias J and Garfield R, Geneva, Switzerland: WHO

United Nation Security Council, Resolution 986 (1995) *On authorization to permit the import of petroleum and petroleum products originating in Iraq, as a temporary measure to provide for humanitarian needs of the Iraqi people.* New York: UN

United Nations World Food Programme (2004) *Baseline food security analysis in Iraq.* Rome, Italy: WFP

United Nations (UN) & World Bank (2003) *Joint Iraq needs assessment.* Geneva: World Health Organization. Available from http://www.who.int [Accessed September 2004]

United States Census Bureau (2010) *International database.* Available from http://www.census.gov/ipc/www/idb/country.php [Accessed 15 December 2009]

Wakai S (2000) Life after sanctions: The fate of Iraq. *The Lancet,* 356: 685

WHO (2010) *World health statistics 2010.* Geneva, Switzerland: WHO

Wilson D (2006) *Where have all the doctors gone? The collapse of Iraq's health care services.* Counter Punch, weekend edition, October 14–15

World Health Organization (2009) *Iraq, country profile.* Cairo, WHO EMRO. Available from www.who.emro.int [Accessed 22 August 2009]

Youssef N (2004) Iraq Ministry says coalition kills more civilians than insurgents do. *Seattle Times.* 6 October 2004

Zarocostas J (2006) WHO returns to Iraq to find major problems among 2.8 million internally displaced Iraqis. *British Medical Journal,* 337: a928

Chapter

26

Summer 2006 War on Lebanon: A Lesson in Community Resilience

Iman Nuwayhid, Huda Zurayk, Rouham Yamout, and Chadi S. Cortas

Editors' note: This chapter appeared in *Global Public Health*, vol. 6:5, (2011) pp. 505–519 (www. tandfonline.com). It is reproduced with permission with minor formatting changes.

In spite of increased concern for issues of human dignity and freedom (Waldam & Martone 1999), disaster relief organizations still view affected communities as vulnerable and fail to integrate their strengths and skills into relief efforts (Manyena 2006; Muecke 1992), thus wasting a valuable resource for alleviating suffering.

The World Disasters Report 2004 has called upon relief organizations to foster the development of resilience in communities in danger, therefore allowing them to define their needs and to find appropriate solutions during disasters rather than having external bodies impose solutions on them (IFRCRCS 2004). Proponents of such an approach propose a process-oriented paradigm of resilience with a programmatic approach that begins during the anticipation of a disaster and is sustained during and after it. The summer 2006 war on Lebanon presents an interesting case study to this effect.

On 12 July 2006, fighters from Hezbollah ("Party of God," a paramilitary Shiite Islamic political movement advocating armed resistance against Israel) killed eight Israeli soldiers and kidnapped two others across the Lebanese-Israeli border, demanding the exchange of Lebanese and Palestinian prisoners detained in Israeli jails. The incident escalated into a major Israeli air and land attack on Lebanese territory, accompanied by a sea and air blockade. On the Lebanese side, the 33-day war resulted in the deaths of over 1200 civilians and the injury of thousands more (*The Daily Star* 2006).

Within one week, nearly one million people, out of a population of four million, were forced to flee their homes. Of these, about 250,000 left the country; approximately 500,000 moved in with relatives and friends in different parts of the country; and the remaining 250,000 took shelter in schools, open spaces, and underground parking lots throughout Lebanon (IDMC 2006a). This latter group of internally displaced persons (IDPs), predominantly Shiite Muslims from South Lebanon and the southern suburbs of Beirut, survived under suboptimal living conditions. From a public health perspective, the worst was expected in such circumstances, be it increased cases of infectious diseases and malnutrition due to crowding and poor food and water quality; violence among the displaced over limited space; and clashes between the displaced and the host communities in light of ongoing political animosities. Yet, there were no reports of major disease outbreaks or social unrest in the displacement centers or the country. The IDPs exhibited a remarkable ability to absorb destabilizing circumstances and to endure the violence of war and its consequences for 33 days.

This paper uses the July 2006 war as a case study to explore the concept of community resilience by examining the manifestations of, and factors contributing to, this resilience. While some aspects of this war and the particularity of the affected community may represent a special case that cannot be generalized, the observed demeanor of this community and the lessons learned may not all be unique. Building on this case study, the authors offer a new model for community resilience that underscores the role of political leadership and ideology and illustrates that community resilience is a *process* rather than an *outcome*. The implications for public health professionals are reviewed at the end of the paper, where a paradigm shift in disaster relief practices is proposed, which focuses on the strengths rather than vulnerabilities of affected communities.

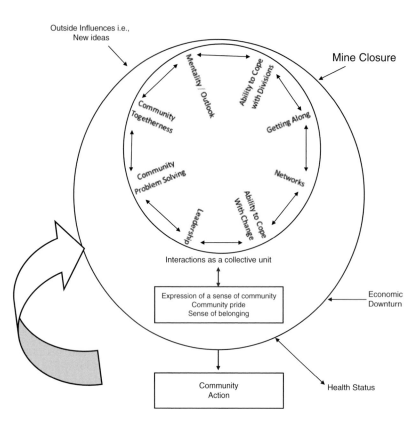

Figure 1. Revised community resiliency model (Kulig et al 2008).

Public health practitioners should be aware of this concept because attributes such as people's willingness to help each other, traditional wisdom, and local capacities are not only crucial in preventing mortality and morbidity during adverse events (WHO 2010), but can also help set relief priorities, direct relief efforts, and save time and costs (Deboutte 2000). Recognizing a community's resilience makes good public health practice as well as economic sense.

What Is Community Resilience?

There exists a large literature on individual resilience, which is not the focus of this paper. In contrast, research on community resilience is rather limited, reflecting a field that is still evolving.

The concept of community resilience was developed particularly in the context of disasters, civil disturbances, and wars, where relief agencies observed that populations reacted differently to similar catastrophes, with some faring better than others under comparable circumstances. It has also been described in the context of economic hardships and in times of financial crisis, such as the shutdown of a main employer to a community (AHPRC 2008).

No single definition of community resilience exists, but it is agreed that community resilience is not the simple summation of individual resiliencies, nor is it simply the reverse of vulnerability; rather, it represents a process in which cultural, political, and social factors interact in the face of adverse conditions to form a cohesive community (Manyena 2006; IFRCRCS 2004; Kulig 2000; Kaplan 1999). According to Manyena (2006), community resilience reflects the ability of a community to withstand stress and has been related to: (1) the magnitude of shock that the community or system can absorb while maintaining a given state; (2) the degree to which the community is capable of self-organization; and (3) the degree to which the community can build capacity for learning and adaptation (ICSU 2002). Community resilience is also described as "a complex of adaptation ... that taps into a nation's social and material strengths" (Schoch-Spana 2008 p. 130).

Several models for community resilience have been proposed, two of which are presented here. The first model was suggested by Kulig et al (2008) based on her research in mining communities in the United States and Canada (Figure 1). The building block in Kulig's model is the behavior of the community under adverse

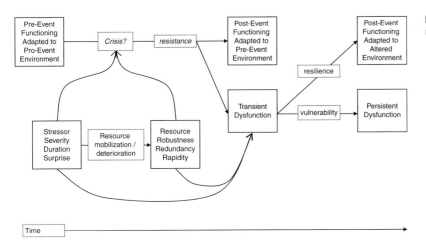

Figure 2. A model for community resilience (Norris et al 2008).

situations as a "collective unit," exemplified by getting along, networking, coping with divisions and adapting to changes, and the presence of a visionary leadership. These elements are decisive for the realization of a "sense of community" that is expressed in a common belonging, spirit, or outlook. This collective feeling and sense of community paves the way to concrete "community action," exemplified by the community's ability to adapt to the change and deal with it positively. Kulig's model also suggests a feedback mechanism whereby experiences accumulate and impact the whole process.

The second model, suggested by Norris et al (2008), is based on an interdisciplinary review of the literature on community resilience to time-delimited disasters of acute onset, but excluding long-term wars and violent conflicts (Figure 2). The model describes the process of community resilience as the balance between disruptions occurring due to the disaster and resources available to the affected community. The characteristics of the stressor and of the resources play a role in determining whether the community will resist, adapt, or become dysfunctional in a post-crisis setting. The model refers to "pre-event functioning adapted to pre-event environment" and to "resources" mobilized during the crisis. Norris et al (2008) identified four sets of networked resources that form the basis of community resilience, namely economic development, information and communication, community competence, and social capital.

The themes common to community resilience can thus be grouped into two categories: (1) the actions taken by the community to absorb the shock of a crisis, in this case war and displacement, and (2) the resources available to help the community act as a "collective unit" and support its resilience. We will examine these themes in our own case study.

Lebanon, Summer 2006

Data on the manifestation of resilience among the IDPs ("community action") and resources that supported this resilience were extracted from direct observations, discussions with key informants, and the review of printed matter. The authors were involved in public health relief efforts during the July 2006 war in Lebanon through the Faculty of Health Sciences (FHS) of the American University of Beirut. They were members of a university-wide voluntary group of public health, medical, nursing and nutrition students and professors who participated in relief efforts provided to more than 16 displacement centers in Beirut. The team met several times a week to evaluate activities and reflect on their experiences. The first author represented FHS on the national Health and Water and Sanitation committees. Two of the authors also contributed to the training and relief efforts of a coalition of non-governmental organizations (NGOs), named *Samidoun*. Observations from these activities were noted on a regular basis and were enriched with the review of written material from different media and Internet sources. After the war, these observations were shared and discussed in public lectures and with small groups of social scientists, public health experts, and individuals who were actively involved in the relief efforts.

This section describes how this community's resilience was manifested throughout the war and then examines the resources that helped build up and sustain this resilience.

Community Action: Manifestations of a Resilient Community

The resilience of the IDPs was manifested throughout the phases of the war in their orderly self-evacuation from threatened and bombarded towns and villages; remarkable ability for self-organization and discipline in displacement centers; phenomenal return to their residences the moment the war stopped; and immediate post-war adaptation.

Orderly Evacuation

The IDPs demonstrated a remarkable ability for self-organized evacuation from dangerous areas in light of the sudden and unexpected disturbance of the war. As soon as the Israeli offensive began, tens of thousands of citizens from regions under attack or threat of attack quickly and efficiently evacuated from locations in danger and found their way to displacement centers throughout the country. People shared vehicles, prioritized individuals to be evacuated and led one another to relatively safer roads and available hosting areas. In a commentary published after the war, David Shearer, the United Nations humanitarian coordinator for Lebanon, wrote, "To my mind, the most intriguing thing about this large-scale migration was just how orderly and without incident it was. [. . .] In my experience, it's simply unprecedented" (Shearer 2006 p. 7).

Self-organization

For most, the selection of a shelter was not a centralized process but rather a personal or family decision based on shared perceptions of the safety of a location and the availability of resources. Spontaneous support groups emerged while IDPs awaited the arrival of humanitarian aid. Those settled in displacement centers managed to survive in crowded and unhygienic environments. The IDPs themselves distributed responsibilities regarding the allocation of resources and cleaning of the premises. One of the authors observed that in some centers IDPs implemented gender-sensitive space organization to provide comfort and privacy for veiled women and nursing mothers. Families with children or elderly members were housed in rooms better suited for their needs. Moreover, discreet measures were taken seemingly to prevent sexual abuse, such as monitoring toilet entry at night and forbidding access to isolated areas in the center.

Disciplined Behavior

No serious clashes within the gathering centers or with the host communities were reported. There was an acceptable adherence to basic principles of hygiene, mostly set by the IDPs themselves, with guidance from the centers' administrative bodies and the health authorities established by the political leadership. Despite the catastrophic hygienic conditions in some centers, there were minimal health impairments among the displaced and no reports of major disease outbreaks. During the period of fleeing, there were no acts of vandalism, such as looting or forceful occupation of homes, contrary to previous mass migrations during the civil war in Lebanon (Lebanese Ministry of the Displaced 2010).

Phenomenal Return

On 12 August 2006, the United Nations announced Resolution 1701, which called for the cessation of all hostilities in Lebanon starting 8 am on 14 August. The post-conflict plans of all national and international relief agencies assumed that the displaced people would delay their return to their towns and villages by about two to four weeks. Accordingly, the plan was to continue relief efforts while the government and relevant agencies cleaned up the ruins and facilitated the return of people to their homes. This impression was further consolidated with the news that over 1.2 million cluster bomblets had been dropped over South Lebanon (Rappaport 2006; *The Lancet* 2006). On 14 August, however, the scene was very different. Hundreds of cars, vans, and mini-buses carrying people, mattresses, clothing, and food began heading south at 8 am sharp, with no consideration for blown-up bridges, cratered roads, or risk of unexploded ordnances. Even those who knew their homes were demolished were jubilant to return to their areas (O'Brien 2006). "I'm so excited to see my home. . . . I'd heard news it was completely destroyed, but even if there's one room intact, I will stay there with my children," stated a returnee mother (Zayan 2006). In a matter of days, the number of IDPs in displacement centers dwindled from between 750,000 and 1 million to a few thousand (UNSC 2006).

Rapid Post-war Adaptation

With the end of the war, the returnees had to worry about shelter, economic opportunities, and schooling for their children. Despite this humanitarian crisis (Fickling 2006), people managed to maintain their unity and improvized housing solutions, counting on the support of relatives above all else. Upon returning to her village the day after the ceasefire, a woman declared, "I don't care if we have to live in tents, but as long as it is on our land" (Zayan 2006).

Resources That Contributed to Community Resilience

Factors that contributed to the resilience exhibited by the IDPs can be grouped in two categories: (1) factors that built up resilience and prepared the displaced communities to endure situations such as those experienced during the war; and (2) factors that helped to sustain this resilience during the war and shortly thereafter.

Building Up Resilience

Three main factors could be grouped under this category, namely: a strong communal identity united around a common cause; "hardiness" developed in reaction to recurrent displacements; and a strong social and political network run by an involved leadership.

First, a common cause provided the affected population with a sense of collective identity. This particular collective ideological framework involved a multitude of interrelated components, including socio-political, economical and historical elements.

The idea of *muqāwamah* or "resistance" regarding the conflict with Israel is deeply inculcated in the psyche of the people of South Lebanon, especially the Shiite community. South Lebanon is the geographical continuation of north Palestine (currently north Israel), and up until 1920 when Greater Lebanon was proclaimed, it was under the administration of the *wilāyat* (province) of Acre in historic Palestine. The residents of South Lebanon traded more commonly with the residents of north Palestine than with those of Mount Lebanon or Beirut. The establishment of the State of Israel in 1948 disrupted these economic, familial, and cultural ties and had a greater impact on the livelihood of the inhabitants of South Lebanon than those in other areas of Lebanon. This might explain the strong support provided by the South Lebanese, with minor exceptions, to all "liberation" and "resistance" movements since 1948, including the Palestinian Liberation Organization and several secular and Islamic Lebanese groups. Accounts from IDPs attest to the importance of this element in building people's resilience. For instance, at the end of the war, one woman told reporters, "It does not matter whether our homes are still standing or not. We have to go back and defend our land. It is all part of the struggle" (Zayan 2006).

The particularity of Shiite religious subculture also contributed greatly to the sense of collective identity in Shiite populations. The martyrdom of Imam Hussayn Bin Ali and his family and companions in the battle of Karbala in AD 680 is focal to this identity. The endurance of the 70 or more victims (Deeb 2006) in the face of hunger, thirst, fear, pain, and murder, as recounted in Shiite accounts of the battle, is commemorated annually during the 10-day *Ashūrah* celebration, and also occasionally at funerals and other religious and political celebrations. This event has taken on a symbolic significance and its persistent celebration reflects its relevance to Shiite culture today (Hamzeh 2004), known for its high religiosity, especially in South Lebanon (Tobin 2000). This religious/cultural rooting almost certainly helped inculcate values of resilience and resistance to oppression among the affected population.

Second, it can be argued that the population of South Lebanon has developed some aspects of "hardiness" (King et al 1998) in its communal culture, in the context of the decades-long Arab-Israeli conflict and as a result of prior instances of displacement that accompanied Israeli incursions into Lebanon (IDMC 2006c).

Third, strong social support, educational and health services networks were established since the mid-1980s on which the Shiite population could rely for assistance (Hamzeh 2004). The Shiite political/spiritual leadership recognized the centrality of the concept of *muqāwamah* in the culture of South Lebanon and helped institutionalize the ideology of a "sacred" Islamic resistance over the past two decades by placing it at the core of its social, economic, and political actions. Shiite organizations, including Hezbollah, thus provided a "helping hand," to use a term used by Cyrulink (2001) in describing resilience, while infusing the ideology of resistance into the curricula of schools they ran and at the party's social, political, and religious events (Hamzeh 2004). In addition, Hezbollah, and to a lesser extent the other main

Shiite political party, Amal, offered job opportunities and economic support to families in South Lebanon and other Shiite regions.

As a result of the above, the Shiite population has rallied around the cause of resistance, incorporating it in its communal subculture, and developed a deep trust in its politico-spiritual leadership (UN-OCHA 2006a). This primed it psychologically to endure hardship by imparting a meaning for the adverse event they came to experience.

Sustaining Resilience

Four factors could be grouped under this category and are also interrelated to the first set of factors.

First was a sense of cohesive community. The Shiites were to a large extent singled out during the war. In addition to targeting infrastructure and other select sites in Lebanon, Israel focused its military attack on the Lebanese Shiite communities in South Lebanon, southern suburbs of Beirut, and parts of the Beqa'a region. The shared destiny and the feeling of being collectively targeted strengthened the communal cohesiveness of the affected community (Greene & Graham 2009). The tendency of population groups to "come together tightly" and undertake collective actions when confronted by a common danger is well documented in the literature (Norris et al 2008). This was reinforced with "good" news from the battleground and the communal sense of victory, later labeled "divine victory."

Second was an active and swift public health response that reassured the affected community and addressed its basic survival needs. Within days of the beginning of the war, hundreds of NGOs – including networks of social and health services run by Hezbollah (UN-OCHA 2006b) – and thousands of volunteers, with the support of the international emergency community, mobilized to supply war victims and IDPs with shelter, food, water, clothing, medical care, hygienic kits, and other urgent necessities.

Third was the support provided by other communities to the affected population. Rather than relying on support from relatives and friends in other Shiite regions, as was the case in previous instances of massive displacement of the South Lebanese, the IDPs had no option but to take shelter in regions inhabited by other religious communities. There was an overwhelming wave of solidarity with the affected community that crossed religious and political divisions. The other Lebanese communities exhibited a sense of "compassion" whereby, " [r]egardless of religion or ethnic background, families, even whole communities, embraced those fleeing the fighting, taking them into their homes and feeding and caring for them" (Shearer 2006 p. 7). This spontaneous support network helped prevent the breakdown of social order.

Fourth was the role of leadership. The support and appeals from Hezbollah leadership specifically seemed to serve to promote resilience within the affected Shiite population. During the war, the group's leadership continuously appealed to a set of deeply held, shared beliefs – which, in previous studies, was shown to be associated with higher resilience among populations in stressful situations of conflict and violence (King et al 1998). The necessity of endurance was emphasized regularly in the speeches of Nasrallah, the leader of Hezbollah. In addition to providing military and political updates, he often made reference to religious beliefs and extolled the "steadfastness" (ṣumūd) of the displaced populations. He addressed the latter explicitly during his speeches, associating their plight with the fight and the cause of the *muqāwamah*, with which they identified. Announcements of military successes, such as hitting an Israeli naval warship off the coast of Beirut, were presented in this light, as well (As-Safir & ACI 2006 p. 235–236). The displaced population was responsive and engaged. A study of mental health of IDPs during the war revealed that, on average, lower anxiety levels were reported by respondents on the day following reported victories against the Israelis than on other days of the war (Yamout & Chaaya 2010).

More pragmatic actions undertaken by the political leadership focused on the dignity of those housed in displacement centers. The health and social arms of Hezbollah and other Shiite political organizations were mobilized within hours of the arrival of the displaced. Delegates were sent to all displacement centers to form local committees jointly run with the IDPs. The relief body of Hezbollah succeeded in centralizing all humanitarian aid within days (Ammar 2009). In addition, the local committees, in coordination with political leadership, implemented activities that contributed to the physical and spiritual welfare of the IDPs. For example, they organized sports activities for children and prayer sessions for adults; would immediately mobilize to offer support to mothers who lost children to the fighting (relying on the support of other women who had also lost their children during this or previous wars), thus building upon the subculture of resilience described above; and would often call upon the people to engage in communal prayers, coordinated across the different displacement centers. These activities provided the affected individuals with a strong spiritual sense of self-worth and reinforced their common identity (UN-OCHA 2006c), enhancing their ability to resist adversity (Greene 2002). During the war, medications were delivered to sick individuals and cash was given to many families. Immediately following the war, Hezbollah encouraged the IDPs to return to their villages, pledging to distribute one year's worth of rent to each affected family and to help finance the reconstruction of destroyed homes (Fickling 2006).

Discussion

Applying Kulig's model to the summer 2006 war, the IDPs formed a cohesive community driven by deep collective cultural beliefs, a unified cause, and hope, leading to a "sense of community." This cohesiveness, nurtured by active and responsive relief and fed by earlier experiences with wars and displacements, was expressed in people's ability to cope with the stressful conditions and their willingness to return to their villages within hours of ceasefire, corresponding with "community action" in Kulig's model. The crucial role of "resources," as presented in the model by Norris et al (2008), was also demonstrated in the experience of the displaced population during this war. More specifically, the communal narratives that provided meaning in the face of adversity, the availability of informal and formal support systems, updates provided by the political leadership, and the financial support provided to the displaced during and after the war illustrate the model's networked "adaptive capacities" (Norris et al 2008).

Although applicable in many ways to the experience of the July 2006 war, both models lack elements that were critical to the community resilience observed among the IDPs during this event. Kulig's model emphasizes the interaction of a community as a collective unit as a condition for its resilience. However, it presents community resilience as a positive reaction to an adverse event at the time of its occurrence rather than as the outcome of a long-term process. The elements of the "collective unit" are naturally nurtured and supported over time; however, the model does not allude to this. Moreover, some of what Kulig refers to as examples of interaction as a collective unit are in reality manifestations of resilience. Finally,

although listed, the critical role of leadership is diluted in Kulig's model. It is our observation that the political and spiritual leadership of the displaced community was a key element in the development of its resilience. In contrast to Kulig, Norris et al (2008) clearly delineate time as a factor in their model of resilience. However, the timeline is presented more to emphasize the phases of an event (before-after) rather than to underscore that community resilience is a process. The findings of our study strongly suggest a period where the community is prepared for the adverse event and the critical role of leadership and collective identity in that phase. It also suggests that community resilience needs to be supported and sustained during and after the event.

The current study reveals the crucial effects of ideological preparedness and mobilization of civilians. These factors may have been decisive in inculcating meaning to the suffering of the IDPs. While the models of both Kulig and Norris et al. underscore community survival as a goal, the IDPs in the summer 2006 war were also united for the survival of an ideology – that of "resistance." This may well be a reflection of the political context of the Lebanese experience and of a political leadership that succeeded over decades in the institutionalization of an already accepted ideology.

A Suggested Model for Community Resilience

Figure 3 incorporates the factors discussed on building up and sustaining community resilience into a comprehensive model. The overlying arrow reflects that community resilience is a process that precedes and follows the adverse event, emphasizing the interaction between the different phases.

This model is applicable to situations other than war. For example, a farming community susceptible to droughts may have built up community resilience based on a sense of collective identity at risk from a common threat, strengthened by experiences with prior droughts and well developed social and economic networks. During and shortly after a drought, continued cohesiveness, immediate intervention, and a "connected leadership" (local or governmental) would help sustain this resilience while also building up more resilience to handle subsequent droughts.

The model is not meant to be rigid, as community resilience is not constant but can fluctuate over time, suggesting a potential limit to its effects (Kulig 2000). Nguyen-Gillham et al (2008) attest to the "fluid

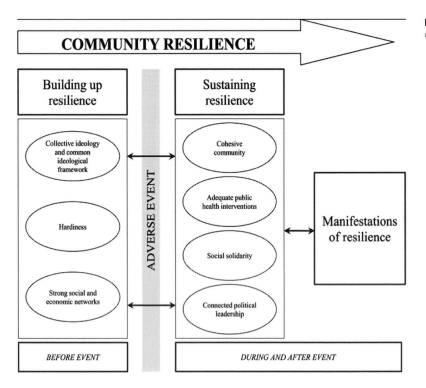

Figure 3. A suggested model for community resilience.

nature'" of resilience as observed among Palestinian youths, and argue that it "does not exist as a static quality or a mechanistic process but in a continuum that varies over time and context" (p. 296). This "fluidity" in resilience is critical to the understanding of this phenomenon, especially in the context of relief and post-crisis activities.

Lessons Learned and Implications for Public Health Professionals

The summer 2006 war experience confirms the need for a paradigm shift in disaster relief efforts to build on communities' resourcefulness and resilience. The new paradigm calls for multilevel action that precedes the onset of a disaster or emergency. This requires the need to address communities rather than individuals in emergency relief research and practice (Nguyen-Gillham et al 2008), and to analyze political and social constructs of the affected populations to help integrate their perceptions and priorities in relief efforts (Schoch-Spana 2008).

The above was not fully implemented by national and international relief efforts during the summer 2006 war. The first two weeks saw several obstacles including access difficulties, lack of coordination, absence of clear public health leadership, and even initial mistrust of relief efforts on the part of the IDPs. These efforts were driven by international expert advice and an assessment of needs and vulnerabilities with minimal, if any, consideration of the affected communities' perceptions of needs and available capacities and resources. These needs and resources were better captured by leaders from the communities themselves, who were appointed by political organizations collaborating with the IDPs to form local committees in displacement centers. These committees addressed issues of community life and did not spare efforts to inculcate and maintain collective optimism. They eventually formed a link between the IDPs and the national and international relief efforts, and their role was critical in alleviating mistrust and improving collaboration between the providers, especially as international aid to Lebanon increased.

As a result, national and international relief agencies came to have full access to all centers, while Hezbollah led the organization of relief efforts. They guided agencies to the neediest centers, organized the overall relief distribution and provided their own minimal services (Ammar 2009). The IDPs showed better knowledge of their priority needs. They addressed issues of potential violence and sexual abuse, while public health groups were focused on provision of basic needs. More strikingly, to reduce injuries, public health experts advised to delay the return of IDPs to clear roads and towns of rubble and unexploded ordinances. In contrast, the Hezbollah leadership encouraged immediate return to towns and villages promising support. The IDPs, responding to their political leadership, elected to take the risk of returning home earlier to claim back their property and declare "victory."

Obviously, attempts to build on the affected community's resourcefulness were complicated by the urgency of emergency relief and legitimate ignorance of the community's cultural and contextual nuances. However, their collective optimism and confidence quickly set the norm for community action itself. Several local and national relief organizations even embodied the communal feeling of pride and confidence. One coalition of NGOs, for example, expressed this by changing its name from the Sanayeh Relief Centre to *Samidoun* (resistant and steadfast). Even the language used by some relief bodies implied the deep respect to people's plight: the displaced were not referred to as the victims or needy, but as "our people," "the steadfast," "the resistant," "victory makers," or "heroes."

To implement this paradigm shift in public health practice, it is necessary to introduce the concept of community resilience into public health education and into the training of relief workers in the preparation for, and response to, disasters. This should not be seen as a request for new curricula. Rather, it is a call for students and practitioners of public health to recognize a community's resources; to value its norms, culture and history; and to recognize its critical role in relief efforts. Communities at risk are the first to react to the calamities of a disaster and are the most informed about their circumstances; it is they who should play a leading role in any emergency relief (Samarasinghe 2005). Understanding how communities cope with disaster is as significant as addressing the needs of the "vulnerable" and ill. Moreover, connecting to existing community resources and organizations moderates suspicion from the affected community as to the motives of international emergency and relief efforts. Such an approach should alleviate, or at a minimum address, concerns of involvement with highly politicized local and regional situations and the ethical considerations of coordinating with political parties, thus enabling them to "demonstrate their power and influence through their access to and distribution of aid" (Shearer & Pickup 2007 p. 346).

Conclusion

Community resilience is a multifaceted and cross-disciplinary concept that transcends the classical public health approach to include analyses of socio-economic, political, cultural, and historical aspects of affected communities. Our model suggests that resilience should be seen as a process whose importance lies not merely in its manifestations but also in factors that contribute to its growth and continuation. Identifying these factors is central in evaluating affected communities' resources and needs. Capitalizing on community resilience should become a substantial component of public health action and relief efforts during crisis. However, this should not undermine the role of public health professionals and their organizations in addressing the root causes of disasters, including the social injustices that lead to wars.

Acknowledgments

We thank colleagues who commented on earlier drafts and presentations of this paper, particularly the Health and Society Group at FHS and Rita Giacaman from Birzeit University.

References

Ammar H (2009) *Experience of Islamic Health Society during summer 2006 war on Lebanon*. Oral presentation. *Understanding the impact of conflicts and wars on health: Bridging research and practice. 18 March*. Center for Research on Population and Health, American University of Beirut

As-Safir & ACI (Arab Centre for Information) (2006) *Diary of Israeli war on Lebanon (Arabic)* Beirut, Lebanon: Bissan li al-nashr wa el-tawzi' wa el-e'lām

AHPRC (Atlantic Health Promotion Research Centre) (2008) *A study of resiliency in communities, Canada's drug strategies*. Available from http://www.hc-sc.gc.ca/hc-ps/pubs/adp-apd/resiliency-enquete/index-eng.php [Accessed 4 April 2009]

Cyrulink B (2001) *Les vilains petits canards* [The ugly ducklings] (In French), Paris, France: Jacob

The Daily Star (2006) *Timeline of the July War 2006*. Available from http://www.dailystar.com.lb/July_War06.asp [Accessed 12 January 2007]

Deboutte D (2000) Good practice in public health: Thinking about the economics of complex emergencies. *Refuge*, 18: 26–30

Deeb L (2006) Lebanese Shi'a women: Temporality and piety. *ISIM Review*, 18: 32–33

Fickling D (2006) *Lebanon facing humanitarian crisis. Guardian Unlimited, 18 August.* Available from http://www.guardian.co.uk/international/story/0,1853533,00.html [Accessed 25 October 2006]

Greene RR (2002) Holocaust survivors: A study in resilience. *Journal of Gerontological Social Work*, 37(1): 2–18

Greene RR, Graham SA (2009) The role of resilience among Nazi Holocaust survivors. A strength-based paradigm for understanding survivorship. *Family Community Health*, 32(Suppl. 1): 75–82

Hamzeh A (2004) *In the path of Hezbollah*. Syracuse, NY: Syracuse University Press

ICSU (International Council for Science) (2002) *Resilience and sustainable development.* Available from http://www.icsu.org/Gestion/img/ICSU_DOC_DOWNLOAD/64_DD_FILE_Vol3.pdf [Accessed 15 January 2009]

IDMC (Internal Displacement Monitoring Centre) (2006a) *Israeli military operations force people to flee their homes in south Lebanon and south Beirut. Global Figures: July-August 2006 conflict.* Available from http://www.internaldisplacement.org/idmc/website/countries.nsf/(httpEnvelopes)/3911CA59193E1263C12572220052111D?OpenDocument#26.3.1 [Accessed 13 July 2007]

IDMC (2006b) *Ceasefire prompts immediate and massive return movements. July-August 2006 conflict.* Available from http://www.internaldisplacement.org/idmc/website/countries.nsf/(httpEnvelopes)/106D505DC30A23DCC125722E003BCE3F?

OpenDocument [Accessed 13 July 2007]

IDMC (2006c) *Israeli troops pull out of South Lebanon (1992–2000).* Available from http://www.internaldisplacement.org/idmc/website/countries.nsf/(httpEnvelopes)/B406F490425604DA802570B8005AAA63?OpenDocument#26.1.1 [Accessed 13 July 2007]

IFRCRCS (International Federation of Red Cross and Red Crescent Societies) (2004) *World Disasters Report 2004: Focus on community resilience.* Available from http://www.ifrc.org/publicat/wdr2004/ [Accessed 15 April 2009]

Kaplan H (1999) Toward an understanding of resilience: A critical review of definitions and models. *In*: M Glantz, J Johnson (Eds.) *Resilience and development* (p. 17–83). New York, NY: Kluwer Academic

King LA, King DW, Fairbank JA, Keane TM, Adams AA (1998) Resilience-recovery factors in post-traumatic stress disorder among female and male Vietnam veterans: Hardiness, post-war social support, and additional stressful life events. *Journal of Personality and Social Psychology*, 74(2): 420–434

Kulig J (2000) Community resiliency: The potential for community health nursing theory development. *Public Health Nursing*, 17(5): 374–385

Kulig J, Edge D, Joyce B (2008) Understanding community resiliency in rural communities through multimethod research. *Journal of Rural and Community Development*, 3(3): 77–94

The Lancet (2006) Yet another country infested with cluster bombs. *The Lancet*, 368(9546): 1468

Lebanese Ministry of the Displaced (2010) *Evacuations and home return.* Available from http://web.archive.org/web/20011011085241/dogbert1.dm.net.lb/displaced/achiev-29.htm [Accessed 10 April 2009]

Manyena S (2006) The concept of resilience revisited. *Disasters*, 30(4): 433–450

Muecke M (1992) New paradigms for refugee health problems. *Social Science & Medicine*, 35(4): 515–523

Nguyen-Gillham V, Giacaman R, Nasser G, Boyce W (2008) Normalizing the abnormal: Palestinian youth and the contradictions of resilience in protracted conflict. *Health and Social Care in the Community*, 16(3): 291–298

Norris FH, Pfefferbaum B, Pfefferbaum R (2008) Community resilience as a metaphor, theory, set of capacities and strategy for disaster readiness. *American Journal of Community Psychology*, 41: 127–150

O'Brien J (2006) *Thousands head home following ceasefire in Lebanon, UNICEF Newsline, 14 August.* Available from http://www.unicef.org/emerg/index_35319.html [Accessed 12 January 2007]

Rappaport M (2006) *IDF commander: We fired more than a million cluster bombs in Lebanon, Haaretz, 9 December.* Available from http://www.haaretz.com/hasen/spages/761781.html [Accessed 12 January 2007]

Samarasinghe D (2005) Disaster management: Lessons from immediate responses to the Tsunami. *Ceylon Medical Journal*, 50(1): 25–27

Schoch-Spana M (2008) Community resilience for catastrophic health events. *Biosecurity & Bioterrorism*, 6(2): 129–130

Shearer D (2006) Lebanon, a unique example of humanitarian solidarity, *The Daily Star*, 26 September 2006

Shearer D, Pickup F (2007) Still falling short: Protection and partnerships in the Lebanon emergency response. *Disasters*, 4: 336–352

Tobin JP (2000) Observations on the mental health of a civilian population living under long-term hostilities. *Psychiatric Bulletins*, 24: 69–70

UN-OCHA (United Nations Office for the Coordination of Humanitarian Affairs) (2006a) *Revised Lebanon crisis flash appeal 2006*. Available from http://www.reliefweb.int/rw/rwb.nsf/db900sid/LSGZ-6T7JH4?OpenDocument [Accessed 12 January 2007]

UN-OCHA (2006b) The many hands and faces of Hezbollah, *Integrated Regional Information Networks (IRIN), 29 March*. Available from http://www.irinnews.org/report.aspx?reportid=26242 [Accessed 12 January 2007]

UN-OCHA(2006c) *We're not just fighters, says Hezbollah, Integrated*

Regional Information Networks (IRIN), 14 August. Available from http://www.reliefweb.int/rw/RWB.NSF/db900SID/LZEG-6SNPGW?OpenDocument [Accessed 12 January 2007]

UNSC (United Nations Security Council) (2006) *Report of the Secretary-General on the implementation of resolution 1701*. Available from http://www.reliefweb.int/library/documents/2006/unsc-lbn-18aug.pdf [Accessed 12 January 2007]

Waldman R, Martone G (1999) Public health and complex emergencies: New issues, new conditions. *American Journal of Public Health*, 89: 1483–1485

WHO (World Health Organization) (2010) *Community resilience in disasters: How the primary health care approach made a difference in recent emergencies in the WHO South-East Asia Region*. New Delhi, India: World Health Organization

Yamout R, Chaaya M (2010) Individual and collective determinants of mental health during wartime. A survey of displaced populations amidst July-August 2006 war in Lebanon. *Global Public Health*, 30: 1–17

Zayan J (2006) *For Lebanon's displaced going back home is a duty, Lebanon Wire, 13 August*. Available from http://www.lebanonwire.com/0608MLN/06081335LAF.asp [Accessed 10 April 2009]

Chapter

27

Introduction: Seeing the Trees, Not Missing the Forest

Samer Jabbour and Salman Rawaf

How best to look at health systems in this region? The five chapters in this section examine five key functions: governance, financing, workforce, delivery, and access to medicines. These are crucial for achieving the health system goals of better health, responsiveness to the needs of people and for financial protection against healthcare costs. Evaluating health systems through the lens of these components is attractive: there is a vast literature upon which to draw; data is commonly available about these functions; and policy makers, practitioners, and academics are readily aware of the importance of these functions that a language of communication is easy to establish. But the functions of a system are not the same as the system itself. Interventions targeted to improving some of the functions may not translate into a better performing system in the presence of serious structural problems. As we look critically at the *overall* health systems in the Arab countries through the published literature and our experiences, we find serious deficiencies. In the first part of this introduction to the section, we focus on examining a few such deficiencies. In the second part, we propose the need to think about new foundations for our health systems, namely the social contract, the health system framework, and linking the health system with broader work on social determinants and protection. We conclude with a brief discussion of health system reforms and the role of health professionals.

Today's Health Systems: The Structural Ills

If, for the lack of better terms, we use "health systems" to describe the current setups in Arab countries, we find diverse arrangements but enough commonalities to allow meaningful comparisons. Our starting point is that a health system should be entrusted with

realizing the comprehensive public health framework (see also Chapter 33). Such a system must meet the needs and expectations of all people and strive to improve population health. A good system ensures equity, universality, comprehensiveness, and free service at the point of delivery. To the extent that most health systems in the Arab world do not meet these criteria, the title of this section is deliberately futuristic. We base this assessment on examining three issues building on the findings of the five chapters in this section and other reviews (Akala & El-Saharty 2006; Pierre-Louis et al 2004; WHO EMRO 2004).

The first issue concerns *health system values and vision*, specifically commitment to equity. Current systems are simply not equitable and chapters in this volume clearly illustrate the lack of commitment of health systems to promoting equity. Despite the lip service paid to the issue by many national health authorities, equity is not a policy priority. There is actually very little recognition or acknowledgement that health systems themselves can be a source of health inequity (Baum et al 2009). Health as a right is enriched in many constitutions in the region but it is neither operationalized nor protected. While health systems in the Gulf countries move toward universal health coverage for their citizens, these systems are not necessarily equitable due to the exclusion of the large expatriate population (see the case study of migrant domestic workers in Chapter 21). Recent health sector reforms in the region suggest a trend away from equity and rights and towards liberalization (see the case study of Egypt in Chapter 37). Governments in several countries, such as Egypt and Syria, are withdrawing from the social protection programs they instituted in the post-independence era (this is discussed in more detail in Chapters 1 and 37). Free health services, free education, and limited pensions are being curtailed through

Public Health in the Arab World, ed. Samer Jabbour et al. Published by Cambridge University Press. © Samer Jabbour et al., 2012.

privatizing, instituting user fees, and creating a double-tier within the public sector. In countries with weak central governments, for example Lebanon, and in countries with highly underdeveloped health systems, for example Somalia and Yemen, the opportunity for equitable health systems is very small. In summary, a majority of Arab countries are either far from having equitable health systems or are not in the position to move in such a direction.

The second issue concerns *health system organization*. A "system" implies harmonic functioning among well-developed and inter-dependent components through the coordinated contributions of various actors. Such a description hardly fits any health system in the region. We are more likely to find a patchwork of momentum-generated services and institutions implemented through various periods that reflect certain socio-economic or political directions and vested interests (see the case studies in Longuenesse [1995] as well as discussion in Chapter 1).

While centralization still dominates, most health systems are still weak at the center. Planning is commonly incremental and demand-led. Command and control is poor and institutions lack the dynamic of modern organizations. Most countries lack the capacity and expertise to carry out essential health system tasks such as accurately assessing and forecasting population health needs; predicting the impact of medical and technological advances; properly regulating both professionals and providers; and controlling corruption, misuse, and waste of public resources.

There are major deficiencies in the three components of a modern health system: public health, primary care, and hospital care. The public health function is especially weak and lacks the mandate, the vision, and the ability to guide and lead the whole system. Public health delivery systems are much weaker than, and consumed by, medical service delivery systems and the two are not well integrated. The international experience in integrating public health into health care delivery is yet to be replicated or critically examined for its relevance in this region (see for example Breton et al 2010). The concept of strong, well-developed, and decentralized public health delivery systems (see for example, Mays et al 2009) has not caught on in the region.

Primary care is patchy, medicalized, and not based on the Alma Ata-inspired social development model. The few experiments around the region of primary care based on family practice and linked with social development, for example community-based initiatives as discussed by Assai et al (2006) and the Health Villages Program, remain limited and have not shown national impact. Primary care is under-staffed and under-appreciated and provides low quality services in the public sector. There are large imbalances in favor of hospital (secondary and tertiary) care, which is becoming increasingly ineffective in addressing the many emerging health challenges in the region. Referral systems from primary care to secondary care are not well established, as discussed in Chapter 31. Poor coordination among the three components is the system's *sine qua non*.

With little investment in the leadership of health system institutions, such leadership is very weak, commonly built around loyalty. Merits, skills, and competence are not adequately (or sometimes not at all) considered in developing leadership. Governance and accountability are also weak (WHO EMRO 2004). Health systems are riddled with bureaucracy, verticalization, and hierarchy. In our experiences, it is very difficult to do *intra*-sectoral collaborative work, let alone to think about *inter*-sectoral work which is even more difficult.

There are two additional aspects of health system organization that deserve to be highlighted. The first concerns the health workforce, an issue that connects Chapters 30 and 31. Many of the practitioners are not trained in structured ways. They might have trained in different countries which have varying standards. Systems for continuing professional development and oversight are weak or not in place at all. The emphasis is on qualifications rather than competencies and quality of practice. This creates important challenges for health service delivery. The second issue concerns the very weak or absent public involvement in virtually all aspects of the health system but especially delivery as this is commonly the interface of the public with the health system. Most systems around the region have not found a space for public involvement and continue to operate in the we-know-what's-best mode. This must and will change with the profound social and political changes under way in the region whereby the public is demanding more accountability and transparency and a greater role in running public affairs.

The third issue, which reflects the first two, concerns *health system performance and effectiveness*. Even by traditional conventions, health systems in the Arab world do not fare well. The 2000 World

Health Report (WHO 2000) showed poor performance in most countries. Efficiency is commonly interpreted to mean cost-reduction, rather than more efficient use of resources. Systems that meet the needs and expectations, both broadly and holistically defined, of people do not exist in this region because the ideas of responding to needs and valuing expectations are not mainstreamed in the thinking and practice of policy makers. The equity gaps in access and utilization are well-demonstrated in Chapter 31. Health service users are commonly left to fend for themselves without adequate protection or reliable legal recourse.

Questioning the Foundations of Health Systems

The problems of our health systems mean that there is a need for a thorough and honest discussion, beyond the technicalities that usually overwhelm "expert" reviews of health systems and thus obscure key issues. We argue that there is a need to re-evaluate the very foundations of such systems. We propose to critically visit three subjects of concern, realizing that they are inter-dependent.

The *first concern* is the social contract that governs the relationship between the state, the different institutions, and the people. If a health system is "the lynchpin of the social role of the national state" as Chiffoleau (2005) correctly notes, then we need to focus on the state not just the system. In the regimes that have dominated the Arab world (at least until the onset of revolutions), unaccountable, idiosyncratic, and poorly functioning health systems reflect the broader systems within which they are embedded. Many Arab states perceive the health system as a burden, a source of financial drain even as they continue to finance and/or provide services. The latter are not seen as rights, investments, and the best method of wealth distribution, but rather as gifts handed by the state. The current social contract has been about providing services in exchange for loyalty.

By focusing on the role of the state we do not mean to excuse health system institutions from their responsibility for promoting good models of health systems. Furthermore, in public eyes, the health system is also commonly perceived as mere services to be used at the time of sickness, which denotes that a health system is merely *reactive*. A new social contract based on rights, accountability, equity, new roles for the state, and new thinking about health, is needed to transform current health systems to assume more *proactive* roles in promotion of health and well-being.

The *second concern* is the framework that has guided the development of health systems over the past decades. There is little hope for real reforms of such systems, beyond mere cosmetic work, if these are to remain predominantly "sickness systems" as they are today. Everyone eventually needs sick care but this is commonly a symptom of adverse health determinants and the failure of the system to promote health and prevent risks to health. A sickness framework gets in the way of examining how health systems help or do not help us address our health needs and secure the health of the entire population. The sectoral nature of current health system thinking creates problems; people do not live in sectors, they live in the community. As their health problems usually originate in social structures and practices, this is where new health system thinking must look for solutions.

Sickness systems have large vested interests to defend them. Even for governments, the sickness model of health systems may be convenient because it transfers the responsibility of ill-health to individuals and communities rather than point to the structures of exclusion, alienation, exploitation, or neglect that cause ill-health. With a sickness model, governments can always provide more services to show that they are responding to people. In turn, they gain more legitimacy and control. The sickness model corresponds well to the deformed social contract to which we have just alluded. The political and ideological basis of this practice, whose translation in health policy is "victim-blaming" and encouraging people to take care of themselves, has been critiqued in other settings for a long time (see for example Crawford 1977).

Some might argue that our health system problems stem not from the models we have adopted but from the ways we have applied the knowledge. We believe the issue is more complex. The test of reality indicates that the application of sickness framework in the region for the past several decades has produced the kind of structures which the five chapters in this section rightly critique. Our health systems, and commonly reform efforts, don't work well because they do not properly address the underlying determinants of failures as Giacaman et al note in the Palestinian case (2003). These determinants are the socio-economic and political conditions that have shaped Arab countries today: Political instability, political exclusion, lack of leadership, the failure of the

359

modernization project following the 1967 defeat, corruption, mismanagement, and wastage of resources, among others.

Linked to the first two issues, the *third* concern is the disconnection of health system work from work on the social determinants. Even as health systems must ensure adequate supplies and services and good technical performance of facilities and providers, they must integrate work on broader determinants of health and ensure protection of health. Ministries of health cannot claim that they have no influence over broader social and economic policies that impact health. Exercising this influence must be integrated as part of their basic mandate. A good measure of how well our future health systems work will be how well they impact the broader policy environment. Indeed, we argue that this line of work is within reach of current systems but is not put to good use because of complacency and fear of confronting vested interests. Parties, not limited to government agencies but including players ranging from global funders to local private investors, are accountable for the health impact of social policies.

Health systems and social determinants are also connected through consequences of ill health. Financial vulnerability in times of sickness and need for services is commonly the most urgent form of the link between the health system and social determinants. Chapter 29 refers to this as social health protection and reviews data on the risks to families from catastrophic health expenditures (see also Elgazzar et al [2010]). That millions of people are impoverished as a result of health care costs each year should no longer be acceptable. It is ironic that health systems that fail to protect from ill health can also impoverish when people get ill. Worse, whatever social protection methods that exist today, efforts have been under way to dismantle them under liberalization reforms.

The comprehensive public health framework of population health goes beyond social protection in times of crisis and into building individual and community assets through work on the social determinants. This should become one of the core functions of future health systems in the Arab world.

Health System Reforms

It may seem far-fetched to think of a new social contract, of re-founding our health systems on the basis of health rather than sickness, and of mainstreaming work on determinants in the core business of a health system. But this is what it would take to address the structural ills of our health systems to which we have alluded earlier. The new realities in the Arab world starting with the regime change in Tunisia and Egypt may offer the rare historical opportunity. This opportunity must be seized. The reforms cannot be realized without a deliberate effort by policy makers and health professionals who join forces with a broader constituency.

As the case study on the fight for health system reform in Egypt (Chapter 37) shows, there have been important efforts of social mobilization to counter efforts at liberalizing and privatizing health care. Such efforts will always be needed. But much more needs to be done to show the possibility of alternatives to existing health systems and even more to develop such alternatives from the structures, services, and workforce that Arab countries already have in place, making the best use of the available resources. The health systems cannot accomplish all the needed changes which require broader political and policy reforms. But change must also happen from within the health systems if health professionals wish to become part of change. This is the real challenge for the near future.

References

Akala FA, El-Saharty S (2006) Public-health challenges in the Middle East and North Africa. *The Lancet*, 367 (9515): 961–964

Assai M, Siddiqi S, Watts S (2006) Tackling social determinants of health through community based initiatives. *British Medical Journal*, 333: 854–856

Baum FE, Bégin M, Houweling TA, Taylor S (2009) Changes not for the fainthearted: Reorienting health care systems toward health equity through action on the social determinants of health. *American Journal of Public Health*, 99(11): 1967–1974

Breton M, Denis JL, Lamothe L (2010) Incorporating public health more closely into local governance of health care delivery: Lessons from the Québec experience. *Canadian Journal of Public Health*, 101(4): 314–317

Chiffoleau S (2005) NGOs and the reform of the Egyptian health system: Realistic prospects of a pipe-dearm? *In*: C Milani, S Ben Nefissa, S Hanafi, N Abd al-Fattah (Eds.) *NGOs and governance in the Arab world* (p. 167–179). Cairo, Egypt: American University in Cairo Press

Crawford R (1977) You are dangerous to your health: The ideology and politics of victim blaming.

International Journal of Health Services, 7(4): 663–680

Elgazzar H, Raad F, Arfa C, et al (2010) *Who pays? Out-of-pocket health spending and equity implications in the Middle East and North Africa. Health, nutrition and population (HNP) discussion paper.* Washington, DC: the World Bank

Giacaman R, Abdul-Rahim HF, Wick L (2003) Health sector reform in the Occupied Palestinian Territories (OPT): Targeting the forest or the trees? *Health Policy and Planning*, 18(1): 59–67

Longuenesse E (Ed.) (1995) Santé médecine et société dans le monde arabe. Lyon-Paris, France: Maison de l'Orient Méditerranéen-L'Harmattan [In French]

Mays GP, Smith SA, Ingram RC, Racster LJ, Lamberth CD, Lovely ES (2009) Public health delivery systems: Evidence, uncertainty, and emerging research needs. *American Journal of Preventive Medicine*, 36(3): 256–265

Pierre-Louis AM, Akala FA, Karam HS (Eds.) (2004) *Public-health in the Middle East and North Africa: Meeting the challenges of the twenty-first century.* Washington, DC: the World Bank

WHO (World Health Organization) (2000) *The World Health Report 2000. Health systems: Improving performance.* Geneva: WHO

WHO EMRO (World Health Organization-Regional Office for the Eastern Mediterranean) (2004) *Health systems priorities in the Eastern Mediterranean Region: Challenges and strategic directions, Technical paper EM/RC51/5.* Cairo: WHO EMRO

Chapter

28

Health System Governance

Sameen Siddiqi and Samer Jabbour

Governance is a key determinant of social, economic, and overall development and of attainment of the Millennium Development Goals in countries in this region (Siddiqi et al 2009). Governance's relationship to health systems and social determinants of health, and consequently to health outcomes, seems obvious; nevertheless how the various attributes of governance influence health is a subject that has received limited attention in the regional public health literature, and only recently has attracted increasing attention in the international literature on low- and middle-income countries (LMICs). Health system governance (HSG) is an increasingly important concern in most such countries, because of the increasing demand to demonstrate results and accountability at a time when increasing resources are being put into health systems and health systems must evolve to adapt to changes in population health, globalization, and unregulated expansion of the private sector.

In this chapter, we start with defining various terms related to HSG and contextualize HSG within the broader regional governance picture. We present findings from a study in six Arab countries that has used a framework developed regionally for assessing HSG. We then examine the response of Arab countries in three areas that present important challenges to health system governance, and conclude with a discussion of recommendations for strengthening HSG.

Terms and Definitions

Defined as the exercise of political, economic, and administrative authority in the management of a country's affairs at all levels, *governance* is not about governments alone. Governance comprises the complex mechanisms, processes, and institutions through which citizens and groups articulate their interests, mediate their differences and exercise their legal rights and obligations (UK Department of Health 1998). *Health system governance* concerns the actions and means adopted by a society to organize itself in the promotion and protection of the health of its population (Dodgson et al 2002). In the broadest sense, HSG includes the formal and informal rules and the organizations that operate within these rules to carry out the key functions of a health system. HSG not only influences all other functions of the health system but ranks above these functions.

Because the government is ultimately responsible for the health of the population and overall health system performance, HSG is primarily a governmental responsibility especially towards achieving the goal of equity (Labonté 2010). As Bennett et al (2009) note, governance "should not only be effective, it also needs to be fair." In addition to improving population health and reducing health inequalities, Bennett et al identify a third key function of governance which is ensuring sustainability of public health solutions. To achieve these functions, governance cannot be merely a technical process; it is also a political process. Governance must percolate through all the levels of the health system in order to maximize health outcomes.

Two other terms overlap with HSG. The first is "stewardship" used in the 2000 World Health Report (WHO 2000). The second is "public health governance," used for example by Bennett et al (2009) and Marks et al (2010). The domains of these terms overlap with those of HSG in many ways although they may not be identical in the minds of many. To avoid confusion we only use the term HSG in this chapter as it has come into wider use recently, has a broader connotation than stewardship, and covers both public health and medical care.

Public Health in the Arab World, ed. Samer Jabbour et al. Published by Cambridge University Press. © Samer Jabbour et al., 2012.

HSG has subcomponents, the most commonly discussed being *health care governance* (Lewis & Pettersson 2009), concerned with improving quality, performance, and outcomes of services. This is important because of the increasingly powerful private sectors and the central role of health services in health systems (UK Department of Health 1998). Health care is commonly discussed in terms of the two dimensions of *clinical* and *financial* governance. Bem (2010) proposes a third dimension, *social* governance, which is concerned with bringing the social dimension of health into delivery. There is now a large literature on clinical governance (see the review by Braithwaite & Travaglia [2008]) and its application in various settings and even health conditions.

Broader spheres of governance also influence health. In a globalized world, *global governance, i.e.* the institutions, rules, state actors, and pressure groups influence transnational rule and authority systems. With the emergence of powerful actors in health, *global health governance* has become the subject of expansive scholarship in recent years (Meier & Fox 2010).

Corporate governance (World Bank 1994), which refers to corporate transparency, accountability, and mechanisms for meeting social responsibility, applies to all the aforementioned levels of governance.

All these spheres of governance can potentially impact public health, depending on a country's macroeconomic and geopolitical situation and the organization of the health system. Countries of the Arab world are not impervious to such influences.

The Broader Governance Picture in the Arab World

Consideration of HSG would be incomplete without contextualizing HSG in the general state of governance in Arab countries (see also Chapter 2). HSG and its reform are as likely to be influenced by the country's overall governance as the health system and its reform are influenced by the broader public sector policies and reforms. The governance picture is not uniform and substantial variations exist among Arab countries in how state governing organs, i.e., executive, legislative, judiciary, civil service, and military/intelligence, operate and interact. But there are many similarities in the architecture and methods of governance. The *executive apparatus*

promotes regime maintenance and ensures centralized control. In many countries such centralization is institutionally guaranteed and vests vast powers in a few people, usually the head of the state. Except in a few countries, *parliaments or shuras*, instead of representing the populace, by enacting independent legislation or providing checks against unrestrained executive power, function as the regime's bureaucratic organs. In many situations, the *judiciary* is subservient to the executive and at times is used by the executive as an instrument to legitimize its political ambitions. The *intelligence apparatus* in many Arab countries is an essential means for sustaining the regime and often has greater say in state decisions than the parliament or the judiciary. Hence, Arab state survival has become increasingly dependent on control and propaganda; on marginalizing elites through scare and promise tactics; on striking bargains with dominant global and regional powers; and on mutually supportive regional blocs to reinforce the status of ruling elites against emerging forces.

This political set-up, which has historical, political, economic, and social determinants related to legacies of colonialism, post-colonial state formation, and complex interactions of global, regional, and local powers, results in major governance deficits, as outlined in Chapter 2. The region has the world's widest governance gap (World Bank 2003). With weak rule of law and constraints of rights, accountability and inclusiveness are especially problematic (World Bank 2003; UNDP 2004). Quality of administration is below developing world average. This governance picture affects all sectors, including health, and thus has a major influence on the performance of the health system. For example, the World Bank (2003) reported that better governance, measured in terms of quality of administration, was associated with higher life expectancy and child immunization and lower maternal and infant mortality.

An Expanded Framework for Assessing Health System Governance: Evidence From a Six-Country Study

Although there are numerous papers and media reports of one or more aspects of HSG such as corruption or lack of accountability, there is very limited regional literature on HSG seen in the comprehensive lens. For example, Tawfik-Shukor & Khoshnaw (2010) explicitly discussed HSG in Iraqi Kurdistan but their analytic framework did not include the typical domains of HSG. The need for a comprehensive evaluation of HSG was a main impetus for a global consultation convened by the WHO's Eastern Mediterranean Regional Office (EMRO) (WHO EMRO 2007). This section reviews the results of an EMRO-sponsored regional study done in six Arab countries, in addition to Afghanistan, Iran, and Pakistan.

Frameworks for Assessing Governance

While there is broad agreement that most Arab countries face enormous HSG challenges (WHO EMRO 2004, 2007), a challenge in itself has been to assess these challenges in as objective a manner as possible, so as to draw the attention of policy makers and other stakeholders. There is limited literature on assessing HSG in LMICs. The four frameworks that have been applied or adapted for the assessment of HSG are (i) World Health Organization's (WHO) domains of stewardship (Travis et al 2002); (ii) Pan American Health Organization's (PAHO) essential public health functions (PAHO 2002); (iii) World Bank's six dimensions of governance (Kaufmann et al 1999); and (iv) UNDP's principles of good governance (UNDP 1997). These frameworks have different but overlapping principles and attributes and have strengths and limitations. The World Bank and UNDP's framework are not specific to health systems. The PAHO framework is more focused on performance of public health rather than on overall HSG. The WHO framework does not carry sufficient detail to capture all relevant attributes of HSG. None of these frameworks have been applied to HSG in the Arab world. It would be useful to use a framework that has been developed regionally. The following case study describes such a framework.

Case Study From Six Arab Countries

Health system governance in six Arab countries – Egypt, Jordan, Lebanon, Syria, Sudan, and Tunisia – was assessed in 2006/07 using an analytic framework developed by the Eastern Mediterranean Regional Office of the World Health Organization. The framework includes 10 HSG principles – *strategic vision, consensus and participation, rule of law, transparency,*

responsiveness, equity and inclusiveness, efficiency and effectiveness, accountability, intelligence and information, and ethics. The explanation of each governance principle is given in Table 1. The framework, case study methodology, and the results of its application in Pakistan have been discussed elsewhere (Siddiqi et al 2009). This analysis of the results in the Arab countries has not been previously published.

The Ministry of Health (MOH) is considered the principal governing body of the health system and has the mandate for health policy making, planning, regulation, monitoring, and evaluation and for ensuring access to essential health services. There are thus two levels – health policy formulation and policy implementation. In some Arab countries, the MOH is responsible for both, while in others implementation of health services falls under the jurisdiction of subnational (state, provincial, district, or local) governments. There is an additional level above the MOH: The national government through its broad social and economic policies, legislative function, civil service reforms, and its political (in)stability influences HSG. The analytical framework thus poses questions for each of the 10 principles at three levels – the national level, the health policy formulation level, and the policy implementation level. The Web Appendix provides the general results of the study in the six countries. We review below selected strengths and weaknesses in the 10 domains.

Strategic vision. Except in Sudan the constitution guarantees universal access to health care and recognizes health as a basic human right to all citizens. All countries have a national health policy, strategy or a medium-term strategic plan that aims at creating a comprehensive health system. The main challenge is the incongruence of objectives between the strategic vision and operational plans, and lack of operational policies, procedures, and protocols to implement strategic vision.

Participation and consensus orientation. The experience among countries is variable. In some countries, e.g., Jordan, there is a higher level health committee which involves other concerned ministries and the non-state health sector. Major decisions regarding the health sector are largely centralized and participation restricted as seen in the case of Sudan, Syria, and also Tunisia. Several countries, particularly Lebanon and Jordan, involve civil society organizations or associations of health professionals. Consumer and community representation in health

Table 1. Framework for Assessing Health System Governance

Governance principle	Explanation
Strategic vision	Leaders have a broad and long-term perspective on health and human development, along with a sense of strategic directions for such development. There is also an understanding of the historical, cultural, and social complexities in which that perspective is grounded
Participation and consensus orientation	All men and women should have a voice in decision making for health, either directly or through legitimate intermediate institutions that represent their interests. Such broad participation is built on freedom of association and speech, as well as capacities to participate constructively. Good governance of the health system mediates differing interests to reach a broad consensus on what is in the best interests of the group and, where possible, on health policies and procedures
Rule of law	Legal frameworks pertaining to health should be fair and enforced impartially, particularly the laws on human rights related to health
Transparency	Transparency is built on the free flow of information for all health matters. Processes, institutions, and information should be directly accessible to those concerned with them, and enough information is provided to understand and monitor health matters
Responsiveness	Institutions and processes should try to serve all stakeholders to ensure that the policies and programs are responsive to the health and non-health needs of its users
Equity and inclusiveness	All men and women should have opportunities to improve or maintain their health and well-being
Effectiveness and efficiency	Processes and institutions should produce results that meet population needs and influence health outcomes while making the best use of resources
Accountability	Decision makers in government, the private sector and civil society organizations involved in health are accountable to the public, as well as to institutional stakeholders. This accountability differs depending on the organization and whether the decision is internal or external to an organization
Intelligence and information	Intelligence and information are essential for a good understanding of a health system, without which it is not possible to provide evidence for informed decisions that influences the behavior of different interest groups that support, or at least do not conflict with, the strategic vision for health
Ethics	The commonly accepted principles of health care ethics include respect for autonomy, nonmaleficence, beneficence, and justice. Health care ethics, which includes ethics in health research, is important to safeguard the interest and the rights of the patients

Source: Siddiqi et al (2009)

boards is weak or absent and their voices not well echoed in decision making or reflected in the decisions taken.

Rule of law. Health laws have existed in most countries for a long time but are often outdated, particularly in Sudan. There is limited capacity in many MOHs to prepare laws due to lack of legal expertise. Mechanisms to monitor or assess enforcement of health-related legislation are generally weak, especially in relation to the private sector. A clear legal recourse for consumers or patients related to unsafe products or medical errors does not function well. Consumer protection laws, consumer rights organizations, or patient safety mechanisms either function sub-optimally or, as in Sudan, do not exist at all.

Transparency. The lack of transparent criteria for public sector resource allocation for the various levels of care is common to all six countries. Formal mechanisms to monitor transparency of administrative decisions such as recruitment, promotion, and transfers to managerial positions often do not exist. MOHs produce information to evaluate access, equity, and quality of health services, as in the case of Tunisia, but this information is not widely shared and often remains internal to ministries or specific institutions.

Responsiveness. of health services and institutions is not regularly assessed. User satisfaction surveys are undertaken occasionally in Jordan, Lebanon, and Tunisia, particularly for public sector facilities. Population health needs are commonly determined by health professionals with little involvement of the public.

Equity and inclusiveness. While equity and universal coverage in health services feature in national policies and strategies, there are gaps between policy and practice. While this is especially evident in Sudan, there are barriers to accessing health services for many vulnerable groups in all other countries. In Egypt, for example, inequities in financing of care exist in terms of high out-of pocket payments although physical access may not be a problem.

Effectiveness and efficiency. Appointment of mid-to senior-level managers is variable and political favoritism and personal preferences are common. Career structures in the MOH are well defined for bureaucrats but not necessarily for technocrats. Figures for staff turnover are not available or reliable. Salaries of public sector staff are unsatisfactory except in Jordan and Tunisia. Except in Jordan, public sector physicians commonly engage in private practice, sometimes during working hours or even within the institution they serve. A system of continuing professional development of staff does not function properly and is not institutionalized. In general, physicians-turned-managers lack understanding of administrative matters, while bureaucrats lack proper understanding of health ones.

Accountability. In this region, this is the area that the public perceives to be the most problematic. Some form of accountability exists in all countries, most commonly being the ability of the cabinet or parliament to question decisions taken by the MOH. Accountability is also theoretically maintained through auditing bureaus, internal auditors, and the media. In reality, due to overall governance structures, internal and external accountability systems, including to the health system beneficiaries, do not function well. Personnel, financial, and procurement systems are managed manually and information is generally not shared. A public health accounts committee exists in some countries but does not function effectively. External auditing by independent firms is practiced only occasionally. The means and measures to monitor the lifestyles and accounts of civil servants are either non-existent or not implemented. Interference by powerful vested interests is a major constraint to promoting accountability. There is limited information about the magnitude of corruption in the health system or measures to control it. The level of engagement of civil society is highest in Lebanon and lowest in Sudan and Syria. The press and media in all countries is playing an increasing role in exposing health system problems. Mechanisms to hold the private health sector accountable are lacking in most countries.

Intelligence and information. This area is especially problematic in Sudan. Other MOHs produce annual or occasional statistical reports that cover several aspects of the health status and health services. But the health information system is not integrated and generally deficient. From a governance perspective, the main challenge is that decision makers do not use information "intelligently" and personal and political considerations override evidence in decision making.

Ethics. Generally, ethics is not considered an important attribute of HSG and is not high on the policy agenda of most MOHs and related institutions.

Building on the Regional Study for Future Research

There is no "gold standard" for HSG against which to assess the framework used in this study. However, the framework has undergone international peer review indicating a level of conceptual rigor. Future research might evaluate a more parsimonious model that retains the ability to capture the key dimensions of HSG as Reidpath & Allotey (2006) did with reducing the six dimensions of the World Bank's governance framework into a single measure using principle factor analysis. At the same time, there is need to explore the local meanings and applications of the various components of HSG. For example, Brinkerhoff (2004) notes that accountability is complex and should have analytic and conceptual clarity "to be more than an empty buzzword." This is consistent with the recommendation of Maddalena (2006).

The framework is designed for cross-sectional analysis. Instruments for tracking HSG need to be developed considering that health systems are dynamic and adaptive and change due to the population's changing demographic and epidemiologic profiles; rising expectations of a more educated and rights-aware clientele; a fast growing private health sector; rapid changes in medical technology; increasing influence of globalization; and the desire to rapidly expand services and achieve universal health coverage.

The data on HSG in individual countries were collected by national researchers and practitioners whose personal experiences and views, closeness to state apparatus (some work in MOH), and access to informants and information sources may have influenced data collection or interpretation. In a sense, the HSG picture may be worse than is assessed here. Future research should validate the findings in the same countries.

The regional study provides useful insights into many areas that need improvement. But which ones are the most critical? This is a subject for future research. We argue that some principles are at the heart of good governance and are key to other governance functions. Good leadership and good governance are inextricably linked. It is less important to debate which governance element to tackle first than to ensure that the leadership is committed to ensuring the desired HSG improvements. In the framework, this is most reflected in three key functions: *Strategic vision, transparency, and accountability*. The country studies demonstrate these areas to be closely intertwined and determine health system performance. Delayed decisions, lengthy procedures, lack of respect for merit, political interference, and "red tape" undermine HSG. Inefficiency and ineffectiveness to a large extent exist due to the lack of *accountability and transparency* which pervades all sectors, including health, in many Arab countries.

The flip side of accountability and transparency is incompetence and corruption. Country studies show numerous examples of both. At the level of service delivery, they take such forms as staff absenteeism, under-the-table payments in public facilities, and kickbacks in private facilities, working in private clinics during public service hours and political interference and nepotism in staff recruitment, promotion, posting, and transfers. At the decision making level, there is inappropriate turnover of policy makers and managers, misallocation of resources based on political influence, kickbacks for large procurements, especially seen in biomedical technology and the pharmaceutical sector, or the lack of monitoring of the assets and lifestyles of

civil servants. These findings validate and add insights to evidence on corruption in the health sector from other reports. In Morocco, for example, 80% of interviewees in surveys of public officials, business executives, and the general public perceived high level of corruption in health; health ranked among the top four most corrupt sectors (Lewis 2006). Delavallade (2006) demonstrated that corruption in health is part of broader corruption in public spending in the Middle East and North Africa. The Global Corruption Report 2006 focusing on corruption and health (Transparency International 2006) shows this problem to be pervasive across regions. Corruption in health adds to the cost of health care and is part of the overall picture of widespread corruption which undermines development in this region (Transparency International 2009). However, the literature on corruption in health is still sparse in this region making this an important area for future research.

The framework does not explore governance outcomes. While the links between overall governance and population health are well demonstrated in the international literature (see for example, the eloquent analysis by Reidpath & Allotey 2006), the literature on the links between HSG and health outcomes is still scant. In stressing the importance of HSG, we agree with Reidpath & Allotey that, in addition to governance, other structural factors, including physical ones such as presence of basic services, must be considered. Future research in this region that explores the structures-overall governance-HSG-health links can make an important contribution to the international literature.

Health System Governance at Work: Responses of Arab Countries to Challenges in a Globalized World

In this section, we examine three examples that illustrate, in practical ways, how HSG is implicitly translated in decision making in public health and health systems.

Trade in Health Services

Under a new global economic order, many trade practices and rules, including the World Trade Organization's (WTO) and its General Agreement on Trade in Services (GATS), pose major challenges to health systems in Arab countries. One such challenge relates to the increasing liberalization of trade in health services (TiHS). A study conducted in 2005/06 in nine Arab countries – Egypt, Jordan, Lebanon, Morocco, Oman, Sudan, Syria, Tunisia, and Yemen – estimated the direction, volume, and value of TiHS; analyzed country commitments; and assessed the challenges and opportunities as a result of liberalization of TiHS (Siddiqi et al 2010).

Consumption of health services abroad and movement of persons were the two prevalent modes. Yemen and Sudan are net importers, while Jordan promotes health tourism. In 2002, Yemenis spent US$80 million out of pocket for treatment abroad, while Jordan generated US$620 million from providing health care to non-Jordanians. Egypt, Sudan, and Tunisia export health workers, while Oman relies on import; 40% of its workforce is non-Omani. The percentage of foreign health workers is even higher in other GCC countries. This was the first organized attempt to look at TiHS in the region. From a governance and public health perspective the assessment showed a lack of policy coherence between ministries of health and ministries of trade and commerce. In trade negotiations it is the officials of the latter ministries that speak on behalf of the MOH; thus their (lack of) understanding of the public health implications is critical. The development of institutional capacity through establishment of trade and health units in MOHs is essential. The most promising is the case in Jordan, which by virtue of being the biggest promoter of medical tourism in the region has a well thought out policy and good capacity in MOH.

Assessing TiHS is particularly relevant for countries in the process of accession to WTO or aspiring to become future members such as Iraq, Lebanon, Libya, and Syria. The decision to liberalize should be based on a sound understanding of the current situation of country needs and the opportunities of TiHS to adequately protect access, equity, and efficiency of domestic health services. Countries are not obliged to liberalize TiHS unless they are convinced that the benefits offset the risks. An important measure in this regard is for countries to update their private health sector regulatory framework prior to inviting foreign direct investments.

Contracting of Health Care Services

Many governments and MOHs commonly contract with the private sector to deliver publicly financed health services that cover some of the population health needs. Contracting has become an important tool in health sector reform proposals and is commonly coupled with policies of economic and social liberalization. Calls within influential international health policy circles for governments to shed their role as service providers and focus on their roles as purchasers and regulators further underline the growing importance of contracting in health systems worldwide (WHO EMRO 2005).

A study sponsored and supported by EMRO in 2004 in seven Arab countries, in addition to Afghanistan, Iran, and Pakistan, has shed light on the contracting experiences (Siddiqi et al 2006). The rationale given by government informants for contracting was the public's disillusion with public health services, improving services, and better targeting of vulnerable populations. In Bahrain and Lebanon, political commitment to the role of the private sector was a main determinant. Contracting was to serve decentralization in Morocco, decrease the cost of treatment incurred on patients sent to foreign countries for treatment in Tunisia, improve utilization of private hospitals and save capital investment on public facilities in Jordan, and to enhance coverage and quality of services and increase access to advanced medical technology available in private hospitals in Egypt.

While contacting may offer a solution to service provision in certain cases, it presents many challenges from a governance and public health perspective. At the policy level, most studied countries do not employ contracting strategically and do not study its broad implications. At the technical level, the public sector has limited capacity to undertake the necessary components of contracting: For example, proper studies of population needs, legal expertise in preparing contracts, and transparent bidding in the pre-contract phase; monitoring the execution of contracts during the implementation phase; and evaluation of outcomes in the post-contract phase. These limitations call on MOHs to approach contracting within a broader health governance perspective.

Capacity for Evidence-Based Health Policy Making

Health policy making is the mechanism by which competing visions for HSG are effectively translated in the health sector. Because of its broad impact on the health system and health outcomes, health policy making, which can be either explicit or implicit (Ham & Coulter 2001), is an essential area for public health scrutiny. While health policy making is fundamentally a political process in any country, policy making also reflects additional considerations such as the capacity of policy makers and resource availability. Furthermore, whether policy making is evidence-based is a key issue for public health. What is the situation in the Arab world?

Policy making can be considered from two aspects – the policy content based on the best available evidence and the participatory policy process. In terms of *policy content*, Arab countries have adopted different approaches; some have clear policy documents to aid in content analysis. For example, in recent years Sudan developed a 25-year national health policy while Morocco has a *Vision 2020 for Health*. Other countries, such as Egypt, have a health sector reform strategy, whereas in Syria, Tunisia, and some Gulf Cooperation Council (GCC) countries, it is the 5-year national health plan that drives policy making. It is difficult to determine the extent to which evidence feeds into any national health policy or strategy in Arab countries. Researching this area is hampered by lack of publicly accessible datasets on health systems in the region (Saleh et al 2009). Anecdotal data and reviews (see for example Jabbour et al 2009) indicate that for whatever evidence that exists, influence on policy making is partial at best with a substantial room for improvement. This is the case even for evidence generated by the governments. For example, in a multi-regional study including five Arab countries, there was variability in how evidence from national health accounts was used to formulate policies (De et al 2003).

Focus on policy content alone diverts attention from understanding the *policy processes*, which explains why desired policy outcomes fail to emerge (Walt & Gilson 1994). Although this has not been sufficiently analyzed in most developing countries (Gilson & Raphaely 2008), there is anecdotal evidence that in most Arab countries this process is not participatory, a measure of weak governance in health and a mirror of the lack of good governance at the broader level. In some countries, e.g., Lebanon and Jordan, there is more debate on health issues among the various stakeholders than in others, e.g., the GCC countries, Syria, or Sudan, where the process is at best restrictive and engagement of non-state actors and academia is minimal.

What are the reasons that undermine evidence-based policy making in the region? Observations point to several key issues. We can look at these issues at three levels. At the national level, in order for evidence

to flow into health policy making, there is a need for high level political commitment to collecting evidence prior to, and using it during, decision making. Such commitment is rarely observed. Many MOHs do not collect the evidence for health policy making and have limited institutional capacity for policy analysis and formulation and cannot reap the full benefits from such policy tools as burden of disease and national health accounts. In many MOHs there are separate policy and planning units, which often lack synergy and coordination. In many countries the final authority with policy decisions in health resides not in MOHs but in the ministries of planning and finance, which adds another layer in the decision-making process.

At the level of social actors, academia's research and practice agendas have not been well aligned with national health agendas (Jabbour et al 2009). Although public health research priorities are slowly changing, the pace of the change has to markedly accelerate to have any influence on policymaking. The published policy research often does not reach policy makers in a timely or effective manner. Civil societies can play an important role in influencing national health policies by being the true voice of the populace and by advocating for policies that promote equity, social justice and benefit the most vulnerable segments of the population. However, this role remains weak.

The third level concerns global factors. In low-income countries such as Yemen and Sudan, there are several development partners and donor agencies without proper harmonization among them or adequate alignment to national health policies, despite the commitments they pronounced to meet these goals through the Paris Declaration on Aid Effectiveness and the Accra Agenda for Action (OECD 2008). This can contribute to derailing instead of streamlining the policy priorities and the entire process itself. Donors also influence health policy and reform directions in other countries such as Egypt and Jordan. In Egypt, the health reform unit was for many years associated with a multi-donor funded project. Global policy developments have influenced national health governance and policies in most Arab countries as they do elsewhere. This is reflected in the opposition of centralized planning vs. reliance on free market approaches seen in the neighbors, Syria and Lebanon, respectively (Siddiqi et al 2009). Similarly, the shift from comprehensive to selective primary health care has had a major influence on health policies with the launch of corresponding vertical and disease-specific prevention and control programs in most

MOHs (Siddiqi et al 2008). These currently constitute the major approaches used by national governments to tackle priority public health problems.

In relation to the third global level, international evidence suggests that influence is more evident in countries with weaker health systems and public health leadership as discussed for example in the case study of Tajikistan (Rechel & Khodjamurodov 2010). This is contrasted with the case study of Thailand (Hanvoravongchai et al 2010) whereby support of the Global Fund to Fight AIDS, Tuberculosis, and Malaria seems to have contributed more positively to an already strong health system. This evidence provides even stronger support for the need to strengthen local and national and even regional health governance and policy making in this globalized era.

There are encouraging signs that things are changing and policy making is receiving more attention. In the area of evidence, the Eastern Mediterranean Regional Health System Observatory (WHO EMRO 2010) is attempting to generate evidence for health policy making. A collaborative regional research project involving 14 countries is now focusing on processes, obstacles, and opportunities in evidence-based policy making as part of a global initiative of the Alliance for Health Policy and Systems Research. New regional forums, such as the Eastern Mediterranean Regional Institutions Network in Public Health (EMRAIN) and the Middle East and North Africa Health Policy Forum, have emerged and aim to mobilize academia and other actors in favor of essential health policy and systems research and will hopefully allow academia to emerge as leaders in this area. There are more NGOs whose work concern health and policy. Even for the public, the word "policy" is no longer the taboo it used to be when confused with "politics" (there is one word in Arabic, *Siyasah*, for both policy and politics), and we see their voices in newspapers and Internet sites.

Toward Better Health System Governance

As HSG assessment tools and instruments get developed, it is important to develop in parallel strategies and interventions for improvement. This can be likened to building a sailing boat and sailing at the same time. Some might ask at the outset whether HSG can be improved without addressing the overall governance in Arab countries. This is an important question that deserves public debate and scholarship. Jabbour et al

(2006) argued that actions in the health domain can contribute to broader social and political reforms. We argue likewise that improving HSG governance might be the harbinger of reforms in broader governance. Research suggests that various components of HSG are high priorities even for policy makers (El-Jardali et al 2010). While such priorities will be different in different contexts, we suggest three areas that potentially have broad implications across the Arab countries.

Building the Evidence Base for Governance in Health and the Role of Non-state Actors

What does not get measured does not get adequately addressed nor effectively managed. The importance of developing tools and instruments for assessing and tracking health governance cannot be overstated. Concerned health professionals can use these tools for awareness-raising among the broader health community and for advocacy with national and health policy makers. Generating the evidence can create the opportunities for opening debates on a subject that is often "pushed under the carpet." This by itself is one step towards more transparency and accountability. If governance is considered as an overarching theme for all health issues, then we can argue that all health research should consider a governance dimension or "variables" as other relevant dimensions. For example, an innovative study by Gaygısız (2010) assessed road traffic fatalities in relation to governance quality and cultural values. Such research brings concrete translation of the notion of governance into public health. To borrow the words of Rashid et al (2005), this helps bring governance down from the "large" and potentially vague to the "small" and concrete.

Non-state actors, especially the civil society and non-governmental organizations, have important roles to play as "watch dogs" over the public sector on matters related to corruption, transparency, accountability, and efficiency. While in some Arab countries these parties have begun to assume this role, as Chapter 33 discusses, in many others they remain weak, unorganized, or too oppressed to rise to the challenge. Policy makers are more inclined to address health governance problems and scandals that appear in the press and television, than those published in the scientific literature. Health advocates can seize a real opportunity here to partner with and use the media to inform the public, hold the policy makers to account, and influence governance in health. Public health training and research institutions, both public and private, enjoy relative academic freedom that they can leverage to generate, synthesize, and disseminate evidence and influence health policy and policy makers. So far such institutions in Arab countries have not been able to play this role effectively due to a multitude of factors including lack of engagement with issues in the public sphere, inadequate or poor channels of communication with policy and decision makers, and pressures of academic work. This situation needs to be remedied as the role of academia is essential (Jabbour et al 2009).

Strengthening the Role of the State and Its Ministry of Health

While the state apparatus can itself be the obstacle to good governance, a stronger role of public sector agencies is the most essential component of improving HSG. The MOHs must find ways to lead this process. If the will for change exists, MOHs can find the means to build their institutional capacity to address many of the aforementioned HSG challenges such as developing a long-term vision for health; improving capacity for policy analysis and formulation; strategic planning; and health legislation, regulation, standard setting, and enforcement. Personnel, financial, procurement, and logistics management systems need to be revamped in many MOHs to reduce bureaucracy, enhance transparency, and improve performance in service of national health goals. The capacity of MOHs to engage and manage non-state actors and development partners, to build partnerships and to successfully undertake intersectoral action for health needs to be particularly strengthened. This is all the more important in countries with weak health systems and those that rely on significant donor support. Many MOHs need to undergo a manner of reorganization or restructuring to better align themselves in the role of stewards of the health system; of financiers, regulators, purchasers, and commonly in this region providers, of health services; and to become robust organizations and more relevant to the changing global and local landscape. This is a major and difficult undertaking that requires commitment at the highest political level but is a necessary step to improve HSG.

A leadership and strong role for national health authorities in HSG can translate across various subcomponents including clinical or health care governance discussed earlier. The benefits are not limited to curative services but can include public health as well. Breton et al (2010) demonstrated this based on a case study from Quebec, Canada. With reorganization of the provincial healthcare system, 95 Health and Social Services Centers were created and entrusted with integrating public health into their local governance structures. In addition to healthcare provision, the Centers gradually assumed population-based responsibilities such as attention to vulnerable groups, health promotion, and social services. Such an innovative model can have important benefits for public health in the Arab countries. This model goes beyond the conventional "decentralization" approach which is more administratively oriented and has shown mixed impact in the Arab countries that have pursued it.

Reducing Corruption to Improve Health Service Delivery

Often, there is reluctance to bring the issue of HSG on the table because it is understood to open the sensitive and difficult issue of corruption. While there is more to governance than just corruption, corruption in health needs to be prioritized and addressed head-on. There are no easy recipes to tackle such corruption. Nevertheless, strategies that have worked in other settings can be used in Arab countries (Transparency International 2006; Vian 2008). Advocates can push for specific health strategies within the broader anti-corruption initiatives in the region, for example the Arab Anti-Corruption & Integrity Network, a part of the UNDP's Programme on Governance in the Arab Region (UNDP 2010).

Conclusions

The road to good governance in health in the Arab world is long and uneven. Assessing health system governance and responses of countries to emerging challenges in a globalized world, as proposed and discussed here, is only the first step. A comprehensive approach to improving governance with the engagement of key actors in government, civil society, academia, and the media is needed. Researchers must be at the forefront to demonstrate impact on improving the performance of the health system and positively impacting public health.

Acknowledgment

Sameen Siddiqi is a staff member of the World Health Organization. The author alone is responsible for the views expressed in this publication and they do not necessarily represent the decisions or policies of the World Health Organization.

References

Bem C (2010) Social governance: A necessary third pillar of healthcare governance. *Journal of the Royal Society of Medicine*, 103(12): 475–477

Bennett B, Gostin L, Magnusson R, Martin R (2009) Health governance: Law, regulation and policy. *Public Health*, 123: 207–212

Braithwaite J, Travaglia JF (2008) An overview of clinical governance policies, practices and initiatives. *Australian Health Review*, 32(1): 10–22

Breton M, Denis JL, Lamothe L (2010) Incorporating public health more closely into local governance of health care delivery: Lessons from the Québec experience. *Canadian Journal of Public Health*, 1(4): 314–317

Brinkerhoff DW (2004) Accountability and health systems: Toward conceptual clarity and policy relevance. *Health Policy & Planning*, 19(6): 371–379

De S, Dmytraczenko T, Brinkerhoff D, Tien M (2003) *Has improved availability of health expenditure data contributed to evidence-based policymaking? Country Experiences with National Health Accounts*, Technical Report No. 022. Bethesda, MD: The Partners for Health Reformplus Project, Abt Associates Inc

Delavallade C (2006) Corruption and distribution of public spending in developing countries. *Journal of Economics and Finance*, 30(2): 222–239

Dodgson R, Lee K, Drager N (2002) *Discussion paper no. 1: Global health governance: A conceptual review.* Centre on Global Change & Health, Department of Health & Development, London School of Hygiene and Tropical Medicine and World Health Organization

Gaygısız E (2010) Cultural values and governance quality as correlates of road traffic fatalities: A nation level analysis. *Accident Analysis and Prevention*, 42: 1894–1901

Gilson L, Raphaely N (2008) The terrain of health policy analysis in low and middle income countries: A review of published literature 1994–2007. *Health Policy and Planning*, 23: 294–307

El-Jardali F, Makhoul J, Jamal D, Ranson MK, Kronfol NM, Tchaghchagian V (2010) Eliciting policymakers' and stakeholders' opinions to help shape health system research priorities in the Middle East and North Africa region. *Health Policy and Planning*, 25(1): 15–27

Ham C, Coulter A (2001) Explicit and implicit rationing: Taking responsibility and avoiding blame for health care choices. *Journal of Health Services Research & Policy*, 6(3): 163–169

Hanvoravongchai P, Warakamin B, Coker R (2010) Critical interactions between Global Fund-supported programmes and health systems: A case study in Thailand. *Health Policy and Planning*, 25: i53–i57

Jabbour S, El-Zein A, Nuwayhid I, Giacaman R (2006) Can action on health achieve political and social reform? *British Medical Journal*, 333: 837–839

Jabbour S, Rashidian A, Shawky S, Zaidi S (2009) *Role of academia in public health and health system development in the Eastern Mediterranean Region.* A background paper commissioned by the WHO EMRO for the "Regional Consultative Meeting on Capacity Development of Academic Institutions to Promote Health Systems and Research based on Primary Health Care" held in Beirut, Lebanon, December 2009

Kaufmann D, Kraay A, Zoido-Lobaton P (1999) *Governance matters, working paper no. 2196.* Washington, DC: World Bank

Labonté R (2010) Health systems governance for health equity: Critical reflections. *Revista de Salud Pública*, 12(1): 62–76

Lewis M (2006) *Governance and corruption in public health systems, Working paper number 78.* Washington, DC: Center for Global Development

Lewis M, Pettersson G (2009) *Governance in health care delivery: Raising performance.* Policy Research Working Paper 5074. Washington, DC: World Bank

Maddalena V (2006) Governance, public participation and accountability: To whom are regional health authorities accountable? *Healthcare Management Forum*, 19(3): 32–37

Marks L, Cave S, Hunter DJ (2010) Public health governance: Views of key stakeholders. *Public Health*, 124: 55–59

Meier BM, Fox AM (2010) International obligations through collective rights: Moving from foreign health assistance to global health governance. *Health & Human Rights*, 12(1): 61–72

OECD (Organization for Economic Co-operation and Development) (2008) *Paris declaration on aid effectiveness and the Accra Agenda for Action.* Available from http://www.oecd.org/dataoecd/11/41/34428351.pdf [Accessed 1 October 2010].

PAHO (Pan American Health Organization) (2002) Essential public health functions. *In: Public health in the Americas: Conceptual renewal, performance assessment and bases for action.* Scientific and Technical Publication no. 589. Washington, DC: PAHO

Rashid S, Savchenko Y, Hossain N (2005) Public health and governance: The experience of Bangladesh and Ukraine. *The Quarterly Review of Economics and Finance*, 45(2–3): 460–475

Rechel B, Khodjamurodov G (2010) International involvement and national health governance:

The basic benefit package in Tajikistan. *Social Science & Medicine*, 70(12): 1928–1932

Reidpath DD, Allotey P (2006) Structure, (governance) and health: An unsolicited response. *BMC International Health and Human Rights*, 6: 12

Saleh SS, Alameddine MS, El-Jardali F (2009) The case for developing publicly-accessible datasets for health services research in the Middle East and North Africa (MENA) region. *BMC Health Service Research*, 29(9): 197

Siddiqi S, Kielmann A, Watts S, Sabri B (2008) Primary health care, health policies and planning: Lessons for the future. *Eastern Mediterranean Health Journal*, 14: S42–S56

Siddiqi S, Masud TI, Sabri B (2006) Contracting but not without caution: Experience with outsourcing of health services in countries of the Eastern Mediterranean Region. *Bulletin of the World Health Organization*, 84(11): 867–875

Siddiqi S, Masud TI, Nishtar S, et al (2009) Framework for assessing governance of the health system in developing countries: Gateway to good governance. *Health Policy*, 90(1): 13–25

Siddiqi S, Shennawy A, Mirza Z, Drager N, Sabri B (2010) Assessing trade in health services in countries of from a public health perspective. *International Journal of Health Planning and Management*, 25(3): 231–250

Tawfik-Shukor A, Khoshnaw H (2010) The impact of health system governance and policy processes on health services in Iraqi Kurdistan, *BMC International Health and Human Rights*, 10: 14

Transparency International (2006) *Global Corruption Report 2006.* London, Ann Arbor: Pluto Press

Transparency International (2009) *Corruption in the MENA region, Working Paper #2/2009.* Berlin, Germany: Transparency International

Travis P, Egger D, Davies P, Mechbal A (2002) *Towards better stewardship: Concepts and critical issues.* Geneva, Switzerland: World Health Organization

UK Department of Health (1998) *A first class service: Quality in the new NHS.* London, UK: Department of Health

UNDP (United Nations Development Program) (1997) *Governance for sustainable human development: A UNDP policy document.* New York, NY: UNDP

UNDP (2004) *The Arab Human Development Report 2004. Towards Freedom in the Arab World.* New York, NY: UNDP

UNDP (2010) *Programme on governance in the Arab Region, Arab Anti-Corruption and Integrity Network.* Available from http://www.pogar.org/resources/ac/ [Accessed 1 October 2010]

Vian T (2008) Review of corruption in the health sector: Theory, methods and interventions. *Health Policy and Planning*, 23(2): 83–94

Walt G, Gilson L (1994) Reforming the health sector in developing countries: The central role of policy analysis. *Health Policy and Planning*, 9(4): 353–370

World Bank (1994) *Governance: The World Bank's experience.* Washington DC: IBRD

World Bank (2003) *Better governance for development in the Middle East and North Africa. Enhancing inclusiveness and accountability.* Washington, DC: World Bank

WHO (World Health Organization) (2000) *The World Health Report 2000, Health systems: Improving performance.* Geneva, Switzerland: WHO

WHO EMRO (WHO Regional Office for the Eastern Mediterranean) (2004) *Health systems priorities in the Eastern Mediterranean Region: Challenges and strategic directions, Technical Paper.* Cairo, Egypt: WHO – Eastern Mediterranean Regional Office (EMRO)

WHO EMRO (2005) *The role of contractual arrangements in improving health system performance. Report on a regional meeting.* Cairo, Egypt: WHO-EM/PHP/034/E

WHO EMRO (2007) *Health system governance for improving health system performance. Report of a WHO global consultation, WHO-EM/PHP/043/E.* Cairo, Egypt: WHO EMRO

WHO EMRO (2010) *Eastern Mediterranean Regional Health System Observatory.* Available from http://gis.emro.who.int/healthsystemobservatory [Accessed 1 October 2010]

Chapter

29

Health System Financing: The Bottleneck of the Right to Health

Belgacem Sabri, Driss Zine-Eddine El-Idrissi, and Awad Mataria

How a health system is financed directly impacts population access to health services, and consequently the right to health. Health system financing (HSF) arrangements determine the amount of resources available for the health sector, how those resources are mobilized, and how they are allocated across competing health and public health priorities. Whether the HSF arrangements prevalent in the Arab world promote or undermine the right to health is the main question that the present chapter aims to answer. We approach this question through analyzing HSF arrangements and policies across income and geographic groups. We intend to show how HSF affects individuals, households, and social protection. The chapter concludes with a vision for health system financing in the Arab world that might contribute to the renewal of the right to health.

The Wider Context

Arab countries are signatories to declarations, such as Universal Declaration of Human Rights, Alma Ata and Qatar Declarations, and world health resolutions that advocate for the right to health and equity, especially through primary health care and universal access (WHO EMRO 2008). The constitutions of most Arab countries recognize the right to health as a basic human right, and highlight government responsibility to protect health – although the scope and coverage are expressed differently across countries. For instance, in some constitutions, citizens are entitled to free health care provided through government services. Many countries incorporate commitments to equity, social justice, and solidarity in their national policies, to guide socio-economic development, including that of the health sector (see also Chapter 5). These commitments are expected to be reflected in financing arrangements for health, which have profound impact on health system performance and health outcomes.

HSF arrangements are influenced by national, regional, and global factors, including social and political determinants. The move toward market economy and some economic reforms have affected health systems and the right to health by weakening the state's role in the social sector. Such situation was worsened by the limited economic growth, particularly in low-income countries, and political instability and civil strife in several countries. In the poorest countries, the average annual economic growth between 1996 and 2005 was close to nil: in Djibouti, 1.3%; Mauritania, 0.1%; and was negative in Somalia. Financial barriers to accessing health care are increasing due to decreasing government spending on health. This shifts the financial burden to individuals and families, negatively affecting equity in access to services.

Methods and Analysis

Our analysis relies on the World Health Organization (WHO)'s framework of health systems that identifies three sub-functions for HSF: mobilizing resources, pooling risk, and allocating resources and purchasing services. Given that national income affects health system functions, including resources for financing, and health outcomes, we examine HSF in three income categories: low-, middle-, and high-income to explore the challenges and draw conclusions about the performance of their HSF policies. We analyze HSF in relation to the level of available financial resources, taking into consideration the structure of total health expenditures. There are different ways of evaluating equity in HSF. We do so through assessing out-of-pocket (OOP) spending, catastrophic health expenditures across income groups, and risk of impoverishment following ill-health. Trend analysis is done for countries where data is available. Inference and extrapolations are made to the various income groups.

Public Health in the Arab World, ed. Samer Jabbour et al. Published by Cambridge University Press. © Samer Jabbour et al., 2012.

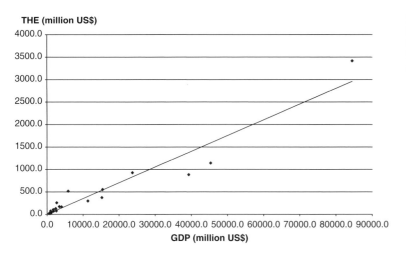

Figure 1. Gross domestic product and total health expenditures in Arab countries. GDP: gross domestic product; THE: Total health expenditures. Sources: WHO – NHA database 2008 and authors' calculations.

Information on HSF is limited and fragmented, particularly in relation to household health expenditures in the private sector; only a few countries have conducted household health expenditures and utilization surveys (Carlson & Douglas 2009). WHO, in collaboration with USAID and the World Bank, has improved data collection and analysis through promoting health-dedicated and population-based surveys, National Health Accounts (NHA), and equity studies (De & Shehata 2001).

Data for the present analysis are collected from country profiles available at the Eastern Mediterranean Health System Observatory of the WHO's Eastern Mediterranean Regional Office (EMRO) Web site, NHA, and various country and regional studies. Eight countries have data on private health expenditures from household surveys: Algeria (MOH-Algeria 2003), Djibouti (El-Idrissi 2006), Egypt (Fouad 2005), Jordan (Al-Halawani et al 2006), Lebanon (Ammar et al 2000), Morocco (MOH-Morocco 2005), Occupied Palestinian Territory (Mataria et al 2009), Tunisia (Boyer et al 2000), and Yemen (MOPHP-Yemen 2006). Such data were used to develop NHA, which are updated regularly in most but not all countries. Where household data on expenditures in the private sector are absent, WHO and other agencies used modeling techniques to provide estimates.

Keys Issues in Health System Financing
Spending on Health

Health spending is highly affected by income in this region as elsewhere. Higher income countries spend more on health (Figure 1). Countries of similar income levels have common characteristics regarding HSF structure and contribution of various financing sources. A challenge is that spending estimates from ministries other than ministries of health are sometimes difficult to consolidate. Estimates from WHO's NHA studies in many countries inform this discussion.

Spending levels are below other developing regions; Arab countries account for 5% of world population but spend less than 1% of global health expenditures. Comparatively, the countries of the Americas and Europe regions of WHO constitute 14% and 13% of the world population but their total expenditure on health amounts to 48% and 35% of global health expenditure, respectively. In 2006 Arab countries spent US$52 billion on health, representing less than 4% of GDP. Spending on health per capita averages US$162 but averages hide inequalities across and within the countries. Most low-income countries cannot secure the US$40 per capita, which is the minimum amount recommended by WHO Commission for Macroeconomics and Health (CMH) to provide essential minimal health services (WHO 2001). WHO now estimates that a minimum of US$60 per capita is needed in 2015 for any health system to perform reasonably (WHO 2010a).

Average government spending on health is less than 5% of total public spending (range, 3–8.5%). This is not enough to support and upgrade government facilities to provide essential health services to the population, especially to the poor and vulnerable groups, much less to meet the growing expectations for good quality preventive, curative, and rehabilitative services. Figure 2 shows the distribution of public

375

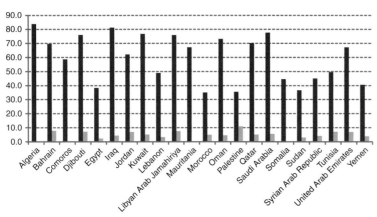

Figure 2. General government expenditure on health as percentage of total heath expenditure. Sources: WHO; NHA database 2008; Countries Ministries of Health; Countries NHA Reports and Documents.

■ General Government Expenditure on Health as Percentage of Total Health Expenditure

■ Ministry of Health budget as % of government budget

expenditure on health as a percentage of total heath expenditure and ministry of health (MOH) budget as a percentage of total government budget.

Structure of Health Expenditures

Financial resources for health typically come from: households as OOP payments; insurance arrangements through contribution mechanisms; government, through public budgets; and external sources, through loans and grants. On average, household OOP contributions amount to 32% (19% in GCC countries, 42% in middle-income countries, 57% in low-income countries). Data on social, private, and community health insurance are scarce and fragmented. Public spending on health through government budgets (ministries of health, higher education, defense, internal security, and others) and through social health insurance represent about 40% of total health expenditures. In view of limited coverage by health insurance, the share of contributive schemes in public spending remains relatively low.

External assistance constitutes a limited share in total spending. Low-income countries and those facing complex emergencies (Somalia, Sudan, Iraq, and Occupied Palestinian Territory [OPT]) receive funding from donor countries and international NGOs. However, this has long-term implications. For example, 87% of budgeted non-salary operating costs of MOH of the Palestinian National Authority in 2003 was covered by donations (US$240 million, US$65 per capita) (Mataria et al 2009). Dependence on external funding for health development threatens

sustainability, particularly if long-term HSF policies are not well articulated.

Social Health Protection

Financing arrangements that ensure increased or universal access to health services reduce financial risks to individuals and families and promote social health protection. Such protection can be eroded within a market-oriented health policy especially if preventive measures are taken and if this happen in a context of poverty and social exclusion due to economic crisis. Since the late 1970s and especially the 1980s, several developments – economic, political, and geo-political – have triggered the adoption of economic reforms towards more economic liberalization in general and of the "health market" in particular in many Arab countries. As a result, only half of the population in Arab countries is now covered by social health protection through taxes or contributions. This average hides inequity as the figure is less than 10% in low-income countries such as Comoros, Somalia, and Yemen and 100% in high-income countries (if expatriates are excluded). Household OOP expenditures are a useful indicator of social health protection. WHO's health expenditures databases suggest that between 1995 and 2007 per capita OOP expenditures increased from US$53 to US$108, while OOP expenditures share from total health expenditures decreased minimally from 38% to 34%. This indicates a slow increase in the share of prepayment schemes.

The composition of OOP expenditures is not well studied. Catastrophic health spending, which occurs when a household's total OOP health expenditure equals or exceeds 40% of a household's capacity to pay on non-subsistence spending, meaning total spending minus expenditure on food, is the most serious. WHO studies in Tunisia (Arfa et al 2008) and Morocco (Ezzrari & El-Alami El-Fellousse 2007) show that 2–4.5% of the population face catastrophic health expenditures and thus risk of impoverishment. In OPT and Jordan, the same figure amounts to 0.82% and 0.60%, respectively. As part of a multi-country study, Xu et al (2003) reported the following figures for proportion of households experiencing catastrophic expenditures: Djibouti 0.32%, Egypt 2.8%, Lebanon 5.17%, Morocco 0.17%, and Yemen 1.66%. In a study of OOP expenditures in five Arab countries (Egypt, Lebanon, OPT, Tunisia, Yemen) in addition to Iran, Elgazzar et al (2010) estimated that 7–13% "face particularly high OOP payments or catastrophic expenditures equal to at least 10 percent of household spending," which is different than the above definition.

By extrapolating various data to the whole Arab world (excluding GCC countries), 5.5 to 13 million individuals face such situations every year. Another WHO study showed that 1–1.4% of households are pushed into poverty when a family member becomes ill, adding 2.5 to 4 million people to the rank of poor in the region. Elgazzar et al (2010) estimated that poverty rates can increase by up to 20% when health care spending is considered.

High OOP payments discourage people from using needed services, which has important implications for population health. For example, in the study by Elgazzar et al (2010) many people forgo health care due to financial costs: 12% in Egypt, 20% in Lebanon, and 37% in Yemen.

Insurance schemes remain weak. Coverage through social health insurance and general government revenue schemes vary across countries of different income levels. Elgazzar et al (2010) reported the following rates for population coverage through social health insurance schemes: Egypt-45%, OPT-48%, Lebanon-52%, and Tunisia-78%. As for private health insurance, coverage data were available for OPT (10.2%) and Lebanon (15%). Existing insurance schemes have important limitations. For example in Egypt, the employment-based scheme reduced OOP expenditure but did not increase utilization (Shawky 2010).

One of the main determinants of coverage remains the status of employment within a country, with the prevalence of high rates of unemployment, and employment in the informal sector, undermining the capacity of a country to expand social health insurance schemes to all citizens. Some forms of mutual insurance have been developed in certain professions and corporations to compensate for the limited coverage by official insurance regimes. Such mutual funds receive subsidies from governments in order to allow for better coverage of health services. Unlike other regions, including sub-Saharan African countries, micro- and community-based health insurance are not well-developed. Private health insurance to cover expatriates is unpopular – except in Lebanon and in some GCC countries. Indeed, insured individuals acquire private insurance to supplement the basic and mandatory package provided by social health insurance and/or through government schemes. Private insurers are forecasting an increase in the potential demand for their services in some middle-income countries.

Policy Implications

Gaps in social health protection have negative implications on the right to health and health equity, particularly for poor and vulnerable groups. More directly, impoverishment due to inadequate social health protection adds to existing poverty in many low- and middle-income countries (LMICs) and contributes to more social exclusion. This challenge is not well appreciated and addressed by Arab social policy makers who design poverty reduction strategies and social safety nets. With some population segments vulnerable to catastrophic health expenditures, urgent measures are needed. The slow growth in insurance coverage is difficult to address, considering the sizeable informal sector of the economy in many LMICs – for instance, more than half of employed men (50.9%) and more than three-quarters of employed women (78.4%) in Egypt are recruited in the informal sector (Chen et al 2005). In Tunisia and Morocco, the share of informal sector in total GDP amounts to 20.3% and 24.9%, respectively (Charmes 2000).

In recent years, social health protection has gained momentum and started to feature high on the political agenda. Achieving universal coverage through health insurance has been in the political manifesto of presidential elections in Egypt, Tunisia, and

Table 1. Level and Structure of Health System Financing in Low-Income Countries, 2006

Country	Population (000)	GDP per capita (US$)	THE per capita (US$)	THE (% of GDP)	OOP (% of THE)	Covered population (% of total)
Comoros	818	493	16	3.2	45	<10
Djibouti	819	925	62	6.7	24	22
Mauritania	3,044	866	19	2.2	31	20
Somalia	8,455	303	8	2.6	55	<10
Sudan	37,708	996	38	3.8	62	20
Yemen	21,732	869	40	4.6	51	<10
Total	**72,576**	**866**	**34**	**3.97**	**57**	**16**

GDP = gross domestic product; THE = total health expenditure; OOP = out of pocket health expenditure.
Sources: WHR 2008; WHO NHA database (2008); WHO EMRO, Mapping health care financing; EMRO countries; Internal WHO EMRO documents.

Yemen. Policy reforms in some countries strive to improve social health protection coverage and harmonize benefit packages of various insurance schemes.

Financing Arrangements and Challenges by Regional Income Groups

Low-Income Countries

Table 1 shows that health systems in most of these countries are under-funded, with health spending averaging 4% of GDP (range, 2.2% in Mauritania to 6.7% in Djibouti) or US$34 per capita. Using the aforementioned minimum US$40 suggested by WHO's CMH, the annual gap is estimated to be US$430 million. Most countries do not have the necessary economic basis to secure the needed resources and require regional and international solidarity. The structure of health spending shows clear iniquities: on average, 57% of resources are generated from households' OOP spending and less than 16% of the population is protected against the financial risk of ill health. Therefore, many families are facing catastrophic expenditures when a member falls sick.

Even the limited resources devoted to health are often inappropriately used as most countries do not have the necessary skills or policy imperatives for allocating resources based on sound analytic methods such as cost-effectiveness. Analyses of NHA demonstrate that curative and hospital care in urban areas consume most of the resources whereas most priority promotion and prevention programs are not properly funded. A high proportion of OOP spending is consumed by purchase of medicines in the private sector (26% in Djibouti (El-Idrissi 2006)) and 39% in Yemen (MOPHP-Yemen 2006).

Middle-Income Countries

These countries spend on average 5% of GDP on health or US$113 per capita (range, US$66 in Syria to US$468 in Lebanon). These figures are credible as seven countries out of the 10 conduct regular household expenditures and utilization surveys followed by NHA studies. In Morocco, Tunisia, and OPT catastrophic health expenditures and risk of impoverishment caused by illness were assessed using household health expenditures data (Arfa et al 2008; Ezzarari & El-Alami El-Fellouse 2007; Mataria & Raad 2009). A study in Egypt and Lebanon found that overall, lower-income groups tended to report having worse health levels and paying more OOP on health as a share of income than did higher-income groups (Elgazzar 2009).

Most countries have mixed financing systems, including tax-based financing through government budgets, contributive arrangements, and private spending (Table 2). Time-trend analysis of patterns of change in each financing source provides useful lessons. Government share in total health spending is most important. In the early 1960s and 1970s, governments of most countries committed to free access to health care. Health budgets increased annually to meet increasing demand for services due to high population growth, rising expectations for quality services, technological development, price-inflation, and the low baseline level of services from

Table 2. Level and Structure of Health System Financing in Middle-Income Countries, 2006

Country	Population (000)	GDP per capita (US$)	THE per capita (US$)	THE (% of GDP)	OOP (% of THE)	Insured population (% of total)
Algeria	33,351	3463	123	3.6	22	87
Egypt	74,167	1460	93	3.2	56	52
Iraq	23,764	1775	67	3.8	28	80
Jordan	5,729	2474	246	9.9	43	75
Lebanon	4,055	5234	468	8.9	40	50
Libya	6,039	8764	255	2.9	30	100
Morocco	30,853	1857	95	5.1	49	31
Palestine	3,952	1247	135	8.6	40	56
Syria	19,408	1693	66	3.9	52	70
Tunisia	10,215	3022	159	5.3	46	85
Total	*211,533*	*2270*	*113*	*5*	*42*	*63*

GDP = gross domestic product; THE = total health expenditure; OOP = out of pocket health expenditure.
Sources: WHO WHR 2008; WHO NHA database; WHO EMRO, Mapping health care financing; EMRO countries; WHO EMRO working papers; Mataria et al 2008.

colonial times. Figures collected by WHO EMRO, however, show that the increase in government per capita spending is accompanied with an increase in per capita OOP spending in most middle-income countries. Adoption of macroeconomic reforms and structural adjustments programs especially since the 1980s strained public spending on social sectors, including health.

Many reasons explain the increase in OOP expenditures in middle-income countries. These include introduction of user fees at various service levels, passive privatization of service delivery, and balanced billing caused by low tariff of reimbursement of private providers. In many countries, below-market tariff rates mean that insured patients pay the difference out-of-pocket as patients usually pay private providers and then submit claims for settlement to the insurance funds, which reimburse but with delays. Reforms that promote private practice in public institutions and drastic reductions in budgets for public facilities have pushed many users entitled to free or subsidized health care into the private sector. In many countries public providers conduct private clinics even during public facility hours, creating distortion by referring patients to their clinics or by accepting under-the-table payments for providing clinical services without delays. Increasing OOP spending is also evident in medicine purchasing from private pharmacies. It is very common to have limited

supply of medicines in public facilities starting in April or May of the fiscal year because of reduced budgets and a weak supply system.

In the case of OPT, a substantial increase in insurance coverage took place due to a presidential decree indicating that all Palestinian victims of the Intifada would be covered by the governmental health insurance scheme and without contributions. From 2000 to 2002, the number of households covered by the new free insurance scheme increased by 205,430 households, whereas revenue from premiums fell from US$29.5 million to US$22 million (Mataria et al 2009). An equity analysis of the health system in the OPT confirms the significant pro-poor characteristic of the governmental health insurance scheme compared to the regressive nature of OOP payments of uninsured individuals (Abu-Zaineh et al 2008).

High-Income Countries

These countries spend, on average, US$620 per capita on health (range, US$325 in Oman to US$2750 in Qatar). These figures were inflated during past years because of increasing oil prices and systematic use of costly curative services and technologies. Most countries, except Bahrain, have not done NHA analyses and thus only estimates as percentage of GDP are presented. However data on health financing is being

Table 3. Level and Structure of Health System Financing in High-Income Countries, 2006

Country	Population (000)	GDP per capita (US$)	THE per capita (US$)	THE (% of GDP)	OOP (% of THE)	Insured (% of total population)
Bahrain	739	21,130	811	3.8	23	100
Kuwait	2,779	36,760	800	2.2	20	100
Oman	2,546	14,160	325	2.3	18	100
Qatar	821	64,190	2750	4.3	19	100
KSA	24,175	14,440	490	3.4	18	100
UAE	4,249	38,400	982	2.6	21	100
Total	*35,309*	*20,360*	*621*	*3.1*	*18.6*	*100*

GDP = gross domestic product; THE = total health expenditure; OOP = out of pocket health expenditure.
Sources: WHO WHR 2008; WHO NHA database; WHO EMRO, Mapping health care financing, EMRO countries; Internal WHO EMRO documents.

improved following analysis of the World Health Survey carried out in five GCC countries.

As welfare states, HSF in high-income countries is mostly provided by governments through budgets of ministries of health, education, defense, interior, etc. Health services are delivered mainly in government facilities, which offer quality services free of charge to all nationals. In some countries, such as Oman, user fees are charged for publicly provided services in order to rationalize their use. Over the past two decades, the private sector has grown with increasing number of private clinics, pharmacies, laboratories, imaging institutions, and private hospitals. Some of the latter have grown into large corporations, for example the Saudi German Hospital Group and Mouwassat Medical Services, and invest in neighboring Arab countries.

As high-income countries rely on oil revenues, fluctuating oil prices raise concerns about HSF sustainability especially with the recent financial crisis. Modeling health spending based on epidemiological and demographic transition indicators suggests growing needs. For example, health spending in GCC countries is expected to increase five-fold in 15 years (from US$12 billion now to about US$60 billion in 2025) (Murshed et al 2008).

In response, high-income countries are revisiting their financing strategies, re-focusing health systems on primary health care with family practice at the center, and planning cost control and containment policies. Rational use of medical technology with focus on medicines, training health professionals in pharmaco-economics, and promoting use of generic medicines are among the latter strategies.

Ways Forward

The commitment to the value of health as a right and to health equity should guide thinking about future directions for improving HSF. Policy makers have indeed taken steps, with support from technical agencies such as WHO, the World Bank and other parties, to address the major shortcomings in current HSF arrangements. Much more needs to be done. We examine four priorities.

Generating Evidence to Support Financing Policies and Strategies

The paucity of HSF data indicates the need to invest in data collection and analysis in Arab countries. National statistical bureaus commonly carry out *general* household expenditure surveys that provide limited data about health utilization and spending. WHO and other partners favor population-based household surveys focusing *specifically* on health expenditures. Such surveys assess spending composition including in the private sector, catastrophic health spending and its impoverishing effect, and provide data to measure financing equity, for example, using WHO's Fairness of Financial Contribution Index which has been considered in the region (Ammar et al 2000) or less commonly used alternatives (Wagstaff 2002). These surveys are uncommon in many Arab countries due to cost and effort-intensiveness and the reluctance of ministries of health to undertake them. Experiences in Egypt, Jordan, Lebanon, Morocco, OPT, and Tunisia are quite promising. In some cases WHO sponsors the surveys with external donors providing the needed resources.

Public expenditure reviews and budget tracking surveys (Brinkerhoff 2009) supplement household surveys. Data from these routine information systems and the aforementioned population-based surveys are used to develop NHA that estimate financial flows within the health system and their contributions to service delivery. Examples from the region show how NHA can provide evidence about HSF strengths and weaknesses and highlight directions for policy reforms.

Across the region, the NHA evidence helped increase awareness of health policy makers about the negative consequences of increasing OOP spending on health and the need to promote social health protection through pre-payment schemes. In Morocco, reforms were introduced to develop mandatory social health insurance for workers in the formal sector, the self-employed, and the poor (El-Idrissi et al 2008). The coverage by social health insurance is supposed to reach more than 60% of the population when the reform matures. Similar reforms have been under way in Egypt, Jordan, and Tunisia to scale up coverage by social health protection to reach special groups including students, children, and some workers in the informal sector.

Health ministers have used NHA evidence to advocate for higher public budgets and to promote investment in health. In Egypt (Fouad 2005), Lebanon (Ammar et al 2000), Morocco (MOH-Morocco 2005), and Tunisia (Arfa et al 2008), NHA have fueled national policy debates on various financing issues, e.g., level of governmental vs. household spending on health, which have included policy makers, parliamentarians, and stakeholders inside and outside the government.

The NHA can help identify gaps or excesses in health spending and expose evidence of inequity. In Morocco, NHA analysis helped identify the financing basis of high maternal mortality (MOH-Morocco 2000). This provided a rationale for advocacy to increase resources to relevant programs, particularly at the primary care level and to invest in human resource development, including provision of incentives to work in rural and deprived areas. In the opposite direction, NHA in Lebanon showed high expenditures on medicines (Ammar et al 2000), leading to an important reform of the pharmaceutical sector focusing on pricing mechanisms, control of quality of registered medicines, rational use of medicines and

promotion of generics. This reform contributed to lowering the OOP expenditures in Lebanon from 60% in 1998 to 44% while health spending as a share of GDP has fallen from 12.4% to 8.4% (WHO 2010b).

In some countries, sub-national and provincial health accounts have been done to assess geographic distribution of financial resources, to understand the determinants of health inequalities, and to look at specific health issues such as mental health subaccounts. Findings have helped improve resource allocation. Efforts are directed towards coupling these analyses with measurement of the burden of diseases in order to advocate the use of cost-effective interventions and programs. So far only four countries (Egypt, Lebanon, Morocco, and Tunisia) have carried out national burden of disease studies and many lack figures about the cost of various health interventions.

Other analytic tools such as costing, actuarial and cost-effectiveness studies are also needed. Generated data should help managers improve financial planning and management, for example through billing the real cost of provided services, and help policy makers devise cost containment strategies at national level, for example by focusing on cost-effective interventions. This way, HSF reforms become evidence based.

Aside from service studies conducted by HSF teams in health ministries, there is also a need for research in key priority areas identified by policy makers, researchers, and other stakeholders (El-Jardali et al 2010). Research is needed to generate evidence about the relative value, effectiveness, and equity implications of financing reform proposals popular in the development literature today such as cash transfers for the poor, pay-for-performance, and results-based financing. Methodological research is also needed to identify the most suitable financing indicators and survey approaches for this region (Lu et al 2009). Lack of publicly available regional health system datasets undermines effective research (Saleh et al 2009).

Increasing Health Investments

The value of increasing health investment in low- and middle-income countries is now widely supported. The 1993 World Development Report, "Investing in Health" (World Bank 1993), demonstrated the added value of health investments in terms of economic return and population well-being particularly when investments are directed towards health protection and promotion.

The WHO's Commission on Macroeconomics and Health (WHO 2001) recommended that, by 2007, health investments in poor countries should reach almost US$66 billion every year. Consequently, each year thereafter, 330 million disability-adjusted life years (DALYs) would be saved, around eight million deaths averted, and US$360 billion generated through direct and indirect economic benefits. The Commission report argued that half of the investments should come from national sources, the other half generated through international solidarity, if the Millennium Development Goals are to be achieved by 2015.

Arab health ministers can use the above arguments and evidence from NHA and other analytic tools in the region to make a strong case for increasing national investments in health during cabinet meetings and budget negotiations with ministries of planning and finance. Health ministers can make reference to benchmarks agreed upon locally and globally, including the minimum US$40 figures of the Commission, to secure at least the primary care components. Interventions such as tuberculosis and malaria control, mother and child health care, control of non-communicable diseases could be costed-out to assess funding gaps to address priority population health needs. Beyond making the argument and showing the evidence, ministries of planning and finance need to be briefed through high level seminars and engaged in policy issues in health systems. The development of a fiscal space, as part of poverty reduction strategies, can be used to increase investment in health, bearing in mind its contribution to economic growth and development.

Designing Appropriate and Sustainable HSF Options

Once evidence is collected, policy makers should devise HSF options, taking into consideration societal values, level of economic growth, epidemiological profile, and the cost trajectory of health services. The ultimate aim is improving equity and financial risk protection. Efforts should address each of the three sub-components: efficient and equitable mobilization of resources; better pooling to secure solidarity in both risks and financing; and the strategic purchasing of needed health services. There is no ready recipe for HSF reform for all Arab countries, but the above discussion suggests different strategies based on national income levels.

In low-income countries, the priority is to mobilize resources from national budgets and from regional and international sources to secure the minimum investments in health and poverty alleviation. Public sector resources should be oriented towards health promotion and scaling up primary health care services. User fees should be dropped as a source of health financing because of their regressive nature. To improve social health protection, policy options should encourage prepayment schemes, including social community-based health insurance (Carrin et al 2005) and tax-based systems.

For middle-income countries with relatively low health investments, these also need to be increased to levels needed to meet population needs. For all countries, social health protection schemes (social health insurance or general revenue-based financing) need to be expanded to improve equitable access to services and reduce OOP, especially catastrophic expenditures. Governments should monitor HSF equity trends through NHA and other operational research activities. As in low-income countries, innovative approaches are needed to channel financing resources towards health promotion (Bayarsaikhan & Muiser 2007).

In high-income countries, governments should remain the major insurers as most funds come from general revenues and taxation. Strategic purchasing of services from service providers based on innovative competition schemes, e.g., pay for performance, can improve results-based financing, management of public-private mix, and overall efficiency. Cost control and containment strategies are obviously needed as is better selection, management, and assessment of health and biomedical technology.

Building Capacity to Support Financing Reform

Regardless of national income, HSF reform requires capacity development of various ministries and many other governmental and non-governmental stakeholders. The ministry of health is expected to lead this effort through such activities as executive courses, policy seminars, and long-term training, which can build experience and research know-how in health financing and economics.

Conclusion

This chapter demonstrates how HSF in the Arab world presents real challenges to policy makers because of the limited coverage by social health protection and limited resources available to health in low- and some middle-income countries. These limitations negatively impact health system performance and reduce equitable access to services. At the same time, inefficient practices in allocating scarce resources undermine health and social outcomes.

We have proposed various HSF reform strategies to reduce risk to people and strengthen social health protection. However, it must be emphasized that financing strategies are not expected to work in isolation. Rather, they need to be coupled with broad public health strategies including addressing social determinants of health, health promotion, strengthening primary health care, population-level prevention, and other health system interventions aimed at strengthening governance, leadership, and policy development.

While the ministry of health is expected to play a leading role in this effort, civil society organizations, professional associations, and academic institutions in the Arab world can play an important role through advocacy to promote investment in health development and to protect equity in access to health services. Such institutions should also be involved in monitoring and promoting the right to health in collaboration with other partners.

Acknowledgments

Belgacem Sabri and Awad Mataria are staff members of the World Health Organization. The author alone is responsible for the views expressed in this publication and they do not necessarily represent the decisions or policies of the World Health Organization.

References

Abu-Zaineh M, Mataria A, Luchini S, Moatti JP (2008) Equity in health care financing in the Palestinian context: the value-added of the disaggregate approach. *Social Science and Medicine*, 66: 2308–20

Al-Halawani F, Banks D, Fardouss T, Al-Madani A (2006) *Jordan National Health Accounts 2001–2002.* Bethesda, MD: The Partners for Health Reformplus Project, Abt Associates Inc.

Ammar W, Fakha H, Azzam O, Freiha Khoury R, Mattar C, Halabi M, et al (2000) *Lebanon National Health Accounts, Ministry of Health.* Beirut, Lebanon: WHO & World Bank

Arfa C, Souiden MA, Achouri N (2008) *Etude relative aux dépenses individuelles catastrophiques et leur impact sur l'appauvrissement des ménages: cas de la Tunisie,* (in French), Cairo, Egypt: WHO EMRO

Bayarsaikhan D, Muiser J (2007) *Financing health promotion, WHO Discussion paper No.4, Department of Health System Financing,* Geneva, Switzerland: WHO

Boyer S, Delesvaux C, Foirry JP, Prieur C (2000) Le risque maladie dans les assurances sociales: bilan et perspectives dans les pays en voie de développement. *In: Direction générale de la coopération internationale et du développement* (p. 31–58). (in French), Paris, France: CREDES, Ministère des Affaires Etrangères

Brinkerhoff DW (2009) *National health accounts and public expenditure reviews: Redundant or complementary tools?* Bethesda, MD: Health Systems 20/20 project, Abt Associates Inc

Carlson K, Douglas G (2009) *Tracking household health expenditures in developing countries through major population-based surveys.* Bethesda, MD: Health Systems 20/20 project, Abt Associates Inc

Carrin G, Waelkens MP, Criel B (2005) Community-based health insurance in developing countries: a study of its contribution to the performance of health financing systems, *Tropical Medicine and International Health,* 10(8): 799–811

Charmes J (2000) *The contribution of informal sector to GDP in developing countries: assessment, estimates, methods, orientation for the future, Paper prepared for the 4th meeting of the Delhi group on informal sector statistics,* Geneva, Switzerland

Chen M, Vanek J, Lund F, Heintz J, Jhabvala R, Bonner C (2005) *Progress of the World's Women 2005, Women, Work, and Poverty.* New York, NY: UNIFEM

De S, Shehata I (2001) *Comparative report of National health accounts, Findings from eight countries in the Middle East and North Africa, Partnerships for Health Reform, Technical Report No. 64.* Bethesda, MD

Elgazzar H (2009) Income and the use of health care: an empirical study of Egypt and Lebanon. *Health Economics, Policy and Law,* 4(4): 445–78

Elgazzar H, Raad F, Arfa C, et al (2010) *Who pays? Out-of-pocket health spending and equity implications in the Middle East and North Africa. Health, Nutrition and Population (HNP) Discussion Paper.* Washington, DC: the World Bank

El-Idrissi DZ (2006) *Consultation on National Health Accounts – Financing options in Djibouti.* Cairo, Egypt: WHO EMRO

El-Idrissi DZ, Miloud K, Belgacem S (2008) Constraints and obstacles to social health protection in the Maghreb: The cases of Algeria and Morocco. *Bulletin of the World Health Organization,* 86(11): 902–904

El-Jardali F, Makhoul J, Jamal D, Kent Ranson M, Kronfol N, Tchaghchagian V (2010) Eliciting policymakers' and stakeholders' opinions to help shape health system research priorities in the Middle East and North Africa region. *Health Policy and Planning*, 25: 15–27

Ezzrari A, El-Alami El-Fellousse A (2007) *Etude relative aux dépenses individuelles catastrophiques et leur impact sur l'appauvrissement des ménages: cas du Maroc* (in French). Cairo, Egypt: WHO EMRO

Fouad S (2005) *Egypt National Health Accounts 2001–02, The Partners for Health Reformplus Project*. Bethesda, MD: Abt Associates Inc

Lu C, Chin B, Li G, Murray CJ (2009) Limitations of methods for measuring out-of pocket and catastrophic private health expenditures. *Bulletin of the World Health Organization*, 87(3): 238–44, 244A–244D

Mataria A, Raad F (2009) *Analyzing health equity in the West Bank and Gaza*. Washington, DC: The World Bank

Mataria A, Khatib R, Donaldson C, Bossert T, Hunter D, Alsayed F, Moatti J (2009) The health care system in Palestine: assessment and reform agenda. *The Lancet*, 373(9670): 1207–1217

MOH-Algeria (Ministry of Health in Algeria) (2003) *Comptes Nationaux de la Santé 2000–2001 (in French)*. Direction de la Planification, Alger

MOH-Morocco (Ministry of Health in Morocco) (2000) *Comptes Nationaux de la Santé 1997–1998,* (in French). Service de l'Economie Sanitaire, DPRF, Rabat

MOH-Morocco (2005) *Comptes Nationaux de la Santé 2001 (in French)*. Service de l'Economie Sanitaire, DPRF, Rabat

MOPHP-Yemen (Ministry of Public Health and Population in Yemen) & National Health Accounts Team (2006) *Yemen National Health Accounts – Estimates for 2003*. Bethesda MD: USAID/PHR plus

Murshed M, Hudiger V, Lambert T (2008) *Health Care: Challenges and opportunities*. Gulf Cooperation Council, McKinsey & Company study

Saleh S, Alameddine M, El-Jardali F (2009) The case for developing publicly accessible datasets for health services research in the Middle East and North Africa (MENA) region. *BMC Health Services Research*, 9: 197

Shawky S (2010) Could the employment-based targeting approach serve Egypt in moving towards a social health insurance model? *Eastern Mediterranean Health Journal*, 16(6): 663–70

Wagstaff A (2002) Reflections on and alternatives to WHO's fairness of financial contribution index. *Health Economics*, 11: 103–115

World Bank (1993) *Investing in health for development, World*

Development Report. Washington, DC: The World Bank

WHO (World Health Organization) (2001) *Macroeconomics and health: investing in health for economic development. Report of Commission on Macroeconomics and Health*. Geneva: WHO

WHO (2008) *National Health Accounts Database*, Geneva available from www.who.int/nha/en/ [Accessed 13 December 2010]

WHO (2010a) *Constraints to scaling up the health Millennium Development Goals: costing and financial gap analysis*. Geneva: WHO

WHO (2010b) *World Health Report 2010. Health systems financing: the path to universal coverage*. Geneva: WHO

WHO EMRO (World Health Organization – Regional Office for the Eastern Mediterranean) (2008) *Progress report on Strengthening primary health care based health systems*. Available from http://www.emro.who.int/rc56/media/pdf/EMRC56INF04en.pdf

WHO EMRO (2009) *Demographic, social and health indicators for countries of the Eastern Mediterranean*. Cairo, Egypt: WHO

Xu K, Evans DB, Kawabata K, Zeramdini R, Klavus J, Murray CJ (2003) Household catastrophic health expenditure: a multicountry analysis. *The Lancet*, 362(9378): 111–117

Chapter

30

The Public Health Workforce and Human Resources for Health

Fadi El-Jardali, Elisabeth Longuenesse, Diana Jamal, and Nabil M. Kronfol

A major challenge to any health system is the availability of a strong, capable, and motivated workforce to support its core functions and advance its goals in advancing population health, promoting equity, and ensuring good quality of services (WHO 2000; Kabene et al 2006). Evidence indicates a strong link between the availability of health workers and population health outcomes (WHO 2006). This is particularly important in low- to middle-income countries (LMICs), which generally have lower health provider densities and associated poorer health outcomes (El-Jardali et al 2007a). Arab countries have started to realize the importance of their public health workforce as a strategic asset and the many challenges that exist in this area. This chapter aims to initiate a discussion about this asset. Because of the inherent difficulties in defining the public health workforce and the implications of different definitions for population health, the chapter emphasizes the need for broad conceptualization of the public health workforce and proposes a framework for the region. The chapter reviews available evidence about the public health workforce, provides a critical reflection on its complex realities and challenges, highlights gaps in knowledge and areas for research, and outlines areas for reform.

What Is the Public Health Workforce? A Proposed Framework for the Arab World

There are several challenges with regard to defining and conceptualizing the public health workforce. There is no universal approach for defining and classifying health workers. Terms such as the "public health workforce," "health workforce," and "human resources for health" are all in use without clear distinctions, thus creating confusion about roles and responsibilities. From a comprehensive public health perspective, there are shortcomings to some of the existing definitions. For example, WHO (2006) defines health workers as "all people engaged in actions whose primary intent is to enhance health" (p. 1). But the definition does not comprehensively encompass the public health workforce. The latter is not simply limited to health service providers; there are a multitude of other professionals that contribute to the health and well-being of the population. For instance, environmental officers provide an indirect type of service. Gebbie et al (2002) described the public health workforce as interdisciplinary "weaving together the various skills, knowledge, attitudes, and worldviews of the multiple professions involved" (p. 57). This definition encompasses some categories of public health workforce, such as biomedical providers, and health and environmental professionals, but not others such as those responsible for occupational safety and health in industries, unions, and governments; individuals involved in population-focused health education in voluntary organizations; and individuals involved in decreasing environmental problems in governmental agencies or other organizations.

There are different frameworks for classifying the health workforce in the literature. A Canadian framework differentiates between regulated (such as physicians and health care specialists) and non-regulated (such as educators, researchers, and support workers) public health workers (Public Health Agency of Canada 2005). The UK health workforce is divided into *specialists*, professionals with higher qualifications in public health and occupy positions focusing on population health, *practitioners*, individuals who have a day-to-day responsibility in influencing population health through front-line and operational interventions, and the *wider workforce*, people from all sectors and at all levels of organizations (Sim et al 2007).

Public Health in the Arab World, ed. Samer Jabbour et al. Published by Cambridge University Press. © Samer Jabbour et al., 2012.

The Commission of the European Communities (2008) considers the health workforce to include many professional cadres including the clinical workforce, social care workforce, informal care providers, complementary individuals, allied health professionals, health management workforce, training workforce, public health and disease surveillance workforce, and administrative and support staff.

There is a general misconception that public health workers are a category within the health workforce. In some countries: "public health workers" refers to the entire workforce rather than a specific component. As Cioffi et al (2003) accurately stipulated "the public health workforce is not a single profession, but rather a fabric of many professions dedicated to a common endeavor" (p. 451).

Existing frameworks and definitions in the literature are not framed within a public health approach and do not distinguish between health and public health, or between preventive and curative care and are commonly outlined based on professions and occupations, not by employment, functional roles, and employment sectors. For example, when referring to health management and support workers, one should consider the structures that offer public health services, such as community centers, and child/maternal, and family planning centers. With regard to physicians, existing definitions and models indicate that they are part of the public health workforce. But is their work public health oriented and by whose definition? Tilson & Gebbie (2004) put it differently by saying "a pediatrician counts in the public health workforce when providing well-child care and immunizations, but does not count when taking care of a baby's ear infection." Therefore, the most important issue is not just their numbers but the type of public health services they provide.

Our review of the existing regional discussions of the public health workforce showed that they focus primarily on direct biomedical care providers and exclude other categories of professionals whose work and actions may directly influence population health. This reflects the unavailability of data for health care providers as compared to other categories of the public health workforce (who they are, their numbers, where they work, and what they do). Nevertheless, the lack of data may itself represent a problem of conceptualization, and therefore of planning, as we will later discuss. In this chapter, we adopt a broad conceptualization of the public health workforce and we use the term to describe individuals providing care for the population (i.e., clinical) and those providing non-personal health services (i.e., core public health activities) (Beaglehole & Dal Poz 2003). We consider the public health workforce to be diverse and complex, and to include people from a wide range of occupational backgrounds. We propose a framework that encapsulates all categories of the public health workforce discussed in the literature and places the health of population at its center (Figure 1).

The framework describes the level and contribution to health improvement rendered by each component of the public health workforce. The purpose of having two layers is to stress the preventive and curative role of each in promoting and protecting health. While each of the professional cadres within the inner layer has a unique role in enhancing population health, the overall role of health workers in this layer is to help improve the health status, thus protecting people from seeking care from providers at the outer layer. There is still limited collaboration and integration between the roles of the different components in the inner layer (horizontal integration). The outer layer of the framework is somehow disjointed. This represents the current status of the workforce whereby there is even less horizontal integration between direct biomedical providers and community health workers and associated care providers than in the inner circle. Even within one category, the direct biomedical providers, there is limited collaboration between physicians, nurses, pharmacists, and dietitians. Vertical integration between the two layers is also needed. For this purpose, the bridges between the different components represent the need for integration and collaboration across and between layers. Such integration will help preserve the continuum of care and improve the health and well-being of the population. Indeed, the key contribution of this framework lies in its emphasis on linkages and relationships among different categories of the public health workforce as improving health and well-being of populations requires inter-professional practice and inter-sectoral action from all categories of the public health workforce.

Types, Density, and Distribution of the Public Health Workforce

While the proposed framework informs our thinking, the available data from the region is generally limited to biomedical care providers and some other components of the outer circle. According to WHO,

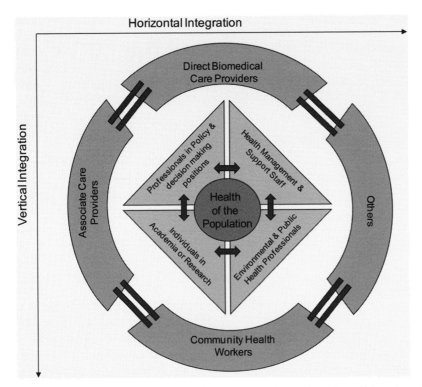

Figure 1. A comprehensive framework for public health workers in the Arab world. Inner layer: * Includes: Business, services and administration managers; Managing directors and chief executives; Lawyers; Accountants; Medical secretaries; Systems administrators; Ambulance workers; Health services managers. ** Includes: Environmental and occupational health and hygiene professionals, Health inspectors. *** Includes: Legislator/Government Minister; Senior government officials; Senior officials of special-interest organization; Policy and planning managers; and Policy administration professionals/policy analyst. ****: Includes: University and higher education teachers; Statisticians; Biomedical researcher; Sociologists, anthropologists and related professionals (including Ethnologists and Geographers) Outer layer: # Includes: Generalist medical practitioners; Specialist medical practitioners; Nursing professionals; Midwifery professionals; Dentists; Physiotherapists; Dieticians and nutritionists; Pharmacists; Medical assistants; Occupational therapists/Podiatrists; Psychiatrists. ## Includes: Nursing aide or Associate professional nurse; Associate professional midwife; Dental assistants and therapists; Pharmaceutical technicians and assistants; Medical and pathology laboratory technicians; Radiographers; Optometrists and ophthalmic opticians; Medical prosthetic technician; and Audiologists and speech therapists. ### Includes: Traditional midwife; Village healer; Community health workers; and Social workers. #### Includes: Volunteers; Trainees and interns; and Journalists.

Human Resources for Health (HRH) are estimated at 2,100,000 in the Eastern Mediterranean Region (EMR), which includes 19 Arab countries. This figure includes only health service providers and health management and support workers. Compared with other regions, the EMR has the second lowest number of health workers after Africa. Three quarters of HRH are health service providers (Table 1). The total number of HRH in the Arab world is difficult to estimate given that some Arab countries, specifically Algeria, Comoros, and Mauritania, are in WHO's African region and some non-Arab countries, specifically Afghanistan, Iran, and Pakistan, are included in the EMR estimates. Although there may be some degree of similarity and comparability in issues pertaining to HRH in the Arab world and the EMR, the

lack of explicit data poses a challenge. We have therefore compiled data from multiple sources, including the EMR Human Resources for Health (HRH) Observatory, established in 2007, the Web site of WHO's African region, WHO Statistical reports and publicly accessible databases on Web sites of WHO and the World Bank. The available data does not cover the broad range of the public health workforce but focuses on specific categories, usually biomedical providers. Table 2 provides density of workers in different categories.

A commonly reported measure of the public health workforce is physician and nurse densities. Figure 2 shows these densities for Arab countries. We observe that the Arab world's average of both densities is below the global average and below the

387

Table 1. Global Health Workforce, by Density (Source: WHO 2006)**

Region	Total health workforce		Health service providers		Health management and support workers	
	Number	Density*	Number	% of total workforce	Number	% of total workforce
Africa	1,640,000	2.3	1,360,000	83	280,000	17
Eastern Mediterranean	*2,100,000*	*4*	*1,580,000*	*75*	*520,000*	*25*
South-East Asia	7,040,000	4.3	4,730,000	67	2,300,000	33
Western Pacific	10,070,000	5.8	7,810,000	67	2,260,000	23
Europe	16,630,000	18.9	11,540,000	69	5,090,000	31
Americas	21,740,000	24.8	12,460,000	57	9,280,000	43
World	59,220,000	9.3	39,470,000	67	19,750,000	33

* Density per 1000 population since this table was adapted from the World Health Report 2006 ** Readers should take note that data provided by WHO is estimated in cases where it is not available. The figures are for "full-time paid health workers."

average for LMICs and that there is large variation in physician and nurse densities across countries. Both observations are concerning since recent evidence shows significant associations between country income, health worker densities, and population health outcomes (El-Jardali et al 2007a). Lower-income Arab countries are generally "donors" when it comes to physicians and nurses. Higher income Gulf countries are "recipients" due to limited production and high dependence on foreign-trained professionals whether from Arab countries or elsewhere (El-Jardali et al 2008d). The social image of physicians is favorable making it a highly sought - after profession in most countries. However, entry into the profession is generally lower in high-income (recipient) countries as nationals are generally more attracted to professions in the business sector which require fewer years of study. The case of nurses is different. In recipient countries, nationals are generally un-attracted to the poor social status of the profession. The exception is Oman, which has been trying to decrease its dependence on expatriates and has successfully encouraged nationals to enter the profession through the establishment of district schools of nursing across the country, thus educating nurses to serve within their own communities.

Data are not available as to how many of the reported physicians and nurses are expatriates, particularly in Gulf countries, making accurate interpretation of national supply challenging. Arab countries have succeeded in developing their human resources within one generation, for example moving from a shortage of physicians in the early 1970s to an overabundance in some countries by the turn of the century (Table 3). This increase is believed to be a direct outcome of establishment of medical schools.

Challenges and Opportunities

The current situation of HRH reflects several challenges specific to the Arab world. Below, we synthesize what is known about those challenges and highlight opportunities for action. Because there is more evidence about challenges facing biomedical providers, we devote more attention to this group while attempting to highlight some of the challenges facing other health workers.

HRH Planning

Weak Planning Capacities and Associated Shortages

Many Arab countries, particularly the poorer ones, suffer from poor capacities, including within their ministries of health, to plan for their country's HRH. One reason for poor institutional capacity is hiring unqualified individuals. In Yemen, young and inexperienced physicians are sometimes hired to fill the positions of heads of districts or departments.

Table 2. Density of Health Workers per 10,000 Population in Arab Countries (2000–2009)

Density of health workers	Physicians	Nursing and midwifery personnel	Dentistry personnel	Pharmaceutical personnel	Environment and public health workers	Community health workers
Algeria	12	19	3	2	1	…
Bahrain	30	58	4	9	4	…
Comoros	2	7	<0.5	1	<0.5	…
Djibouti	2	6	1	1	<0.5	…
Egypt	24	34	3	12	1	…
Iraq	5	10	1	1	1	<0.5
Jordan	26	32	8	14	3	…
Kuwait	18	37	3	5	…	…
Lebanon	33	13	11	11	…	…
Libya	12	48	2	2	…	…
Mauritania	1	7	<0.5	<0.5	1	…
Morocco	6	8	1	2	<0.5	…
Oman	18	39	2	5	1	…
OPT	11	13	1	1	…	…
Qatar	28	74	6	13	…	…
Saudi Arabia	16	36	2	6	…	…
Somalia	<0.5	1	…	<0.5	<0.5	…
Sudan	3	9	<0.5	<0.5	1	1
Syria	5	14	1	5	…	…
Tunisia	13	29	3	3	1	…
United Arab Emirates	15	46	4	7	…	…
Yemen	3	7	<0.5	1	<0.5	1
African Region	*2*	*11*	*<0.5*	*1*	*<0.5*	*…*
Region of the Americas	*23*	*55*	*12*	*7*	*…*	*…*
South-East Asia Region	*5*	*11*	*<0.5*	*4*	*…*	*1*
European Region	*33*	*68*	*5*	*5*	*…*	*…*
EMR	*10*	*14*	*2*	*3*	*1*	*3*
*Arab Countries**	*13*	*25*	*3*	*5*	*2*	*1*
Western Pacific Region	*14*	*21*	*2*	*4*		
Global	*14*	*28*	*3*	*4*		

* This figure is calculated from above list of countries, other regional figures were reported in the World Health Statistics Report, Data was extracted from the World Health Statistics Report 2010.
OPT: Occupied Palestinian Territory.

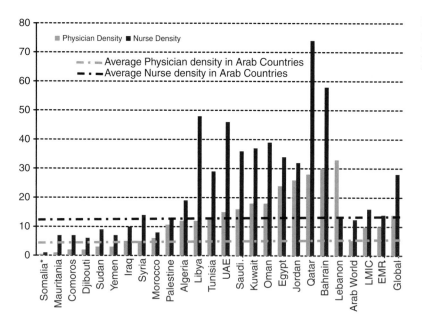

Figure 2. Average density per 10,000 population of physicians and nurses across Arab countries (based on data extracted from the World Health Report 2010). *Somalia has a physician density <0.5 per 10,000 population.

This undermines team building and leadership (EC-MOPHP 2003).

Poor planning results in growing shortages and attrition of health workers along with lack of financial and non-financial incentives and poor satisfaction of consumers with care (El-Jardali et al 2008a). Shortages are not only in overall number of professionals, but also in specialties (El-Jardali et al 2007a). Shortages can result from low entry into the profession, poor job satisfaction, or poor retention and management capacities. Shortages affect all Arab countries: Higher income countries report shortages in health facilities, despite having provider densities exceeding the regional average. Addressing the shortages requires a multi-pronged approach including needs assessment, national observatories that can provide accurate estimates of the existing workforce, and future forecasting, as was done by Al-Jarallah et al (2010) for Kuwait, and staff training in planning techniques (El-Jardali et al 2008a). Strategic planning requires the integration of input of multiple disciplines in addition to public health.

Learning from HRH strategies in Oman

Arab countries with similar contextual factors can learn a lot from the experience of other countries with regard to specific HRH challenges. Oman is one such country whose experience can be mimicked by similar countries in the region.

Oman was highly dependent on foreign-trained health workers to meet its needs. To respond to growing dependence on expatriates, the "Omanization" initiative was launched to achieve self-sufficiency. One strategy was strengthening the health education infrastructure. Through opening schools of nursing in most regions, Oman increased production of nurses and made nursing a socially accepted profession. Educational facilities and programs for medicine, public health, and allied professions were also created. In 2001, the MOH launched a national human resources development strategy to better plan for its HRH including computer models for manpower planning (staffing), which are now being regularly used by hospitals and primary health care centers (Oman MOH 2006). "Omanization" led to increasing the stock of the Omani workforce in the MOH by 52% and increasing employment opportunities for nationals and reduced reliance on expatriate workforce (Oman MOH 2006). The number of health personnel recruited from abroad, which included physicians, decreased from 1054 in 1997 to 702 in 2002. Such an achievement sets a precedent for countries of similar income status and HRH challenges to engage in similar activities.

While the experience of Oman can provide lessons for other countries, we need to pay closer attention to the socio-economic factors that explain why Oman has partially succeeded in "Omanizing" their HRH, at least when it comes to nurses.

Table 3. Ratios of Physicians to Population 1970–2005 by Country

	MD per 10,000 population (1970)	MD per 10,000 population (1990)	MD per 10,000 population (1995)	MD per 10,000 population (2000)	MD per 10,000 population (2005)	Ratio physicians (1970 over 2005)
Bahrain	5.56	13.0	11.1	13.2	27.6	**5.0**
Djibouti	4.55	2.05	2.0	1.3	1.8	**0.4**
Egypt	5.0	17.3	20.2	21.8	24.3	**4.9**
Iraq	1.67	5.8	5.1	5.5	6.6	**4.0**
Jordan	2.86	18.3	15.8	19.8	24.5	**8.6**
Kuwait	10.0	14.8	17.8	16.0	18.0	**1.8**
Lebanon	6.67	8.9	19.1	29.2	28.4	**4.26**
Libya	4.55	13.7	13.7	14.0	12.5	**2.75**
Morocco		1.6	3.4	4.6	5.6	
Oman	0.4	8.6	12.0	13.5	17.9	**44.75**
OPT			0.9	9.4	10.7	
Qatar	8.33	18.2	14.3	20.1	27.6	**3.32**
Saudi Arabia	1.0	18.8	16.6	17.1	20.0	**20.0**
Somalia	0.56	0.6	0.4	0.4		
Sudan	0.53	1	1.0	1.5	2.9	**5.47**
Syria	2.86	8.6	10.9	13.1	14.8	**5.17**
Tunisia	1.25	5.7	6.7	7.0	9.5	**7.6**
UAE		17.5	16.8	17.8	16.1	
Yemen	0.16	1.4	2.6	3.5	3.6	**22.5**

Source: Data retrieved from the annual reports of the regional director EMRO for the respective years.
OPT: Occupied Palestinian Territory

Mal-distribution of the HRH

There is gross mal-distribution of health workers across specialties, regions, and sectors (Table 4). In Egypt, the majority of physicians are specialized (88%); only 12% are general practitioners (Nandakumar et al 1999). In Lebanon, over 70% of physicians are specialists (Mohammad-Ali et al 2005). Unsurprisingly then, HRH is concentrated in urban areas leaving rural areas, where health workers are greatly needed but have limited salaries and career incentives to work and stay, underserved (El-Jardali et al 2008a). In Yemen, approximately 70% of all health workers are concentrated in three main cities (Sana'a, Aden, and Taiz) where only 35% of the population resides (EC-MOPHP 2003).

Internal migration of providers contributes to geographic misdistribution as documented in Lebanon (Mohamad Ali Osseiran et al 2005) and is commonly feared as a step toward eventual external migration. Geographic mal-distribution may also be an indirect outcome of the concentration of medical and nursing schools in urban areas. One manifestation of sectoral misdistribution is dual employment of many health workers in both the public and private sectors. While in many countries the public sector employs a majority of health workers, dual employment is common (El-Jardali et al 2008a; Iraq CCS 2006). The reasons for variations in employment of workers across countries deserve further examination. The various types of mal-distribution reflect poor

Table 4. Proportion of Total Health Workers in Urban Areas and Public Sector in Selected Arab Countries

	Yemen		Iraq		Morocco		Egypt
	Urban (%)	Public (%)	Urban (%)	Public (%)	Urban (%)	Public (%)	Public (%)
Physicians	87.54	74.95	80.17	86.44	69.49	57.25	68.91
Nurses	69.97	71.10	68.30	90.53	80.64	95.56	97.07
Midwives	59.70	49.44	80.57	37.78	71.41	94.95	99.49
Dentists	91.18	70.71	64.65	42.54	92.01	92.01	75.06
Pharmacists	75.74	71.99	79.19	52.70	95.85	95.81	83.73
Physiotherapists	100.00	100.00	77.57	100.00	97.35	100.00	100.00
Medical assistants	69.81	47.55	76.13	97.22	100.00	100.00	
Laboratory	76.41	65.34	80.03	87.04	99.64	100.00	100.00
Radiographers	64.40	61.84	80.82	90.61	99.69	100.00	100.00
Environmental and Public Health Officers	94.32	50.88	86.01	100.00	86.43	100.00	
Other Technicians and Health Care Cadres	22.82	84.97	76.99	100.00		100.00	100.00
Administrative and support staff	65.22	100.00	79.28	97.48	100.00	100.00	100.00
Date of data	2003–2004		2004		2004		2004

Source: Dr. Ghanim Alsheikh, Human Resource for Health, WHO Regional Office for the Eastern Mediterranean.

planning but possibly other factors such as policy choices in development and in health systems that have not favored rural areas and primary health care, social values, and prestige attached to urban life and high tech specialization, or professional interests. More research can help understand the causes and possible solutions to the mal-distribution issues.

Lack of Data and Limitations of Existing Data

Many countries lack data on HRH beyond the categories in the outer layer of our framework (Figure 1). Data are sparse about important attributes such as overall workforce size, composition, skills, training needs, functions, and performance; this hinders action on population health (Rawaf 2004). Estimates from international organizations such as WHO may be different than those from their regional offices. There are no centralized data registries that researchers can use to estimate available supply and future needs of public health workers (El-Jardali et al 2008a). Data collected by professional syndicates and in some instances the Ministry of Health may not be accurate.

For example, in Lebanon two Orders of Physicians, one in Beirut and another in Tripoli, exist. Physicians may register in one, both, or neither. The databases of both Orders as well as that of the Order of Nurses are not regularly updated (Mohammad Ali Ossseiran et al 2005). Although 6026 nurses were registered in 2006, many have yet to register (El-Jardali et al 2007b). Ammar (2009) reports that 5.3% of nurses in Lebanon are non-nationals, yet there is no documentation relating to where they work, their qualifications, and other vital information. Some countries completely lack information about HRH not employed within organizations. For example, community health providers are not recognized as providers in many countries. But even in countries such as Iraq and Sudan where community health workers are legitimate and significant care providers, in-depth data about these providers was not documented.

Lack of data forces researchers to resort to annual reports of international organizations which are vague about sources, and thus the reliability is not clear, and scope, i.e., who they include. It is rarely specified whether the health workers include foreign-trained professionals as well as nationals, and unemployed workers. Types of professionals are also rarely indicated. For instance, having the number of total nurses for a specific country may not be as important as knowing how many are university trained, technically trained, nurse aids, or practical nurses. In the few cases where data from an Arab organization exist, discrepancy with data from international organizations (El-Jardali et al 2007a) leaves researchers in a quandary.

To remedy all these problems, better data collection methods are needed (El-Jardali et al 2008a). Establishing a national well-functioning HRH observatory is a first step (WHO EMRO 2008). With the support of WHO EMRO, Sudan has pioneered a National Human Resources for Health Observatory (can be accessed at http://www.hrhobservatory.sd).

Gender Inequities

Literature indicates that the gender distribution of biomedical care providers varies according to profession. Medicine was a generally male oriented profession and entails potential travel and examining male patients, making it less desirable for females. Furthermore, the primary care giving role of women in their families leaves them with less time for study and work in medicine. Having a male-dominated medical profession has setbacks. In many Arab countries, it is culturally unacceptable or uncomfortable for women to be examined or seen by a male doctor (Winslow & Honein 2007). Failure to communicate information and gender bias often affects women's willingness to use services, which impacts their health (Winslow & Honein 2007). These gender stereotypes are changing, and the worldwide trend of female entry into medical schools is being observed in the region as well. In fact, the proportion of female physicians in Lebanon has been steadily increasing (Mohammad Ali Osseiran et al 2005), which is a trend that is also expected in many other Arab countries.

By contrast, women dominate nursing and midwifery in most Arab countries, as elsewhere, despite recent changes in a few countries. These two professions have always been socially perceived as "female-oriented," which is why males are generally reluctant to venture into them. Nursing has historically been perceived as a "natural gift" requiring little or no education, which has falsely given it a poor social image and also influenced the quality of candidates enrolling in the profession (Al-Kandari and Ajao 1998). This has

decreased entry into nursing and made nurses leave the profession altogether or migrate to countries where nursing conditions are better (Winslow & Honein 2007). The poor social image of the profession is documented in several Arab countries, including Egypt, Jordan, Kuwait, and Saudi Arabia (Mansour 1992; AbuGharbieh & Suliman 1992; Meleis 1980). In Kuwait, lack of support from family and social network (91.6% and 84%, respectively) were barriers to entry into nursing schools. The heavy academic load (77%), poor salary (77%), and possible night duty (75%) were other barriers to retaining nursing students (Al-Kandari and Ajao 1998).

Most health managers are males; 72% according to a WHO EMRO assessment in six Arab countries including 100% in Yemen (Abubaker et al 2008).

Policy, Leadership, and Partnership
Coordination Between Ministries

Partnerships are crucial for HRH development. This requires coordination between all relevant bodies, which does not happen in many Arab countries as there is no shared vision, common policies, or proper coordination of activities between different ministries and agencies. Human Resource Development departments in ministries of health, whenever available, are weak in many countries and cannot lead the way. The communication lines between the ministries of health and education are not always well functioning. The latter may continue to build or license medical and nursing schools without needs assessment. The ministries of health and finance rarely discuss the budget allocated to health care, a large portion of which finance HRH salaries. Several countries struggle with the legal aspects of HRH such as scope of practice, job description, licensing, and performance evaluation. These challenges require political decisions to place HRH development at the top of the national agenda, and leadership to build effective partnerships and collaboration among various actors. Such actors are not limited to policy makers in various ministries but also include academic institutions, researchers, professional associations, community organizations, civil society groups, NGOs, and international organizations working in Arab countries.

Capacity Building and Financing

Building HRH capacity is a process of improving its ability to meet its objectives and perform better

(Beaglehole and Dal Poz 2003). This is no longer a matter of choice, but one of strategic necessity (WHO EMRO 2008). Human resources development has not received adequate attention in the region. Strengthening HRH requires preparing enabling work environments; recruiting and training a sufficient number of staff; and involving all stakeholders (WHO EMRO 2008). Funds, preferably from national budgets, are needed for various human resource development initiatives, especially for adjusting salary structures and continued capacity development of existing workforce (WHO EMRO 2008).

HRH Management

Recruitment and Retention

The recruitment and retention of HRH with appropriate skills is a major challenge (Rawaf 2004). Many countries lack clear strategies in this area, for example incentives for entry into the health profession or job satisfaction for those in it (El-Jardali et al 2008a; El-Jardali et al 2009b). Poor recruitment and retention is due to low status, for example of nursing, and income; undeveloped infrastructures; lack of career development opportunities for most health workers; and lack of data, data collection capacities, and skills to interpret available data (Rawaf 2004). Some people shift away from entering the medical profession given that it requires many years of study. In UAE, nationals prefer professions in the business sector as they require fewer years of study and can secure them more profit in less time (El-Jardali et al 2008d).

Few studies have assessed recruitment and retention practices and strategies. In a study targeting nursing directors in Lebanon, the majority of sampled hospitals reported challenges in retaining nurses due to unsatisfactory salary and benefits (81%); unsuitable shifts and working hours (38%); better opportunities abroad (30%) and within the country (30%). Additional factors included workload (27%) and political instability (16%). Turnover rates ranged from 13% in 2004 to 16.8% in 2006 (El-Jardali et al 2009a). In response, many hospitals offered incentives such as financial rewards and benefits (63%); a salary scale (48%); flexible schedules (31%); and staff development (30%). The detrimental work conditions for some HRH categories are widely recognized in the Arab world, particularly for frontline care providers. Work environment is especially difficult under armed

conflict as in Sudan, Iraq, and Palestine (See Web Appendix). More research is needed in this area.

Job Satisfaction

Job satisfaction is a key to performance (Kennedy & Moore 2001). It predicts successful recruitment and retention of health providers but influences entry into the profession. There is more research in this as compared with other HRH areas. Studies have been conducted in Egypt, Iraq, Jordan, Kuwait, Lebanon, Occupied Palestinian Territory (OPT), Saudi Arabia, and UAE. While most studies focus on nurses, a few explore physicians and other providers. Satisfaction levels vary among studies but most report significant gaps. Various factors are associated with satisfaction among nurses, for example salaries and financial rewards in Jordan (Mrayyan 2007) and professional opportunities and rewards in Kuwait (Al-Enezi et al 2009). Job satisfaction, less job stress, and support from supervisors and coworkers were associated with the intent to stay at the job (Mrayyan 2007; AbuAl-Rub et al 2009; El-Jardali et al 2009a; El-Jardali et al 2010). Job satisfaction was a strong predictor of nurses' performance in Saudi Arabia and was also linked to organizational commitment (Al-Ahmadi 2009). Satisfaction levels seem to differ between physicians and nurses. For example, in a primary care setting in Saudi Arabia 67% of nurses and 53% of physicians were dissatisfied (Al Juhani & Kishk 2006). This may reflect differential opportunities, control, and other factors.

Much can be done to improve the working conditions and job satisfaction of HRH and particularly biomedical care providers. Sources of job dissatisfaction and resources and strategies for addressing them may be different in different contexts, for example, between countries in conflict or post-conflict and those with higher incomes in the region. Incentive structures are crucial in this process and would lead to better retention. While financial incentives rank high (Younies et al 2008; El-Jardali et al 2009b), non-financial incentives, such as career development programs and paths, recognition, improving the work environment, and recruitment and retention strategies, are also very important as previously discussed.

External Migration

HRH migration, a global phenomenon, is on the rise in this region. Within the region, the direction is generally from low to high-income countries. Several factors account for this phenomenon. Rapid development in the Gulf countries created an increasing demand for qualified expatriate health professionals since local production is insufficient to meet needs (El-Jardali et al 2008b). The main exporters of HRH are Egypt, Iraq, Jordan, Lebanon, Morocco, Sudan, Syria, and Tunisia. Wars, deprivation, and social unrest (El-Jardali et al 2008b) also drive migration. Better wages and working conditions abroad along with hampered prospects for social mobility within institutions at home, which hinder professional advancement and rarely reward people according to their skills, are also important (Fargues 2006).

Emigration streams are generally in the direction of countries of higher economic standing in North America, Europe, and Australia. HRH shortages in such countries create opportunities. Young physicians often emigrate to seek specialty training since opportunities are limited at home (El-Jardali et al 2008b; Akl et al 2008). Lebanese physicians rank second (after Grenada) among expatriate physicians in the United States after controlling for country population size (Akl et al 2007). Only a quarter of Lebanese new medical graduates intend to return home after training (Akl et al 2008). Conflict plays an important role in emigration. Physician emigration from Lebanon intensified after the civil war broke out in 1975. Of all graduates from the American University of Beirut over the period 1935–1974, only 33.2% were practicing in Lebanon in 1977 (Kronfol 1979) and only 16.5% in 1984 (Kronfol et al 1992). In the OPT, 31% of physicians intended to emigrate due to unrest or to pursue self-development (Mataria et al 2008).

Within-region migration and emigration patterns are also significant. Aggressive recruitment by employers from Northern countries facing nursing shortages is an important drive. Many Jordanian nurses choose to migrate to the Gulf, Canada, or the United States for better salaries and working conditions (AbuAlRub 2007). In Lebanon, one in five nurses emigrate within 2 years of receiving their degree (El-Jardali et al 2008c). Nurses with university training were preferred. In a national study, 68% of nurses reported an intent to leave, 37% of whom disclosed plans to leave (El-Jardali et al 2009a). As opportunities for expatriate career advancement are limited in the Gulf, many expatriate nurses use Gulf countries as a stepping stone for migration to countries in Europe and North America where they acquire citizenship in addition to benefits (El-Jardali et al 2008b).

HRH Production

Investments in HRH education promote competency and skill development and are linked with improved health outcomes (Cioffi et al 2004). There is a wide variation in production of health professionals across the region. As expected, low-income countries with low densities and high mortality had much fewer medical and nursing schools than higher income ones (Joint Learning Initiative 2004). There is a limited number of public health schools and existing ones are not always oriented in the population health framework (see Chapter 34). Production of allied specialties such as nutrition, radiography, community health work, and social work is low compared with demands.

Poor educational programs and outdated curricula cripple the production of competent and market-ready HRH in many countries. The quality of teaching staff in some programs is poor (El-Jardali et al 2008a, 2008b). In Yemen, competency of some professional cadres is poor as a result of poor training programs (EC-MOPHP 2003). Even in a high-income country such as UAE, variation in the quality of educational programs may lead to multiple standards and adversely affect service delivery (El-Haddad 2006). The EMR Advisory Panel on Nursing suggested that over a period of 15 years, member states should combine all their nursing programs into one standard, 4-year Bachelor of Science program (WHO EMRO 1998 as cited in El-Haddad 2006). This was endorsed by the Scientific Association of Arab Nursing (Gulf News, 2002 as cited in El-Haddad, 2006). UAE now encourages and supports Emirati nurses with diplomas in nursing to enroll in BSN bridging programs. There are similar programs in other countries such as Jordan and Lebanon.

There is also limited information on the competencies of graduating health workers. Accreditation of schools and educational programs can promote competency-based learning (El-Jardali et al 2008a). This experience was learned in the Graduate Public Health Program (GPHP) at the Faculty of Health Sciences in the American University of Beirut, which received accreditation from the Council on Education for Public Health in 2008.

The Complex Reality and Entry Points to Change in Policy and Practice

Understanding the needs and realities of the public health workforce is central to our ability to shape and affect change. Despite the challenges we have described, entry points to change do exist, with the most important being collaboration of all relevant actors, for example, through policy dialogues of governmental and non-governmental actors, on an agenda of priorities in policy, action, and research.

Because any discussion of the workforce comes down to defining this workforce, a first crucial need is to invest in data collection and analysis on all aspects of the public health workforce as described in this chapter. This requires that different categories be clearly defined and their public health role recognized as legitimate. The proposed public health workforce framework can serve as a starting point for initiating discussions and mapping exercises of different categories. If done within the framework of developing a national observatory of public health workforce, this can build the basic blocks to inform a critical review of existing policy decisions and help guide future policies.

At the governmental level, better coordination among ministries of health, education, planning, and financing is needed on a comprehensive national public health workforce vision and strategy. Because of the regional dimensions of public health workforce migration, regional coordination is also needed. How ministries dealing with public health functions prepare public health managers, particularly those involved in policy- and decision-making processes and who have tremendous impact on public health, is an understudied issue. As many health managers come from medical backgrounds, this often necessitates investing time and resources to introduce them to the public health issues they need to address. What is needed is a clear policy for allocating and training workforce in ministries to assume their public health role.

Policy dialogues should be held to help update and identify core competencies required to deliver essential services in all public health program areas and explore whether public health workforce credentialing can create a competent and fully functional workforce. A related area is promoting and expanding public health educational and training programs and supporting them to move from a biomedical to a population health focus. The public health curricula need to be somewhat unified and modernized to meet population health needs, and should be developed in partnership with the communities.

The many gaps we have identified in this review indicate the need for rigorous research to support evidence-based policies. Research is needed in areas such as the educational profile of the public health workforce, their public health functions, the work environments, and the dynamics behind the education, recruitment, retention, and deployment. Research should explore attrition and migration patterns, turnover, causes, practices and consequences, working conditions, job satisfaction, and quality of care (and how it might be impacted by re-licensing of health professionals). The situation of health professions should be examined from quantitative as well as qualitative perspectives and this should be shared in publicly supported scientific forums to synthesize evidence and agree on directions. Research evidence can complement and feed into information systems in ministries of health and national workforce observatories. Obviously, researchers and research institutions must be encouraged and given resources to pursue workforce research questions of most interest to policymaking. While we emphasize the importance of primary research, this chapter has already presented enough evidence for action in many areas. Existing knowledge translation to action is a joint responsibility of researchers and policy makers. A window of opportunity in the policymaking process, such as new strategic plans or health system reform plans, etc., can offer the right condition for such translation.

The various priorities we have proposed require devoting public resources, both financial and non-financial, to workforce development. Such investment must have a broader scope as improving the public health workforce and strengthening its impact on population health would be difficult without addressing broader public health and health systems, issues such as governance, financing, and delivery, described throughout the chapters in this section. More focus on population health would stir health systems away from disease-focus and curative care and create the demands for a workforce with a strong public health mandate. This is imperative for health sector reform in this region (Alwan & Hornby 2002).

There is no doubt about the importance of a well-developed public health workforce in achieving all the goals of public health. It is quite evident in this chapter that the public health workforce plays a crucial role in improving population health outcomes and strengthening public health system functions. This chapter has justified the need for reform and we are confident that the health of populations will gain immensely from reform. This is our challenge – why don't we rise to it?

Acknowledgments

We thank Dr. Huda Zurayk for providing useful insights into the proposed conceptual framework and critical review of its content. We are grateful to Dr. Ghanim Alsheikh for providing data on several Arab countries. We thank Ms. Farah Amro, Mr. Razmig Markarian, and Ms. Hiba Abu Sweid for their assistance with literature search and Ms. Maha Jaafar for her assistance in compiling data and conducting part of the literature review.

References

AbuAlRub RF, Omari FH, Al-Zaru IM (2009) Support, satisfaction and retention among Jordanian nurses in private and public hospitals. *International Nursing Review*, 56(3): 326–332

Abubaker W, Alsheikh G, Gedik G, Dal Poz M, Dovlo D (2008) *Health management workforce in selected countries of Eastern Mediterranean Region*. Presented at the first Global Forum on Human Resources for Health, 2–7 March 2008, Kampala, Uganda

AbuGharbieh P, Suliman W (1992) Changing the image of nursing in Jordan through effective role negotiation. *International Nursing Review*, 39(5): 149–152

Akl EA, Maroun N, Major S, et al (2008) Post-graduation migration intentions of students of Lebanese medical schools. *BMC Public Health*, 8: 191

Akl EA, Maroun N, Major S, Chahoud B, Schünemann HJ (2007) Graduates of Lebanese medical schools in the United States: An observational study of international migration of physicians. *BMC Health Services Research*, 7: 49

Al-Ahmadi H (2009) Factors affecting performance of hospital nurses in Riyadh Region, Saudi Arabia. *International Journal of Health Care Quality Assurance*, 22: 40–54

Al-Enezi N, Chowdhury RI, Shah MA, Al-Otabi M (2009) Job satisfaction of nurses with multicultural backgrounds: A questionnaire survey in Kuwait. *Applied Nursing Research*, 22(2): 94–100

Al-Jarallah K, Moussa M, Figen Al-Khanfar K (2010) The physician workforce in Kuwait to the year 2020. *International Journal of Health Planning and Management*, 25: 49–62

Al Juhani AM, Kishk NA (2006) Job satisfaction among primary health care physicians and nurses in Al-madinah Al-munawwara. *Journal of the Egyptian Public Health Association*, 81(3–4): 165–180

Al-Kandari FH, Ajao E (1998) Recruitment and retention of nursing students in Kuwait. *International Journal of Nursing Studies*, 35: 245–251

Alwan A, Hornby P (2002) The implications of health sector reform for human resources development. *Bulletin of the World Health Organization*, 80: 56–60

Ammar W (2009) *Health beyond politics*. Beirut, Lebanon: World Health Organization, Eastern Mediterranean Regional Office

Beaglehole R, Dal Poz MR (2003) Public health workforce: Challenges and policy issues. *Human Resources for Health*, 1: 4

Cioffi JP, Lichtveld MY, Thielen L, Miner K (2003) Credentialing the public health workforce: An idea whose time has come. *Journal of Public Health Management Practice*, 9(6): 451–458

Cioffi J, Lichtveld M, Tilson H (2004) A research agenda for public health workforce development. *Journal of Public Health Management and Practice*, 10(3): 186–192

Commission of the European Communities (2008) *Green Paper on the European Workforce for Health*. Brussels: COM 725/32

El-Haddad M (2006) Nursing in the United Arab Emirates: An historical background. *International Nursing Review*, 53: 284–289

El-Jardali F, Jamal D, Abdallah A, Kassak K (2007a) Human resources for health planning and management in the Eastern Mediterranean region: Facts, gaps and forward thinking for research and policy. *Human Resources for Health*, 5: 9

El-Jardali F, Dimassi H, Jamal D, Dumit N, Mouro G (2007b) *Developing country specific retention strategies for nurses in Lebanon, final research report – Eastern Mediterranean Regional Office*. Special Grants for Research in Priority Areas of Public Health. Published at the WHO EMRO Human Resources for Health Observatory

El-Jardali F, Makhoul J, Jamal D, Tchaghchaghian V (2008a) *Identification of priority research questions related to health financing, human resources for health, and the role of the non-state sector in low and middle income countries of the Middle East and North Africa Region*. Research Report Submitted to Alliance for Health Policy and Systems Research

El-Jardali F, Jamal D, Jaafar M, Rahal Z (2008b) *Analysis of health professionals migration: A two-country case study for the United Arab Emirates and Lebanon*. Report prepared for the World Health Organization, Geneva

El-Jardali F, Dumit N, Jamal D, Mouro G (2008c) Migration out of Lebanese nurses: A questionnaire survey and secondary data analysis. *International Journal of Nursing Studies*, 45(10): 1490–1500

El-Jardali F, Makhoul J, Jamal D (2008d) *Lebanon case study on the identification of priority research questions related to health financing, human resources for health, and the* role of the non-state sector. Research Report Submitted to Alliance for Health Policy and Systems Research

El-Jardali F, Dimassi H, Dumit N, Jamal D, Mouro G (2009a) A national cross-sectional study on nurses' intent to leave and job satisfaction in Lebanon: Implications for policy and practice. *BMC Nursing*, 8: 3

El-Jardali F, Dimassi H, Jamal D, Tchaghchaghian V (2009b) Comparing reasons for nurse migration against predictors of intent to leave Lebanon: A two-hospital case study. *Middle East Journal of Nursing*, 3(1): 26–33

El-Jardali F, Alameddine M, Dumit N, Dimassi H, Jamal D, Maalouf S (2010) Nurses' work environment and intent to leave in Lebanese hospitals: Implications for policy and practice. *International Journal of Nursing Studies*, 48: 204–214

European Commission – Ministry of Public Health and Population, Human Resources Development (EC-MOPHP) (2003) *Policies that provide incentives for better performance of health staff in rural and remote areas*. Support to Health Sector Reform in the Republic of Yemen

Fargues P (2006) *International migration in the Arab region: Trends and policies'*, Expert Group Meeting on International Migration and Development in the Arab Region: Challenges and Opportunities. Beirut: ESCWA, 15–17 May 2006. Available from www.un.org/esa/ population/publications/ EGM_Ittmig_Arab/P09_Fargues. pdf [Accessed 15 December 2010]

Gebbie K, Merrill J, Tilson HH (2002) The public health workforce. *Health Affairs(Millwood)*, 21(6): 57–67

Joint Learning Initiative, Human Resources for Health: Overcoming the Crisis (2004) Available from http://www.healthgap.org/camp/ hcw_docs/JLi_Human_Resources_ for_Health.pdf [Accessed 15 December 2010]

Kabene SM, Orchard C, Howard JM, Soriano MA, Leduc R (2006) The importance of human resource management in health care: A global context. *Human Resources for Health*, 4: 20

Kennedy V, Moore F (2001) A Systems approach to public health workforce development. *Journal of Public Health Management and Practice*, 7 (4): 17–22

Kronfol N (1979) *The migratory patterns of the AUB medical graduates, 1935–1974*. Doctoral dissertation. Boston: Harvard School of Public Health

Kronfol NM, Sibai AM, Rafeh N (1992) The impact of civil disturbances on the migration of physicians: The case of Lebanon. *Medical Care*, 30 (3): 208–215

Mansour AA (1992) Nursing in Saudi Arabia as perceived by university students and their parents. *Journal of Nursing Education*, 32: 45–46

Mataria A, Abu-Hantas I, Amer W (2008) *The "Brain Drain" of the Palestinian Society: With an exploratory study of the health and higher education sectors*. Ramallah, Palestine: Palestine Economic Policy Research Institute (MAS)

Meleis Al (1980) A model for establishment of educational program in developing countries: The nursing paradoxes in Kuwait. *Journal of Advanced Nursing*, 24: 289–293

Mohamad Ali Osseiran A, El Jardali F, Kassak K, Ramadan S (2005) *Harnessing the private sector to achieve public health goals in counties of the Eastern Mediterranean: Focus on Lebanon*. Department of Health Management and Policy. Faculty of Health Sciences. American University of Beirut

Mrayyan M (2008) Jordanian nurses' job satisfaction and intent to stay: Comparing teaching and non-teaching hospitals. *Journal of Professional Nursing*, 23(3): 125–136

Mrayyan MT (2007) Nursing practice problems in private hospitals in Jordan: Students' perspectives. *Nurse Education in Practice*, 7: 82–87

Nandakumar AK, Berman P, Fleming E (1999) *Findings of the Egyptian Health Care Provider Survey, Technical Report No. 26*. Bethesda, MD: Partnerships for Health Reform Project, Abt Associates Inc.

Oman Ministry of Health (2006) *The human resources development plan: 7th Five-Year Health Development Plan 2006–2010*. Muscat, Oman: Ministry of Health Directorate General of Planning

Public Health Agency of Canada (2005) *Building the public health workforce for the 21st Century: A Pan Canadian Framework for Public Health Human Resources Planning, The Joint Task Group on Public Health Human Resources, Advisory Committee on Health Delivery and Human Resources*. Advisory Committee on Population Health and Health Security, October 2005

Rawaf S (2004) Public health functions and infrastructures in MENA/EM Region. In: AM Pierre-Louis, FA Akala, HS Karam (Eds). *Public health in the Middle East and North Africa: Meeting the challenges of the twenty-first century* (Ch 2; p. 25–39). Washington, DC: World Bank Publications

Sim F, Lock K, McKee M (2007) Maximizing the contribution of the public health workforce: the English experience. *Bulletin of the World Health Organization*, 5: 935–938

Tilson H, Gebbie KM (2004) The public health workforce. *Annual Review of Public Health*, 25: 341–356

WHO (World Health Organization) (2000) *The World Health Report 2000: Health Systems: Improving performance*. Geneva, Switzerland: World Health Organization

WHO (2006) *Working together for health: The World Health Report 2006*. Geneva, Switzerland: World Health Organization

WHO Eastern Mediterranean Regional Office (WHO EMRO) (2008)

Health Workforce Development Series 1, Strengthening national and subnational departments for human resources development

Winslow WW, Honein G (2007) Bridges and barriers to health: Her story – Emirati women's health needs. *Health Care for Women International*, 28: 285–308

Younies H, Barhem B, Younis MZ (2008) Ranking of priorities in employees' reward and recognition schemes: From the perspective of UAE health care employees. *International Journal of Health Planning and Management*, 23(4): 357–371

Chapter

31

Health Care Delivery: The Missing Links

Nabil M. Kronfol and Samer Jabbour

The WHO framework for health systems (WHO 2000) highlights the central role of health care delivery as the final common pathway for inputs into the health care system (HCS). As delivery is just one aspect of this system; assessing it must consider the many complex issues around health care, and indeed the broader health system, discussed throughout this section, such as governance, financing, and workforce. To avoid overlap with, and further inform the discussions in, other chapters, we will attempt a focused review in this chapter. After discussing how to approach delivery actors and structures, we provide a basic description of health services focusing on ambulatory and primary care and hospitals. We then review barriers in access to and utilization of health services. Lastly, we discuss selected issues and initiatives in reforming delivery systems and conclude with a few recommendations.

Approaching Delivery Structures and Actors

Delivery systems around the region are diverse and can be examined along multiple domains (Table 1). Understanding the system in each country requires a consideration of national income, level of development, policies, and, importantly, history. Conflict has a profound impact on delivery as discussed in Section 5. In the Occupied Palestinian Territory (OPT) there are *de facto* two ministries, one in West Bank and another in Gaza with parallel delivery systems (Giacaman et al 2009); because of the legacy of occupation, the delivery system has unique features with NGOs contributing 31.8% of hospital beds and 28.2% of primary care facilities. The major concern is ensuring delivery in light of restrictions on movement, widespread poverty, unemployment, and recurrent violence. The situation is expectedly different

Table 1. Domains of Health Care Delivery

Levels of care	Primary, secondary, tertiary
Nature of care	Promotion, prevention, cure, rehabilitation, palliative
Facility	Ambulatory, inpatient, long term, emergency, traditional home care, treatment abroad
Types of utilization	Preventive, pharmaceuticals, diagnostics, dental, mental
Providers	Various providers in public and private sectors
Attributes	Access, coverage, quality, efficiency, equity
Barriers to utilization	Geographical, cultural, social determinants, cost, organizational
Responsiveness	Utilization reviews, satisfaction, quality

in another national context. In Saudi Arabia, Walston et al (2008) identified rising costs, privatization, quality of services, and the expansion of insurance coverage to expatriate workers as the main delivery concerns.

Acknowledging the diversity, there are common features of delivery systems around the region. All are pluralist with a public–private mix, and commonly fragmented with multiple sub-systems belonging to the ministry of health (MOH), other ministries, "uniformed" medical services, and the private sector. Except in Lebanon, the public sector dominates provision. The private sector, including for-profit providers and non-profit organizations, captures a significant and growing share, even in poorer countries. This is due to deteriorating public health services, the governments' encouragement of the private sector to increase its investments, and public perception of better quality

---

and more efficiency and privacy in the private sector. Public–private partnerships, especially through public contracting of private services, have gained momentum over the past two decades and are now important components of health systems in several countries (Siddiqi et al 2006).

Ambulatory and Primary Care

The public sector has tried to play a key role in developing ambulatory care. At the turn of the twentieth century, governments opened dispensaries, staffed by employed physicians, to provide free care and dispense medicines, mainly for infectious diseases. These evolved over time based on the health priorities of the state. In the 1950s maternal and child health clinics developed. Later school health clinics and specialty clinics emerged to complement general clinics. Ambulatory care followed, then a "vertical" approach to address defined population groups or selected diseases. It was not until 1978 and the Alma Ata conference that the primary care model gained momentum with many countries building large networks of primary care centers to cater to the needs of different age groups. By 2008, Syria, for example, had built up almost 1800 public-sector primary care centers (WHO EMRO 2009a). Saudi Arabia had 17,000 such centers. Ambulatory care availability (Table 2) varies among countries. Generally, public primary care services are either free or require small user fees. Government health centers are either managed by the state or by contracted non-governmental organizations. In some countries, international NGOs and charity have established clinics to attend to the needs of populations under duress.

Public investments in primary care have not yet achieved the objectives of universality and affordability. Much of ambulatory care today is provided through office-based private physicians, mainly in solo fee-for-service practices. This is the case even in countries with wide primary care networks. In Egypt, Nandakumar et al (2000) reported that 49.7% of treatment seekers see private physicians. Hospitals, both public and private, also provide primary care through outpatient departments, walk-in clinics, emergency departments, and recently urgent care centers. The proportion of hospital visits of total outpatient visits is much higher than the global average, ranging from around 20% in Jordan to around 40% in Qatar and 50% in Syria (WHO EMRO 2009c). This raises questions about cost-efficiency, the effectiveness of referral systems,

and public perception of quality in the ambulatory sector. In a number of countries, especially where state provision is weak such as in Lebanon and in conflict such as OPT, non-governmental, charity/civil society, politically affiliated, and international organizations also provide services. Although these organizations fill important gaps, they commonly act as private providers and their goals are not aligned with those of public delivery.

The contribution of primary care to the gains in health and human development cannot be denied. Oman is often highlighted as a success story (Abdullatif 2008; WHO 2008), having built up a strong primary care, based on *welayat* (governorate) health systems. Oman increased the number of health centers and dispensaries from 22 in 1970 to 175 in 2006, and achieved substantial improvement in life expectancy and health indicators, for example reducing infant mortality rate from 118 to 10.5 (per 1000 live births) in the same period. Several countries, especially North African ones, have also made similar progress. Although it is difficult to quantify the contribution of primary care to these improvements, it has played a key role (Abdullatif 2008). While health indicators have improved in all countries, progress has been uneven; the poorest countries, especially if affected by conflict and instability such as Somalia and Yemen, show the least progress.

Further development of primary care faces many challenges (Abdullatif 2008; Siddiqi et al 2008; WHO 2008). We review some of these challenges in four areas.

Efficiency

Inefficiencies are substantial, especially in the public sector. Wastage of resources is common. In Jordan, health providers in public primary care centers spent 48.7% of their work day as down time (Mawajdeh et al 2004). As personnel represent 43.8% of recurrent costs, this amounted to an annual loss of US$13.7 million. The lack of a gate-keeping system leads consumers to use specialists and hospitals directly rather than primary care. Referral systems are commonly inefficient. In Egypt, referral from general practitioners (GPs) to specialists varied 6.6-fold among clinics and 54.6-fold among individual GPs (Abdel-Wahab et al 2004). In Saudi Arabia, a referral system was established in 1989 (Qureshi et al 2009) but has many problems including higher than desired rates (Abdelwahid et al 2010). There is anecdotal evidence

Table 2. Selected Indicators of Health Services Availability and Utilization

	Hospital beds/10,000 pop.	PHC units/10,000 pop.	Population with access to local health services (%)		Antenatal coverage/ attendance (%)	Births attended by skilled personnel (%)	1-year-old immunized DPT3 (%)
			Urban	Rural			
Algeria	...	0.5*	...	...	79*	92	86
Bahrain	19.7	0.2	100	...	99	99	97
Comoros	...	...	...	...	...	62	76
Djibouti	...	...	...	...	76	57	89
Egypt	20.8	0.7	100	100	60	81	97
Iraq	12.6	0.6	96	87	54	80	80
Jordan	18	2.4	...	...	99	99	97
Kuwait	18	0.4	100	na	100	100	99
Lebanon	34.3	...	...	...	96	98	93
Libya	37	2.6	100	100	93	99	98
Mauritania	...	...	...	...	63*	57	70
Morocco	11	0.8	66	77	68	63	99
Oman	20.2	0.9	100	95	99	99	99
Palestine	12.8	1.8	100	100	100	100	96
Qatar	25.2	2.7	100	...	100	100	97
S. Arabia	22.1	0.8	...	...	96	96	98
Somalia	...	4.8	15	50	26	33	31
Sudan	7.3	1.6	...	...	70	49	93
Syria	15.4	1	100	90	84	93	98
Tunisia	20	2	...	...	96	95	99
UAE	18.6	0.3	100	100	100	100	92
Yemen	7	2	80	25	45	36	87

... data not available.
Sources: For all countries WHO EMRO (2009d) except for Algeria, Comoros, and Mauritania where data was obtained from WHO Regional Office for Africa's Country Health System Fact Sheet 2006 for each country.
* At least one visit. The number of visits is not indicated for countries within WHO EMRO.

from many countries on over-referral and associated kickbacks as well as under-referral for fear of losing patients to specialties.

Quality of Care and User Satisfaction

There is variability in reports from various countries of quality of primary care. Because most studies are not national and do not use similar methodologies

and indicators, it is difficult to synthesize studies and compare findings. There is more evidence on quality of care in the public and affiliated sector than on the private sector, which is rarely studied.

Important gaps in quality are usually documented through satisfaction surveys and documented practices. Al-Ahmadi & Roland (2005) synthesized 31 studies in Saudi Arabia. Access and effective care was good in basic areas such as immunization, maternal health, and epidemic control but poor in chronic disease management, prescribing patterns, health education, referral patterns, and some aspects of interpersonal care. Correlates of good quality were management and organizational factors, implementation of evidence-based practice, professional development, use of referrals to secondary care, and organizational culture. Studies published after this review document similar findings. Well-baby care was mostly satisfactory with the exception of documenting breastfeeding duration (Al-Saigul & Al-Alfi 2009); there was low adherence to a national protocol for managing asthma (Abudahish & Bella 2010); diabetic and hypertension care is sub-optimal (Al-Homrany et al 2008; Al-Hussein 2008); and problems remain in referrals (Abdelwahid et al 2010). Problems with prescribing were also common in other high-income countries, for example, Bahrain (Otoom et al 2010) and Kuwait (Ayyad et al 2010) as well as in low- and middle-income countries, Sudan (Mannan et al 2009), Syria (Barah & Gonçalves 2010), and Yemen (Bashrahil 2010).

Even within the area of maternal and child health, which has traditionally received important attention and funding, there are major quality gaps. For example, in Tunisia after the introduction of seven quality criteria for mother and child care in 2005, El-Mhamdi et al (2010) showed that only 21% of women who received care met all quality criteria. In Egypt, Hong et al (2006) reported that 32.2% of women reported low quality of family planning services; Zaky et al (2007) also reported non-satisfaction of beneficiaries with the quality of reproductive health services including those attending a "model" facility in the health sector reform initiative. An older study of reproductive health services in Egypt, Jordan, and Tunisia documented multiple problems with quality in the domains of woman-provider relationship, continuity and follow-up, management, and information exchange (Al-Qutob et al 1998). Health facility-based surveys of quality of child care in Egypt (2002), Morocco (2007), and Sudan (2003) show important deficiencies. For example, in Morocco (WHO EMRO 2009b) basic tasks such as weight and temperature taking were "often" done incorrectly; only 55% of children with low weight-for-age, anemia and/or persistent diarrhea were assessed for feeding; and only 28% of anemic children were prescribed iron. Considering that health providers in surveyed facilities had already received training in Integrated Management of Childhood Illnesses means that the situation may be worse in contexts without such training.

Studies show variability in patient satisfaction with primary care. There are correlates to dissatisfaction and perceived good quality of care, which form targets for future interventions. For example, in the study by Zaky et al (2007) sources of dissatisfaction were waiting time, interior furnishings, cleanliness of the units, and consultation time. In Saudi Arabia, Al-Sakkak et al (2008) reported a 64% satisfaction rate with the main sources of dissatisfaction being accessibility and continuity of care; Mahfouz et al (2004) reported a 79% overall satisfaction among the elderly with dissatisfaction caused by inadequate audiovisual means for health education, long time spent in the health centers, and not enough specialty clinics. In Oman, women were highly satisfied with antenatal care services with laboratory services and crowding being the leading causes of dissatisfaction (Ghobashi & Khandekar 2008).

Utilization

Increased availability of primary care services is important because it promotes desired utilization (Steele et al 1999). However, availability, accessibility, and affordability may not be enough to increase utilization of public services if the actual or perceived quality is low. In Egypt, Hong et al (2006) showed that family planning service quality was correlated with IUD use among women in public facilities. Accommodation is another factor of utilization. Zaky et al (2007) found that many women expressed intention to seek private physicians because of more flexible working hours and availability of specialties. In Saudi Arabia, the physician's communication skills, Arabic-speaking health team, and free service were the factors most encouraging of primary care utilization (Saeed & Mohamed 2002). The dual employment of physicians, whereby many users are directed to private offices, may also compromise utilization of public services. In Lebanon, up to 80% of ambulatory encounters occur in private offices, even by lower income groups, although public primary care centers have been remodeled and equipped (Kronfol 2004). Many visit the public centers to receive medications for chronic diseases and other essential drugs dispensed only through public facilities. Preference for private providers was also reported in Egypt (Nandakumar et al 2000). Underuse of public facilities wastes national and household resources.

Responsiveness to the Changing Population Needs

Al-Ahmadi & Roland's findings of poor care quality in such areas as chronic disease management, health education, and interpersonal care, have profound implications for the whole region. Primary care networks were started with focus on issues such as maternal and child health. With changing population needs due to demographic and epidemiological transitions and increasing public expectations of health services, the question arises as to whether primary care is equipped to address current and emergent challenges such as health inequities, smoking cessation, obesity, assessment and treatment of chronic diseases, care of older people, and mental health. Al-Ahmadi & Roland's review and reports from other countries (see for example Ammar 2009; WHO 2008) suggest that this may not be the case. This raises the need to re-examine primary care, including the basic benefit packages which have been adopted in some countries such as Egypt, Oman, and Syria, and assess their continued relevance to population health needs.

Hospital Care

In 1974, hospital availability was limited: less than one bed per 1000 population in Jordan, Somalia, Sudan, Syria, and Yemen; one bed per 500–999 in Oman and Saudi Arabia; one bed per 200–499 in Bahrain, Egypt, Iraq, Libya, Tunisia, Qatar, and UAE. Only Lebanon had one bed per less than 200 population. The period of 1970–1995 witnessed an impressive expansion and construction of predominantly public, but also private, hospitals in all countries. This improved the availability of hospital care, nearing 100% population coverage in some countries. Today, hospitals account for 50%–70% of government health expenditures (WHO EMRO 2009c). Hospitals are important politically and socially because they provide concrete and visible health achievements for the political class in the eyes of the public and employ half the physicians and two-thirds of nurses. In most countries, except Lebanon, government-owned hospitals provide the bulk of services, which are free or subsidized. In Lebanon, private hospitals provide the bulk of the care but public patients account for 70–80% of private bed occupancy. In Egypt, nearly 85% of all inpatient stays occurred in public facilities. Nevertheless, hospital care still suffers from important gaps.

Inequalities

Despite improved availability of hospitals (Table 2), important regional disparities persist. Hospital beds per 10,000 population varies from 37 in the highest income countries to 4.2 in the lowest income countries (Abdullatif 2008). Hospitals concentrate in large cities creating sub-national access inequalities. In Egypt, beds per 1000 population range from 4.5 in Cairo to 0.88 in Kena with a 5:1 differential between wealthier urban and poor rural governorates (WHO EMRO 2007). Increasing cost of care is an additional source of inequalities. Private, for-profit and nonprofit, hospitals are proliferating due to active and passive privatization policies and now account for a variable proportion of total beds: 80% in Lebanon, 43% in Jordan, 8% in Yemen, and 6% in Sudan (WHO 2009c). Private care is potentially problematic, because it is not just the rich who use it; all population segments, including the poor, have to use it especially if public care is perceived to be of low quality and the medical condition life threatening.

Public hospitals, especially teaching ones, are the reference places for service excellence, tertiary care, training of human resources and research and have somewhat of an equalizing effect. In Jordan, for example, the difference in report of hospital use in the past year between the poorest and the richest in use of MOH public hospitals (8.4% vs. 5%) and Royal Medical Services (5.7% vs. 7.5%) is much smaller than the use of public primary care (59.1% vs. 13.5%) (Halasa et al 2010). In most countries, teaching hospitals fall within the purview of the Ministry of Higher Education with very little coordination with the MOH.

Efficiency

Bed occupancy is around 80% in higher income Gulf countries but only around 45% in low- and middle-income countries (WHO EMRO 2009c). Occupancy is commonly low in peripheral and rural hospitals but high in major centers. In Egypt, this creates excessive bed capacity (WHO EMRO 2007). As many public hospitals around the region receive block grants for care based on beds, they have little incentive for improvement (WHO EMRO 2007). In Lebanon, fee-for-service arrangements for hospital care, and absence of public coverage for outpatient care, favor over-utilization of hospital care (WHO EMRO 2007). Length of stay is also higher than global averages due to quality, efficiency, reimbursement modalities, and human resource factors. There are only a limited number of costing studies. Estimated cost of stay per day depends on a country's income and hospital level, for example Algeria (US$14.8–26.3) vs. UAE (US $111.3–197.9) (Adam & Evans 2006). Fixed costs and salaries accounted for 70% and 62% of hospital costs in the OPT, respectively.

Management and Accountability

This section is mostly based on WHO EMRO (2009c). Hospital management capacity is low, especially in low-income countries; less than 25% of managers are trained in management in Sudan and Yemen compared with over 80% in Jordan, UAE, and Lebanon. Working conditions in most middle- and low-income countries are not conducive to quality or efficiency due to "staff motivation, lack of management tools and limited transparency and accountability." Clinical governance has not been introduced to hospitals. Quality programs are sporadic rather than system-wide and rarely institutionalized. A culture of patient rights is weak. Hospital autonomy initiatives have been introduced in many countries. However, there is very limited information about successes and lessons from autonomy experiences.

Quality of Care

While countries collect various service data about hospitals, peer reviewed research on hospital is limited considering the resources devoted to them. One area that has received considerable research attention is quality and outcome of care. Both research and service data indicate important deficiencies. A WHO regional study of adverse events based on record review in 27 hospitals in six countries (Egypt, Jordan, Morocco, Sudan, Tunisia, and Yemen) showed a regional average of 8% (range, 2.5%–18%) (WHO EMRO 2009c) Published research from around the region confirms variability in incidence. In a retrospective cohort study of 620 inpatients in Tunisia, adverse events occurred in 10% (55% were surgery related and 21% related to therapeutic errors): 21% led to death and 60% were highly preventable. This death rate is very high as compared with the 2.5% death and permanent disability rate for the region, which is the highest such figure globally (WHO EMRO 2009c). Reports of medication errors were filed in only 0.15% of admissions in Saudi Arabia (Sadat-Ali

et al 2010) suggesting possibly under-reporting, a common problem in this region and elsewhere. In Jordan, only 42.1% of nurses reported medication errors (Mrayyan et al 2007). There were gaps in safety culture in Lebanese (El-Jardali et al 2010) and Saudi (Al-Ahmadi 2010) hospitals.

Safety concerns are not just about adverse events but also over-utilization, over-medicalization, and lack of use of evidence-based care. Childbirth is one area where these concerns have been investigated. In Lebanon, cesarean rates are very high (40.8% according to DeJong et al 2010). Kabakian-Khasholian et al (2007) suggest that the policy and practice environment, specifically health care organization and the dominance of the private sector, lack of physician accountability, and the limited role of midwives in the process, contribute to this situation. Carayol et al (2008) documented that having insurance and practice in large urban areas were correlates of more cesarean sections. Similarly, in Egypt non-medical factors, such as urban status, more education, and private hospital, led to more cesarean sections (Khawaja et al 2004).

As with the case for primary care, user satisfaction with hospital care is usually a correlate of quality of care. There is limited nationally representative data on this. In Jordan, there was general satisfaction with care among patients in MOH hospitals (Banks & Halasa 2005). In users of private hospitals in Yemen, only 28.6% reported good quality and satisfaction while 34.2% and 37.2%, felt quality was poor or acceptable (Anbori et al 2010). Considering how common it is to find reports of patient dissatisfaction with hospital care in various media outlets in many countries, quality and safety of, and satisfaction with, hospital care need continued examination.

Other Health Care Services
Emergency Medical Services (EMS)

These are essential to a properly functioning HCS, especially with the high rates of road traffic and other injuries (see Chapter 16). EMS are provided in most countries in major public hospitals through internists or family physicians as the specialty of emergency medicine is not well developed. The pre-hospital phase, usually delegated mainly to the Police and Civil Defense organizations except in Lebanon where it is provided by the Lebanese Red Cross or lately by private for-profit organizations, is neither well developed nor effective (Kronfol 2000). Lack of reimbursement for EMS has inhibited their development. A large proportion of emergency department (ED) visits in many countries are non-urgent (Abdallat et al 2000; Al-Hay et al 1997; Rehmani & Norain 2007). Many countries are considering lengthening the service hours of primary care centers or establishing walk-in clinics within ED staffed by trained family physicians, to serve non-urgent needs while triaging urgent cases to the ED. The Rafik Hariri University Hospital in Lebanon is remodeling its ED with this service in mind.

Long-term Care and Home Care

Long-term facilities have existed for a century in most countries but generate limited policy or research interest. Many facilities were originally sanatoria for treating tuberculosis, mental illnesses, and special needs but serve today as hospices or provide care for the dependent older population that family caregivers cannot support (Sinunu et al 2009). Hospice and palliative care services are only now beginning to emerge in the region and still have a long way to go (Abu-Saad Huijer et al 2009; Stjernswärd et al 2007). Long-term institutions are usually operated by voluntary, not-for-profit, charitable religious associations. They are supported by community donations and, commonly, by the ministries of health and social affairs, as in Lebanon. House calls by general practitioners have all but vanished in the region. Recently, such calls have been reported by family physicians and by organizations providing emergency care in Lebanon As the population ages, home care will become more important in the future.

Health Care Technology

There are limited data on technology, whose importance can be inferred from the sheer volume of existing and new health services, in terms of magnitude and appropriateness of and controls on investments, modes of management and maintenance, cost-effectiveness, and impact assessment. One important issue is ensuring availability of essential health technology especially for the poor. A second issue is controlling over-supply of high technology, especially in the private sector where it is exploited as signifying high quality care. With a dominant private sector, Lebanon has more CT scans and MRIs per population than many OECD countries and supply is continuing to increase (Figure 1 and Table 3). Lebanon is

Table 3. Growth of Medical Technology, Lebanon

	1997	2001	2006
Open heart surgery	12	19	22
Cardiac catheterization/Lab	19	30	31
CT scanners	54	70	90
MRI	12	28	28

Source: Kronfol (2006).

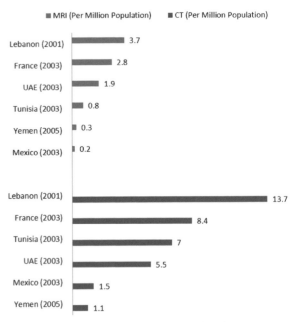

Figure 1. Comparison of technological availability between Lebanon and selected countries. Source: WHO EMRO (2006).

considering legislation such as the "certificate of need" and "carte sanitaire" to rationalize the acquisition of sophisticated technologies. Pharmaceuticals, as a special case of technology development and use, are discussed in Chapter 32.

Traditional and Alternative Care

The existence of traditional medicine and healing is well recognized (Azaizeh et al 2010), especially in traditional communities. In Saudi Arabia, 42% of people in a large representative sample in Riyadh reported consulting traditional healers including 24% in the past year (Al-Rowais et al 2010). Failure or dissatisfaction with medical care is a commonly reported reason for seeking traditional and alternative care. Graz (2005, 2010) carried out the only studies on effectiveness that we can find and reported that traditional healing was effective and can be complementary to Western medicine. Use of herbal medicine is common across the region, aided by use of mass media by profiting industries, and probably dominates the alternative care market. This area is not well regulated and the public health consequences, including of known side effects, are not well studied.

Barriers to Access and Utilization

In addition to inter-country inequalities in access and utilization (Table 2), there are important within-country inequalities not captured in national averages (see Chapter 5). These inequalities may increase with the current trends toward liberalization and introduction of cost-sharing and co-payment. We examine barriers at three levels.

Policy and Governance Barriers

Since the early 1980s, the move towards market economies and diminishing government budgets allocated to health as compared with growing population needs, have undermined efforts to increase access through building more hospitals and primary care facilities. Reduction in government health spending meant more care in the private sector and thus more cost to users. This is done through passive privatization, as public institutions increasingly lack the necessary medicines, functioning technology, and motivated human resources, and fail to provide quality care, encouraging users to shift to private providers. Double employment of providers in many countries contributes to this phenomenon.

Healthcare System-Related Barriers

A reasonable supply of primary care facilities and hospitals exists in most countries, except the poorest. But existing structures do not seem to promote good access and utilization. Quality-of-care-related barriers discussed under primary care are probably relevant to all services. In hospitals, quality improvement and accreditation has yet to be institutionalized due to factors such as lack of political commitment, limited partnerships and public oversight, and insufficient resources. In ambulatory care, there are many other barriers such as complex and bureaucratic procedures, long wait times, inadequate opening hours, lack of an appointment system and poor referral systems. This is compounded by language barriers, low general health literacy level, and lack of public understanding of primary care and the role of family physicians. The result is diversion of many users to the private sector and increased emergency and inpatient utilization. Some health care systems present disincentives to proper utilization. In Lebanon, the MOH covers hospitalization, but not outpatient care, for citizens not covered by one of the public or private insurers. This provides incentives for some users to access inpatient facilities even for services such as testing, which can be done on an outpatient basis.

Social and Structural Barriers

Socio-economic barriers are the most obvious. Inequalities in delivery are commonly patterned according to indicators of exclusion. In Egypt, the number of outpatient visits per capita per year varied according to residence and wealth (Abdullatif 2008): 4.48 in urban vs. 2.75 in rural areas and 5.11 for the higher vs. 2.32 in the lowest income quintiles. In Sudan, utilization of antenatal health care was approximately 5 times and application of TT-vaccination was 3.7 times higher in urban than rural women (Ibnouf et al 2007). As elsewhere, education and health literacy are related to utilization, for example of antenatal care (El-Sherbini et al 1993). These two attributes were positively correlated and may at least partially explain the urban/rural divide in utilization (Kishk 2002).

Financial barriers are among the most important, if not *the* most important, barriers. Current high levels of out-of-pocket (OOP) expenditures (see Chapter 29) and the withdrawal of the state from public provision might reduce access for many or make utilization a source of financial stress. High OOP expenditures are a problem not just for inpatient care; in Lebanon only 13% of household expenditures on health is for inpatient care and the rest goes to ambulatory care and medicines (Figure 2). Lack of strong social protection systems and high proportions of informal employment in many countries (this is discussed in Chapter 2) leave many workers and their families without health insurance. Even pre-paid schemes, e.g., insurance premiums, can present a cash flow problem for families since payments are often paid up front but data on the impact on access is limited.

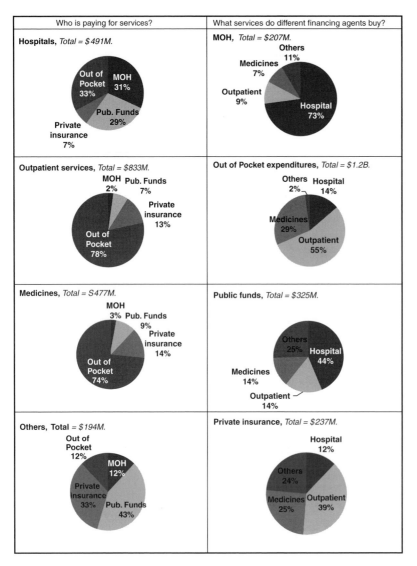

Figure 2. Services and sources of financing, Lebanon. Source: Lebanon National Health Accounts (1998); MOH/WHO/World Bank 2000; MOH-Lebanon 2011.

Gender differentials in utilization are complex. In Lebanon, women in all household income categories use more outpatient services (average 4.1 vs. 3.1 visits for women vs. men, respectively, per capita per year). There is limited data on patterns in more traditional settings. There is concern that in some settings less availability of financial resources for health care for women vs. men, less literacy, including health literacy, among women, lack of gender-sensitive health care, and lack of empowerment of women in health care decision making may undermine utilization (WHO EMRO 2007). There are gender differentials in seeking care, for example, for heart attacks in Lebanon (Nour-eddine et al 2008), or compliance and outcome of care,

for example, for tuberculosis in Syria (Bashour & Mamaree 2003). These are isolated reports and the generalizability of findings is not clear. Gender differentials in specific health care measures are explored in Chapter 7 and in chapters of Section 4.

The Arab world has many stateless and marginal groups. For example, Bedouins in Lebanon face financial barriers. Since many do not have citizenship, they do not qualify for MOH coverage making hospitalization inaccessible to most. Bedouin women complain of discrimination by service providers (CRPH 2008); although this did not prohibit women from seeking care, it compromised its quality. Palestinian refugees in OPT, Jordan, Lebanon, and Syria follow a separate health care system administered by a UN agency, UNRWA, and do not have access, except through self-pay, to the regular system of the host country. Nationality is also important in delivery for migrant workers. The Gulf countries have large expatriate populations and delivery is segregated by nationality; many migrant workers have limited access to health care. While expatriate facilities have good standards, the segregation by nationality compromises the rights-based foundation of health care. There are also utilization differentials by nationality. In Kuwait, 92% of nationals were registered at primary care centers compared with only 62% of Arabs and 39% of Asians. Nationality was the most important correlate of lack of registration and this correlated with excess use of emergency services (Al-Hay et al 1997). The health care access of the two or so million foreign domestic workers from Asia and Africa working in Arab countries commonly depends on the will of employers. Chapter 21 explores this in more details.

There are socio-cultural attributes that might undermine delivery. Some Arab countries, e.g., Sudan, Maghreb countries, and GCC, have racially mixed populations. We could not find studies of race and ethnicity differentials. However, there are public perceptions that such differentials exist. Religion and traditions play important roles in Arab countries and can affect delivery. Health practices, such as male and female circumcision, and beliefs, such as the role of fate and destiny, impact utilization. But institutional structures and interpretations and macro-level policies are perhaps more crucial. The area of regulation of abortion, which happens in 1 in 10 pregnancies in the region, is illustrative (Hessini 2007). Progressive interpretations of Islam have resulted in laws allowing for early abortion on request in two countries; six others permit abortion on health grounds and another three allow abortion in cases of rape or fetal impairment.

Delivery Reform Issues and Initiatives

Health sector reforms in the region in the past two decades have prioritized delivery. Reform projects, many funded externally as in Egypt (USAID and others), Syria (EU), and Lebanon and Yemen (World Bank), typically pronounce the goals of improving cost effectiveness, responsiveness, efficiency, quality, and equity. However, these reforms bring up a number of issues, the most contentious

of which concern the *role of the state*. There are proposals for reducing public sector provision, which now dominates delivery, in favor of a greater private sector role, and for refocusing state efforts on financing and regulation. Public sector advocates, however, maintain that the state is too weak to regulate a private sector where reports of regressive and informal payments and poor quality abound, and that a better strategy is to address the chronic problems of the public sector, such as salary scale, civil service regulation, poor governance, unaccountability, and corruption. Chapter 37 discusses the contentious issues around liberalization reforms.

In several countries, public provision contributes to market regulation for both pricing and quantity of services. This has been the rationale behind the recent development of public hospitals within the health sector reform program in Lebanon (Kronfol 2000). Public provision is essential to ensuring equity, particularly in rural, impoverished, and remote areas where the private sector does not identify niches for profit-making. Where the state makes a real effort in improving delivery, results are encouraging. In Lebanon, the number of patients treated in public hospitals has risen dramatically over the period 2007–2009 (Ammar 2009). Some countries, such as Jordan and Lebanon, have espoused the principle that services could be purchased from the private sector and that the government could contract for goods and services that it can buy and focus instead on the provision of goods that are not "buyable." In this process, the MOH secures services without the need to own physical assets.

Arab countries are grappling with how to *finance* delivery. Chapter 29 examines financing in more detail. Suffice it to say that private financing, especially through OOP expenditures, should be reduced. Private health insurance is not an efficient or equitable way of funding delivery. Lebanon has reduced OOP health expenditures from 60% in 1998 to 44% in 2005 through increasing efficiency, reducing spending on medicines, and increasing utilization of public facilities (WHO 2010). Whatever financing reforms are pursued, it is essential that this does not lead to the evolution of the public sector into a "poor service for the poor."

Decentralization as an instrument for improving delivery is another challenge. In 1986, WHO highlighted decentralization within the district health system approach for Health for All following the 1978 Alma Ata Conference. Decentralization was meant to improve access and community participation, improve quality, transparency, efficiency, and accountability, and thus greater equity, and promote democratization. Arab countries are at different stages and levels of decentralizing delivery. However, the outcomes are not clear. For example, Sudan has adopted decentralization since the 1990s, when it adopted the federal system, but this has been marred by problems such as lack of clear policies, regulations, and operating standards and lack of allocation of needed resources (World Bank 2003).

Improving management, especially in hospitals, is another delivery reform priority. Lebanon, Tunisia, Oman, and lately Syria, have introduced initiatives to increase the autonomy of public hospitals. Although legislative arrangements differ, the intent is to promote community involvement and decrease the centrality of decision making. There is a need to review the performance of autonomous hospitals and to ascertain whether autonomy experiments have improved access, quality of care, managerial practices, and cost containment. Syria is in the stage of evaluating its recent experience in hospital autonomy and developing national guidelines.

Quality assurance and improvement is high on most reform agendas. Egypt and Jordan initiated quality assurance programs in the 1990s with USAID assistance. Other countries, such as Lebanon and Oman, implemented performance reforms commonly patterned after the WHO EURO PATH model. Several countries have introduced systems for accrediting health facilities and guidelines for quality assurance and improvement. This is done by either international or national bodies. Accreditation can uncover important gaps: Lebanon initiated national accreditation for hospitals in 2000 but over 40% failed the third round in 2004 (Ammar et al 2007). In addition to hospitals, efforts are under way to implement accreditation in ambulatory and primary care centers and diagnostic facilities but there is limited data on impact. In Egypt, accreditation of NGO health centers improved user satisfaction and overall performance (Al-Tehewy et al 2009).

Priorities for Action

Improving delivery is connected with reforming other health system components and attributes such as governance, financing, and workforce. Based on this review, we can identify many opportunities for delivery-focused interventions. Considering regional experiences and literature on reforming delivery, we focus on a few actionable priorities.

Foremost is ensuring access especially for the poor and vulnerable groups. This should include services currently excluded from benefit packages such as dental and mental care, Improving access requires addressing multiple barriers such as increasing availability of decent services including in rural and remote areas, improving quality and addressing organizational barriers, but removing financial barriers is probably the most important intervention. Evidence from a few Arab countries and elsewhere supports this strategy especially in low-income countries. User fee exemption for malaria treatment in Sudan increased utilization, improved treatment-seeking behavior, and promoted early diagnosis (Abdu et al 2004). In 2008, North Sudan started providing free care for under-5 children and cesarean section. In Mauritania, exempting poor women from paying the US$21.60 premium for the MOH's Obstetric Risk Insurance increased utilization (Renaudin et al 2007). Hotchkiss et al (2005) showed the need to exempt poor and rural households from maternal health services in Morocco. Some have argued that exemption is not enough and abolishing user fees, as the government of South Sudan has done, is needed.

Expanding primary care networks, building on the work over the past three decades, to improve population coverage is important but ensuring that primary care is the basis for our health systems takes more than numbers (Abdullatif 2008). Countries have reaffirmed their commitment to this latter goal (Qatar Declaration 2008). This must be translated with redirecting health investments, reorganizing services towards integrated delivery, changing professional attitudes and public expectations towards preventive vs. curative services, and building a strong primary care workforce. Many countries, including Egypt and Gulf countries, are adopting the family practice model. The challenge is that well-trained family practitioners are in limited supply around the region and current training programs cannot meet the needs. Interim and innovative mechanisms relying on existing workforce, including nurse practitioners and midwifes, may prove useful.

Improved quality of care is another priority. Some reform efforts have already shown improvement as in Egypt (Gadallah et al 2010). In Lebanon, there is perception that hospital accreditation has contributed to improving quality of care but this needs to be demonstrated through patient outcome measures (El-Jardali et al 2008) especially that hospitals may focus their accreditation efforts on meeting standards to secure contracts rather than on sustaining improvements in quality of care (Ammar et al 2007; El-Jardali 2007). Engaging the community in health care decisions and clinical governance can improve accountability and hopefully quality but this has not yet been picked up by either consumer groups or policy makers. Such engagement would require a move away from centralized decision making and a greater degree of democratic practices. Workforce retraining and development strategies may help heighten the importance of quality but the impact on improving quality would be limited with the current incentive and regulatory structures around the region. These structures must change.

The public sector has dominated delivery around the region mainly in provision of care, not in the governance function. It is difficult to imagine meaningful reforms without stronger leadership. This means difficult decisions in a complacent public sector and regulating the private sector.

The ethical basis for leadership in delivery is the right of people to health care. The research community can uphold this right by identifying critical gaps in knowledge, supplying the evidence for change, and advocating for it.

Still, any major advancement in the development of health systems needs to be anchored on the "rights" of the population, irrespective of its economic status, geographical location, religion, ethnicity, or any other factor. Government must understand, support, and uphold health care as a right of the citizen. This will require stronger political commitment and a new vision of the state toward its population, a new social contract, and only then can real development in the health sector, as in all others, be achieved.

References

Abdallat AM, al-Smadi I, Abbadi MD (2000) Who uses the emergency room services? *Eastern Mediterranean Health Journal*, 6(5–6): 1126–1129

Abdel-Wahab MM, Nofal LM, Guirguis WW, Mahdy NH (2004) Statistical analysis of referral by general practitioner at health insurance organization clinics in Alexandria. *The Journal of the Egyptian Public Health Association*, 5(6): 332–361

Abdelwahid HA, Al-Shahrani SI, Elsaba MS, Elmorshedi WS (2010) Patterns of referral in the Family Medicine Department in Southeastern Saudi Arabia. *Saudi Medical Journal*, 30(8): 925–930

Abdu Z, Mohammed Z, Bashier I, Eriksson B (2004) The impact of user fee exemption on service utilization and treatment seeking behaviour: The case of malaria in Sudan. *The International Journal of Health Planning and Management*, 19(Suppl. 1): S95–S106

Abdullatif AA (2008) Aspiring to build health services and systems led by primary health care in the Eastern Mediterranean Region. *Eastern Mediterranean Health Journal*, 14(Suppl.): S23–S41

Abudahish A, Bella H (2010) Adherence of primary care physicians in Aseer region, Saudi Arabia to the National Protocol for the Management of Asthma. *Eastern Mediterranean Health Journal*, 16(2): 171–175

Abu-Saad Huijer H, Abboud S, Dimassi H (2009) Palliative care in Lebanon: Knowledge, attitudes and practices. *International Journal of Palliative Nursing*, 15(7): 346–353

Adam T, Evans DB (2006) Determinants of variation in the cost of inpatient stays versus outpatient visits in hospitals: A multi-country analysis. *Social Science and Medicine*, 63: 1700–1710

Al-Ahmadi HA (2010) Assessment of patient safety culture in Saudi Arabian hospitals. *Quality & Safety in Health Care*, 19(5): e17

Al-Ahmadi H, Roland M (2005) Quality of primary health care in Saudi Arabia: A comprehensive review. *International Journal for Quality in Health Care*, 17(4): 331–346

Al-Hay AA, Boresli M, Shaltout AA (1997) The utilization of a paediatric emergency room in a general hospital in Kuwait. *Annals of Tropical Paediatrics*, 17(4): 387–395

Al-Homrany MA, Khan MY, Al-Khaldi YM, Al-Gelban KS, Al-Amri HS (2008) Hypertension care at primary health care centers: A report from Abha, Saudi Arabia. *Saudi Journal of Kidney Diseases and Transplantation*, 19(6): 990–996

Al-Hussein FA (2008) Diabetes control in a primary care setting: A retrospective study of 651 patients. *Annals of Saudi Medicine*, 28(4): 267–271

Al-Qutob R, Mawahdeh S, Nawar L, Saidi S, Raed F (1998) *Assessing the quality of reproductive health services, The Policy Series in*

Reproductive Health, No.5. Cairo, Egypt: The Population Council

Al-Rowais N, Al-Faris E, Mohammad AG, Al-Rukban M, Abdulghani HM (2010) Traditional healers in Riyadh region: Reasons and health problems for seeking their advice: A household survey. *Journal of Alternative and Complementary Medicine*, 16(2): 199–204

Al-Saigul AM, Al-Alfi MA (2009) Audit of well-baby care in primary health care centers in Buraidah, Saudi Arabia. *Saudi Medical Journal*, 30(7): 956–960

Al-Sakkak MA, Al-Nowaiser NA, Al-Khashan H, et al (2008) Patient satisfaction with primary health care services in Riyadh. *Saudi Medical Journal*, 29(3): 432–436

Al-Tehewy M, Salem B, Habil I, El-Okda S (2009) Evaluation of accreditation program in non-governmental organizations' health units in Egypt: Short-term outcomes. *International Journal for Quality in Health Care*, 21(3): 183–189

Ammar W (2009) *Health beyond politics*. Beirut, Lebanon: WHO and Ministry of Public Health

Ammar W, Wakim R, Hajj I (2007) Accreditation of hospitals in Lebanon: A challenging experience. *Eastern Mediterranean Health Journal*, 13(1): 138–149

Anbori A, Ghani SN, Yadav H, Daher AM, Su TT (2010) Patient satisfaction and loyalty to the private hospitals in Sana'a, Yemen. *International Journal for Quality in Health Care*, 22(4): 310–315

Ayyad S, Al-Owaisheer A, Al-Banwan F, Al-Mejalli A, Shukkur M, Thalib L (2010) Evidence-based practice in the use of antibiotics for respiratory tract infections in primary health centers in Kuwait. *Medical Principles and Practice*, 19(5): 339–343

Azaizeh H, Saad B, Cooper E, Said O (2010) Traditional Arabic and

Islamic medicine, a re-emerging health aid. *Evidence-Based Complementary and Alternative Medicine*, 7(4): 419–424

Banks DA, Halasa Y (2005) *Patient satisfaction and pain management in Ministry of Health Hospitals in Jordan*. Bethesda, MD: The Partners for Health Reform plus Project, Abt Associates Inc

Barah F, Gonçalves V (2010) Antibiotic use and knowledge in the community in Kalamoon, Syrian Arab Republic: A cross-sectional study. *Eastern Mediterranean Health Journal*, 16(5): 516–521

Bashour H, Mamaree F (2003) Gender differences and tuberculosis in the Syrian Arab Republic: Patients' attitudes, compliance and outcomes. *Eastern Mediterranean Health Journal*, 9(4): 757–768

Bashrahil KA (2010) Indicators of rational drug use and health services in Hadramout, Yemen. *Eastern Mediterranean Health Journal*, 16(2): 151–155

Carayol M, Zein A, Ghosn N, Du Mazaubrun C, Breart G (2008) Determinants of caesarean section in Lebanon: Geographical differences. *Paediatric and Perinatal Epidemiology*, 22: 136–144

CRPH (Center for Research on Population and Health) (2008) *CRPH News, Issue No 8*. Beirut, Lebanon: Faculty of Health Sciences, American University of Beirut

DeJong J, Akik C, El Kak F, Osman H, El-Jardali F (2010) The safety and quality of childbirth in the context of health systems: Mapping maternal health provision in Lebanon. *Midwifery*, 26(5): 549–557

El-Jardali F (2007) Hospital accreditation in Lebanon: Its potential for quality improvement. *Lebanese Medical Journal*, 55(1): 39–45

El-Jardali F, Jamal D, Dimassi H, Ammar W, Tchaghchaghian V (2008) The impact of hospital

accreditation on quality of care: Perception of Lebanese nurses. *International Journal for Quality in Health Care*, 20(5): 363–371

El-Jardali F, Jaafar M, Dimassi H, Jamal D, Hamdan R (2010) The current state of patient safety culture in Lebanese hospitals: A study at baseline. *International Journal for Quality in Health Care*, 22(5): 386–395

El-Mhamdi S, Soltani MS, Haddad A, Letaief M, Ben Salem K (2010) Les nouveaux critères et la qualité des services de soins de santé dans le gouvernorat de Monastir (Tunisie). *Eastern Mediterranean Health Journal*, 16(1): 107–112

El-Sherbini AF, el-Torky MA, Ashmawy AA, Abdel-Hamid HS (1993) Assessment of knowledge, attitudes and practices of expectant mothers in relation to antenatal care in Assiut governorate. *Journal of the Egyptian Public Health Association*, 68(5–6): 539–565

Gadallah MA, Allam MF, Ahmed AM, El-Shabrawy EM (2010) Are patients and healthcare providers satisfied with health sector reform implemented in family health centres? *Quality & Safety in Health Care*, 19(6): e4

Ghobashi M, Khandekar R (2008) Satisfaction among expectant mothers with antenatal care services in the Musandam region of Oman. *Sultan Qaboos University Medical Journal*, 8(3): 325–332

Giacaman R, Khatib R, Shabaneh L, et al (2009) Health status and health services in the occupied Palestinian territory. *The Lancet*, 373: 837–849

Graz B (2005) Assessing traditional healers: An observational clinical study of classical Arabic medicine in Mauritania, with comparison of prognosis and outcome. *Tropical Doctor*, 35(4): 217–218

Graz B (2010) Prognostic ability of practitioners of traditional Arabic medicine: Comparison with Western methods through a relative patient progress scale. *Evidence-Based*

Complementary and Alternative Medicine, 7(4): 471–476

Halasa Y, Nassar H, Zaky H (2010) Benefit–incidence analysis of government spending on Ministry of Health outpatient services in Jordan. *Eastern Mediterranean Health Journal*, 16(5): 467–473

Hessini L (2007) Abortion and Islam: Policies and practice in the Middle East and North Africa. *Reproductive Health Matters*, 15(29): 75–84

Hong R, Montana L, Mishra V (2006) Family planning services quality as a determinant of use of IUD in Egypt. *BMC Health Services Research*, 6: 79

Hotchkiss DR, Krasovec K, El-Idrissi MD, Eckert E, Karim AM (2005) The role of user charges and structural attributes of quality on the use of maternal health services in Morocco. *The International Journal of Health Planning and Management*, 20(2): 113–135

Ibnouf AH, van den Borne HW, Maarse JA (2007) Utilization of antenatal care services by Sudanese women in their reproductive age. *Saudi Medical Journal*, 28(5): 737–743

Kabakian-Khasholian T, Kaddour A, DeJong J, Shayboub R, Nassar A (2007) The policy environment encouraging C-section in Lebanon. *Health Policy*, 83(1): 37–49

Khawaja M, Kabakian-Khasholian T, Jurdi R (2004) Determinants of caesarean section in Egypt: Evidence from the demographic and health survey. *Health Policy*, 69(3): 273–281

Kishk NA (2002) Knowledge, attitudes and practices of women towards antenatal care: Rural-urban comparison. *Journal of the Egyptian Public Health Association*, 77(5–6): 479–498

Kronfol N (2000) *Report of the Inter-Ministerial Commission for Health Reforms*. Beirut, Lebanon: Office of the Prime Minister (unpublished internal document)

Kronfol N (2004) *Review of the Primary Health Care Program*. Beirut, Lebanon: WHO and Ministry of Public Health (Unpublished internal document)

Kronfol N (2006) *Beyond Reconstruction: A national strategy for health system development in Lebanon, in preparation for the donors' meeting for the reconstruction and development of the health sector of Lebanon*. Beirut, 21 October 2006

Mahfouz AA, Al-Sharif AI, El-Gamal MN, Kisha AH (2004) Primary health care services utilization and satisfaction among the elderly in Asir region, Saudi Arabia. *Eastern Mediterranean Health Journal*, 10(3): 365–371

Mannan AA, Malik EM, Ali KM (2009) Antimalarial prescribing and dispensing practices in health centres of Khartoum state, 2003–04. *Eastern Mediterranean Health Journal*, 15(1): 122–128

Mawajdeh S, Khoury SA, Yoder R, Qtaishat M (2004) Reducing health care costs by rationalizing staffing in primary care settings. *Eastern Mediterranean Health Journal*, 10(3): 382–388

MOH (Ministry of Public Health)-Lebanon (2001) *National household expenditures and utilization survey*. Lebanon: MOH

Mrayyan MT, Shishani K, Al-Faouri I (2007) Rate, causes and reporting of medication errors in Jordan: Nurses' perspectives. *Journal of Nursing Management*, 15(6): 659–670

Nandakumar AK, Chawla M, Khan M (2000) Utilization of outpatient care in Egypt and its implications for the role of government in health care provision. *World Development*, 28(1): 187–196

Noureddine S, Arevian M, Adra M, Puzantian H (2008) Response to signs and symptoms of acute coronary syndrome: Differences between Lebanese men and women.

American Journal of Critical Care, 17(1): 26–35

Otoom S, Culligan K, Al-Assoomi B, Al-Ansari T (2010) Analysis of drug prescriptions in primary health care centres in Bahrain. *Eastern Mediterranean Health Journal*, 16(5): 511–515

Qatar Declaration (2008) *Health and wellbeing through health systems based on primary health care*. Signed by health ministers in the Eastern Mediterranean Region. Doha, Qatar

Qureshi NA, van der Molen HT, Schmidt HG, Al-Habeeb TA, Magzoub ME (2009) Criteria for a good referral system for psychiatric patients: The view from Saudi Arabia. *Eastern Mediterranean Health Journal*, 16(5): 1580–1595

Rehmani R, Norain A (2007) Trends in emergency department utilization in a hospital in the Eastern region of Saudi Arabia. *Saudi Medical Journal*, 28(2): 236–240

Renaudin P, Prual A, Vangeenderhuysen C, et al (2007) Ensuring financial access to emergency obstetric care: Three years of experience with obstetric risk insurance in Nouakchott, Mauritania. *International Journal of Gynaecology and Obstetrics*, 99(2): 183–190

Sadat-Ali M, Al-Shafei BA, Al-Turki RA, Ahmed SE, Al-Abbas SA, Al-Omran AS (2010) Medication administration errors in Eastern Saudi Arabia. *Saudi Medical Journal*, 31(11): 1257–1259

Saeed AA, Mohamed BA (2002) Patients' perspective on factors affecting utilization of primary health care centers in Riyadh, Saudi Arabia. *Saudi Medical Journal*, 23(10): 1237–1242

Siddiqi S, Kielmann A, Watts S, Sabri B (2008) Primary health care, health policies and planning: Lessons for the future. *Eastern Mediterranean Health Journal*, 14(Suppl.): S42–S56

Siddiqi S, Masud T, Sabri B (2006) Contracting but not without caution:

Experience with out-sourcing of health services in countries of the Eastern Mediterranean Region. *Bulletin of the World Health Organization*, 84: 867–875

Sinunu M, Yount KM, El Afify NA (2009) Informal and formal long-term care for frail older adults in Cairo, Egypt: Family caregiving decisions in a context of social change. *Journal of Cross-Cultural Gerontology*, 24(1): 63–76

Steele F, Curtis SL, Choe M (1999) The impact of family planning service provision on contraceptive-use dynamics in Morocco. *Studies in Family Planning*, 30(1): 28–42

Stjernswärd J, Ferris FD, Khleif SN, et al (2007) Jordan palliative care initiative: A WHO Demonstration Project. *Journal of Pain and Symptom Management*, 33(5): 628–633

Walston S, Al-Harbi Y, Al-Omar B (2008) The changing face of healthcare in Saudi Arabia. *Annals of Saudi Medicine*, 28(4): 243–250

World Bank (2003) *Sudan stabilization and reconstruction-Country economic memorandum.* Washington, DC: the World Bank

WHO (World Health Organization) (2000) *The World Health Report 2000. Health systems: Improving performance.* Geneva, Switzerland: World Health Organization

WHO (2007) *The performance of hospitals under changing socioeconomic conditions. A global study on hospital sector reform.* Geneva, Switzerland: WHO & International Hospital Federation

WHO (2008) The World Health Report 2008. *Primary health care: Now more than ever.* Geneva, Switzerland: WHO

WHO (2010) World Health Report 2010, *Health systems financing: The path to universal coverage.* Geneva, Switzerland: WHO

WHO EMRO (Regional Office for the Eastern Mediterranean)(2006) *The role of medical devices and equipment in contemporary health care systems and services, Technical discussions EM/RC53/Tech.Disc.2.* Cairo, Egypt: WHO EMRO

WHO EMRO (2007) *Cross-cutting gender issues in women's health in the Eastern Mediterranean Region.* Cairo, Egypt: WHO EMRO

WHO EMRO (2009a) *Progress report on strengthening primary health care based health systems, Document: EM/RC56/INF.DOC.4.* Cairo, Egypt: WHO EMRO

WHO EMRO (2009b) *National Health Facility Survey on the quality of outpatient primary child health, Care Services, IMCI Health Facility Survey.* Morocco October–December 2007, Cairo, Egypt: WHO EMRO

WHO EMRO (2009c) *Improving hospital performance in the Eastern Mediterranean Region, Technical Paper EM/RC56/5.* Cairo, Egypt: WHO EMRO

WHO EMRO (2009d) *Demographic, social and health indicators for countries of the Eastern Mediterranean.* Cairo, Egypt: WHO EMRO

Zaky H, Khattab HA, Galal D (2007) Assessing the quality of reproductive health services in Egypt via exit interviews. *Maternal and Child Health Journal*, 11: 301–306

Chapter

32

Access to Essential Medicines: Impediments and the Way Forward

Rana Khatib, Zafar Mirza, and Awad Mataria

This chapter focuses on essential medicines as one form of health technology. We view access to such medicines as a basic human right. While this right is enshrined in the constitution of several Arab countries (Perehudoff 2008), gross inequities persist due to challenges of availability and affordability (WHO-EMRO 2009a). Lack of access, irrational prescribing, non-adherence, and misuse are common. Arab governments spend 10%–40% of total health expenditures on pharmaceuticals and consumables, yet a large proportion of the population buys medicines out-of-pocket, indicating a lack of financial protection especially for the poor. In analyzing the regional situation, we use WHO's framework of accessibility (WHO 2004a), which addresses four components: the rational selection and use of medicines, affordable prices, sustainable financing, and reliable health and supply systems. This framework, part of WHO's medicines strategy (WHO 2004b) facilitates the understanding of the complexity of issues and the role of various stakeholders and highlights possible interventions at various levels. We bring examples and case studies and propose a way forward, taking into account the regional and country contexts.

The Medicines Situation

Accessibility includes physical accessibility (distance, quantity, and quality), financial accessibility (affordability), and appropriate utilization (Frost & Reich 2008). Even if medicines are available and affordable, access might be affected by inappropriate storage and usage (Sawalha 2010; Sweileh et al 2010). Seen through the lens of the WHO framework, accessibility remains a main challenge in the region with problems in all four components.

Rational Selection and Use of Medicines

Rational selection of medicines is based on developing and implementing a National Medicines Policy (NMP) for the pharmaceutical sector. "Essential medicines" is an important pillar of NMP as it enables health systems to use limited resources to select and procure the most needed medicines without compromising effectiveness, safety, or quality. Medicines on the Essential Medicine List (EML), mostly generic, should be available at all times in adequate amounts and in appropriate dosage forms. Provision of essential medicines is one of the eight components of a primary health care strategy. Countries develop their own national EML (NEML), in line with local disease patterns, priorities, and resources. The WHO (2009d) has published model EML for both adults and children.

Lists for over the counter (OTC) medicines, prescribed only medicines (POM), medications used for public health interventions (e.g., vaccines, and medications for prevention of CVD), and for herbal and traditional medicines are also necessary. These lists should be publicly available and widely distributed. Moreover, there is a need to ensure transparency in developing the NEML and prohibit additions of non-essential medicines through unethical promotion or conflict of interest of responsible parties.

Thirteen countries (Djibouti, Egypt, Jordan, Iraq, Lebanon, Morocco, Oman, Somalia, Occupied Palestinian Territory (OPT), Sudan, Syria, Tunisia, and Yemen) have NEMLs; however, these are irregularly updated. Most high-income countries do not have NEMLs; but with the introduction of health insurance schemes, lists of medicines eligible for reimbursement are being developed (Mirza 2008). While an NEML alone is not enough to ensure proper prescribing,

Public Health in the Arab World, ed. Samer Jabbour et al. Published by Cambridge University Press. © Samer Jabbour et al., 2012.

dispensing, and use, it can promote better prescribing practices as reported in the OPT (Younis et al 2009).

Essential medicines, however, are commonly limited to the public sector, which has low availability of these medicines due to limited public financing and erratic supply systems. In addition, NEML is not always institutionalized, nor regularly reviewed by national committees – if those exist – or strictly adhered to in procurement. Only a few countries provide legal protection to NEML. Medicine procurement is not always rational because it is dependent on the trade and tariff regime of the country, and is affected by insurance systems and reimbursement mechanisms.

Multiple sources of supply can undermine rational selection. This is especially challenging in chronic emergency situations as in Iraq, Lebanon, OPT, and Sudan. Governments, private, national and international NGOs, UN organizations, and donors overlap, each has its own mechanisms for procurement with varying adherence to WHO (1999) Guidelines for Drug Donations. Some countries lack systems to monitor donations. Often non-EML items enter a country as "donations," or undergo fast track registration, leading to availability of substandard and counterfeit medications, as well as corruption and waste.

Corruption affects the selection criteria (quantity, quality, and source). Good governance and political commitment can undermine corruption (Frost & Reich 2008; Transparency International 2006). WHO launched the Good Governance for Medicines program in 2004 and the International Products Anti-Counterfeiting Taskforce (IMPACT) in 2006–2007 to support countries in fighting corruption and counterfeit medicines. Governance assessment studies carried out in Jordan, Lebanon, Syria, and Morocco showed vulnerabilities in policy, structures, and procedures (individual countries, reports are available in WHO-EMRO 2009b) with lessons synthesized in a global report by Baghdadi-Sabeti & Serhan 2010).

After good selection, the rational use of medicines, i.e., "the therapeutically sound and cost-effective use of medicines by health professionals and consumers" (WHO 2004b), is crucial. Up to half of medicines may be incorrectly prescribed – too little or too much – or misused, resulting in wastes and health hazards. Surveys using WHO's Medicine Use Indicators (WHO 2003) reveal variability but also major gaps in use across the national income spectrum (Table 1).

Problems in this region are common as elsewhere (WHO 2009c): low use of generics; limited availability of medicines from the EML; poor availability of EML and Formulary; over-prescribing, especially of antibiotics and injections; misuse; polypharmacy; short consulting and dispensing times; inadequate counseling and labeling; and absence of educational materials and continuing professional development programs. Comparing results across countries should be done cautiously due to differences in time frame and sampling procedures. These indicators do not explain the processes leading to irrational practices, making it difficult to develop specific interventions to rationalize use (Irshaid et al 2004, Otoom & Sequeira 2006, Awad et al 2007, Khatib et al 2008, Cheraghali & Idries 2009, Otoom et al 2010, Ayyad et al 2010; Al-Tawfiq et al 2010).

Prescribing has received considerable attention in pharmaceutical research. Good prescription writing is scarce, affecting the type and amount of dispensed medications and creating medical errors and poor adherence to treatment (Awad et al 2007; Irshaid et al 2005; Al-Khaja et al 2006, 2007; Yousif et al 2006; Sawalha 2010). Studies from Bahrain, Jordan, OPT, Saudi Arabia, and Syria document wastage associated with inappropriate prescribing (Irshaid et al 2004; Khatib et al 2006; Otoom & Sequeira 2006; Al-Khaja et al 2008; Otoom et al 2002, Sweileh et al 2010). Poor prescribing is described in primary care and in hospitals. The area of antibiotic prescribing is especially problematic (Khatib et al 2006, Ayyad et al 2010; Al-Tawfiq et al 2010). Overuse and inappropriate use of antibiotics lead to alarming increases in microbial resistance, such as the use of broad spectrum and second-generation antibiotics for viral or self-limiting infections.

Physicians' specialty, place and quality of training, and availability of continuing education affect prescribing (Otoom & Sequeira 2006; Khatib 2003). Specialized physicians tend to prescribe expensive, branded second and third-line medications, while GPs tend to prescribe generic, cheaper, and first-line medications. However, GPs prescribe more antibiotics (Irshaid et al 2004; Awad et al 2007; Al-Khaja et al 2008) and engage in more polypharmacy (Otoom et al 2010).

Education of prescribers and pharmacists in rational use, both at undergraduate level and through continuing education programs, is the key to rationalizing use. There are severe shortcomings on both

Table 1. Medicine Use Indicators in Selected Arab Countries

Indicator	Country/year						
	OPT 2008	Jordan 2006	Syria 2006	Sudan 2009	KSA 2004	Bahrain 2010	Yemen 2010
Core drug use indicators							
Average number of drugs per encounter	1.9	2.8	2.5	2.3	2.0	3.3	2.8
Percentage of drugs prescribed by generic name	24	17.5	NA	48	33	10.2	39.2
Percentage of encounters with antibiotics prescribed	59	55	45	66		45.8	66.2
Percentage of encounters with an injection prescribed	16	15	25	27		9.2	46.0
Percentage of drugs prescribed from essential drugs list	NA	82.5	NA	74			81.2
Patient care indicators		2002					
Average consultation time (min)	4.6	4 ± 4		1.4			
Average dispensing time (seconds)	102	29 ± 24		33			
Percentage of drugs actually dispensed %				85			
Percentage of dugs adequately labeled %	60			50			
Patient's knowledge of correct dosage %		77		77			

Sources: OPT (Khatib et al 2008), Jordan (Otoom et al 2002, Otoom & Sequeira 2006), Sudan (Awad et al 2007, Cheraghali & idries 2009); KSA (Irshaid et al 2004), Bahrain (Otoom et al 2010), Yemen (Bashrahil 2010).

accounts (Otoom & Sequeira 2006; Al-Wazaify et al 2006; Kheir et al 2008). Even as pharmacy programs and number of graduates increase, rational use has not improved. This reflects the quality of education and the environment of practice. In some Gulf countries, new programs aim to increase the number of nationals working in pharmaceutical settings to fulfill national requirements only (Kheir et al 2008). Studies show that a skill mix could contain costs while providing better counseling and dispensing (WHO 1998). Investment in education, research, and development is still inadequate compared to other regions (WHO 2009c). Academic–private sector partnership is weak. The inability to link research findings to practice is compromising independent policy formulation efforts. Moreover, the produced research is mostly published in English, limiting access.

Promotional activities by pharmaceutical companies negatively impact rational use, as they are often unethical, contravening internationally recognized guidelines. Studies in Syria, Lebanon, and Jordan showed high vulnerability to corruption in promotional activities emphasizing lack of clear regulations and conflict of interest (WHO EMRO 2009b).

Self-medication, especially of antibiotics, is another major challenge. Studies commonly documenting poor knowledge of implications of self-medication, multiple doctoring, and attempt to save costs by direct purchasing, repeated use of unfinished stored medications, exchange of medicines between families and friends, and poor compliance (Abasaeed et al 2009; Awad et al 2007; Sallam et al 2009; Sawair et al 2009; Sawalha 2008). There is evidence of considerable wastage associated with use and storage patterns (Sawalha 2010). In many countries, consumers can easily obtain prescription medicines from pharmacies without a prescription. Prescribers often blame patients for their medicine demands as consumers may shop around for doctors to prescribe, especially where health care is provided by various sectors, as in Lebanon and OPT, or where the private sector is dominant, as in Lebanon and Jordan.

Inadequate information systems and lack of pharmaco-epidemiologic, -economic, and -vigilance

417

studies undermine policy development and decision making. Qualitative research into causes of irrational prescription and use of medicines is limited. There is limited availability of technology in clinics; when available, utilization is inadequate. Available databases in most countries tabulate number of visits (reflecting the workload) and number of medications prescribed (reflecting financial burden and procurement polices), without linking these two variables. Data collected on pharmaceuticals reflect gross consumption but not its rationality, thus limiting interventions to cost-containment rather than cost-effectiveness.

Efforts to improve rational use at various levels exist but remain isolated and unsustainable. Countries that have developed standard treatment guidelines rarely link these with selection of medicines, nor monitor adherence. Prescribers' education is seldom assessed in terms of changes in practice. Only Oman (Box 1) has attempted to tackle this problem in an institutionalized, comprehensive, and systematic way.

Affordable Prices

"Medicines Prices, Availability, and Affordability" surveys in 10 countries (Algeria, Jordan, Kuwait, Lebanon, Morocco, Sudan, Syria, Tunisia, United Arab Emirates (UAE), Yemen) as part of a global survey of more than 50 countries indicate both positive and negative aspects along with remarkable variations (Cameron et al 2008; WHO EMRO 2009a). Large differences exist between private and public sector prices within the same country (UAE, Syria, Yemen), and between neighboring countries (Syria, Lebanon). Some countries paid more for generics than others (Jordan, Sudan, and UAE). Some bought expensive brands (Morocco, UAE, Kuwait). Essential medicines were poorly available in the public sector in some countries (Yemen) and poorly affordable in the private sector in others (UAE, Yemen, Lebanon, Kuwait). Procurement policies and add-on prices in the supply chain – in the form of taxes and import regimes (custom duty, taxes, and mark-ups) – vary between countries, ranging between 30% and 70%.

Affordability is a major challenge in many countries. Catastrophic health expenditures on medicines could lead to impoverishment (Wagner et al 2011; Niëns et al 2010). A medicine is considered unaffordable if the cost of standard treatment for a specific condition is more than one day's wage of the lowest unskilled governmental worker. In the public sector

Box 1. A Comprehensive Approach to Promoting Rational Use of Medicines: Oman

A 1995 study of prescribing and dispensing practices showed that 60% of prescriptions contained antibiotics, and much polypharmacy. A team was formed under the Directorate General of Pharmaceutical Affairs & Drug Control to monitor rational drug use. In 2000, an independent Directorate on Rational Drug Use (DRDU) was established in the Ministry of Health (MoH) and given sustainable financing and required human resources.

Human Resource Management and Development: Qualified key personnel were recruited including a Director and a Pharmacist, with clinical pharmacology background; a Primary Care Physician, with research experience in RDU; an experienced Senior Clinical Pharmacist; a Senior Clinical Pharmacologist, with academic and industrial experience; and an Auditor. The pharmacy curriculum was changed to reflect drug management principles and concepts. In collaboration with the College of Medicine at Sultan Qaboos University and the teaching hospitals, the Directorate initiated a program on RDU for medical interns. Key pharmacists are routinely trained in field research and drug management. All new GPs in MoH are tested for knowledge of RUM.

Information: The Directorate continuously undertakes both quantitative and qualitative investigative and intervention research and these findings guide policy formulation. DRDU acts as a "Rapid Response Unit" when serious problems of irrational use of medicines are identified. A knowledge, attitude, and practices survey has been conducted throughout the Sultanate to establish the major problems associated with public use of health facilities. A regular newsletter dedicated to rational drug use principles and research is being published.

Training programs in RDU were initiated for all cadres resulting in reduction in antibiotic consumption and other key drugs. Oman National Formulary and Pharmacotherapy Charts 2003 & 2004 were published and new guidelines issued for NSAIDs and atypical anti-psychotics. Drugs and Therapeutics Committees and a national network on RDU were established involving universities, colleges, the private sector, and other major stakeholders. Some health regions are conducting their own Promoting Rational Drug Use workshops and a public education program was initiated. Apparent is a gradual increase in awareness and acceptance of the importance of the RDU role in the health care system in Oman.

Source: WHO 2005

in Sudan, treatment with metformin for type II diabetes is equivalent to 4.1 days' wage (WHO EMRO 2009b). In Jordan and Kuwait, the originator brand of amoxicillin for treating acute respiratory tract infection costs 2.4 and 2.3 days' wages, respectively (WHO EMRO 2009b). Studies do not usually include costs for consultation, diagnostics, transportation, and time lost from work, which further undermines affordability. Affordability is especially important in medicines for non-communicable diseases, given the increased prevalence (Van Mourik et al 2010), and for controlling infectious diseases of the poor and vulnerable, such as malaria, TB, and HIV, especially in low-income countries, as the coverage is still low despite the existing Global Fund mechanisms. The focus should not only be on the number of cases, but the cases seen in practice, which are drug resistant, mainly for malaria and TB – even in high-income countries.

Some countries have begun to implement recommendations made in pricing and affordability studies. Jordan removed selected markups on pharmaceuticals, which reduced market prices (WHO-HAI 2007). The civil society and the Pharmacists Association have advocated abolishing sales tax on medicines, but the Ministry of Finance opposed this idea because of the estimated annual revenue loss of around six million JD. Lebanon distributed its first formulary in 2007 and revised the pricing mechanism, thereby reducing prices in 2008 (Box 2). In OPT, generic procurement and prescribing has been enforced in the public and NGO sectors since 2000 (Khatib et al 2008); however, high poverty and unemployment and heavy dependency on donors financing undermine affordability (Mataria et al 2009). These examples show that it is insufficient to focus solely on pricing and total costs. Addressing accessibility within the geopolitical, socioeconomic, and environmental context of each country is necessary.

Understanding country-specific pricing components is crucial when addressing affordability. Lowering or removing add-ons could be difficult for low-income countries as those are a source of revenue. Nevertheless, it is still necessary for policy makers to improve affordability for vulnerable populations. Removing certain add-ons, such as the "wound tax" in Sudan, the "professional organization tax" in Lebanon, and "sales taxes" in most countries would definitely decrease prices. Syria has implemented a regressive mark-up to lower incentives

---

Box 2. Acting on Evidence and Improving Access to Medicines in Lebanon

A MOH survey in 2004 found that medicine availability in public sector facilities, where they are provided for free, was poor. Consumers paid high prices for both originator brands and generics in the private sector. The government responded quickly. Procurement prices of 2200 imported medicines were compared to prices in Saudi Arabia and Jordan. Large discrepancies led the government to reduce prices by 20%–30% for 1100 medicines, one-quarter of Lebanon's registered medicines. Concurrently, the government increased the budget for purchasing cancer, HIV, and other specialized medicines, from US$14 million to $55 million. In 2005, the government implemented regressive margins for importers, wholesalers, and pharmacies. This was expected to decrease patient prices for imported medicines by 3%–15%. By 2007, the MOH had reviewed the price of all medicines registered between 2000 and 2006. Across 1037 medicines, prices were lowered by an average of 14%. Currently, the prices of 833 medicines registered between 1996 and 2000 are being reviewed. By March 2008, 116 had been reviewed resulting in price reductions for 67 medicines. To improve transparency, in 2006 the MOH commenced publishing patient prices and pharmacy margins on its Web site and published the first edition of the *Lebanon National Drug Index*. Product information includes the active ingredient, dosage form and strength, ATC, MOH code and registration number, importer, manufacturer and country of origin, whether it is a generic or originator brand, the patient price, and whether the product is covered by the National Social Security Fund.

Source: WHO 2008

---

for selling high-priced products. Lower prices, however, could affect RUM by encouraging pharmacists to sell more to make up for the loss of unit profit. Selling promotes misuse while dispensing encourages rational use.

Developing rational pricing policies is difficult. Pricing committees are not always separate from registration committees, undermining transparency. In some countries, policy makers are inclined to decontrol the prices of medicines. Price determination mechanisms generally remain piecemeal and disjointed, and are not based on comparison with independent sources of information. The prices of branded medicines are high in Morocco, which uses the reference prices in European countries, rather than those in countries of the same economic development. In the case of generic medicines, the cost-plus formulas have not been fully utilized. Some countries have curtailed generic competition by limiting the number of generics, e.g., to five in Egypt.

International trade agreements impact medicine pricing. World Trade Organization agreements that concern intellectual property and patents affecting medicines; e.g., TRIPS, contribute to rising prices and diminish access to medicine, especially in low- and middle-income countries (LMICs). Patent owners can raise prices without ceilings or regulations. Knowledge of these agreements, use and flexibilities for protecting public health is still limited in the health community (Smith et al 2009). Some Arab countries have either already ratified (Morocco, Jordan, Bahrain) or in the process of developing bilateral Free Trade Agreements with the US, which invariably calls for more stringent patent protection than TRIPS, making it more difficult for countries to access patent-protected essential medicines except at producer-set prices. Some multinational companies have developed mechanisms to keep patented medicines in the market, rather than introduce generics. These strategies increase market prices, not only affecting international bidding, but also restrict countries to update their NEML with less expensive off-patent medications.

Large international pharmaceutical companies play an important role in pricing and thus impact access. Now in its second edition, the Access to Medicine Index (2010) indicates how such companies impact access. This should hopefully stimulate awareness about the need for a socially responsible role for companies in securing access. Some companies have made "out-license" and "transfer agreements" with many LMICs, mostly for essential medicines identified according to national burden of disease studies. Positive partnerships are being documented to improve access to essential medicines, mainly for tuberculosis, HIV/AIDS, and malaria. Arab countries could benefit from such partnerships, locally, regionally, and internationally, if they are based on reliable information on disease burden; and if local pharmaceutical companies have the needed infrastructure and human resources to handle the new lines of production, with robust quality assurance systems.

Local production is expanding. However, only a few countries can cover the large share of their needs; e.g., around 90% in Syria. Most markets are patent driven, especially in Lebanon, UAE, Bahrain, and Morocco, and are mostly still dependent on imports (Kuwait, Lebanon, and Bahrain import >90% of their needs). Hopefully, developing local industries (Box 3) should improve affordability and accessibility of essential medicines, while ensuring quality, and competitive pricing.

Box 3. The Pharmaceutical Industry in the Arab World

- Number of pharmaceutical companies varies between countries based on population size, level of investments, and the role of international companies in each country. Egypt has 74 companies, Syria 45, Morocco 35, Saudi Arabia 27, Jordan 18, Lebanon 9, UAE 8, Palestine 7, Algeria 5, Bahrain 4, and Kuwait 1.

- In some countries companies produce under license and generics with international companies steering the inputs, processes, and outputs of production. Egypt has (8), Jordan (2), Morocco (2), Palestine (1) and UAE (1). These experiences should be evaluated further before embarking further on this scheme.

- All products are generics with a focus on basic items. However, Syria and Egypt produce vaccines and Morocco produces insulin under license.

- Some regional companies are opening factories in other neighboring countries to override national regulations and restrictions on business in their countries.

- Local consolidation took place in Jordan and in OPT to increase market share and to improve competition possibilities. Exports of generics are strong in Jordan, Egypt, and Morocco but weak in OPT.

- Main challenges facing the local industries: National rules and regulations for trade and economy and pricing mechanisms; inadequate qualified human resources in the area of pharmaceutical production; weak Research and Development activities; small local markets and high costs; inability to meet the GMP and ISO requirements leading to weak international competition; uncertain quality and public mistrust for generics; political instability; and reliance on imports of active pharmaceutical ingredients and raw materials.

Sources: BMI 2008; WHO-HAI 2004–2007; Saleh 2003

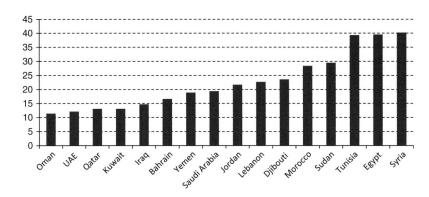

Figure 1. Total expenditure on pharmaceuticals as percentage of their Total Health Expenditure, 2009 (Iraq – 2006, Sudan – 2000). Source: WHO (2010).

Sustainable Financing

This is the responsibility of governments. Most Arab governments spend between 10% and 40% of their health budgets on pharmaceuticals and consumables (see Figure 1), the second largest category of health expenditure after salaries, but this is still low compared to industrialized countries and some high-income Gulf countries. With poverty, unemployment, and ongoing conflicts, sustainable financing is a daunting challenge for many governments and out-of-pocket expenditures on medicines remain extremely high. In Egypt and Morocco, up to 54% and 75% of medicines are purchased directly by households, respectively (WHO EMRO 2009a), although both countries, unlike many others, provide social protection in the form of health insurance to a sizeable portion of the population.

Cost sharing schemes, such as user charges to support health facilities, have been used to sustain financing. This has been shown to increase irrational prescribing and polypharmacy aimed at augmenting revenues (Uzochukwu et al 2002) and impact utilization by the most vulnerable groups (Witter 2007). Using the Revolving Drug Fund as a financing mechanism, medicine supplies are replenished, and paid for, with monies collected from medicine sales, as in Sudan (Ali 2009) (Box 4).

Global Funds can help finance the fight against major diseases such as HIV/AIDS, tuberculosis, and malaria and help secure medicines for those most in need. However, vertical programs can undermine existing health systems and exacerbate health inequity. External funds can be useful if countries integrate them within existing structures and needs. In conflict zones, donors focus on relief and emergency rather than long-term development, limiting effectiveness,

Box 4. The Revolving Drug Funds (RDF) in Sudan Over 20 years

By Ali GKM, PhD, Federal Pharmacy and Poisons Board, Secretary General, Khartoum-Sudan

Revolving Drug Funds (RDFs) is a leading method of community financing. A successful example is in the Ministry of Health, Khartoum State (KS)-Sudan. The KS-RDF started with the technical and financial support of Save the Children Fund-UK in 1989 to improve the quality of services by providing quality medicines to the KS population, especially in rural areas, at affordable prices. The project – the largest of its kind in the world – has remained viable for more than 20 years. It has achieved a high level of availability of essential medicines at affordable prices. The number of health facilities, where the RDF operated, grew from 13 in 1989, to 186 including 130 health centers, 24 hospitals, and 32 community pharmacies. Most households are now located less than 5 km from the nearest RDF facility.

The RDF users used to pay the actual cost of prescriptions plus operating costs (mark-up up to 38%) and still often considered the cost affordable. The average cost of a prescription at RDF health facilities is SDG4 (US$2), only 3% of the lowest monthly government salary. For 30% of the population covered by the health insurance, users only pay 25% of the prescription cost. However, 6% of patients at RDF health facilities still reported that they did not have enough money to purchase the prescribed medicines. In 2008, the contribution of users was reduced to only 50% of prescription cost and only 25% for children under 5. The monthly average number of users who filled prescriptions at the RDF facilities increased by 40% and the RDF revenue increased by 44%. Monthly subsidy from the KS government is needed to cover the increased utilization.

Factors leading to KS-RDF's success include: the substantial investments and phased implementation;

Box 4. (*cont.*)

leadership and RDF management style; commitment of the Federal and KS governments; availability of hard currency through Currency Swap Agreement; design and selection of RDF medicine list; regular revision of RDF medicines prices; constant availability of low cost medicines; community acceptance and confidence in the RDF; focus on common health problems faced by communities; and strength of KS economy. While the success of the KS-RDF model remains context specific, it could be successfully replicated in other settings.

duplicating efforts, and sometimes undermining previous progress. In these cases, dependence on external funding compromises sustainability and future self-sufficiency, such as the case of OPT (Mataria et al 2009). Coordination between donors and governments, based on good governance and transparency, is imperative and should lead to more effective, efficient, and equitable use of donor funding.

Reliable Health and Supply Systems

Supply systems must be timely and reliable. Managing the supply cycle is complex as many parties in the public, NGO, and private sectors are involved. The elements of the system include: selection and forecasting of essential medicines; efficient procurement from reliable suppliers; negotiating appropriate contracts for timely delivery at agreed sites; good transport system; and inventory management, storage, and warehousing. The Ministries of Health, through their national regulatory organizations, set norms and standards for ensuring and maintaining the quality of medicines during procurement, storage, and transportation. This is applicable in both the public and private sectors.

In most countries, the government procurement and supply department is linked with the central medicine store except in Tunisia where the supply agency can only procure medicines, which are mostly imported, and then supplies them to both the private and public sectors (Ratanawijitrasin & Wondenagegnehu 2002). Some countries have created autonomous supply agencies, such as the Central Medical Supply Agency in Sudan. Decentralization poses challenges to medicine supply. Devolution of power and functions weakens central involvement and can lose the economies of scale. Governance of autonomous supply

agencies is challenging because these can easily become too commercial in their outlook to the detriment of the public good. For these reasons, these agencies have to serve the public sector primarily, and government must have direct input to their policies and operations.

Other challenges in public sector supply agencies include outdated and opaque procurement systems; lack of computerized procurement and inventory management; collusion among suppliers and lack of international bidding; low salaries and morale of supply officials; sub-standard storage and transportation facilities; and lack of trained human resource with no opportunities for capacity building. Regular assessment of the structure and function of these organizations seldom happens in most countries. The tools in the transparency studies in Jordan, Lebanon, and Syria (WHO EMRO 2009b) can be used to affect policy change.

The private sector supply chain also requires improvement. Here, one finds an abundance of sub-standard or counterfeit medicines, inadequate storage and transport, lack of availability of pharmacists at different levels of the supply chain, and lack of adherence to regulations regarding prescription and over-the-counter medicines. All need to be addressed.

Pooled and joint procurement can be useful; however, not always feasible because of political and administrative incompatibility. This has worked successfully in the Gulf Cooperation Council (GCC) since 1976 (Khoja & Bawazir 2005) and in Jordan (Al-Abbadi et al 2009). In the GCC, the first tender was completed in 1978, included 32 items, and awarded to nine companies totaling US$1.1 million. In 2005 the total value of tenders for pharmaceuticals and other medical supplies reached US$580.9 million for 7617 items. In Jordan, savings were around 8.9% in 1 year due to central procurement. Unfortunately, a pooled procurement initiative between Maghreb countries had to be abandoned.

In high-income countries, the large lists of generic and branded medications burden the logistic chain to procure, store, and transport. In low-income countries, the logistic chain is often compromised because of lack of essential resources such as qualified staff, transport vehicles, and infrastructure for storage. The situation is worse in countries in conflict, where the supply system is interrupted and is overburdened by donations as has been the experience in Iraq, Lebanon, OPT, and Sudan (Box 5).

Box 5. Conflict and Medicine Supply: Gaza Strip (GS) – Occupied Palestinian Territory

The GS blockade imposed by Israel since 2007, compounded by an internal Palestinian rift and the suspension of international aid, resulted in a devastating impact on the 1.3 million inhabitants. The coordination for the entry of medical supplies was daunting, affecting medicine availability. According to WHO, "the central drug store (CDS) in GS reported that at the end of October 2008, 94 (22.6%) drug items out of the 473 EML were at zero level; as compared to 63 (15.0%) items at mid September." Moreover, "no pharmaceutical supplies have been delivered by the MoH CDS in Ramallah to the Gaza CDS since 1 Sep 2008, except for few shipments facilitated by WHO." On the eve of the carnage on Gaza on December 27, 2008, the MoH reported that 105 items of EML were at zero stock level at the CDS.

The Ministry of Health, with support from UN and international organizations, launched an "Operation Room" to coordinate logistics for donations and supplies. Focus was on emergency supplies to respond to war injuries. Guidelines and procedures for logistics were developed with the support of the UN pipeline. Inventory lists of needed medicines, and other supplies, was prepared, updated daily, and shared with donors. However, donations were not always in line with selected items, nor adequately labeled or packed, leading to delay and inefficiency in responding to needs. Provision of lists of donated drugs in brand names rather than generic names caused much delay in monitoring drug supplies. It was not possible to maintain good storage practices due to the huge amounts received and destroyed buildings. Despite all efforts, the logistic chain could not secure regular supply, mainly due to Israeli blockade.

Sources: OCHA report (17/11/2008); WHO: Health Situation Report (27/12/2008); WHO: Gaza Strip. Initial Health Needs Assessment (2/2009); MoH: Ministry of Health Emergency Operation Room reports (19/2/2009)

Lessons Learned and the Way Forward

The experiences reviewed herein provide valuable lessons for this and other regions. While access and affordability have improved in many countries, rates are not yet satisfactory and many challenges exist. Improving access using the accessibility framework is contingent on committed participation of all stakeholders along with regular monitoring to sustain successes. It is essential to link all components and processes leading to access. Just having, for example, an NMP or an EML, does not assure regular supply, e.g., OPT; local pharmaceutical production does not always guarantee better affordability, e.g., Egypt and Jordan; availability of financing may not lead to full coverage of the population, e.g., GCC countries. This calls for concerted efforts that consider the geopolitical situation and socio-economic conditions and resources in each country. The income levels and public spending on health, arrangements of social protection, levels of development of local production of medicines, and state of national regulatory and supply organizations are some of the key overarching factors which largely determine the medicine situation. The suggested opportunities for action are on two levels.

Strategies at the Country Level

The priorities for action depend on the national context. There are opportunities for improving access even within current levels of health system investments, including in poorer countries with low spending on health. Pharmaceutical reform does not happen in a vacuum. Such reform should be addressed within the comprehensive health system framework with a focus on inter-sectoral collaboration among all relevant stakeholders and engaging the community in affecting policy change. Little can be achieved without political commitment to equitable access. Such commitment will mobilize the needed resources and people.

Each Arab country has to identify its own priorities for action. Unavailability of medicines in the public sector and unaffordability in the private sector, especially for marginalized and vulnerable groups, are common problems in several countries and will become problematic for many more with the rising prevalence of non-communicable diseases. Often these challenges reflect not just weak financing but also irrational selection and use, inefficient procurement and supply systems, and a poor regulatory environment. Addressing these system constraints should be done before embarking on new interventions. For example, establishing an NEML and enforcing generic procurement and prescribing is necessary not only to contain costs, but also to ensure efficient supply, education, and incentives for health professionals, transforming public attitudes toward generics and toward reducing polypharmacy, and controlling the marketing propaganda of pharmaceutical companies. Increasing trust in and use of generics necessitates ensuring the quality of generics purchased or locally manufactured by establishing robust registration and quality assurance systems.

Improving rational use is a key strategy for all countries. Building capacity of personnel can be efficient in improving practices, albeit intense and costly as reported in Sudan and OPT (Awad et al 2007; Khatib et al 2007). The cost-effectiveness of various interventions in capacity building has not been explored (le Grand et al 1999). "Knowledge transfer" of improved practices is another potentially useful approach. In the OPT, use of injections at the public primary health care centers was prohibited. This experience was then transferred to NGO clinics, resulting in lowering national injection use (Khatib et al 2008).

The need for revising price components and comparing international prices, which are readily available, applies to all countries. This will allow countries more leverage in price negotiations as has been the case with Brazil, Jordan, and Lebanon (OECD 2008). The WHO EMRO initiative to establish a pricing database can be very useful. In some countries, e.g., Australia and Canada, pharmaco-economic analysis as a requirement for medicine registration has reduced prices of branded medicines (Birkett et al 2001; OECD 2008). Arab countries can benefit from this experience.

The role of the public and civil society is essential in influencing policy change. In Brazil and India, public outcry to access HIV/AIDS medicines, in the face of dire need, resulted in medications locally produced and available at reduced prices. Examples from the region include civil society lobbying against sales tax in Jordan (WHO-HAI 2009) and the campaigns for the "right to access to medicines" in Egypt and Jordan. Civil society mobilization is limited by low awareness of consumer rights, except perhaps in Lebanon, Egypt, and Morocco, and the lack of platforms for the public's input in national dialogues, when they exist, on pharmaceutical issues. This creates an opportunity for public health professionals and activists to mobilize public opinion, and create platforms for discussions and debate, with a focus on the "right to access" concept. A public "Access Monitoring System" can help assess progress toward improving access.

Equitable access to and rational use of essential medicines concern all health professionals and need to be mainstreamed in public health, medical, and pharmacy education in the region. Various professional associations must come together to work toward a common agenda that engages the wider public. Academic institutions can contribute the evidence needed to inform policy change, for example, with regard to the cost effectiveness of different treatment protocols, and advocate for such change.

Regional Action to Improve Access

There are many opportunities for collective action by Arab countries to improve the medicines situation. We focus on four such opportunities:

Cooperation and partnership among countries, many of which have large cash reserves or investors looking for opportunities, to strengthen local industries can improve quality production and affordability and lead to pharmaceutical security, even "sovereignty," for the region. When needed, partnerships with international pharmaceutical companies, including those in the South, can be built to support national and regional efforts and investments to build a regional industry.

If extended regionally or to other sub-regions, the GCC and national experiences in pooled procurement can improve access to essential medicines. This should be tried again, taking into consideration the lessons of why it did not work before as in Maghreb. Regional coordination in procurement can prove crucial with regard to low-income countries with relatively small populations such as Djibouti. Governments within these countries need more flexible but reliable procurement systems and policies to improve access to medicines.

The large variations in prices and affordability of medicines across the region indicate the need for coordinated effort in this area. Countries can share information and knowledge on pricing components and international price indices. In addition, cross-country surveys of prices and pricing components and mechanisms would lead to better understanding of the situation in any one country and hopefully inform interventions.

Quality assurance (QA) of medicines requires long experiences, institutionalization, and resources beyond the capacities of many countries. Regional cooperation to establish accredited QA centers can lower costs of QA and improve quality of generics produced locally or purchased internationally.

Assurance work can be aided by regional resource centers for research and interventions. There are existing capacities in various parts of the region that can form the core for resource centers. These are best hosted by academic institutions and should have the mandate to carry out cross-country essential research on access and support countries in work on access. Technical agencies, such as WHO, can provide support, but funding and logistic support can only be secured through commitments of countries in the region.

In conclusion, this chapter has attempted to provide a picture of the access to essential medicines situation in the region with the focus on "Right to Health," outlined the challenges that remain, and highlighted a few areas for future action. It is hoped that the future will bring more realization of this right.

Acknowledgments

Zafar Mizra and Awad Mataria are members of the World Health Organization. The author alone is responsible for the views expressed in this publication and they do not necessarily represent the decisions or policies of the World Health Organization.

References

Abasaeed A, Vlcek J, Abuelkhair M, Kubena A (2009) Self-medication with antibiotics by the community of Abu Dhabi Emirate, United Arab Emirates. *Journal of Infection in Developing Countries*, 3(7): 491–497

Access to Medicine Index (2010) Available from http://www. accesstomedicineindex.org [Accessed 15 December 2010]

Al-Abbadi I, Qawwas A, Jaafreh M, Abosamen T, Saket M (2009) One-year assessment of joint procurement of pharmaceuticals in the public health sector in Jordan. *Clinical Therapeutics*, 31(6): 1335–1344

Al-Khaja KA, Al-Ansari TM, Damanhori AH, Sequeira RP (2006) Rational use of antimicrobials in infants in primary care of Bahrain. *Journal of Tropical Pediatrics*, 52(6): 390–393

Al Khaja KA, Al Ansari TM, Damanhori AH, Sequeira RP (2007). Evaluation of drug utilization and prescribing errors in infants: A primary care prescription-based study. *Health Policy*, 81(2–3): 350–357

Al-Khaja K, Sequeira R, Damanhori A, Ismaeel A, Handu S (2008) Antimicrobial prescribing trends in primary care: Implications for health policy in Bahrain. *Pharmacoepidemiology and Drug Safety*, 17(4): 389–396

Ali GK (2009) How to establish a successful revolving drug fund: The experience of Khartoum state in the Sudan. *Bulletin of the World Health Organization*, 87(2): 139–142

Al-Tawfiq J, Stephens G, Memish Z (2010) Inappropriate antimicrobial use and potential solutions: A Middle Eastern perspective. *Expert Review of Anti-Infective Therapy*, 8(7): 765–774

Al-Wazaify M, Matowe L, Albsoul-Younes A, Al-Omran O (2006) Pharmacy education in Jordan, Saudi Arabia, and Kuwait. *American Journal of Pharmaceutical Education*, 70(1): 18

Awad AI, Ball D, Eltayeb I (2007) Improving rational drug use in Africa: The example of Sudan. *Eastern Mediterranean Health Journal*, 13(5): 1202–1211

Ayyad S, Al-Owaisheer A, Al-Banwan F, Al-Mejalli A, Shukkur M, Thalib L (2010) Evidence-based practice in the use of antibiotics for respiratory tract infections in primary health centers in Kuwait. *Medical Principles and Practice*, 19(5): 339–343

Baghdadi-Sabeti G, Serhan F (2010) *WHO Good Governance for Medicines programme: An innovative approach to prevent corruption in the pharmaceutical sector. Compilation of country case studies and best practices.* Geneva, Switzerland: WHO

Bashrahil KA (2010) Indicators of rational drug use and health services in Hadramout, Yemen. *Eastern Mediterranean Health Journal*, 16 (2): 151–155

Birkett DJ, Mitchell AS, McManus P (2001) A cost-effectiveness approach to drug subsidy and pricing in Australia. *Health Affairs (Millwood)*, 20(3): 104–114

BMI (Business Monitors International) (2008) *Pharmaceuticals and health care, report Q4 2008.* London: Business Monitors International LTD

Cameron A, Ewen M, Ross-Degnan D, Ball D, Laing R (2008) Medicine prices, availability, and affordability in 36 developing and middle-income countries: A secondary analysis. *The Lancet*, 373: 240–249

Cheraghali A, Idries A (2009) Availability, affordability, and prescribing pattern of medicines in Sudan. *Pharmacy World & Science*, 31: 209–215

Frost L, Reich M (2008) *Access: How do good health technologies get to poor people in poor countries.* Cambridge, MA: Harvard Center for Population and Development Studies

HAI (2009), *Civil Society Perspective: Repeal of sales tax on medicines to improve treatment affordability.* Available from http://www.haiweb. org/medicineprices/20072009/PDF

%20sales%20tax%20english.pdf [Accessed 15 December 2010]

Irshaid Y, Al-Homrany M, Hamdi AA, Adjepon-Yamoah K, Mahfouz AA (2004) A pharmacoepidemiological study of prescription pattern in outpatient clinics in Southwestern Saudi Arabia. *Saudi Medical Journal*, 25(12): 1864–1870

Irshaid Y, Al Homrany M, Hamdi AA, Adjepon-Yamoah K, Mahfouz AA (2005) Compliance with good practice in prescription writing at outpatient clinics in Saudi Arabia. *Eastern Mediterranean Health Journal*, 11(5–6): 922–928

Khatib R (2003) *A review of antibiotic use and policy development before and during the Palestinian uprising "Intifada" in Ramallah District-Palestine, RGU.* PhD Thesis. Aberdeen, UK

Khatib R, McCaig, D, Giacaman R (2006) Treatment of infection: A cross-sectional survey of antibiotic drug utilization in the Ramallah district of Palestine. *International Journal of Pharmacy Practice*, 14(3): 211–217

Khatib R, Mataria A, Daoud A, Abu-Rmeileh N (2007) *Implementing rational drug use practices at the primary care level: The importance of in-field intensive transformative supervision.* Report. Birzeit University, OPT: Institute of Community and Public Health,

Khatib R, Daoud A, Abu-Rmeileh N, Mataria A, McCaig D (2008) Medicine utilisation review in selected non-governmental organizations primary healthcare clinics in the West Bank in Palestine. *Pharmacoepidemiology and Drug Safety*, 17(11): 1123–1130

Kheir N, Zaidan M, Younes H, El Hajj M, Wilbur K, Jewesson P (2008) Pharmacy education and practices in 13 Middle Eastern countries. *American Journal of Pharmaceutical Education*, 72(6): 132

Khoja TA, Bawazir SA (2005) Group purchasing of pharmaceuticals and medical supplies by the Gulf

Cooperation Council states. *Eastern Mediterranean Health Journal*, 11 (1–2): 217–225

le Grand A, Hogerzeil HV, Haaijer-Ruskamp FM (1999) Intervention research in rational use of drugs: A review. *Health Policy and Planning*, 14(2): 89–102

Mataria A, Khatib R, Donaldson C, et al (2009) The health-care system: An assessment and reform agenda. *The Lancet*, 373(9670): 1207–1217

Mirza Z (2008) Thirty years of essential medicines in primary health care. *Eastern Mediterranean Health Journal*, 14(Special issue): s74–s81

Niëns LM, Cameron A, Van de Poel E, et al (2010) Quantifying the impoverishing effects of purchasing medicines: A cross-country comparison of the affordability of medicines in the developing world. *PLoS Med* 7(8): e1000333.

OECD (Organization for Economic Co-operation and Development) (2008) *Pharmaceutical pricing policies in a global market.* Health Policy Studies: OECD

Otoom S, Batieha A, Hadidi H, Hasan M, Al-Saudi K (2002) Evaluation of drug use in Jordan using WHO patient care and health facility indicators. *Eastern Mediterranean Health Journal*, 8(4–5): 544–549

Otoom S, Sequeira R (2006) Health care providers' perceptions of the problems and causes of irrational use of drugs in two Middle East countries. *International Journal of Clinical Practice*, 60(5): 565–570

Otoom S, Culligan K, Al-Assoomi B, Al-Ansari T (2010) Analysis of drug prescriptions in primary health care centres in Bahrain. *Eastern Mediterranean Health Journal*, 16 (5): 511–515

Perehudoff SK (2008) *Health, essential medicines, human rights & national constitutions.* Geneva, Switzerland and Amsterdam, the Netherlands: WHO

Ratanawijitrasin S, Wondemagegnehu E (2002) *Effective drug regulation:*

A multicountry study. Geneva, Switzerland: World Health Organization

Saleh AA (2003) *The Arab drug industry. Challenges and future potential.* Cairo, Egypt: WHO EMRO

Sallam S, Khallafallah N, Ibrahim N, Okasha A (2009) Pharmaco-epidemiological study of self-medication in adults attending pharmacies in Alexandria, Egypt. *Eastern Mediterranean Health Journal*, 15(3): 683–691

Sawair F, Baqain Z, Abu Karaky A, Abu Eid R (2009) Assessment of self-medication of antibiotics in a Jordanian population. *Medical Principles and Practice*, 18(1): 21–25

Sawalha A (2008) Self- medication with antibiotics: A study in Palestine. *The International Journal of Risk and Safety in Medicine*, 20(4): 213–222

Sawalha A (2010) Extent of storage and wastage of antibacterial agents in Palestinian Households. *Pharmacy, World & Science*, 32: 530–535

Smith RD, Correa C, Oh C (2009) Trade, TRIPS, and pharmaceuticals. *The Lancet*, 373: 684–691

Sweileh W, Sawalha A, Zyoud S, Al-Jabi S, Bani Shamseh F, Khalaf H (2010) Storage, utilization and cost of drug products in Palestinian households. *International Journal of Clinical Pharmacology and Therapeutics*, 48(1): 59–67

Transparency International (2006) *Global corruption report.* Ann Arbor, MI: Pluto

Uzochukwu BS, Onwujekwe OE, Akpala CO (2002) Effect of the Bamako-Initiative drug revolving fund on availability and rational use of essential drugs in primary health care facilities in south-east Nigeria. *Health Policy and Planning*, 17(4): 378–383

Van Mourik M, Cameron A, Ewen M, Laing R (2010) Availability, price and affordability of cardiovascular medicines: A comparison across 36 countries using WHO/HAI data.

BMC Cardiovascular Disorders, 10: 25

Wagner AK, Graves AJ, Reiss SK, Lecates R, Zhang F, Ross-Degnan D (2011) Access to care and medicines, burden of health care expenditures, and risk protection: Results from the World Health Survey. *Health Policy*, 100: 151–158

WHO (1998) *The role of pharmacist in self-care and self medication in the prevention and treatment of diseases.* Geneva, Switzerland: WHO

WHO 1999 *Guidelines for drug donations – Revised 1999.* Available from http://apps.who.int/ medicinedocs/en/d/Jwhozip52e [Accessed 15 December 2011]

WHO (2003) *How to investigate health facilities: Selected drug use indicators.* Geneva, Switzerland: WHO

WHO (2004a) *Equitable access to essential medicines: A framework for collective action.* Geneva, Switzerland: WHO

WHO (2004b) *WHO medicines strategy – Countries at the core – 2004–2007.* Geneva, Switzerland: WHO

WHO (2005) *Country situation analysis.* Geneva, Switzerland: WHO

WHO (2008) *Medicine pricing matters.* Report No 3: HAI Global-WHO

WHO (2009c) *Medicine use in primary care in developing and transitional countries. Fact book summarizing results from studies reported between 1990 and 2006.* Geneva, Switzerland: WHO

WHO (2009d) *Model lists of essential medicines.* Available from http:// www.who.int/medicines [Accessed 15 December 2010]

WHO (2010) *National health accounts, database, Geneva.* Available from http://www.who.int/nha/en/ [Accessed 15 December 2010]

WHO EMRO (Eastern Mediterranean Region office) (2009a) *Medicine prices, availability, affordability and price components, A synthesis report of medicine price surveys undertaken in selected countries of the WHO EMR.* Cairo, Egypt: WHO EMRO

WHO EMRO (2009b) *Measuring transparency to improve good governance in the public pharmaceutical sector in Lebanon/Jordan/Syria.* Cairo, Egypt: WHO EMRO

WHO-HAI (World Health Organization- Health Action International) (2004–2007) *Pricing surveys, 2004–2007.* WHO-HAI

WHO-HAI (2009) *Medicines prices, availability and affordability in Jordan.* Geneva: Switzerland: WHO–HAI

Witter S (2007) Achieving sustainability, quality and access: Lessons from the world's largest revolving drug fund in Khartoum. *Eastern Mediterranean Health Journal*, 13(6): 1476–1485

Younis M, Hamidi S, Forgione D, Hartmann M (2009) Rational use effects of implementing an essential medicines list in West Bank, Palestinian Territories. *Expert Review of Pharmaco-econmics and Outcomes Research*, 9(3): 243–250

Yousif E, Ahmed AM, Abdalla ME, Abdelgadir MA (2006) Deficiencies in medical prescriptions in a Sudanese hospital. *Eastern Mediterranean Health Journal*, 12(6): 915–918

Chapter

33

Graduate Education in Public Health: Toward a Multidisciplinary Model

Huda Zurayk, Rita Giacaman, and Ahmed Mandil

The public health workforce today includes many types of professionals whose work contributes to influencing population health, such as physicians and nurses caring for individual health, engineers managing water systems, social workers helping vulnerable families, and even journalists writing on health (Sim et al 2007; Tilson & Gebbie 2004). This chapter will focus on one key component of this workforce, the public health professional in the Arab world whose work is directly aimed at improving population health outcomes. This definition is consistent with contemporary usage elsewhere. In the United Kingdom, for example, public health "specialists" are those with "higher qualifications in public health and who occupy positions exclusively or substantially focused on population health" (Sim et al 2007 p. 936). In the United States, the public health professional is "a person educated in public health or related discipline who is employed to improve health through a population focus" (Gebbie et al 2003 p. 29).

Educating public health professionals has traditionally been undertaken by schools of medicine, nursing, or health sciences. However, beginning in the early twentieth century, this type of education began to be offered by newly established, independent public health schools. These aimed to provide a comprehensive, multidisciplinary education beyond the focused biomedical framework, and to teach the notion of health as produced in, and determined by, society. Focusing on independent public health schools, this chapter argues that this educational model is much needed in the Arab world and is complementary to public health training offered in medical and nursing schools. While we recognize the need to introduce the comprehensive public health approach into traditional community medicine and public health programs in schools of medicine and

nursing, elaborating on the conditions and needs of these programs would require a separate investigation. Nevertheless, for comparative purposes, we begin with a brief review of graduate public health education programs in the Arab world as they currently exist.

Graduate Public Health Education in the Arab World

Approach to Identifying Graduate Public Health Programs

To identify programs offering higher education in public health in the region, we first reviewed the Health Professions Education Directory produced by WHO's Eastern Mediterranean Regional Office (EMRO) (2009), which provides information on universities offering various types of health degrees throughout the region. We then searched the Web for a list of universities in each Arab country, and used the keywords "public health" and "country name" to identify universities offering public health programs. For all universities identified, we reviewed Web sites to locate higher education programs in public health. Our search included public health specializations in departments of public health or community medicine; graduate public health programs outside medical schools leading to the MPH, MSc, or DrPH degrees; and undergraduate programs in public health or in one of its specializations.

Because a Web search might miss universities without Web sites and those not included in the EMRO Directory, we also sought information directly from knowledgeable colleagues from countries in the region. We believe that our search has identified most programs in the region but recognize that a few may have been missed.

A Brief Review

In the Arab region, public health is most commonly taught in medical schools: at the undergraduate level to medical students and at the graduate level as a specialty track in departments of community medicine leading to master or doctoral degrees in community medicine and public health. We have identified 66 departments offering these programs. Independent academic schools (we use this term broadly to also include faculties or institutes) of public health, of which there are seven, offer the MPH program; some also offer MSc/Master and Doctoral degrees in public health disciplines, and/or undergraduate programs. Graduate public health education is also provided in non-medical and non-public health academic schools or departments such as administration or management. The ministries of health or national health authorities in several countries in the region have also set up graduate educational programs in public health, typically for their staff, in collaboration with international agencies and institutions.

All in all, 15 programs offer MPH degrees, 18 offer MSc/Master degrees, and one program offers a DrPH degree (See Table 1 and Appendix I). Twenty universities offer BSc degrees in public health or one of its specialties.

A few notes are worth making regarding our findings. Egypt has the most programs in graduate public health and thus educates the largest number of public health professionals. However, there is only one independent graduate public health program at the High Institute of Public Health (HIPH) of the University of Alexandria and it offers the only doctoral program in public health outside medical schools in the Arab world. On the other hand, there are five countries that do not have a medical specialization in community medicine and eight countries that do not have a graduate public health education program outside medical schools. The Occupied Palestinian Territory (OPT) is an exception with three universities – Birzeit, al-Najah, and al-Quds – offering the MPH degree, while there is no specialization in public health within the one medical school (al-Quds) in the country. The increasing number of undergraduate programs in public health perhaps reflects an emerging appreciation of country needs for intermediate levels of public health specialization. These undergraduate programs as well as programs in

medical schools deserve dedicated reviews which are beyond the scope of this chapter.

Implications for Public Health Education and Practice

With public health professionals in the Arab world still largely trained in medical schools, and the tendency of ministries of health and other health institutions to employ physicians or nurses to undertake public health functions (see Chapter 30), we can surmise that such professionals continue to operate mainly within a biomedical paradigm. While necessary, this paradigm represents only one approach to health and health improvement, and is not sufficient for addressing population health the way we understand it today. Classical biomedical frameworks adopt an interpretation of health that remains largely attached to a disease-specific perspective and the main concern is with disease risk factors and emphasizing medical, environmental, and individual behavioral lifestyle factors. The focus is on the delivery of a narrowly viewed set of health services as the main intervention (Hunter 2008).

Within such a focus, the social determinants of health are viewed through the lens of biomedicine. However, as other chapters in this volume show (see chapters in Section 2), key determinants of individual and population health lie in the circumstances in which people live, and those circumstances are affected by the social and economic environment, causing premature disease and suffering (CSDH 2008). Poverty, unemployment, bad housing and working conditions, poor social policies, unjust economic arrangements, and inequitable power relations are among the factors that need to be addressed by public health professionals of the twenty-first century.

The Comprehensive Public Health Approach: A Conceptual Framework

The comprehensive public health approach, developed within the context of independent public health schools and programs, began in the United States in the early twentieth century and has spread around the world in recent decades (Bhopal 1998; El Ansari et al 2003; Ijsselmuiden et al 2007; Gebbie et al 2003; Mokwena et al 2007; Foldspang 2008; Petrakova & Sadana 2007; Tangcharoensathien & Prakongsai 2007; Thorpe et al 2008). These schools

Table 1. Number of Universities Providing Specialization/Degree in Public Health and Related Fields in the Arab World

	Medical specialization: community medicine	Graduate degree			Under-graduate degree
		MPH	MSc/Master	DrPH	BSc
Algeria	9[e]	–	2	–	1
Bahrain	1	–	2	–	
Comoros	–	–	–	–	–
Djibouti	–	–	–	–	–
Egypt	18	1[a]	–	1[a]	–
Iraq	7	–	–	–	1
Jordan	2	2[b]	1	–	1
Kuwait	1	–	–	–	1
Lebanon	1	2[a]	3	–	3
Libya	2	–	–	–	–
Mauritania	–	–	–	–	–
Morocco	4	1[c]	1	–	–
Oman	1	–	1	–	2
Palestine	–	3[a]	1	–	–
Qatar	–	–	–	–	1
Saudi Arabia	4	1[a]	3	–	2
Somalia	1	–	–	–	–
Sudan	4	1[b]	–	–	4
Syria	1	2[b,c]	–	–	–
Tunisia	3	–	2	–	–
UAE	3	2[c,d]	2	–	3
Yemen	4	–	–	–	1
Total	**66**	**15**	**18**	**1**	**20**

[a] offered by an independent school or program.
[b] offered by the Faculty of Medicine.
[c] offered by the Ministry of Public Health.
[d] offered by the University.
[e] specialization in Epidemiology and Public Health.

have gradually evolved from a biomedical emphasis to incorporate disciplines that reflect the comprehensive nature of population health. They have expanded the pool of public health professionals beyond the physician, whose basic training is in caring for individuals, not populations (Gebbie et al 2003; Mokwena et al 2007). Students from diverse backgrounds, including physicians, study public health together and develop a multi-professional team approach to public health. Estimated by WHO at around 400 operating in the world today (Petrakova & Sadana 2007), these schools and programs produce researchers and academics through MSc and PhD/DrPH degree programs, and public health practitioners mainly through MPH degrees.

A leading advocate of the comprehensive approach has argued that placing public health education outside medical schools "liberated public health to pursue its proper goal" (Susser 1993). In other words, independent schools of public health have reinforced the multidisciplinary approach to public health, a perspective now adopted by WHO, among others. The comprehensive public health approach was advanced further by debates on the scope of public health, especially in the past couple of decades and in the UK (Berridge 2007; Goraya & Scrambler 1998; Gray et al 2006; Heller et al 2003). It is time then to turn to what this approach entails.

The comprehensive public health approach considers the multifaceted influences on health, and views health as a human right and societal goal (Goraya & Scrambler 1998). Public health is thus "values-laden" (Raphael & Bryant 2002), joining cross-disciplinary perspectives and action to achieve the goal of "health for all" (Wills & Woodhead 2004). This approach can be summarized in five key facets:

1. *The ecological model*: This model provides an overarching framework for analysis and action. The model considers health determinants at various levels, including individual biological and behavioral factors, social and family factors, living and working conditions, as well as other broader societal factors influencing health (Gebbie et al 2003). The emphasis is on linkages and relationships among these multiple determinants (Gebbie et al 2003), in contrast to a static view that considers each determinant separately as operating at the individual level. The model underscores "the role of structural forces, especially power, in the organization of societies and the effects these structures have on health determinants" (Raphael & Bryant 2002 p. 193). This critical perspective inserts social sciences strongly into public health, reinforcing it as a multidisciplinary field. It calls for adherence to the primary health care strategy which supports both health and social action.

2. *Multisectoral public health practice*: To improve population health, public health professionals must work with a plurality of agents and stakeholders in governmental, non governmental and private agencies, and across multiple sectors

(Gray et al 2006; Hunter, 2008; Goraya & Scrambler, 1998). Multi-sectoral practice requires the development of standards and domains of practice (Gray et al 2006; Thorpe et al 2008; Gebbie et al 2003) that are compatible with the conceptual framework for action of the new public health. It also requires graduate public health programs to produce a different kind of graduate, one grounded in the realities of public health practice linking what "they know" with what "they are able to do." (Gebbie et al 2003).

3. *People and communities at the center*: The approach brings the "public" back into public health by situating populations in their community context (Heller 2008; Raphael & Bryant 2002). Individuals and communities become active participants in the public health system, not passive recipients of services (Kohatsu et al 2004 p. 419). Communities have a right to health, but also a right to be fully engaged in research, intervention, and policy making aimed at improving their overall health.

4. *Different ways of knowing*: Research and the generation of evidence use a range of methods and approaches from disciplines as diverse as sociology, psychology, anthropology, economics, and political science, in addition to the traditional medical and public health disciplines (Baum 1995; Raphael & Bryant 2002). Recognizing that improvements are best achieved through "initiatives that are embedded in local knowledge and have local support" the new public health approach also values lay knowledge emanating from people's lived experiences (Baum 1995 p. 462). Community-based participatory research is particularly relevant because it incorporates community resources, and integrates research and intervention (Kohatsu et al 2004).

5. *Values*: The values of social justice and ethics are at the foundation of the approach (Raphael & Bryant 2002; Krieger 2003), and its central goal of addressing inequities in health. Whereas researching and understanding health inequities serve to advance awareness of the social justice framework, addressing these inequities requires also the "frank engagement with the politics of public health" (Krieger 2003 p. 1990). The new public health is thus committed to social and political action – through collaboration,

participation, and empowerment – to bring about change in the distribution of health and health resources of communities nationally and globally.

By addressing the root causes of ill health, the comprehensive public health approach is particularly relevant to the Arab world: where many countries lag in indicators of human development; are undergoing rapid demographic and epidemiological transitions; and where war, conflict, violence, and political instability can be part of daily life. Public health professionals can contribute to bring about health improvements in these complex environments. However, to become leaders and guardians of a comprehensive approach to public health, professionals must be trained in and adopt that approach.

To what extent does graduate public health education in independent schools and programs in our region produce this kind of public health professional? What are the issues and challenges involved in bringing these schools closer to the comprehensive public health approach?

Three Case Studies From the Arab World

We examine these questions through case studies of three independent schools of public health attached to leading universities in the region. The schools are the aforementioned HIPH at the University of Alexandria in Egypt founded in 1956, the Faculty of Health Sciences (FHS) at the American University of Beirut (AUB) in Lebanon founded in 1954; and the Institute of Community and Public Health (ICPH) founded in 1978 at Birzeit University in the OPT (Table 2).

Box 1. HIPH Case Study

Historical Background

The Egyptian Ministry of Health founded the High Institute of Public Health (HIPH) in Alexandria in 1956 to prepare needed cadres in public health disciplines. In 1963, the HIPH joined the University of Alexandria to become a leading academic institution in the Middle East and Africa for graduate public health education, research, and community service. Since its inception, the HIPH has had strong ties with many sectors of the Egyptian government and with regional and international agencies including WHO and FAO. Its graduates continue to serve the Arab region and beyond as public health professionals and decision makers.

HIPH: A Mission of Various Dimensions

The HIPH mission to prepare public health professionals to face the health and environment challenges of the twenty-first century is achieved through multidisciplinary programs, including: inter-disciplinary *education and training*; community-oriented *research; partnerships* with health care providers, academic institutions, health and environment-related sectors and agencies; and the *provision of consulting services* from the local to international level. The HIPH publishes its own scientific Journal, the *Bulletin of the HIPH*, which plays a pivotal role in achieving its mission.

The HIPH offers graduate degrees in public health at three levels, namely: *Diploma programs* as Diploma in Public Health (DPH); *Master's programs* as Master's in Public Health (MPH for physicians), and Master's in Public Health Sciences for others; and *Doctoral Programs* as Doctor in Public Health (DrPH for physicians) and Doctor in Public Health Sciences for others. Doctoral programs strengthen the research mission of HIPH, allowing the rigorous and in-depth analysis of problems of major public health significance in Egypt and the region.

Such programs (DPH, MPH, DrPH) are offered in nine different public health disciplines, including: epidemiology, biostatistics, family health, occupational health, microbiology, environmental health, nutrition, public health administration, and tropical health, as well as 23 sub-specializations of such disciplines.

MPH: A popular cross-cutting program

The HIPH Masters of Public includes the classical requirements of any MPH program worldwide, plus a thesis. Like other programs at the HIPH, the MPH has evolved over the past 50 years. Recent revisions were made to accommodate the newly introduced credit hour system and the possibility of taking electives in other disciplines. The MPH has been flexibly structured to suit the needs of part-time post-graduate students.

The following features characterize the HIPH-MPH program:

– *Local orientation and multidisciplinarity.* Lecture courses are given typically by instructors from different departments and with the participation of local health professionals. Community-based fieldwork training requires students from different majors to work together, and often with involvement of vulnerable populations, such as squatters or pregnant women in rural areas. Candidates also conduct fieldwork for theses on local community health priorities.

Box 1. (*cont.*)

– In a process that transformed the substance and approach of the MPH curriculum, the Institute recently defined 36 *Intended Learning Objectives* (ILOs) or competencies now required of program graduates. These specify the knowledge, attitudes, and professional skills expected.

– *Comprehensive training* on *research methodology* enables students to design their thesis projects following bioethical standards and using a mix of methods appropriate for answering environmental and health questions.

Students

During AY 2008–09, the student body included 529 Masters (19 non-Egyptians); 113 Doctoral (13 non-Egyptians), and 126 Diploma students. Most Egyptian students are supported by their public sector employers (such as the Ministry of Health, the health insurance organization, the armed forces); most non-Egyptians are supported by international organizations.

Admission criteria vary by specialization. For example, the specializations of epidemiology, microbiology and environmental health are restricted to health professionals (physicians, nurses, dentists, and veterinarians.) Only physicians may register for programs involving clinical applications as tropical health, family health, primary health care, and occupational medicine. Those with baccalaureate degrees in non-health fields may apply to the other HIPH programs including: biostatistics, food control, food analysis, health planning, hospital administration, health education, and environmental engineering.

Graduates: where are they working?

HIPH graduates work in the Arab region and Africa in technical, professional, applied, administrative and consulting capacities. They work in the public sector, the private sector and in non-governmental and international organizations such as UN (WHO, UNICEF), NAMRU-3, and the Population Council. HIPH is currently developing a database to facilitate follow-up with Institute alumni.

Faculty

The great majority of the 118 faculty members began their appointment at the HIPH as fresh graduates of the University of Alexandria, entering the academic system as instructors and progressing to higher ranks through their careers. Some specializations hire only physicians (epidemiology, family health, tropical health, primary health care,

microbiology), while other departments or units recruit biologists, engineers, and professionals with training in social and behavioral sciences.

Faculty are expected to balance their time between teaching, research, service, and consulting. Community service and related research are usually conducted in collaboration with national agencies responsible for health, development, and the environment. Recent examples include salt iodization (to prevent goiter), oral rehydration solution (to manage diarrhea), and new vaccine trials.

Evaluation and Planning

Programs are evaluated internally and externally. Internally, this includes course evaluation of students (by instructors, according to specific methods), faculty evaluation by students (implemented for many courses), and peer evaluation (planned for). Externally, external examiners sit on theses defences and some comprehensive and oral examinations.

To pave the way for the academic accreditation of its programs, HIPH is applying quality control through the monitoring and evaluation of all HIPH programs.

Box 2. FHS Case Study

Historical Background

Public health activities at the American University of Beirut (AUB) began within the School of Medicine shortly following its opening in 1867. An independent School of Public Health was established in 1954, and continued to provide public health education to medical students while developing its own undergraduate and graduate programs, with the MPH program initiated in 1971. In 1978 the name of the School was changed to Faculty of Health Sciences (FHS) for possible wider inclusion of health science disciplines. FHS has chosen to remain focused on public health, driven by the commitment of its faculty to advancement of the public's health in Lebanon and the region. FHS was actively engaged in addressing public health issues in Lebanon during the civil war, evolving greater emphasis on public health practice together with research and teaching. Following emergence from the war and its aftermath, an intensive effort was made in the past decade to review and improve the graduate program under new leadership.

The Graduate Public Health Program

The core public health program of FHS is the Graduate Public Health Program (GPHP) which consists of the MPH program and three MSc programs

Box 2. (*cont.*)

(in Environmental Sciences major Environmental Health, in Epidemiology, and in Population Health).

Mission and values: The Graduate Public Health Program at FHS provides advanced training in public health to prepare professionals, both practitioners and academicians, who can competently assess, research, and respond to health needs and current public health issues in Lebanon and the region. The Program promotes multidisciplinary and community-based research as well as community service as means to improve instruction, advance knowledge, and address public health issues and needs of relevance to the population served. Teaching, research, and service are guided by core values. These values derive from our context as a school of public health in a developing world setting and from basic principles of professional conduct and human rights.

The GPHP received accreditation from the US Council for Education on Public Health (CEPH) in 2006. It is the first program to be accredited by CEPH outside the North American Continent.

The Master of Public Health Program (MPH)

The MPH is the main program offering of the GPHP. Major revisions to the program in the past 10 years have aimed at establishing excellence internationally with relevance to the region. The program adheres to the multidisciplinary ecological framework for health, incorporating the multiple determinants of health.

The program offers three concentrations including Epidemiology and Biostatistics, Health Promotion and Community Health, and Health Management and Policy, as well as a general program with no concentration. The MPH normally takes 18 months of full-time study, but can be completed in 12 months of full-time intensive study for students with experience. In addition to core, concentration, and elective courses, as shown in Table 2, MPH students undertake a research project and a practicum experience. They also attend during their last semester a culminating experience seminar, involving case study discussions and theoretical wrapping up, which all graduating students must take irrespective of concentration with faculty representing all departments.

The program is led by a coordinator who works closely with departments. MPH courses are located in departments and they all, to varying degrees, emphasize the multidisciplinary approach. An attempt to integrate courses across departments was not successful, however, pointing to difficulties in breaking boundaries between disciplines. Courses reinforce one

another so that knowledge is integrated as students move through the program.

Following accreditation activities at AUB and FHS, the MPH program adopted a competency framework defining learning outcomes and competencies for its core program and concentrations with reference to guidelines from CEPH and the Association of Schools of Public Health in the United States while emphasizing local relevance. Important cross-cutting competencies relate to critical thinking and to ethics. Assessment tools are being developed to evaluate the extent to which competencies and learning outcomes are achieved by students.

The program is moving towards integration of teaching with research and practice, as each of these functions is strengthened. Through the establishment of the Center for Research on Population and Health in 2002, faculty were encouraged to work in multidisciplinary research teams forming programs of research on key issues influencing health research in Lebanon and the region such as urban health, tobacco practice and control, healthy child-bearing, youth mental health among others. The civil war and the many crises that followed encouraged faculty to participate in community-based as well as institution based practice activities in partnership with a diverse body of stakeholders in active relief and development projects. Through these activities, students are exposed to research and practice experiences in partnership with communities and major stakeholders. An appreciation for social justice issues and for ethics are instilled in students through these experiences, preparing them for potential to act as agents of change.

Students

FHS admits about 45 graduate students per year primarily from Lebanon. Through securing funding to offer scholarships to qualified regional students, in recognition of the great regional need for preparing public health professionals, FHS has recently attracted 4 to 5 students annually from the region (36 over the past 8 years from 12 different countries). Diversity of students is also sought by the University of previous degrees and majors including backgrounds in health, the sciences, business and engineering, and the social sciences. Many study on part time basis, working at the same time in the public health workforce.

Faculty

Currently FHS faculty are 31 in number, with 26 at professorial ranks. FHS faculty have diverse public health specializations which are mostly earned in the US, Europe, and Australia. A special effort was

Box 2. (*cont.*)

made in the past decade to recruit social science faculty, yielding several social scientists who have greatly contributed to enrich the multidisciplinary perspective, and have expanded the range of research methods strengthening qualitative approaches to public health evidence. There are three MDs currently among full-time faculty but practicing physicians on a part time basis and from the Faculty of Medicine contribute to teaching in most departments.

Given that AUB promotion guidelines emphasize research and teaching and impose an up or out policy with strict time limits, faculty find little time for practice activities despite their high level of commitment. Efforts have started at FHS to revise guidelines for faculty reward and advancement to include faculty contributions to public health practice.

Evaluation and Planning

A system for evaluation and planning has been recently developed. Indicators have been established that enable assessment of process and outcome measures related to the MPH, allowing an annual systematic evaluation. A more qualitative process of soliciting input from students, alumni, and stakeholders, as well as periodic surveys, have contributed significantly to the continuous improvement of the MPH program.

Since its initiation, FHS graduated over 900 from its Graduate Public Health Program. A recent review of alumni of the graduate program (2005) stretching back 30 years revealed a substantial number (111) currently occupying key positions in the Lebanese health and related sectors, with 14 percent of them in the public sector, and the great majority in the private sector, non-governmental organizations, and international agencies. Given the dominance of the private sector in Lebanon, these graduates are no doubt influencing public health in Lebanon, and creating a presence for the public health professional. They form a resource that must be better utilized in FHS activities and networking, to include regional graduates, expanding outreach and outcomes.

Future Directions

Current initiatives are aimed at studying the feasibility of adding three concentrations to the MPH program in health policy, population and reproductive health, and occupational health. An initiative to examine the feasibility of establishing an executive MPH is also ongoing. Development of doctoral degrees is considered important and an initiative in that direction is expected to begin soon.

Box 3. ICPH Case Study

Mission and Goals

ICPH was established informally as Palestinian social action was emerging at the end of the 1970s, then as a university unit, a department, and an institute in 1998. Its mission and goals were primarily defined by the extra-ordinary conditions of Israeli military occupation of the West Bank and Gaza Strip. In line with Birzeit University's three pillared mission entailing teaching, research, and community development, ICPH's main aim is to assist in improving health conditions and services in the Occupied Palestinian Territory.

Programs

Programs run in cycles, beginning with research/needs assessment to inform action; teaching and training; field experimentation and implementation, monitoring, advocacy, and evaluation, which guide new programming. Active involvement with communities ensures that the link between theory and practice is maintained. ICPH's programs are almost entirely supported by fund raising from international bodies.

MPH

ICPH began to offer post-graduate degrees in 1996 following the signing of the Declaration of Principles on Interim Self-Government Arrangements in 1993 (the Oslo Accords). With the handing over of selected spheres to the Palestinian Authority, it became necessary to assist in capacity building so that Palestinians could build a health system with capable human resources as a foundation. Two degrees are offered: the Diploma in Primary Health Care, and the Master in Public Health (MPH). In 2008, a concentration in Health Economics and Management was launched. Concentrations vary depending on health system needs, and the availability of faculty with the relevant specialties. This accommodates the conditions in the country where the system is closed to the outside world.

ICPH courses combine essential public health competencies with the concepts, skills, and practices needed in the local context. Other than the required core and elective courses (see Table 2), students must either submit a thesis, or complete two graduating seminars, engaging students in more elaborate field research than what they experienced up till then, and applying in practice the combined knowledge gained in courses. The multidisciplinary approach is integrated as much as possible into all courses and is reflected in syllabi and how courses are taught. When necessary, courses are taught by a team of specialists from within and outside the

Box 3. (*cont.*)

University, and coordinated by an ICPH faculty. However, integrating some courses, notably methodologies, has proven to be a challenge.

Students

Students have different backgrounds, including medicine and any allied health profession, statistics, engineering, economics, education, and sociology among others. The majority are employed part time in Palestinian ministries and other health institutions. Part-time enrollment while working is sometimes challenging to students and has resulted with variable rates of attrition. However, this is the best way to build capacity of staff who are unable to leave their jobs because they must earn family income, or because the health system cannot afford to release them for full-time studies because of the scarcity of personnel. The advantage of this arrangement is that ICPH can follow up students in their places of work. Regular field visits to students in their workplace are conducted to monitor and evaluate, assist in the application of knowledge in practice, highlight structural constraints to the implementation of what has been taught in class, and work with students to solve some of these problems. With about 230 graduates to date, ICPH also follows up alumni in their workplaces to evaluate the longer term effects of teaching on performance. Overall, about one third are promoted to key positions during or after receiving the MPH, another third leave their original places of work for better jobs, and the last third remain in the job held before joining the MPH program.

Teaching

The involvement of faculty in research and model building at the community levels has an important influence on the teaching process. Information from the field is regularly fed back to the classroom for discussions, and keeps teaching grounded in reality. Ongoing research and visits to students in their workplace are used to assess overall system progress, and alerts faculty to the changes taking place in the system – which can be rapid – requiring adjustment or revision of curricula. Course content is therefore modified regularly in line with systemic changes.

History and Context

The most striking differences among the three schools concern the national context in which they have developed and worked and their relationship to the state. HIPH was founded by the Egyptian Ministry of

Table 2. Case Studies: Curriculum of MPH Programs

Core area courses and credits	FHS	ICPH	HIPH
Epidemiology	3	2	
Biostatistics	3	3	
Epidemiology & biostatistics			3.5
Social and behavioral foundation	3		
Social epidemiology		2*	
Behavioral sciences for public health			1
Introduction to environmental health	2		
Environmental health		2*	
Man and the environment			4.5
Health care systems	3		2
Primary health care		3	
Health planning and management		3	
Communication skills	2		
Communication and training skills		2	
Research design	3		
Research methodology			3*
Health surveys			2
Total core area credits	**19**	**20**	**16**
Number of concentrations (other than general)	3	1	9
Concentration courses	12–13	10	13
Research project	3		
Practicum	2		
Culminating experience	1		
Graduating seminars or thesis		6	
Field survey			2
Special studies			2
Thesis			6
Total concentration credits	**18–19**	**16**	**23**
Total elective credits	**4–5**	**10**	**6**
Grand Total	**42**	**36**	**45**

* Required course but not considered core.

Health and has maintained strong ties to the Ministry and other organs of the Egyptian government after it joined the University of Alexandria, by producing public health professionals closely linked to the classical biomedical framework primarily for Egypt. These professionals have also responded to the unfulfilled needs for public health in the Arab world and those of regional and international organizations working in public health and development. Like all Lebanese institutions, FHS was profoundly affected by the civil war (1975–1990) and the period of reconstruction that followed, where public health by necessity required engagement with a multiplicity of stakeholders beyond the weakened state sector. Responding to the needs of war propelled the FHS graduate program toward an early recognition of the non-biomedical factors affecting health. ICPH was established informally as Palestinian social action was emerging at the end of the 1970s, then as a university unit, a department, and an institute in 1998. Social action for survival and resistance under the Israel occupation in the context of absent state structures have shaped the development of ICPH, cementing its practical understanding of the social and political determinants of health. ICPH has had to confront the war-like conditions under occupation, with continuing military incursions and restricted movement from checkpoints and closures (Giacaman & Halilel 2003).

Graduate Degree Programs

With 123 regular full-time faculty members, and an additional 66 faculty members above 60 years of age, HIPH offers graduate degrees in nine public health disciplines at three levels, namely: Diploma programs; Master's programs (MPH for physicians and a Master's in Public Health Sciences for others); and Doctoral Programs (DrPH for physicians and Doctor in Public Health Sciences for others). During AY 2009–10, these programs enrolled 842 students (139, 598, and 105, respectively). Most Egyptian students are supported by their public sector employers, such as the Ministry of Health, the health insurance organization, the armed forces; most non-Egyptian students (who constitute approximately 4%) are supported by international organizations.

FHS full-time faculty amount to 34 in AY 2009–10. In addition to the MPH program, initiated in 1971,

MSc programs in three different disciplines are offered. These programs form the Graduate Public Health Program (GPHP), which has been admitting between 40 and 70 students per year over the past decade, mostly in the MPH program. Enrollment in the GPHP in AY 2009–10 amounted to 155 students, 131 in the MPH program and 24 in the MSc programs. The GPHP has gone through several cycles of revisions and rigorous self study leading to accreditation from the US-based Council for Education on Public Health in 2006 and was the first such accredited program outside the North American continent. The GPHP emphasizes student-centered learning outcomes and competencies and the integration of instruction, research and practice.

ICPH began to offer post-graduate degrees in 1996 following the signing of the Declaration of Principles on Interim Self-Government Arrangements in 1993 (the Oslo Accords). With the handing over of selected spheres to the Palestinian Authority, it became necessary to assist in capacity building so that Palestinians could build a health system with capable human resources as a foundation. In addition to the MPH program, a Diploma in Primary Health Care is also offered. Enrollment in the MPH and Diploma programs amounted to 39 students, supported by 8 faculty members for AY 2009–10. A unique feature of ICPH is that because of the extra-ordinary circumstances in OPT, program concentrations vary depending on health system needs, and the availability of faculty with the relevant specialties.

Progress Toward Comprehensive Public Health

Multidisciplinarity and the Ecological Model

While each of the three institutions has made progress toward incorporating multidisciplinary perspectives in teaching, research, and practice, meaningful change at both theoretical and methodological levels requires often difficult collaborative work among scientists with different perspectives. Multidisciplinarity is part of the HIPH mission statement, and emphasizes interdepartmental collaboration in training and research. Yet, multidisciplinarity at HIPH differs from that at FHS and ICPH; it means work across the biomedical and hard sciences, and less about incorporating the theoretical perspectives of the social sciences. HIPH maintains a privileged place for physicians as faculty and students, and hires other scientists, engineers, and professionals with training in social and behavioral sciences as teaching staff. Most HIPH faculty members are products of the University of Alexandria, entering as instructors and remaining for their professional lives. Physicians only may register as students for concentrations involving clinical health care applications, and only health professionals may study epidemiology, microbiology, environmental health, and occupational medicine. Biostatistics, health planning, hospital administration, food control, environmental engineering, occupational health, and health education are open to students from other backgrounds.

FHS has made steady progress in improving its graduate programs during the past decade, following the country's gradual emergence from the civil war years and their aftermath, and the recruitment of a new leadership in the late 1990s. Considerable efforts were made to attract PhD-level social scientists to faculty positions, as well as young well-trained faculty in all disciplines. The social science faculty members have been instrumental in broadening frameworks for research and encouraging critical thinking. The adoption of the ecological framework for health to guide program development reinforced the multidisciplinary approach. Experience to date suggests that the multidisciplinary approach is easier to achieve in research than in teaching as breaking down disciplinary boundaries through the development of integrated courses requires time and considerable effort. Qualified students from any field showing interest in public health may join FHS programs.

ICPH is more geographically isolated than the other two institutions and has developed different strategies for integrating social action with research, teaching, and public health services practice. ICPH is organized into flexible units, not departments, which facilitates multidisciplinary and team teaching. The small full-time faculty covers the essential public health specialties and is complemented by faculty from other departments and institutes at Birzeit University, especially from sociology, psychology, history, women's studies and political science. Students come from health and other professions, and the hard and social sciences.

Multi-sectoral Public Health Practice

Public health practice also varies across the three institutions. At HIPH, faculty consultations and service projects apply evidence-based interventions to improving the health care delivery system and the environmental determinants of disease. Faculty members are expected to balance their time between teaching, research, and service. Recent examples include iodization of salt to prevent goiter, oral rehydration therapy for diarrhea, and new vaccine trials. Faculty work with a range of health providers and policy makers in national, regional, and international health agencies.

During the process of program revision in the aftermath of a long civil war – and while undertaking the self-study for CEPH accreditation – FHS began to question its marginalized approach to public health practice and this led to expanding multi-sectoral public health outreach, and linking practice more closely to research and teaching. Recognizing the need to reward practice in order to strengthen its contribution as an academic pillar, discussions have considered how practice can be evaluated in performance appraisals and promotion decisions, an issue which also must be addressed at the highest levels of AUB.

Theory and practice are strongly linked at ICPH. Since its inception ICPH has collaborated with local health care institutions and community-based groups, following part-time students and alumni to their workplaces. Faculty consultations reinforce those connections inside and outside health services. Research, teaching, and interventions are labor-intensive, and given the substantial difficulties in moving around the West Bank, ICPH faculty have less time to write for publication than what is required for academic promotion (promotion does not have a strict timeframe at Birzeit University).

Different Ways of Knowing: Restating Values

The three institutions also vary in their approaches to evidence creation, and the explicit values that underlie their work. HIPH strength lies primarily in its use of quantitative, especially epidemiological, methods, although faculty and students also use qualitative methods in research. Lack of PhD-level social scientists at HIPH, however, limits the types of social questions asked and analyzed. The values that underline HIPH work are ethics, as defined by the biomedical tradition, and a concern with inequities in health that are reflected in some core public health courses, offered to all HIPH graduate students. Community-based fieldwork training requires students from different majors to work together, and often with involvement of vulnerable populations, such as squatters or pregnant women in rural areas. Candidates also conduct fieldwork for theses on local community health priorities.

FHS has been profoundly influenced in recent years by pioneering participatory research by faculty undertaken among some of Lebanon's most disadvantaged communities, and the relief and rehabilitation work during and following the July 2006 War on Lebanon. These experiences, together with the use of explicitly eclectic research methods, have reinforced the value of different sources of knowledge. The establishment of the Center for Research on Population and Health in 2002 has led to programmatic multidisciplinary team research on key public health issues. Faculty in several departments are now making conscious efforts to instill in students the values of ethics and social justice and a commitment to social action.

ICPH faculty uses various forms of knowledge in building evidence, relying on both quantitative and qualitative methods in research. The values that guide teaching, research, and practice at ICPH have emerged from over three decades of work to resist occupation and survive war-like conditions, and out of partnerships with the popular movements and other community-based groups. The necessary focus on addressing periodic emergencies has allowed ICPH to make a real contribution to understanding health in war-like conditions, but has limited the development of other research that is important for public health teaching and intervention. The values embedded in the ICPH program – ethics, social justice, empowerment – encourage their graduates to defend health as the right of all people, and to work for change.

Outcomes: Our Graduates

In 54 years, HIPH has produced a large number of graduates, many of whom hold key technical, administrative, and leadership positions in Egypt, the region and beyond. They typically work in the health care delivery system in the public and private sectors, and in non-governmental and inter-governmental organizations. In their work in Egypt and the region, HIPH graduates make an impact within a traditional public health approach. FHS has also been producing graduates for over 50 years, but it

is in the last 5 years that it has taken strides to prepare them in a comprehensive multidisciplinary approach to public health. Alumni have reached leadership positions in private, nongovernmental, and international organizations, and some in the public sector, in Lebanon and abroad. Recent graduates are now working for a broader spectrum of organizations particularly at the community level. The challenges of the biomedical health system and the unstable political situation in which graduates work are daunting, but their influence is being felt especially in Lebanon and can be enhanced by stronger Alumni networks. Over the years, ICPH has produced a critical mass of graduates trained in comprehensive public health, sharing values, knowledge, and competencies that are needed to bring about change. Some have reached key leadership positions and are creating facts on the ground in the highly challenging context of war and dependence on international aid.

Realizing the Educational Vision of Comprehensive Public Health

Our experiences and those of our graduates indicate that national and local public health and development organizations increasingly recognize the importance of the public health professional who is well educated in the comprehensive framework and strongly anchored in the social realities of their contexts. Recent regional and international developments converge with this national/local need to create an opportunity for pushing the comprehensive approach forward. Public health practitioners from the region have called for a stronger role for academia (Mahgoub 2000). A meeting organized by WHO/EMRO in Beirut in December 2009 of academic institutions to explore their potential contributions to health system development identified the establishment of new independent schools of public health, and strengthening existing ones, as key priorities for strengthening public health in the region (WHO-EMRO 2009). This was also a key recommendation of a review by academic public health professionals from various public health academic institutions in the Eastern Mediterranean region (Jabbour et al 2009). At the global level, numerous initiatives, for example, the recently established Commission on Education of Health Professionals for the twenty-first century (Bhutta et al 2010), support the push for more independent schools of public health.

To realize the opportunities, we must address the obstacles. The case studies, our experiences with academic public health in the region, and recent reviews (Jabbour et al 2009) point to various challenges facing the implementation of comprehensive public health in upcoming and already established independent programs. We examine these challenges in three domains.

Challenges Facing Universities

Leadership for change: Public health schools or programs require strong and committed leadership to adopt the comprehensive multidisciplinary approach; to develop the educational, research, and outreach programs correspondingly; and to gain support within the university. In specific contexts, an independent leadership for the graduate public health programs, working closely with departments, may be needed to support the new approach.

Multidisciplinary faculty: Recruiting a faculty that includes public health disciplines, physicians, and social scientists is a necessary but not sufficient condition for adopting a comprehensive approach. Multidisciplinary collaboration and engagement are difficult, particularly in teaching, when departments are organized along disciplinary lines. Doing this requires time and effort to break disciplinary boundaries, encourage collaboration, emphasize issues rather than specialties, and create a shared perspective on education, research, and practice. Promotion policies must also support multidisciplinary collaboration for even the evaluation of multi-authored research papers resulting from large multidisciplinary research programs can produce difficulties in assigning credit to any one individual. Rewards and salary differentials that favor some disciplines, especially physicians, over others at the same academic rank work against an atmosphere supportive of multidisciplinary collaboration.

Enhancing the value of practice: Integrating teaching, research and practice is at the heart of the comprehensive approach. However, academic rules and regulations do not encourage the involvement of public health faculty with practice, particularly in community interventions and social action which require considerable time and effort. Teaching and research are prioritized in promotion assessment.

The contribution of practice activities to teaching and research is not well understood by university bodies. Although the case studies have provided examples of efforts to recognize practice in promotion, more needs to be done to change the way in which university administrations conceptualize and implement promotion policies.

Student backgrounds: Students are generally not well prepared by their prior education for the demands of the comprehensive approach. The case studies show that efforts are being made to encourage students from diverse backgrounds to work together. However, collaboration and team spirit do not come naturally, as students have been segregated by discipline in undergraduate education. Thus, they must be supported to develop an appreciation of the roles different disciplines can play in public health practice, to learn from each other and to collaborate as a team. Our experiences indicate that the patriarchal and conservative environments in which many students have been raised and the rigid nature of their prior education limit their ability to think critically, and to systematically absorb, analyze, synthesize, and integrate what they are learning. While attention may already be given to building English language skills, strengthening classical Arabic abilities is also needed for better student integration in their future work environments. These realities indicate the need to develop context-specific competencies.

Resources: Limited resources constrain the establishment of new schools and programs, attracting qualified and diverse faculty, conducting quality research and organizing practice programs. Both public and private universities face this challenge. The dearth of national funding for research prompts academic institutions to seek international funding, which is often driven by donor agendas. This can weaken the comprehensive approach where local public health priorities should guide the research agenda.

The support of university leaders: The highest levels of university administration may not understand the comprehensive approach to public health and its requirements. Yet their support is essential to allocate resources, facilitate fundraising for research and practice, and provide scholarships to create a diverse student body. The support of leadership in other university faculties, for example, in medicine and social sciences, is important when

441

establishing an independent school of public health, and for facilitating mutually beneficial collaborative relations later. Once established, the school of public health should have equal status to other schools and faculties to ensure independence and ability to introduce change.

Competition with imported programs: We have recently witnessed aggressive initiatives by various reputable US universities in setting up offshore/satellite campuses, particularly in the Gulf region, and offering a range of programs, including graduate public health education. Such programs seem to merely replicate frameworks, curricula, indeed, "the wholesale adoption of the American university model as the sole standard" (Coffman 2003), rather than learn from and involve local partners to adapt teaching to the local context and priorities. These initiatives have so far not demonstrated any regional capacity building in public health, and appear to be motivated by financial considerations (Silvergate 2008).

Health System Constraints and Challenges

In many Arab countries, health systems have not moved beyond the disease-focused biomedical model to the broader conceptualization of public health and remain biased toward curative services, especially the hospital, and the employment of physicians and nurses. Preventive activities are usually confined to those offered in the health services, and broader health protection and promotion are afforded modest attention, if any. This leaves little room for the expansion of public health functions to include community involvement, inter-sectoral collaboration to solve health problems, or key preventive/promotive activities such as anti-smoking and accident prevention campaigns. Because of the absence or limited inclusion of these functions, resources and positions for the employment of public health professionals other than physicians and nurses are limited. This dilemma faces not only the graduates of independent public health programs, but also other needed health personnel such as counselors, psychologists, community health workers, and mobilizers.

Thus faculty, students, and graduates learning and adopting the comprehensive public health approach may find themselves frustrated in attempting to integrate this model into existing systems if and when employed in such constraining settings.

These challenges call for strong advocacy and support of health sector reforms, which include a re-conceptualization of health as going beyond disease and into healthy states, of illness as culturally constructed, and of quality of life and well-being as ultimate health objectives. This necessarily calls for restructuring systems to incorporate varied functions beyond services, and the employment of new human resources relevant to population health needs of this day and age. Such restructuring must include a new national vision, and corresponding strategies, for public health education, which is now rarely considered in health professional development strategies.

Because the comprehensive public health approach questions the status quo, and in particular the inequities in living that create inequities in health, it is potentially threatening to the existing power structures. While working with communities along the classical approach of health education and disease prevention is generally supported in Arab countries, it is not clear that collaboration with communities in consciousness-raising and empowerment for communal action on health would be allowed or supported.

Collective Action to Meet the Challenges

This third force may offer both universities and health systems the necessary push to sustain or accelerate needed change. Collective action could take the shape of regional networks composed of leading academics and public health professionals, that bring different disciplinary perspectives and sectoral and institutional experiences to bear in formulating a comprehensive public health agenda. Remarkably too few such regional forums exist where public health researchers and practitioners in the region can meet to debate the pressing issues, mentor young scholars, plan collaborative research to generate needed evidence, and advocate for change. Together, people of influence could press for establishing independent schools of public health in countries with evident need, such as Egypt, Syria, and Sudan; support health sector reform; push for community-based public health functions outside health services; and work with medical colleagues to develop a mutual understanding of priorities and to strengthen the commitment to improving population health in the Arab region.

References

Baum F (1995) Public health in the graduate medical curriculum at Flinders University. *Australian Journal of Public Health*, 19: 525–526

Berridge V (2007) Multidisciplinary public health: What sort of victory? *Public Health*, 121: 404–408.

Bhopal R (1998) The context and role of the US school of public health: Implications for the United Kingdom. *Journal of Public Health and Medicine*, 20: 144–148

Bhutta ZA, Chen L, Cohen J, et al (2010) Education of health professionals for the 21st century: A global independent commission. *Lancet*, 375: 1137–1138.

Coffman J (2003) *Higher education in the Gulf: Privatization and Americanization international higher education*. Available from http://www.bc.edu/bc_org/avp/soe/cihe/newsletter/News33/text009.htm [Accessed 15 December 2010]

CSDH (The Commission on Social Determinants of Health) (2008) *Closing the gap in a generation: Health equity through action on the social determinants of health. Final report of the CSDH*. Geneva, Switzerland: World Health Organization

El Ansari W, Russell J, Wills J (2003) Education for health: Case studies of two multidisciplinary MPH/MSc public health programmes in the UK. *Public Health*, 117: 366–376

Foldspang A (2008) Public health education in Europe and the Nordic countries: Status and perspectives. *Scandinavian Journal of Public Health*, 36: 113–116

Gebbie K, Rosenstock L, Hernandez LM (Eds.) (2003) *Who will keep the public healthy? Educating public health professionals for the 21st century*. Committee on Educating Public Health Professionals for the 21st Century, Washington, DC: Institute of Medicine and the National Academies Press

Giacaman R, Halilel S (2003) Maintaining public health education in the West Bank. *Lancet*, 361: 1220–1221

Goraya A, Scrambler G (1998) From old to new public health: Role tensions and contradictions. *Critical Public Health*, 8(2): 141–151

Gray S, Pilkington P, Pencheon D, Jewell T (2006) Public health in the UK: Success or failure? *Journal of the Royal Society of Medicine*, 99: 107–111

Heller RF (2008) The Peoples-uni: Public health education for all. *The Medical Journal of Australia*, 189: 189–190

Heller RF, Heller TD, Pattison S (2003) Putting the public back into public health. Part I. A redefinition of public health. *Public Health*, 117: 62–65

Hunter DJ (2008) The state of the public health system in England. *Public Health*, 122: 1042–1046

Ijsselmuiden CB, Nchinda TC, Duale S, Tumwesigye NM, Serwadda D (2007) Mapping Africa's advanced public health education capacity: The African health project. *Bulletin of the World Health Organization*, 85: 914–922

Jabbour S, Rashidian A, Shawky S, Zaidi S (2009) *Public health academia and health system development in the Eastern Mediterranean Region*. A background paper commissioned by the WHO Eastern Mediterranean Regional Office

Kohatsu ND, Robinson JG, Torner JC (2004) Evidence-based public health: An evolving concept. *American Journal of Preventive Medicine*, 27: 417–421

Krieger N (2003) Latin American social medicine: The quest for social justice and public health. *American Journal of Public Health*, 93: 1989–1991

Mahgoub E (2000) Role of academia and professional associations in support of health for all. *Eastern Mediterranean Health Journal*, 6(4): 788–790

Mokwena K, Mokgatle-Ntabhu M, Madiba S, Lewis H, Ntuli-Ngcobo B (2007) Training of public health workforce at the national school of public health: Meeting Africa's needs. *Bulletin of the World Health Organization*, 85: 949–954

Petrakova A, Sadana R (2007) Problems and progress in public health education. *Bulletin of the World Health Organization*, 85: 963–965

Raphael D, Bryant T (2002) The limitations of population health as a model for a new public health. *Health Promotion International*, 17: 189–199

Sadana R, Petrakova A (2007) Shaping public health education around the world to address health challenges in the coming decades. *Bulletin of the World Health Organization*, 85: 902–903

Silvergate H (2008) *Are universities selling out to oil nations? 25 September 2008, The Boston Phoenix*. Available from http://thephoenix.com/Boston/News/68865-Are-universities-selling-out-to-oil-nations/?page=4#TOPCONTENT [Accessed 13 March 2009]

Sim F, Lock K, McKee M (2007) Maximizing the contribution of the public health workforce: The English experience. *Bulletin of the World Health Organization*, 85: 935–940

Susser M (1993) The bell tolls for a school of public health – and for thee? *American Journal of Public Health*, 83(11): 1524–1525

Tangcharoensathien V, Prakongsai P (2007) Regional public health education: Current situation and challenges. *Bulletin of the World Health Organization*, 85: 903–904

Thorpe A, Griffiths S, Jewell T, Adshead F (2008) The three domains of public health: An internationally relevant basis for public health education? *Public Health*, 122: 201–210

Tilson H, Gebbie KM (2004) The public health workforce. *Annual Review of Public Health*, 25: 341–356

WHO EMRO (World Health Organization-Eastern Mediterranean Regional Office) (2009) *Regional consultative meeting on capacity development of academic institutions to promote health systems and research based on primary health care*. Beirut, Lebanon: WHO EMRO

Wills J, Woodhead D (2004) 'The glue that binds . . .': Articulating values in multidisciplinary public health. *Critical Public Health*, 14(1): 7–15

Chapter

34 Participatory Community Interventions: A Case Study Approach

Rima Afifi, Iman Nuwayhid, Mayssa T. Nehlawi, and Mohammad Assai

Health intervention, such as education for behavioral change, addressed to the individual and development projects distanced from the communities they mean to serve are being challenged by participatory and community-based interventions. The latter are based on the premise that solutions to public health problems must be multi-faceted and broad-based, involve a variety of stakeholders, and be more responsive to community needs (Cargo & Mercer 2008). To the degree that the community owns programs, they will be more sustainable. In this chapter, we review the literature and present selected community-based participatory interventions in the Arab world; and assess their validity and impact.

Background

The term "participatory community interventions" (PCI) covers a variety of approaches that engage beneficiaries, users, and organizers and researchers of public health interventions in an equitable manner through development, implementation, and evaluation (Cargo & Mercer 2008; Minkler & Wallerstein 2008). PCI aims to organize the community to bring about social change through multiple interventions targeted at various ecological levels. The term "community" describes either a geographic area, or people bonded relationally, such as communities of women or public health practitioners (Butler et al 1999).

PCI are grounded in mutual respect and trust as well as capacity building of, and ownership by, community members (Cargo & Mercer 2008). The historical basis for these approaches is rich and includes both theoretical and practical paradigms (Wallerstein & Duran 2008; Rifkin 1996). The listening-dialogue-action approach of the notable educator and theorist Paulo Freire form a foundation for the basic social justice tenets of PCI (Wallerstein & Duran 2008). PCI is based on three principles: social justice, autonomy/self-determination, and enhancing the interface between science and practice (Cargo & Mercer 2008; Wandersman & Florin 2003).

Some schools of public health in the United States have adopted the PCI approach in public health education and training and have promoted community-based participatory research (CBPR) and community-campus partnerships (CCP) in professional practice. Both CBPR and CCP integrate research, action, and education (Wallerstein & Duran 2008), and require the engagement of academics with community members in needs assessment and solution building for community change. "Participatory research is fundamentally about who has the right to speak, to analyze and to act"

> **Box 1. Principles of CBPR**
> 1. Recognizes community as a unit of identity
> 2. Builds on the strengths and resources within the community
> 3. Facilitates collaborative equitable partnerships in all research phases and involves an empowering and power-sharing process that attends to social inequities
> 4. Promotes co-learning among all partners
> 5. Integrates and achieves a balance between research and action for the mutual benefit of all partners
> 6. Emphasizes public health problems of local relevance and also ecological perspectives that recognize and attend to the multiple determinants of health and disease
> 7. Involves systems development through a cyclical and iterative process
> 8. Disseminates findings and knowledge gained to all partners and involves all partners in the dissemination process
> 9. Requires a long-term process and commitment to sustainability.

Public Health in the Arab World, ed. Samer Jabbour et al. Published by Cambridge University Press. © Samer Jabbour et al., 2012.

(Minkler & Wallerstein 2008). CBPR is built on nine principles (Israel et al 2008 – see Box 1). These principles apply equally to participatory interventions that are not research based.

International agencies are also adopting participatory approaches. The World Health Organization (WHO) has developed a practitioner model of PCI as evident in the Community Based Initiative (CBI) effort. This effort in the Eastern Mediterranean Region embodies the WHO definition of health (Assai Ardakani 2007) and aims "to improve health in poor populations through action on social determinants" (Assai et al 2006). More specifically, CBI has been defined as "an integrated bottom-up community development concept, which is based on full community involvement supported through intersectoral collaboration. It is a "self sustained people-oriented strategy" (Assai Ardakani 2007 p. 1244). CBI includes the Healthy Cities and Healthy Villages as well as the Basic Developmental Needs (BDN) approaches (Assai Ardakani 2007). The Canada-based International Development Research Center (IDRC) has supported an EcoHealth approach to health and environment research at a global level. This approach promotes participatory and action-oriented, policy-linked approaches to research (Lebel 2004). In the Arab world, research activities were supported in Egypt (two), Jordan (one), Lebanon (one), and Morocco (two).

Recently, analysis of common features of success in PCI suggest five key components: (i) assessment and collaborative planning, (ii) targeted action and intervention, (iii) community change, (iv) widespread behavior change, and (v) improvement in population level outcomes (Institute of Medicine 2002; Watson-Thompson et al 2008). Critical processes for community change and improvement have also been identified such as establishing a mission and vision, developing a framework of change, developing leadership, arranging for community mobilizers, implementing effective intervention, documenting progress, and sustaining the work (Watson-Thompson et al 2008).

Why Community Participation?

A complex set of social, economic, and political factors influence health (WHO 2008). As such, it is difficult to expect individual behavioral change without changing the social environment and context (Merzel & D'Afflitti 2003). As resources, strengths

and skills to effect change are located within communities themselves (Israel et al 2001), there have been increasing calls for participatory interventions in health, and even demands for participation as a "right" of people (Chilaka 2005). Participation, "a process in which individuals take part in decision making in the institutions, programs and environments that affect them" (Florin & Wandersman 1990 p. 43), provides a variety of health and social benefits (Florin & Wandersman 1990; Zakus & Lysack 1998; Campbell et al 2004). When successful, participatory interventions are more sustainable as they are more relevant (Rifkin 1996; Schwab & Syme 1997; Zakus & Lysack 1998). There is added value of using participatory approaches at every stage of interventions (planning, implementation, and evaluation) (Cargo & Mercer 2008).

There are challenges to PCI (Berkowitz 2001; El Ansari 2005; Israel et al 2008; Roussos & Fawcett 2000; Zakus & Lysack 1998). Participation has been used too liberally as a panacea (Taylor et al 2006). Some have criticized it as a "tyranny" that reinforces power relations under the guise of change (Sultana & Abeyasekera 2008). The very natures of community and of participation may be limiting factors in the success of PCI (Zakus & Lysack 1998). In relation to the former, unless the conditions are favorable, most importantly a political and socio-cultural climate that "supports individual and collective public awareness, knowledge acquisition and discussion of issues and problems affecting individual and community well-being" (Zakus & Lysack 1998), PCI may not be effective in impacting health.

In relation to participation, few people within a community actually participate (Kapiriri et al 2003; Wandersman 2009), promoting some to call it a "minority sport" (Blakeley & Evans 2009 p. 17). Achieving wide participation is difficult (Taylor et al 2006). Evidence suggests that participation of individuals is more likely in communities that are smaller with strong social networks and rootedness, where trust exists between governments and the people, and where individuals exhibit personal and collective efficacy and control. Poverty diminishes participation (Blakeley & Evans 2009; Coakes & Bishop 1998, Wandersman 2009). Women who have "status" in the community and who have children are more likely to participate (Coakes & Bishop 1998). The strongest motivators for participation are purposive – betterment of the community – and social interactions with others (Coakes & Bishop 1998). PCI is also time consuming, with outcomes clear only over the long term. Whether PCI can change the social conditions that are the root causes of ill health is uncertain.

Community participation has been discussed and practiced both as a means to an end, i.e., health improvement, and as an end in itself, i.e. empowerment (Rifkin 1996). The former denotes top-down approaches where participation is seen as a "magic bullet" to achieve a change in health status (Morgan 2001). The latter is linked to bottom-up approaches where the outcome is community empowerment. Rifkin argues that we should use both approaches. Doing so requires public health workers to be able to adapt to the changing role of partner, listener, facilitator, and must be ready to advocate for community-identified, rather than professionally oriented needs and priorities. Health workers must be willing to accept that the solutions to similar problems must be local and cannot be identical (Rifkin 1996; Schwab & Syme 1997).

Community participation often requires the establishment of community coalitions comprising "individuals representing diverse organizations, factions, or constituencies ... who agree to work together to achieve a common goal" (Butterfoos & Kegler 2002 p. 157). Evidence suggests that effective coalitions must have attributes that may be weak or absent from underprivileged and marginalized communities such as: (i) formalized rules, roles, structures, and procedures; (ii) strong leadership; (iii) high involvement of people from diverse backgrounds representing all community sectors; (iv) having benefits of participation outweigh costs; (v) ability to pool member resources; and (vi) group cohesion (Butterfoos & Kegler 2002; Zakocs & Edwards 2006). Additionally, coalitions must have internal and external resources and visible outputs (Wandersman 2009). A recent review of CBPR partnerships that resulted in policy change suggest key facilitating factors including: the presence of strong and autonomous community-based organizations prior to the development of the CBPR partnership; a high level of mutual respect and trust among the partners; commitment of all partners to solid scientific data as a necessary prerequisite to making the case for policy action; commitment to "doing your homework"; facility for building strong collaborations and alliances with numerous and diverse stakeholders beyond the formal partnership; knowledge and facility for attending to a variety of "steps" in the policy process (Minkler 2010).

In what follows, we describe selected regional case studies of PCI and use the international literature to critically examine the extent that such interventions are being applied effectively. We conclude with a discussion for the way forward for PCI in our region.

Case Studies From the Arab World

Participatory interventions can be initiated by governments, international agencies, non-governmental agencies, donors, academic institutions, or communities themselves. They also follow various methodologies, and focus on a variety of outcomes. Several PCIs have been or are currently being implemented in the region. We have already discussed WHO/EMRO's Community Based Initiative program which includes past or ongoing demonstration projects in several countries (WHO 2009). Several CBPR projects have been completed or are under way, some of which were critically discussed in a 2009 international workshop at the American University of Beirut's Faculty of Health Sciences (AUB/FHS). Overall, little formal documentation and critical assessment of these initiatives through peer-reviewed publications exist.

For this chapter, we have selected four case studies from different sub-regions. Two of the four are WHO/EMRO CBI projects, one is part of the IDRC EcoHealth research projects (IDRC 2011), and the last is a community based participatory research project initiated by AUB/FHS. The cases were developed based on reading various documents about these initiatives, including previously written case studies, and site visits. These case studies vary by the type of community (urban/rural), size of its population, extent of poverty, initiator of the project (university, government, community, WHO, international NGO), and the health issue(s) of concern. All programs were initiated within the same period (2001 to 2005). We use the Framework for Collaborative Public Health Action by Communities recommended by the Institute of Medicine (2002) in its landmark follow-up report: "The Future of the Public Health in the 21st Century" to describe each of the cases.

Batn al Baqara and al Fawakhir: Old Cairo, Egypt

Description of the community: Batn al Baqara and al Fawakhir is a poor urban neighborhood crowded with small and impoverished dwellings and shops.

447

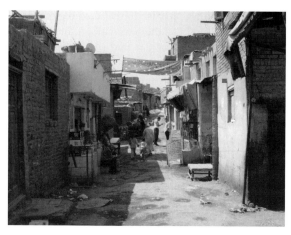

Figure 1. Walking around Batn El Baqara area, shops and dwellings.

Assessing, prioritizing, and planning: Following public complaints from the community in 2004 about foul smell and environmental hazards, a WHO team visited the governor, approached key leaders in the area and proposed a BDN program to the community in 2005. Several stakeholders participated in an initial meeting, including WHO, the Ministries of Health and Education, two NGOs, and key leaders and volunteers from the area. A "community development committee," which included key leaders and community volunteers, identified three main problems: lack of clean water supply, lack of a sanitation system, and the large garbage dumps spread about on the streets. The WHO suggested adding income-generating projects to the agenda. A baseline health survey was completed in coordination with the Ministry of Health in 2005.

Implementing targeted action: Based on the results of the survey and environmental scan, intervention focused on four overarching themes: (i) enhancing living conditions and maintaining a healthy environment, (ii) increasing health awareness, (iii) building the capacity of women and youth, and (iv) promoting entrepreneurship. With respect to the second theme, several actions were taken including organizing awareness sessions around health-related issues. With respect to the third theme, educational classes and vocational trainings were organized.

Changing community conditions and systems: With respect to the first theme, garbage dumps were cleared out, dwellings provided with access to water, and a sanitation system established in the community. With respect to the final theme, income generating activities were provided to women supervised by a subcommittee of the development committee.

Achieving widespread change in behaviors and risk factors: There are no data on changes in behaviors or risk factors. Sustainability of the project was enhanced by the participatory aspect of the interventions. As an example, community members participated in the water network project by donating part of the money, volunteering as workers, following up on progress and taking care of maintenance. The community development committee evolved into an NGO called *Toyour al Salam* (Birds of Peace) supported by WHO and New Horizon, an active NGO in the area. Toyour al Salam helped the community feel ownership of the initiative and employ their own resources in implementing and monitoring developmental activities.

Improving population health and development: The observed community changes enhanced community development, but no data are available to document changes in health status.

In conclusion, the health problem that motivated this PCI was environmental, as defined by community members. Citizen participation was relatively high as was NGO participation but the involvement of the Ministry of Health and overall government support was low. Action resulted in activities aimed at individuals, and at changing community conditions. Changes in risk factors or health status have not been officially documented, although they are obviously present.

Al-Sehel Healthy Village – Syria

Description of the community: Around 7000 people live in al-Sehel village (64 km^2); most are either employees or shop owners, or work in agriculture and shepherding animals. Houses, mostly made of cement, are scattered across the village. There are two schools, and various shops offering a variety of products and services. Most services are available with good quality; electricity provision is sufficient and residents obtain drinking water from artesian wells.

Assessing, prioritizing, and planning: The Healthy Village Program (HVP), initiated by the Syrian ministry of health with the support of international and local entities, reached al-Sehel village in 2002. A Development Committee, comprising mostly men, manages the program, and partially finances it. A baseline survey in 2004 identified two major goals: improving the quality of life within the village, and enhancing the health of its inhabitants.

Implementing targeted action: A field coordinator assisted by cluster representatives, mostly female volunteers, supervised the implementation of activities. They were trained to conduct a baseline survey, visit households and check for any occurring health conditions, remind families of routine checkups, and communicate health problems to the field coordinator. They were also trained to promote awareness about health generally, and reproductive and child health specifically. Empowering citizens included encouraging residents to enroll in free literacy classes and vocational trainings; but only women attended such classes.

Changing community conditions and systems: Improving the infrastructure consisted of building a nursery and a primary school; enhancing the phone network; improving the sewage system; and paving the main road between the village and the nearby city. A medical laboratory and a room for women's gynecological exams were added to the health center. A medical file was opened for each woman and child in the village to follow up on their health status.

The program also encouraged and assisted villagers, especially women, to obtain loans and carry out small economic projects. The seed money was provided by WHO and other partners, and is managed by the HVP directorate. The loans are interest free; however, there are some administrative fees.

The program included unique activities. The "child-healthy home" promoted providing the child with a healthy environment, both physically and psychologically. The "community school initiative" introduced changes into schools to let children acquire healthy habits at an early age, and communicate these habits to their families. The "a nurse in every house" trained cluster representatives on basic nursing skills and taking care of sick people in their families.

Achieving wide-spread changes in behavior or risk factors and improving population health and development: Implemented activities were varied and aimed at changing community conditions. No evaluation was conducted to measure the output, impact, and outcome of this project.

As an indication of commitment and potential for sustainability, financial support for this project has shifted from WHO to donations from expatriates and well-off villagers.

In conclusion, no specific health problem motivated this intervention as the decision to engage in the Healthy Villages project was taken by the government of Syria. Once the village was selected, the planning, prioritizing, and implementation of the activities were conducted by a local coalition. There is a relatively high level of citizen participation, but NGO participation is low. Ministry of Health involvement is very high, and political support for the Healthy Villages program is high. Interventions were aimed both at individuals and at changing community conditions. Changes in risk factors or health status have not been officially documented, although they are clearly present.

The Qaderoon Project in Burj El Barajneh Palestinian Refugee Camp: Beirut, Lebanon

Description of the community: This camp is the sixth largest of the 12 official camps established in Lebanon after 1948 to house Palestinian refugees. Approximately 14,000 to 18,000 people live in an area of 1.6 km^2 (Makhoul 2003). Palestinian refugees in Lebanon live under dire environmental and social conditions, among the worst for refugees in the region. Employment is limited, economic resources scarce, and access to basic health and social services limited. These conditions are exacerbated by state-imposed restrictions on employment and education (Jacobsen 2000).

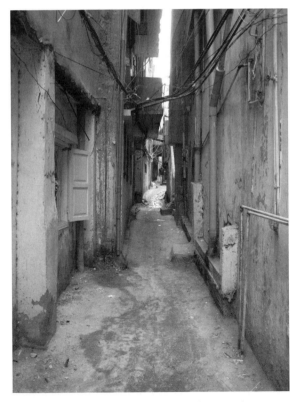

Figure 2. No place to walk; Burj El Barajneh Palestinian refugee camp.

Assessing, prioritizing and planning: A 2003 survey (Makhoul & Nakkash 2009) conducted by American University of Beirut researchers of 482 never married adolescents (13–19 years) in the camp revealed the need for interventions to improve the lives of these youth. Using a community-based participatory research approach, an intervention program was developed, designed, planned, and implemented by a community youth committee which includes representatives (not necessarily leaders) of NGOs that work in the camp; UNRWA (United Nations Relief and Works Agency – which provides health and educational services to Palestinian refugees); adult and youth residents; and researchers from AUB/FHS. The committee discussed and ranked in priority a number of health issues that affect Palestinian youth, and which could be addressed by an intervention. The two that received the highest ranking were school dropout and adolescent mental health; the coalition chose to focus on the latter as a main objective.

Implementing target action: An intervention, informed by data, collected through a randomized controlled trial, was implemented. It included 45 sessions with children aged 10–14 years, 15 sessions with their parents, and 6 workshops with their teachers. Several conceptual frameworks guided the project: the ecological model, positive youth development, social cognitive theory, and positive mental health. The project was named "Qaderoon" meaning "we are capable of" in Arabic, to indicate intent to empower young persons (Afifi et al 2011).

Changing community conditions and systems: The intervention took place in an UNRWA school with support from UNRWA and community NGOs. Activities were coordinated by a resident of the community, and carried out by 6 facilitators, and 23 mentors. The mentors are young persons, 17–25 years old, from the camp, who were recruited through community NGOs. The intent is to build their job-related skills while achieving the objectives of the project.

Achieving widespread changes in behavior and risk factors: Monitoring and evaluation extended throughout all phases of the project and included pre- and post-tests. A thorough process evaluation assessed the extent to which the project was executed as planned and with a high degree of fidelity. The combined children's satisfaction score for all sessions was more than 90% (Afifi et al 2010). Measured risk factors include the intermediate outcomes of communication

skills, problem solving skills, interaction with parents and teaching, interactions with peers, school achievement among others. Data are currently being analyzed.

Improving population health and development: Mental health was measured at pretest, posttest, and follow-up (6 months after completion of the intervention); the results are still being analyzed, but preliminary results suggest that despite the scope of the intervention, the intervention and comparison groups had equivalent mean mental health scores at all measurement time points (Afifi et al 2010).

In conclusion, concern over youth health and social issues motivated this participatory intervention. There is high community involvement – including youth – in defining the problem, and developing intervention activities. NGO participation is high, but government involvement is low. Activities aimed at individuals and at changing community conditions. Extensive documentation will provide the evidence regarding changes in both risk factor and health status. Conducting randomized controlled trials with complex interventions in disadvantaged community settings is challenging owing to the difficulty of "controlling" confounding factors and ensuring adherence to protocol. Also, in contexts of high poverty, high stress, and high disadvantage, determinants of mental health for children may be more structural than individual or interpersonal.

Cleaner Water in Settat, Morocco

Description of the community: Settat, located 60 km south of Casablanca, is a center for production and trade of agricultural products, thanks to its rich soil.

Assessing, prioritizing, and planning: Industrialization of towns surrounding Settat caused pollution of water supplies by wastewater and chemicals leading the government to ban the growth of agriculture products for human consumption. This adversely affected the income of farmers who grow traditional crops, and also did not solve the health problems related to the polluted water. Businesses in the nearby industrialized town employed thousands of locals and therefore enjoyed considerable clout. They threatened to shut down if the government required them to treat effluents. A water treatment plant established in 2006 has solved 80% of the wastewater problem, but will be unable to meet the demands of continued industrial expansion.

A multidisciplinary research team was formed to work with the community at finding a solution for the wastewater problem, while preserving the ecosystem. The team included health and environment experts, and representatives of the Ministries of Agriculture, Health, and Education, in partnership with the National Institute for Agricultural Research. At first, the villagers refused attempts to engage with the team. Several town wells had already been closed down and villagers wanted to preserve whatever water supply was left. In addition, as relayed by project researchers, "research fatigue" was evident, villagers "tired of folks from the city coming to them, asking questions, raising expectations, and then never coming back".

Implementing targeted action: Several activities were implemented and began to allay villagers' mistrust. A key entry point was the focus on clean water needed for religious purposes. Villagers agreed to have their water tested to ensure that it was suitable for cleaning before prayer. Open discussions were conducted with villagers and village priorities identified. The research team provided heath examinations and free medication and treatment when needed. These activities began to establish trust, and issues originally not identified as priorities began to be discussed by the community with the research team.

Changing community conditions and systems: A community development association was established and has taken over dealing with government and non-government actors to address needs. Electricity is not available to the village but a source of treated potable water has been secured.

Achieving widespread change in behavior and risk factors: Although access to safe water has increased, mosquito breeding has also increased confirming the need for a continued ecosystem approach to health. Changes in behaviors and risk factors have not been documented.

Improving population health and development: The activities clearly influence health and development outcomes, although they are not specifically documented.

In conclusion, concern over wastewater, as identified by researchers, motivated this participatory intervention. Community involvement in decision making was originally low, but has increased with time. NGO participation is low, while government involvement is high. Activities aimed at individuals and at changing community conditions. Documentation in this project is high but specific changes in risk factors or health status have not been officially documented, although they are clearly present.

A Critical Analysis of the Case Studies

A critical analysis of these cases suggested that there are circumstances in which PCI works better, confirming what has been found elsewhere. Community commitment and participation seem most likely when the issue being addressed is related to basic needs – water and sanitation – rather than higher order needs such as lifestyle. Success is more likely at the local level, in neighborhoods and villages, than at the provincial level. Participation in activities is more likely if rules are flexible and facilitators are provided: for example, providing child care or allowing children to accompany their mothers to attend literacy sessions. Participation is enhanced if the project responds to needs identified by community members. Involvement of university academics leads to more robust research and stronger evidence.

To synthesize the lessons learned from the four cases, we use the same framework employed in describing the cases. The framework has 12 processes distributed over four phases.

Assessing, prioritizing, and planning: This phase includes the following processes: (i) Analyzing information about the problems, goals, and factors affecting them; (ii) establishing a vision and mission; (iii) developing a framework or model of change; and (iv) developing and using strategic plans. The four cases use available data to analyze the problem. No specific mission or vision statements were specified in these projects. Such statements can rally individuals and organizations with potentially different agendas around one mission for a specified time. Priorities were based on the analysis of the problem. The case projects use broad frameworks or models of change, for example EcoHealth or community-based initiatives. Specific theoretical models are rarely specified. One recommendation for future PCI is to specify the hypothesized pathways of change, using theory as applicable, which would assist in evaluating the interventions. As none of the cases specified a strategic long-term plan of action, a second recommendation is to develop strategic plans early in the life of the project. This would enhance the probability of sustainability.

Implementing targeted action: This phase includes the following processes: (i) developing organizational structure and operating mechanisms, (ii) arranging for community mobilization, (iii) developing leadership, and (iv) implementing effective interventions. All the case studies developed organizational structures such as the development committees or coalitions. However, there is no clear discussion of the extent to which the operating mechanisms proven to be critical for coalition effectiveness have been applied. For example, have these organizational structures set formal rules for decision making and communication? Are the roles of each member of the coalition clear? Is the leadership strong? Are those involved in the coalition representative of various sectors of the community? A recommendation for future PCI is to apply lessons learned from prior coalition building projects.

The discussion of community mobilization brings back the concern raised earlier about the scale of participation. Communities are heterogeneous. The four cases describe the participation of selected individuals in the planning and implementation of activities. The WHO documents describing the desired process of BDN projects and setting up of community development committees clearly insist on democratic representation of various community segments. The characteristics of the individuals serving on the community development committees in the case studies are not specifically delineated; one must question whether, in fact, they were accessed and chosen to participate due to their advantaged position. By working only through a small group of individuals, who might be committed, there is a risk of perpetuating power differentials present even within disadvantaged communities (Zakus & Lysack 1998). Research suggests that participation is most likely among the more privileged of society – having the "unintended consequence of increasing social inequalities rather than reducing them" (Campbell et al 2004 p. 315).

The conscious attempt to include all layers of the community is critical and determines "which realities will be revealed and which realities will remain hidden" in the analysis of community issues (Wallerstein & Duran 2008 p. 33). As an indicator of the above, of the CBI projects of WHO EMRO, those that showed evidence of success and program expansion had high levels of community involvement. It is a challenge and probably an impossibility to aim at full representation of the community. Public health professionals should be aware of this limitation and use creative ways to ensure listening to the voice of the weak and marginalized subgroups. One possible

solution, used in all the case studies to some extent, is first to understand and map the social fabric of the community, then engage subgroups (defined by neighborhood, socio-economic status, education, and other) in planning and decision making; once each subgroup has clearly defined their needs and solutions, one can bring them together.

Leadership was another challenge in the case studies. A recent paper summarizing the experience of WHO EMRO CBI projects stated that "full ownership by community" is a major challenge in community participatory projects; one may thus question who the true leader is of these intervention projects. Is it the community coalition, community development committees, WHO, university, or the research group? If it is the community, is the leadership capable of being sustained? Leadership was found to be a distinguishing feature of community projects that were sustained after funding ended (Nkansa & Chapman 2006).

All four projects implemented effective interventions. However, except for Qaderoon and the Eco-health project, evidence was not relied on to identify potentially effective interventions. This may be due to the fact that much of the "evidence" comes from contexts vastly different from the communities included. Still, using evidence to inform, if not base, interventions, is recommended for future community participatory projects.

Changing community conditions and systems: Processes in this phase include: (i) ensuring technical assistance, and (ii) documenting progress and using feedback. Technical assistance was available in all case studies as a result of links to WHO, universities, research institutions, or international NGOs. All projects have resulted in at least some change in community conditions and systems. The process of gathering and using feedback is less clear. This is partially a result of lack of systematic plans for monitoring and evaluation. Often termed process or implementation evaluation, monitoring entails measuring the reach of the intervention, the activities provided as well as satisfaction of participants (and the wider community) with intervention activities. Future PCI are encouraged to establish plans for monitoring intermediate outcomes and using data to inform project activities.

Achieving widespread change in behavior and risk factors: This phase includes two processes: (i) making outcomes matter, and (ii) sustaining the work. "Making outcomes matter" is dependent on the presence of a conceptual or logic framework (Afifi et al 2011) that identifies hypothesized relationships between intervention activities, intermediate impacts, and intended outcomes and thus guides all phases of intervention planning, development, implementation, and evaluation. Robust evaluation designs are critical to our ability to ascribe impact to the intervention activities and thus to accumulate enough evidence on the effectiveness of community-based interventions in the region. A recommendation for future PCI is to apply rigorous evaluation designs including assessment pre and post intervention and, when possible, comparison against a non-intervention community.

Several of the case studies have made initial strides in sustaining the work, either through the establishment of NGOs in the communities to carry on the work, known as an indicator of sustainability (Kiyu et al 2006), or through the training of community members to implement the intervention. However, ultimate sustainability of PCI is dependent on changing government interactions with citizens, and diminishing of political and socio-economic oppression. Until such a time that wide participation of various sectors and populations is a reality – until participation becomes an end in itself or both an end and a means, transfer of leadership to community will remain piecemeal and problematic; and risks sustaining power differentials.

The intent of participatory community interventions is to bring about social change. The case studies make a clear intent to change lives, for example through focusing on basic needs and supporting income generating activities. However, it remains unclear to what extent the projects have lifted the selected communities out of poverty, and closed the equity gap between the haves and have-nots. Each of these projects has aspects of the top-down paradigm. We believe that bottom up and top down are not dichotomies but rather a continuum; perhaps both are needed to efficiently and effectively achieve health outcomes using participatory interventions. However, changing social determinants requires changes in structures and systems of practice linked to the status quo, as described below.

Ethical Considerations and Politics in the Case Studies

Community participatory projects must adhere to basic principles of ethical conduct for research such as beneficence, respect for persons, and justice (Belmont Report 1979), which apply to public health work more generally. Attention to ethical issues is

vital in our work with communities in the region. Field experiences reveal barriers to applying ethical principles. A recent publication from the Qaderoon project reviews these barriers and highlights some of the ethical issues that arose while working in communities (Nakkash et al 2009).

Public health ethics are broader than the three principles of the Belmont report and include human rights (Mann 1997). In the ideal, work with communities is only ethical if it advocates for human rights of its people. It is in this broader sense, that PCI, by engaging individuals in dialogue about their social and health conditions, and in determining health priorities as well as strategies for action, can be seen to be "more" ethical than individual interventions. Individual interventions put the onus of change squarely on individuals. At a time when social conditions are increasingly recognized to influence health, this can lead to "blaming the victim."

The issue of human rights is linked to broader issues of governance in the region. The degree of community participation is linked to the social, political, economic, and cultural environment, and to individual and community empowerment (Kapiriri et al 2003). Many scholars have noted that voiced commitment to participation is insufficient; it must be accompanied by support systems and structures that promote participation (Butler et al 1999; Chilaka 2005; Kapiriri et al 2003). These systems and structures include decentralization, reductions in bureaucracy, and an emphasis on strengthening local infrastructure. Years of scholarship on the issue of community participation has resulted in the conclusion that "participation in health care development cannot be isolated from the general level of people's participation in other spheres of human endeavors, especially governance." (Chilaka 2005 p. 992). For example, youth and women cannot "participate" unless political and cultural structures allow them to do so (Kapiriri et al 2003). Underprivileged communities are equally disadvantaged. In this region where participation in governance is restricted by existing power structures, is there hope for participation in health?

Conclusions and the Way Forward

The extent to which community participation as an approach is effective in achieving health outcomes – internationally, and more specifically, in our region – remains a contested issue. Several reviews of community-based health promotion, coalition effectiveness, and collaborative partnership effectiveness more generally, have been inconclusive (Berkowitz 2001; Merzel & D'Afflitti 2003; Roussos & Fawcett 2000; Wandersman & Florin 2003). Nonetheless, the authors of these reviews remain firm in their support for community participation but suggest that methods need refinement; the use of best practices need to be strengthened; measures need more specificity; and theories of change need to be described more clearly (Wandersman & Florin 2003). Most recently, a "conceptual logic model of community based participatory research" has been developed, which suggests the pathways of influence from context through group dynamic and interventions, to outcomes (Wallerstein & Duran 2010), and indicates particular factors which may be critical for impact.

Community participatory programs are one and not the only method to achieve community, national, or global health goals. In their commitment to giving voice to people in communities, they exemplify a rights-based approach, and work towards equity. By engaging people in the prioritization of health problems and their solutions, PCI ensure more relevant research and practice. In creating bridges between academics and community members, government and community members, NGOs and community members, funders and community members, PCIs begin to break the barriers between haves and have-nots, and increase compassion and understanding between people; at the core, it is doing the right thing. For that alone, it can and should be practiced. With the information we have, and our commitment to giving voice to persons living in disadvantaged circumstances, we recommend that this method be implemented more often in our region, in more communities, and with diverse populations and health issues.

In the four case studies and others we know about, there is a clear sense of change, or bettering of lives. The challenge is to be able to measure this "sense." We thus recommend that future projects be based on clear theoretically driven logic models (Kapiriri et al 2003); be implemented carefully; be evaluated through rigorous designs; and be provided with system and resource support to enable the above (Wandersman 2009). While we work on establishing more evidence for the impact of community based interventions, we concur with the suggestion that these interventions should be paired with one-on-one interventions for high risk individuals and policy level interventions to change social and political environments (Merzel & D'Afflitti 2003). This three-pronged approach maximizes potential for health outcomes.

Not all practitioners or researchers are able or willing to engage in community-based participatory practice and research. This methodology requires a specific attitude – a passion and a willingness to be patient and spend time on the process of community building; a willingness to be an activist rather than a pragmatist (Morgan 2001); a willingness to be a facilitator of a process, rather than an expert; as such a willingness to engage in a process of co-learning where all stakeholders, including practicing professionals and researchers, learn. We therefore recommend that formal (degree) and informal (continuing education) programs of public health provide competencies for skill building related to community participatory interventions. Specific values that need to be instilled include those of social justice, equity, and ethics. Specific skills needed include "group process, communication, conflict resolution, ability to be self-reflective and admit mistakes … working within different power structures" (Israel et al 2001 p. 190).

Based on our critical analyses, PCIs generally do more good than harm in the short run. However, unless we are willing to critically examine and dissect our successes and failures, and take up the challenge of changing systems of governance – then, in promoting this model, we may be acting as agents of the system rather than agents of change (Shuftan 2008).

Acknowledgment

Mohammad Assai is a staff member of the World Health Organization. The author alone is responsible for the views expressed in this publication and they do not necessarily represent the decisions or policies of the World Health Organization.

References

Afifi RA, Nakkash R, El Hajj T, Mahfoud Z, Hammad S, Makhoul J, et al (2010) Qaderoon youth mental health promotion programme in the Burj El Barajneh Palestinian refugee camp, Beirut, Lebanon: A community-intervention analysis (online abstract). *The Lancet*, Abstract published online July 2, 2010. Available from http://download. thelancet.com/flatcontentassets/ pdfs/palestine/S0140673610608471. pdf [Accessed 2 December 2010]

Afifi RA, Nakkash RT, Makhoul J, El Hajj T (2011) Developing a logic model for youth mental health: Participatory research with a refugee community in Beirut. *Health Policy and Planning*, 26(6): 508–517

Assai M, Siddiqi S, Watts S (2006) Tackling social determinants of health through community based initiatives. *British Medical Journal*, 333: 854–856

Assai Ardakani M (2007) Community-based initiatives and their relation to poverty reduction and health development: Experiences in the Eastern Mediterranean Region. *Eastern Mediterranean Health Journal*, 13(6): 1242–1248

Belmont Report (1979) *Ethical principles and guidelines for the protection of human subjects of research.* Washington, DC: Department of Health, Education and Welfare

Berkowitz B (2001) Studying the outcomes of community-based coalitions. *American Journal of Community Psychology*, 29(2): 213–227

Blakeley G, Evans B (2009) Who participates, how and why in urban regeneration projects? The case of the new 'city' of East Manchester. *Social Policy & Administration*, 43(1): 15–32

Butler C, Rissel C, Khavarpour F (1999) The context for community participation in health action in Australia. *Australian Journal of Social Issues*, 34(3): 253–265

Butterfoos FD, Kegler MC (2002) Towards a comprehensive understanding of community coalitions. *In:* RJ DiClemente, RA Crosby, MC Kegler (Eds.) *Emerging theories in health promotion practice and research* (p. 157–193). Francisco, CA: Jossey-Bass

Campbell C, Cornish F, McLean C (2004) Social capital, participation and the perpetuation of health inequalities: Obstacles to African-Caribbean participation in 'partnerships' to improve mental health. *Ethnicity and Health*, 9(4): 313–335

Cargo M, Mercer SL (2008) The value and challenges of participatory research: Strengthening its practice. *Annual Review of Public Health*, 29: 325–350

Chilaka MA (2005) Ascribing quantitative value to community participation: A case study of the Roll Back Malaria (RBM) initiative in five African countries. *Public Health*, 119: 987–994

Coakes SJ, Bishop BJ (1998) Where do I fit in? Factors influencing women's participation in rural communities. *Community, Work and Family*, 1(3): 249–271

El-Ansari W (2005) Collaborative research partnerships with disadvantaged communities: Challenges and potential solutions. *Public Health*, 119: 758–770

Florin P, Wandersman A (1990) An introduction to citizen participation, voluntary organizations, and community development: Insights for empowerment through research. *American Journal of Community Psychology*, 18(1): 41–54

IDRC (International Development Research Center) (2011) *Eco-Health research projects.* Available from www.copeh-mena.org [Accessed 3 January 2011]

Institute of Medicine (2002) *The future of the public's health in the 21st Century.* Washington, DC: National Academies Press

Israel BA, Schulz AJ, Parker EA, Becker AB (2001) Community-based participatory research: Policy recommendations for promoting a partnership approach in health research. *Education for Health*, 141(2): 182–197

Israel BA, Schultz AJ, Parker EA, Becker AB, Allen AJ III, Guzman JR (2008) Critical issues in developing and following CBPR principles.

In: M Minkler, N Wallerstein (Eds.) *Community-based participatory research for health: From process to outcomes* (2nd ed., p. 47–66). San Francisco, CA: Jossey-Bass

Jacobsen LB (2000) *Finding means: UNRWA's financial situation and the living conditions of Palestinian refugees. Summary Report, FAFO report 415.* Norway: Interface Media

Kapiriri L, Norheim OF, Heggenhougen K (2003) Public participation in health planning and priority setting at the district level in Uganda. *Health Policy and Planning*, 18(2): 205–213

Kiyu A, Steinkuehler AA, Hashim J, Hall J, Lee PF, Taylor R (2006) Evaluation of the Healthy Village program in Kapit District, Sarawak, Malaysia. *Health Promotion International*, 21(1): 13–18

Lebel J (2004) Ecohealth and the developing world. *Ecohealth*, 1(4): 325–236

Makhoul J (2003) *Physical and social contexts of the three urban communities of Nabaa, Borj el Barajneh Palestinian Camp and Hay el Sullum.* Unpublished report, CRPH, American University of Beirut

Makhoul J, Nakkash RT (2009) Understanding youth: Using qualitative methods to verify quantitative community indicators. *Health Promotion Practice*, 10(1): 128–135

Mann JM (1997) Medicine and public health, ethics and human rights. *Hastings Center Report*, 27(3): 6–13

Merzel C, D'Afflitti J (2003) Reconsidering community-based health promotion: Promise, performance and potential. *American Journal of Public Health*, 93(4): 557–574

Minkler M, Wallerstein N (2008) Introduction to community-based participatory research: New issues and emphases. *In:* M Minkler, N Wallerstein (Eds.) *Community-based participatory research for* health: From process to outcomes (2nd ed., p. 5–23). San Francisco, CA: Jossey-Bass

Minkler M (2010) Linking science and policy through community-based participatory research to study and address health disparities. *American Journal of Public Health*, 100: S81–S87

Morgan LM (2001) Community participation in health: Perpetual allure, persistent challenge. *Health Policy and Planning*, 16(3): 221–230

Nakkash R, Makhoul J, Afifi RA (2009) Obtaining informed consent: Observations from community research with refugee and impoverished youth. *Journal of Medical Ethics*, 35: 638–643

Nkansa GA, Chapman DW (2006) Sustaining community participation: What remains after the money ends? *Review of Education*, 52: 509–532

Rifkin SB (1996) Paradigms lost: Toward a new understanding of community participation in health programmes. *Acta Tropica*, 61: 79–92

Roussos ST, Fawcett SB (2000) A review of collaborative partnerships as a strategy for improving community health. *Annual Reviews of Public Health*, 21: 369–402

Schwab M, Syme SL (1997) On paradigms, community participation, and the future of public health. *American Journal of Public Health*, 87(12): 2049–2051

Shuftan C (2008) An ethical question: Are health professionals promoters of the status quo or of social change? *Promotion and Education*, 15(3): 30–33

Sultana P, Abeyasekera S (2008) Effectiveness of participatory planning for community management of fisheries in Bangladesh. *Journal of Environmental Management*, 86: 201–213

Taylor J, Wilkinson D, Cheers B (2006) Is it consumer or community participation? Examining the links between 'community' and 'participation'. *Health Sociology Review*, 15: 38–47

Wallerstein N, Duran B (2008) The theoretical, historical, and practice roots of CBPR. *In:* M Minkler, N Wallerstein (Eds.) *Community-based participatory research for health: From process to outcome* (2nd ed., p. 25–46). San Francisco, CA: Jossey-Bass

Wallerstein N, Duran B (2010) Community-based participatory research contributions to intervention research: The intersection of science and practice to improve health equity. *American Journal of Public Health*, 100(S1): S40–S46

Wandersman A (2009) Four keys to success (Theory, implementation, evaluation and resource/system support): High hopes and challenges in participation. *American Journal of Community Psychology*, 43(1–2): 3–21

Wandersman A, Florin P (2003) Community interventions and effective prevention. *American Psychologist*, 58(6/7): 441–448

Watson-Thompson J, Fawcett SB, Schultz JA (2008) A framework for community mobilization to promote healthy youth development. *American Journal of Preventive Medicine*, 34(3S): S72–S81

WHO (World Health Organization) (2008) *Closing the gap in a generation: Health equity through action on the social determinants of health. Final report of the Commission on the Social Determinants of Health*. Geneva, Switzerland: WHO

WHO (2009) *Community-based initiatives: Success stories 2*. Cairo, Egypt: WHO EMRO (Regional Office for the Eastern Mediterranean)

Zakocs RC, Edwards EM (2006) What explains community coalition effectiveness? A review of the literature. *American Journal of Preventive Medicine*, 30(4): 351–361

Zakus DJ, Lysack CL (1998) Revisiting community participation. *Health Policy and Planning*, 13(1): 1–12

Chapter

35

Reflections on the De-politicization of Health and Scholarship

Livia Wick

This chapter engages scholarly work on health and culture in the Arab world. I hope to illuminate ways in which our scholarship is part of the world we live in, not just about it or outside it. To do so, I reflect first on the context of this review in relation to my work and formative studies. I then review some of the dominant themes in medical anthropology. The literature revolves around two approaches to studying health, one focused on the meaning of illness and disease and the second focused on inequalities. This has impacted not only the way we look at health in the Arab world but consequently the way we understand the Arab world itself. Lastly, as a case study of scholarship on health in the Arab world, I examine the themes that have been reflected in papers about this region in one prominent journal, *Social Science and Medicine*, which sits at the intersection of health and social studies. I show a diversity of themes and topics. The largest proportion of articles focus on the biomedical aspects of health and less so on in-depth exploration of the politics and political economy of health. While my case study has the obvious limited scope of focusing on one journal, I argue that the observation may reflect a broader trend and hence the need for a more comprehensive synthesis of research on health in the Arab world.

Why This Review?

This text is the product of the places, personal, intellectual, political, social, and historical in which I am situated. Among these is the institution where I work, the American University of Beirut. Because many scholars at this university contribute to policy reports or receive funding to do research on topics with a policy application, I come across a number of articles, meet researchers, and am often doing research on questions about health in various places of the Arab world. Scholarship needs to pay attention to this production of texts and through them, of knowledge itself. Of course, research is much more than an article, a book, or a report. The process of fieldwork, observations, surveys, questionnaires, and practices within universities, including lectures, seminars, and conferences, and the very funding of research together constitute objects of study. Writing and publishing are nonetheless important components. Through this exposition of work here and abroad, I want to argue that writings in public health and medical anthropology contribute to shaping a culture as well as a notion of health, employing and molded by disciplinary conventions, American (at some universities French or British or a mixture) standards of scholarship, exigencies of academia, the funding of research, as well as political and economic concerns. Influential medical anthropologists in the region, for example, Morsy (1981) and Sholkamy & Ghannam (2004), have commented on the influence of these different factors and how they are reflected in the medical anthropology literature on this region.

In Middle Eastern Studies, Edward Said's *Orientalism* (1978) opened up fields of questioning to scholarly discourse on the Arab world, and it is from this site that this chapter wishes to begin as it traces some of the topical and historical patterns of scholarship on health and culture. On the one hand, it focuses on health as a changing object of study and on the other hand, it studies the Arab world as a place in medical anthropology and public health. I focus on three areas, asking the following questions: Why do particular areas of health receive more interest than others? What historical, political, and economic forces shape these areas? What kinds of thinking are excluded and silenced by these interests?

Public Health in the Arab World, ed. Samer Jabbour et al. Published by Cambridge University Press. © Samer Jabbour et al., 2012.

Scholars in science studies, sociology, anthropology, and public health have vital interests in scientific production, fundamental to their legitimacy as intellectuals. Scholarship is intrinsically connected to the invisibility of these vital interests and is perpetuated by the naturalized routines of its production. The first question concerns the way in which "the Arab world" has been constituted in works about health, and "health" has been constituted in works about the Arab world.

After discussing some of the books and articles I read as a student and scholar, I shall proceed, by way of a case study, to an evaluation of the public health literature through the prism of the articles on the Arab world that have appeared in one prominent journal, *Social Science and Medicine*, since its inception.

Recent Themes of Medical Anthropology

In medical anthropology, although the literature is varied, there are essentially two areas of theorizing on health, and its relation to culture, in the Arab world: one on meaning-making and another on inequalities.

Let us begin with a recollection of the way students recently learned the discipline of medical anthropology in the Arab world. From the 1980s, I read the works of Evelyn Early (for example, Early 1982 and 1988) and Janice Boddy (for example Boddy 1988) on spirit possessions and spiritual healing systems. The mode of analysis is based on phenomenological narrative studies which Byron and Mary-Jo Good had been doing in Iran during the 1970s (see for example Good 1977). Early's and Boddy's research was carried out in Egypt and Sudan.

That generation of medical anthropology was influenced by the work of Clifford Geertz, who reintroduced a Weberian concern with "meaning," "culture" and interpretation into American anthropology (see for example, Geertz 1973, for some of his influential essays). Geertz had worked with the metaphor of cultures as texts to be read and linked the methods to those of literary criticism, seeing the anthropologist's role as interpreting people's actions in terms of systems of shared symbols and analyzing how these symbols influence people's worldviews and emotions. The idea was to access what Bronislav Malinowski called "the native's point of view" (Malinowski 1961 p. 25) by describing social action in detail and understanding what it means to the

actors (and to others), a method he came to name "thick description" (a term borrowed from philosopher Gilbert Ryle). Geertz's own work on cultural systems was, one should add, based on fieldwork he conducted in Morocco in the 1960s (Geertz 1968). Geertz's theory and methods, in other words, strive to infer meanings for individuals and groups and raise questions about who is doing the interpreting. This then became a central concern of the following generation of anthropologists.

In medical anthropology more specifically, scholars have emphasized the need to tease out the difference between biomedical categories and the subjective experiences of illness, which have major consequences for the well-being of patients. Good's concept of a "semantic illness network" (Good 1977 p. 40) in which popular illness categories are interpreted as part of networks of words, metaphors, and images that concentrate on specific events has widely been used. Rosen et al (1982) have thus attempted to counter the pathologizing approach of clinical literature which often medicalizes as "somatization" certain widely disseminated cultural categories (such as nerves/*nervos*). These scholars argue that such categories can usefully be interpreted as pointing to the relationship between the incidence of the bodily state and structural inequalities in society.

Bodily distress and its cultural meanings are important to individuals and they can also possess political possibility. Aihwa Ong (1988), for example, analyzes attacks of spirit possession on the shop floor of multinational factories in Malaysia as part of a complex negotiation in which young women respond to violations of their gendered sense of self and difficult work conditions. Nancy Scheper-Hughes (1992), in her analysis of impoverished shantytown dwellers in Northeast Brazil, interprets an epidemic of *nervos* having multiple meanings: at times a refusal of men to continue demeaning and difficult labor, at times a response of women to a violent shock and also in part a response to the ongoing state of emergency in everyday life. She suggests that *nervos* has been used as a metaphor for hunger and child malnutrition in northeast Brazil because of the dangers of openly discussing malnutrition and its causes. Exceptional in both ethnographies are the detailed descriptions of the everyday experiences of labor in factories and on sugar plantations.

Inspired by Geertzian anthropology as well as other theorists, Early and Boddy explored the meanings of subjective experiences of illness during the 1970s and 1980s in Egypt and Sudan. But this was a time of tremendous change in the Arab world with strong political and social movements, civil wars, and social upheaval. These developments did not receive real attention in the anthropological literature. The detailed descriptions of economies and the everyday infrastructures of labor and lives were usually a background element of the ethnographic work, rather than a central one.

One of the critiques of Geertz's work has been that he is less concerned with political, economic, and historical forces that create particular cultural systems than with sheer reading, meaning, and interpretation. In influential articles, Soheir Morsy (1979, 1981) criticized medical anthropology for emphasizing the relevance of people's culturally constructed experiences of disease while failing to account for the conditions that produce ill health. She called attention to the relationship between health and power, understood illness as an expression of powerlessness, and reintroduced social class and power relations as an important factor in the processes of diagnoses and treatment.

Concurring with these critiques of medical anthropology, Marcia Inhorn and Sandra Lane's early work (Inhorn & Lane 1988) called for a reintegration of history and in particular the history of medicine into the works on culture and health in the Middle East. In their article, "Ethno-Ophthalmology in the Egyptian Delta," they followed the history of treatment of eye ailments from Pharaonic medicine, through prophetic medicine to colonial and contemporary medical systems, embedding the beliefs and treatments in their ethnographic data of a village in the Egyptian Delta in the history of ideas regarding eye ailments.

Also interested in the social relations and structures that produce distributions of ill health, its treatments and their influence on the health experiences and problems of individuals and communities, is the work of Rita Giacaman. Although pertaining to the field of public health, her *Life and Health in Three Palestinian Villages* (1988) is ethnographic in its descriptions of ways of life, focuses on local meanings and connections made to macro-level processes including occupation and poverty. It is noteworthy that the work of these scholars concerns what is sometimes referred to as "critical medical anthropology," focused on villages and rural life.

"Village studies" were a trend in anthropology of the Arab world more generally since the 1960s (see for example, Antoun 1972; Ayoub 1970; Sweet 1974). As Michael Gilsenan noted, the village seemed like a self-evident unit. The Middle East was imaged as a village society or at least predominantly rural; the village was a classical element of social organization, kin terminology could be traced from Morocco to Iraq in lineage and clan terms, "norms and values" – usually Islamic – were seamlessly present. It could thus be both richly particular, small-scale, bounded, apparently self-selecting, *and*, although in rather shifting, ambiguous and uncertain ways, "typical" (Gilsenan 1990 p. 231). In addition, villages had a particular rhythmic and slow way of life, which suited a certain disregard for analyses of history and change on the part of anthropologists.

Morsy, Giacaman, and Inhorn and Lane's early works took the village unit and inserted macro-level conditions, focusing on the connection between poverty and ill health. After the defeat of 1967 and the passing of Nasser, Sukarno, Nkruma, and the non-aligned movement, the 1970s and 1980s were decades of a different kind of social activity and energy. In the Occupied Palestinian Territory, where Giacaman's team was doing research, it was the period of popular committees, forms of social and political organization created during the decade of grassroots mobilization preceding the First Intifada of 1987, and the popular health movement of doctors and other health practitioners who organized to decentralize Palestinian health services and provide care to rural, refugee, and underserved populations in the occupied Territory during the late 1970s and throughout the 1980s. These works and their critiques of the field reflected a wider social interest in labor and social inequalities and shifted the lens to the effects of history, politics, and economies on local understandings of illness and health.

Toward the late 1980s, Morsy and Giacaman published articles about recent changes in the health infrastructure (Barghouthi & Giacaman 1990; Morsy 1988). But it is well into the 1990s that the medical anthropology literature takes biomedicine as its central object of study, trying to situate biomedicine in the world and thinking about biomedicine as a cultural system. Thus, Inhorn's work moves to the sites of high-tech reproductive technologies and in vitro fertilization clinics (2004) where she analyzes medical practices and traditions as well as the meanings of child-bearing and childlessness in a poor urban setting in Alexandria, Egypt. Sherine Hamdy analyzes how poor Egyptian kidney-disease patients in the context of dialysis clinics understand their illness in terms of larger social, economic, and political problems (Hamdy 2008). During the same time-period, other scholars started studying doctors as professional and social actors (Longuenesse 1995; Dewachi 2008; Wick 2008).

In the region today, many medical anthropologists work for at least certain periods of their career in health and development projects and/or agencies such as the UN. I argue that this proximity to policy and practice work may have contributed to directing some of the research toward thinking about the meanings and experiences of medical disease categories and illnesses once again, rather than emphasizing living conditions, labor, and economies. I explore this question through a case study.

A Case Study: Social Science and Medicine

Has scholarship on public health in the Arab world explored the same themes as medical anthropology? Has this scholarship also embraced some of the changing paradigms that I have outlined in the previous section? Many might argue, probably correctly, that the mainstream of such scholarship has narrowly focused for a long time on issues of mortality and morbidity to the detriment of considering the spectrum of issues ranging from lived and subjective experiences at the individual level to the macro level issues of politics and economy. Examining the entirety of public health scholarship is not my aim. Rather, in this section, I attempt to explore the directions of scholarship at the intersection of the disciplines of public health and other social sciences. To do this, I examine articles on the Arab world from one prominent journal, *Social Science and Medicine*, from its inception in 1981 to the present. This journal has positioned itself at the intersection of health sciences, medicine, and social sciences and has been successful in attracting important scholarship on health in the Arab world, as I show, which presents a useful case study of my subject.

In examining the articles on the Arab world in *Social Science and Medicine*, I aim to understand how public health knowledge is constructed, what is being conveyed as expert knowledge on public health issues, what factors in past decades have shaped this knowledge, and how themes from social sciences are integrated in public health. While a search of articles in only one journal has obvious limitations, it does present an opportunity to understand the presentation and representation of illness, culture, and inequalities. I approach this with many questions: what illnesses and conditions are portrayed? What disciplines and methods are used to portray them? Why were they selected and what was left out? What has been identified as health risks? What strategies are recommended to improve health conditions? In whose interest is the change directed? For what purpose was the research undertaken? In the words of Aronowitz (2008), I attempt to understand how this scholarship portrays what he called the "social patterning" of health and disease. In brief, I ask what counts as "health" in the Arab world. In search of answers, I do not restrict my readings to this journal but also draw on scholarship from other sources in public health.

Out of 67 articles found in the journal on health in the Arab world (the Maghreb was not included in the search) between 1981 and 2010, 12 were directly related to child health, 22 to maternal health and women's role in society, 9 to war and mental health, 11 to various aspects of health services and quality of care, 6 to adult health and the elderly, 2 to youth and adolescent health, 2 to disability, and 3 to the history of disease and its transmission. Thirty of the articles were from Egypt, 13 from Lebanon, 7 from Palestine, 7 from Kuwait, 3 from Saudi Arabia, 3 from Jordan, 2 from Yemen, 1 from Syria, and 1 from the United Arab Emirates. More than half of the first authors are women, and most of the anthropologists in these articles are women. Several of the Egyptian studies are funded by USAID, but most of the articles do not mention their source of funding.

While the themes of these articles are quite diverse, they are not random. To understand these themes, we must situate them in relation not only to evolving paradigms in social sciences, the focus of the previous section, but, perhaps more importantly, to evolving themes in the development literature and influential public health circles. I turn to this issue first.

Different approaches to health have had a strong influence on the choice and conduct of research topics in the Middle East. As Belgin Tekçe (1990) noted 20 years ago, much public health research tended to focus narrowly on assessing a specific intervention and how it affected health outcomes, without taking into consideration the specific cultural and historical context. Development programs, on the other hand, have tended to consider "one size fits all" approaches (Mohindra & Nikiema 2010 p. 551). Such programs are influential as research agendas, including in public health. Mohindra and Nikiema show the evolution of development paradigms from economic growth in the 1950s and 1960s, to growth with redistribution in the 1970s and 1980s focusing on basic needs, equality, and anti-poverty programs, to structural adjustment and efficiency in the 1980s and to human development, human rights, empowerment, and a new poverty agenda from the 1990s to the present (Mohindra & Nikiema 2010 p. 547).

Research topics throughout the decades have reflected these broad paradigms as well as other economic and political trends. Within a framework of equity, community participation and health for all in the Alma-Ata Declaration of 1978, the World Health Organization and UNICEF promoted the expansion of basic health services. However, the critique that comprehensive primary health would be too costly soon led to selective primary health care with cost-effective interventions targeting mainly child health (immunizations, diarrhea control, breastfeeding) (Mohindra & Nikiema 2010 p. 553). Thus as international funding focused on themes of child survival and population control, many studies, from this region as from other "third world" or "developing" regions, assessed the outcomes of maternal child health interventions and the role of cultural factors in disease causation, prevention, and control. For example, between 1977 and 1983 USAID alone allocated $87 million to the Egyptian family planning program and pressured the government of Egypt to adopt its own approach of fertility control, which continued to be heavily funded into the next decade (Ali Kamran 2002 p. 32). The national political discourse of the time linked overpopulation with poverty, underdevelopment, and the inability of parents to look after the health and welfare of their children (Ali Kamran 2002 p. 36). Rhoda Kanaaneh has shown how Palestinian women in the Galilee have internalized the ideology behind family planning and linked the small family to modernization and consumerism (Kanaaneh 2002 p. 87).

The recommendations resulting from assessments of child survival and family planning programs were framed within the biomedical model of the programs themselves including training of physicians in technical and interpersonal skills, and respect for the patient, raising knowledge and awareness among women of the risk of large families and the importance of self-regulation for child health and the development of the nation, and improving the utilization and efficiency of services. The production of data was necessary for the evaluation of such programs, for establishing norms and marking "progress" and for the surveillance of the populations (Petersen & Lupton 1996).

In addition, in the 1980s the increasing influence of the World Bank and neo-liberal economic policies focused attention on the cost-effectiveness of health interventions and promoted cheap basic packages of care. Women's health, whether viewed as contributing to biological or social reproduction, tended to be instrumentalized as a means to reach child survival and economic goals, rather than as an end in itself (Mohindra & Nikiema 2010 p. 561).

The articles on the Arab world in *Social Science and Medicine* of the 1980s reflect these topics and frameworks. Afaf Meleis (1982) focused on women's roles in Kuwaiti society and their effects on stress and mental health. Theresa El-Mehairy (1984) studied the attitudes of a group of Egyptian medical students towards family planning. Louise Weidner et al (1985) explored sanitation and water usage practices in a village in the Nile Delta and called for community education. Hassan Abu-Zeid and William Dann (1985) studied health services utilization and cost in Ismailia, Egypt. The Private Practitioner Family Planning Project explored the effects of rumor and misinformation about oral contraceptives in Egypt (DeClerque et al 1986). In the *Social Science and Medicine* articles, women are studied as the caretakers of children, the educators, the consumers of health services, the objects of domestic violence (Diop-Sidibe et al 2006; Clark et al 2010), the perpetrators of child abuse (Maziak et al 2002), and the victims of trauma during war. Men's bodies are rarely part of the research gaze, except as soldiers in time of war (Petersen & Lupton 1996 p. 85; Saab et al 2003). As all these examples show, many of the articles of the 1980s focus on the effects of cultural factors (such as women's roles or physicians' attitudes or beliefs or people's misinformation about health interventions) on health and well-being as well as the efficiency and cost effectiveness of services.

The 1990s witnessed a broadening of focus in international health agendas from family planning, antenatal care' and child survival to include reproductive and sexual health and women's rights. This culminated in the 1994 International Conference on Population and Development in Cairo. Several factors influenced this development: the growth of the international feminist movement, a reaction to population control programs for poor women, the urgency of the HIV/AIDS pandemic, and the rising awareness of the complexity of reproductive health issues which cannot be adequately addressed by simple and cheap primary health care interventions (Dudgeon & Inhorn 2004). Some of the topics of the *Social Science and Medicine* articles of the 1980s continue to reappear in the 1990s. In addition, however, reflecting a change in the field, Sandra Lane and Afaf Meleis (1991) shift the focus of attention from motherhood and fertility to work and family responsibilities. Inhorn (1994) brings the topic of infertility to the discussion of reproduction in the Arab world. Sandra Lane and colleagues (1998) discuss the costs, access, and methods of abortion in Egypt. Catherine Panter-Brick writes about parents' responses to consanguinity and genetic disease in Saudi Arabia (Panter-Brick 1991).

Another important theme in this journal is the relationship between the loss and violence of war and mental health outcomes. These studies have come from Lebanon and Palestine for over 25 years now (see for example, Armenian et al 1981; Hourani et al 1986; Bryce et al 1989; Khamis 1997; Farhood et al 1993; Al-Eissa 1995; Saab et al 2003). Lebanon and Palestine, in particular, have experienced long periods of conflict, where psychosocial stressors have been studied in relation to physical and mental disease outcomes, and the role of social support and the extended family in mediating this relationship. Laila Farhood and colleagues (1993) have shed light on the stressful context of everyday life (the "daily hassles" as they were called) involving the structural violence of poverty, displacement, malnutrition, and the destruction of social networks. Reducing these daily stressors following conflict has more recently been identified as having a long-term effect on the capacity of the individual to recover, which has important implications for the type of psychosocial interventions and support, which might be effective in treating traumatized populations (Miller & Rasmussen 2010). The region has been fertile ground for constructing the new domain of humanitarian psychiatry (Fassin & Rechtman 2009 p. 215).

Researchers writing on the Arab world in *Social Science and Medicine* were, in some cases, pioneers in the region in exploring new themes and topics. Some of the innovative themes and approaches to public health research, included thinking about hegemonic ideas about health and illness (Myntti 1988), social and political determinants of health and access to resources (Morsy 1981; Myntti 1993; Tekçe 1990); women's lived experiences of illness and well-being (Early 1982); studying marginal groups (Yount 2003; Khawaja 2004; 2006); the role of modern medical services in legitimizing the state (Gallagher & Searle 1985); a life cycle approach to women's health and their multiple roles within households (Lane & Meleis 1991; Doan and Bisharat 1990); a historical systems and gender approach to health (Inhorn and Lane 1988, Inhorn 1994, 2003; Lamb 1997; Yount 2003; Yount et al 2004); and the causes, consequences, and political implications of infertility in the region (Inhorn 1994, 2003). Not only a broader conception of women's health is reflected in the studies, but also an interest in other age groups, generating research on youth and adolescent health (Khawaja et al 2006) and the elderly (Sibai et al 2007; Lamb 1997).

Most of the articles use a quantitative epidemiological study design. Perhaps in this region the political and cultural sensitivities favor what is widely viewed as an "objective" statistical approach, deemed more effective in influencing policy makers and donors and in evaluating programs. The use of quantitative vs. qualitative procedures in research is not a random phenomenon and has profound implications as Gingrich (2011 p. 171) argues. Inhorn, however, calls for combining epidemiology and anthropology and uses the two disciplines to understand why certain patterns of behavior exist in specific contexts and the socio-cultural and politico-economic reasons for their continuation (Inhorn & Buss 1994). Most of the articles combining the two disciplines have used what has been called "parallel" collaboration, with researchers working in their own disciplines but on common projects (Trostle & Sommerfeld 1996 p. 258). Such approaches have contributed to greater contextual knowledge in the region on, for example, disease risk and behavior (Inhorn & Lane 1988), infant feeding and child nutrition (Sukkary-Stolba 1987; Harrison et al 1993; Lewando-Hundt & Forman 1993), cultural and political understandings of reproductive morbidities (Lane et al 1998; Inhorn 1994), and the complex role of extended families in intimate partner violence (Clark et al 2010).

In spite of the tendency to apply multidisciplinary approaches to public health issues, the overview of these articles suggests that the dominant thread has been an ever-greater biomedicalization of the life cycle (Morsy 1995) and of social suffering in the region by pointing towards the reliance on science and technology to alleviate these problems. Aside from the rare critique, improving health services and raising awareness are represented as the way forward to modernization and to reducing mortality (see for example, El-Mehairy 1984; Weidner et al 1985; Abu-Zeid & Dann 1985; DeClerque et al 1986). While these are significant issues in public health in the Arab world, other important topics, such as class differences and rising inequalities between rich and poor, dependence on aid, the privatization of health services, the high consumption of medications, and the dwindling social and economic protection programs, have received much less attention.

Conclusion: The Dearth of Political and Socio-economic Studies of Health

Based on this review, I argue for the need to integrate several aspects of analysis as we examine health in the Arab world. The first concerns the need to acknowledge and understand how our institutional realities, political, economic, and social contexts, both global and local, and international health and development literature impact what we study and how we write about health and thus shape ways of understanding an Arab world. Few works explore the production of scholarship and research in relation to dominant institutional, political, and economic contexts.

While a review of one journal does not allow wholesale generalization about the field of studies on health, my preliminary reflections should perhaps be explored in more depth and with a broader scope in future research. Such research might not only cover a larger number of journals but also other outlets for scientific production, such as the vast gray literature on public health that exists in the region. Because *Social Science and Medicine* has founded its niche at the intersection of medicine, public health, and social studies, one might argue that published work in this journal tends to integrate social aspects of health better than one might see in more mainstream medical or public health journals. This needs to be validated in future research.

Although the articles examined in this overview of *Social Science and Medicine* have covered a variety of public health topics, few of the articles explore critically the socio-economic and political causes of the widespread poverty and inequities underlying the violence and ill health in the region. Many of the primarily social problems in the articles are viewed through the biomedical lens, and thus call for improving various components of health services, which cannot bridge the widening gaps or reduce the inequalities. As Nancy Scheper-Hughes argues, when clinically applied medical anthropology is used to investigate public health issues, it may serve the interests of expanding the domains of biomedical knowledge and expertise and medicalizing ever more life's suffering (Scheper-Hughes 1990). In her own words, "the social relations contributing to illness and other forms of disease are in danger of being medicalized and privatized rather than politicized and collectivized." (Scheper-Hughes 1990 p. 192). The policy implications for interventions will be individualized, superficial, and inadequate. What was published in this same journal two decades ago, rings all the more critical today.

References

Abu-Zeid H, Dann W (1985) Health services utilization and cost in Ismailia, Egypt. *Social Science and Medicine*, 21(4): 451–461

Al-Eissa Y (1995) The impact of the Gulf armed conflict on Kuwaiti children. *Social Science and Medicine*, 41(7): 1033–1037

Ali Kamran A (2002) *Planning the family in Egypt. New bodies, new selves*. Austin, TX: University of Texas Press

Antoun R (1972) *Arab village: A social-structural study of a trans-Jordanian peasant community*. Bloomington, IN: Indiana University Press

Armenian H, Chamieh M, Baraka A (1981) Influence of wartime stress and psychosocial factors in Lebanon on analgesic requirements for postoperative pain. *Social Science and Medicine*, 15: 63–66

Aronowitz R (2008) Framing disease: An underappreciated mechanism for social patterning of health. *Social Science and Medicine*, 67: 1–9

Ayoub V (1970) Conflict resolution and social reorganization in a Lebanese village. *In*: L Sweet (ed.) *Peoples and cultures of the Middle East* (vol. 1., p. 137–154). Garden City, NY: The Natural History Press

Barghouthi M, Giacaman R (1990) The emergence of an infrastructure of resistance: The case of health. *In*: J Nassar, R Heacock (Eds.) *Intifada: Palestine at the crossroads* (p. 73–90). New York, NY: Praeger

Boddy J (1988) Spirits and selves in northern Sudan: The cultural therapeutics of possession and trance. *American Ethnologist*, 15(1): 4–27

Bryce J, Walker N, Ghorayeb F, Kanj M (1989) Life experiences, response styles and mental health among mothers and children in Beirut, Lebanon. *Social Science and Medicine*, 28(7): 685–695

Clark CJ, Silverman J, Shahrouri M, Everson-Rose S, Groce N (2010) The role of the extended family in women's risk of intimate partner violence in Jordan. *Social Science and Medicine*, 70: 144–151

DeClerque J, Tsui AO, Abul-Ata MR, Private Practitioner Family Planning Project (1986) Rumor, misinformation and oral contraception use in Egypt. *Social Science and Medicine*, 23(1): 83–92

Dewachi O (2008) *The professionalization of the Iraqi medical doctor in Britain: Medicine, citizenship, sovereignty and empire*. Unpublished PhD dissertation. Harvard University

Diop-Sidibe N, Campbell J, Becker S (2006) Domestic violence against women in Egypt–wife beating and health outcomes. *Social Science and Medicine*, 62: 1260–1277

Doan RM, Bisharat L (1990) Female autonomy and child nutrition status: The extended family residential unit in Amman, Jordan. *Social Science and Medicine*, 31(7): 783–789

Dudgeon M, Inhorn M (2004) Men's influences on women's reproductive health: Medical anthropological perspectives. *Social Science and Medicine*, 59: 1379–1395

Early E (1982) The logic of well being: Therapeutic narratives in Cairo, Egypt. *Social Science and Medicine*, 16: 1491–1497

Early E (1988) The baladi curative system of Cairo, Egypt. *Culture, Medicine and Psychiatry*, 12: 65–83

El-Mehairy T (1984) Attitudes of a group of Egyptian medical students.

Social Science and Medicine, 19(2): 131–134

Farhood L, Zurayk H, Chaya M, Saadeh F, Meshefedjian G, Sidani T (1993) The impact of war on the physical and mental health of the family: The Lebanese experience. *Social Science and Medicine*, 36(12): 1555–1567

Fassin D, Rechtman R (2009) *The empire of trauma. An inquiry into the condition of victimhood*. Princeton, NJ: Princeton University Press

Gallagher E, Searle M (1985) Health services and the political culture of Saudi Arabia. *Social Science and Medicine*, 21(3): 251–262

Geertz C (1968) *Islam observed: Religious development in Morocco and Indonesia*. Chicago, IL: University of Chicago Press

Geertz C (1973) *The interpretation of cultures*. New York, NY: Basic Books

Giacaman R (1988) *Life and health in three Palestinian villages*. London, UK: Ithaca Press

Gilsenan M (1990) Very like a camel: The appearance of an anthropologist's Middle East. *In*: R Fardon (Ed.) *Localizing strategies: Regional traditions and ethnographic writing* (p. 222–239). Edinburgh, UK: Scottish Academic Press

Gingrich A (2011) Anthropological comparison as a research method in Arabia: Concepts, inventory, and a case study. *In*: R Heacock, E Conte (Eds.) *Critical research in the social sciences. A transdisciplinary east-west handbook* (p. 165–189). Birzeit: Ibrahim Abu-Lughod Institute of International Studies, Birzeit University and the Institute for Social Anthropology, Austrian Academy of Sciences

Good B (1977) The heart of what's the matter: The semantics of illness in Iran. *Culture, Medicine and Psychiatry*, 1: 25–58

Hamdy S (2008) When the state and your kidneys fail: Political etiologies

in an Egyptian dialysis ward. *American Ethnologist*, 35(4), 553–569

Harrison G, Zaghloul Z, Galal O, Gabr A (1993) Breastfeeding and weaning in a poor urban neighborhood in Cairo, Egypt: Maternal beliefs and perceptions. *Social Science and Medicine*, 36(8): 1063–1069

Hourani L, Armenian H, Zurayk H, Afifi L (1986) A population-based survey of loss and psychological distress during war. *Social Science and Medicine*, 23(3): 269–275

Inhorn M (1994) Kabsa (A.K.A. mushahara) and threatened fertility in Egypt. *Social Science and Medicine*, 39(4): 487–505

Inhorn M (2003) Global infertility and the globalization of new reproductive technologies: Illustrations from Egypt. *Social Science and Medicine*, 56: 1837–1851

Inhorn M (2004) Privacy, privatization and the politics of patronage: Ethnographic challenges to penetrating the secret world of Middle Eastern, hospital-based in vitro fertilization. *Social Science and Medicine*, 59: 2095–2108

Inhorn M, Buss K (1994) Ethnography, epidemiology and infertility in Egypt. *Social Science and Medicine*, 39(5): 671–686

Inhorn M, Lane S (1988) Ethno-ophthalmology in the Egyptian Delta; an historical systems approach to ethnomedicine in the Middle East. *Social Science and Medicine*, 26(6): 651–657

Kanaaneh R (2002) *Birthing the nation. Strategies of Palestinian women in Israel*. Berkeley, CA: University of California Press

Khamis V (1997) Psychological distress and well-being among traumatized Palestinian women during the Intifada. *Social Science and Medicine*, 46(8): 1033–1041

Khawaja M (2004) The extraordinary decline of infant and childhood mortality among Palestinian refugees. *Social Science and Medicine*, 58: 463–470

Khawaja M, Abdelrahim S, Afifi R, Karem D (2006) Distrust, social fragmentation and adolescents' health in the outer city: Beirut and beyond. *Social Science and Medicine*, 63: 1304–1315

Lamb V (1997) Gender differences in correlates of disablement among the elderly in Egypt. *Social Science and Medicine*, 45(1): 127–136

Lane S, Jok JM, El-Moulhy MT (1998) Buying safety: The economics of reproduction, risk and abortion in Egypt. *Social Science and Medicine*, 47(8): 1089–1099

Lane S, Meleis A (1991) Roles, work, health perceptions, and health resources of women: A study in an Egyptian delta hamlet. *Social Science and Medicine*, 33(10): 1197–1208

Lewando-Hundt G, Forman M (1993) Interfacing anthropology and epidemiology: The Bedouin Arab infant feeding study. *Social Science and Medicine*, 36(7): 957–964

Longuenesse E (1995) Les médecins syriens, des médiateurs dans une société en crise. *In: Santé, Médecine et Société dans le Monde Arabe* (p. 219–243). Paris, France: L'Harmattan

Malinowski B (1961) *Argonauts of the Western Pacific*. New York, NY: Dutton and Co

Maziak W, Asfar T, Mzayek F, Fouad FM, Kilzieh N (2002) Socio-demographic correlates of psychiatric morbidity among low-income women in Aleppo, Syria. *Social Science and Medicine*, 54(9): 1419–1427

Meleis A (1982) Effect of modernization on Kuwaiti women. *Social Science and Medicine*, 16(9): 965–970

Miller K, Rasmussen A (2010) War exposure, daily stressors, and mental health in conflict and post-conflict settings: Bridging the divide between trauma-focused and

psychosocial frameworks. *Social Science and Medicine*, 70: 7–16

Mohindra KS, Nikiema B (2010) Women's health in developing countries: Beyond an investment? *International Journal of Health Services*, 40(3): 543–567

Morsy S (1979) The missing link in medical anthropology: The political economy of health. *Reviews in Anthropology*, 6: 349–363

Morsy S (1981) Towards a political economy of health: A critical note on the medical anthropology of the Middle East. *Social Science and Medicine*, 15(2): 159–163

Morsy S (1988) Islamic clinics in Egypt: The cultural elaboration of biomedical hegemony. *Medical Anthropology Quarterly*, 2(4): 355–369

Morsy S (1995) Deadly reproduction among Egyptian women: Maternal mortality and the medicalization of population control. *In: F Ginsburg, R Rapp (Eds.) Conceiving the new world order. The global politics of reproduction* (p. 162–177). Berkeley, CA: University of California Press

Myntti C (1988) Hegemony and healing in rural North Yemen. *Social Science and Medicine*, 27(5): 515–520

Myntti C (1993) Social determinants of child health in Yemen. *Social Science and Medicine*, 37(2): 233

Ong A (1988) The production of possession: Spirits and the multinational corporation in Malaysia. *American Ethnologist*, 15: 28–42

Panter-Brick, C (1991) Parental responses to consanguinity and genetic disease in Saudi Arabia. *Social Science and Medicine*, 33(11): 1295–1302

Petersen A, Lupton D (1996) *The new public health: Health and self in the age of risk*. London, UK: Sage Publications

Rosen G, Kleinman A, Katon W (1982) Somatization in family practice: A biopsychosocial

approach. *Journal of Family Practice*, 14: 493–97

Rubinstein, R (1998) "Breaking the bureaucracy": Drug registration and neocolonial relations in Egypt. *Social Science and Medicine*, 46(11): 1487–1494

Saab B, Chaaya M, Doumit M, Farhood L (2003) Predictors of psychological distress in Lebanese hostages of war. *Social Science and Medicine*, 57: 1249–1257

Said E (1978) *Orientalism*. New York, NY: Vintage Books

Scheper-Hughes N (1990) Three propositions for a critically applied medical anthropology. *Social Science and Medicine*, 30(2): 189–197

Scheper-Hughes N (1992) *Death without weeping: The violence of everyday life in Brazil*. Berkeley, CA: University of California Press

Sholkamy H, Ghannam F (2004) *Health and identity in Egypt: Shifting frontiers*. Cairo, Egypt: Cairo University Press

Sibai A, Yount K, Fletcher A (2007) Marital status, intergenerational co-residence and cardiovascular and all-cause mortality among middle-aged and older men and women during wartime in Beirut: Gains and liabilities. *Social Science and Medicine*, 64: 64–76

Sukkary-Stolba S (1987) Food classifications and the diets of young children in rural Egypt. *Social Science and Medicine*, 25(4): 401–404

Sweet L (1974) *Tell Toqaan: A Syrian village*. Ann Arbor, MI: Museum of Anthropology, University of Michigan

Tekçe B (1990) Households, resources and child health in a self-help settlement in Cairo. *Social Science and Medicine*, 30(8): 929–940

Trostle J, Sommerfeld J (1996) Medical anthropology and epidemiology. *Annual Review of Anthropology*, 25: 253–274

Weidner L, Nosseir N, Hughes C (1985) A need for community education in development: An Egyptian village. *Social Science and Medicine*, 20(12): 1259–1268

Wick L (2008) Building the infrastructure, modeling the nation: The case of birth in Palestine. *Culture, Medicine and Psychiatry*, 32(3): 328–357

Yount K (2003) Provider bias in the treatment of diarrhea among boys and girls attending public facilities in Minia, Egypt *Social Science and Medicine*, 56(4): 753–768

Yount K, Agree E, Rebellon C (2004) Gender and use of health care among older adults in Egypt and Tunis. *Social Science and Medicine*, 59: 2470–2479

Chapter

36

Toward a Regional Perspective on Health and Human Security

Omar Dewachi, Samer Jabbour, Nasser Yassin, Iman Nuwayhid, and Rita Giacaman

Since the mid 1990s human security has become a buzzword in the international development literature and an analysis tool used by several international organizations working in the Arab region. In 2009 the Arab Human Development Report (AHDR) devoted its general theme to *Challenges to Human Security in the Arab Countries* (UNDP 2009). Sponsored by the United Nations Development Programme (UNDP), the AHDR series published over the last 8 years – each tackling a theme – is meant to provide leading Arab scholars with a platform to examine human development challenges in the region. Local scholars involved in the writing of the most recent report argued for the adoption of human security as the framework for a better understanding of the social, political, and economic conditions in the Arab world. Human security was proposed to examine indicators of development not only in terms of human capabilities and opportunities, but also in terms of *threats* to the everyday, through "enabling people to avert threats to their lives, livelihood and human dignity" (AHDR 2009 p. 2). The report was prompted, at least partly, by concerns over the everyday life conditions of millions of individuals living under precarious security conditions under occupation and perpetual state of conflict, be it in Iraq, the Occupied Palestinian Territory (OPT), or other Arab countries. The 2009 AHDR explored crucial issues pertaining to health and development, especially within the context of political conflict and other forms of structural violence. While the report received considerable attention, it ignited controversy in Arab newspapers and media outlets, mostly concerning the identification of priorities of human security in many parts of the Arab world (Nafaa 2009a). Still, this brief debate about the relevance of human security to the region, especially in terms of both development and health, died out very quickly in the public sphere.

Recognizing the lack of comprehensive regional scholarship on the theoretical and practical significance of human security, this chapter attempts to examine the implications of the human security concept and framework on public health research and advocacy in the Arab world. By problematizing the notion of human security, we suggest a careful exploration of the concept within regional and local contexts, particularly in terms of the social and political meanings associated with the notion of "threats" to human security and protection. More specifically, we consider how human security could be deployed as a critical concept and framework by advocates of public health and social protection in the region. As we attempt to build on human security in addressing structural threats to the health of individuals, communities, and populations, we aim to foreground the alleviation of social suffering and address the long-term social and economic determinants of health as a priority for national and global agendas.

Our interest as scholars in human security originates in our engagement with this concept in various forms. Both Jabbour and Nuwayhid were commissioned to write a background paper on *Health and Human Security* for the AHDR 2009, which prompted them to raise questions regarding the relevance of human security to the research and practice of public health in the region. Giacaman and her colleagues from Birzeit University have deployed human security as a framework to develop indicators of quality of life, distress, and health in the specific context of the Israeli military occupation and ongoing colonization of the OPT (Batniji et al 2009). Yassin's interests in human security started during his association with the Institute for Environmental Security in London and have continued in relation to his work on development and urban conflict. Dewachi's interest stems from an anthropological critique of human security as it relates to the displaced Iraqis both inside and outside Iraq.

In debating health and human security within the context of the region, our views converged on three main issues: First, pervasive threats to human security in the region constitute important health determinants in areas of conflict but are also important in non-conflict areas, pertaining to forms of structural violence. Second, there is insufficient understanding of the relationship between health and the concept of human security in our region. Finally, the application of the human security framework needs to be sensitive to local, national, and global contexts. Its use and value would depend on a better understanding of where threats are coming from, whose security we are talking about, and who is providing this security.

We begin this chapter by first tracing the shift in political and international development discourses of the concept from a focus on national to human security. We then review the various ways of defining and measuring human security and examine the relevance of the framework to understanding public health in our region. Through the unpacking of the aforementioned problems and their link to public health practice and research, we propose outlines for the careful deployment of human security within our regional context.

From National to Human Security?

Human security has represented a paradigm shift in the West from conventional thinking of security as a state-centered model concerned with threats to the nation-state to a notion of security embedded in the everyday life of individuals and communities (UNDP 1994; CHS 2003; Jolly & Ray 2006; Günter Brauch 2009; Makaremi 2010). This shift does not necessarily mean that national security became replaced by human security, rather human security introduced new ethics of engagement and intervention which can simultaneously exist with the traditional understanding of national security, mostly through broadening the scope of actors and interventions involved in the provision of security.

After the end of the Cold War and the collapse of the Soviet Union as a global military power, the concept began appearing in international literature as a way of rethinking an increasingly globalized world. Different forms of social, economic, and political *threats*, to citizens and populations within conflict settings were seen

as requiring interventions, both in terms of their effects on these populations and their potential impact beyond national boundaries. This globalization of threats raised the question of what to do when states "fail" to provide basic security conditions for their citizens or vulnerable populations. In 1995, the Commission on Global Governance proposed revising the UN Charter to allow "an international response to violation of human security on humanitarian grounds" (Meddings 2001 p. 1553). This meant extending the responsibility of the provision of security beyond state institutions to incorporate non-state actors, both local and global. Critics have questioned this formulation and its role in justifying humanitarian and military interventions (Meddings 2001; Chandler 2004). An example of this "responsibility to protect and intervene", *despite* the objection of the state, is illustrated during NATO's intervention in Kosovo in the 1990s – which was also one of the logics given for the invasion of Iraq in 2003. Here human security was given a political value compromising state sovereignty, which in turn justified the military intervention in Kosovo (Meddings 2001). It is almost like an interventionist logic was built into the human security framework. The responsibility to protect eventually became institutionalized and sanctioned within the UN system and promoted by many emerging human security centers in the North in accordance with the UN World Summit in 2005 (Schütte & Kübler 2007; UN General Assembly 2005). While the global geopolitical landscape was being redefined after the Cold War, international interventionism was transcending "limitations" of state sovereignty.

Meanwhile in the development circles, the emergence of the human security framework coincided with another paradigm shift from a focus on purely *economic* development concerned with national income and growth to a focus on development attuned to threats, choices, and attainments of people, (Duffield 2001, 2006). The coupling of the concept and framework of human security with development was most visibly outlined in the UNDP's World Development Report (WDR) of 1994, which defined it as the freedom from economic, environmental, personal, social, community, food, and health threats (UNDP 1994). Through seeing threats within the everyday life of individuals and communities, the WDR and several initiatives that followed have attempted to incorporate security dimensions within social and economic indicators employed in the analysis of development. Building on this report, the

Commission on Human Security (2003) promoted the mandate of protecting people from critical and pervasive threats and situations, building on their strengths and aspirations.

Critics such as Mark Duffield (2001), however, saw in this coupling of security and development a radicalization of the politics of development. Duffield argues that, "In attempting to promote direct social change, development has increasingly come to resemble a series of projects and strategies to change indigenous values and modes of organization and replace them with liberal ones" (Duffield 2001 p. 42). Within such proposition, underdevelopment and poverty are seen as sources of threats such as fundamentalism and thus dangerous. This would allow global powers and governments to contemplate the transformation of societies as a whole, and implement various forms of interventions. Such interventions aim to promote behavioral and attitudinal change and institutional reform toward accepting Western liberal principles, while disseminating a global form of liberal governance.

While much of the critics and critiques of human security have raised very crucial and important questions that we need to keep at hand when addressing relevance to public health, this type of critique assumes that interventions are unidirectional, dismissing the role of local agency. In other words, it does not consider or show how communities, professionals, activists, and institutions have managed to utilize and co-opt the discourse on human security and how they have realigned this discourse with their own social and economic agendas in an attempt to address the urgent needs and threats at the local level.

The reality on the ground is that human security discourse and framework has become the *modus operandi* for foreign policy and aid programs in many donor countries, such as Japan, Canada, and Norway. In turn many international organizations working on various development and relief projects in the region – particularly in conflict areas – have adopted this framework to attract funding from such donors. This represents an important factor in defining how public health researchers and practitioners in the region will be engaging with both local and international organizations in defining their strategies and agendas.

Measures of Human Security

It is safe to say that after more than two decades of debates, there is no agreement on a universal definition or measures of human security (Günter Brauch 2009). Several definitions have addressed certain angles and focuses of the concept. For example, the Human Security Report has adopted a narrow focus on threats to life measured as deaths caused by armed conflict and criminal violence (Human Security Report 2009). Here, threats to human security are seen as a mere result of conflict situations and settings. In contrast, the Index of Human Insecurity (Lonergan et al 2000) adopts a broader scope and uses four indicators, from the social, environmental, and institutional domains. However, such measures do not account for the human insecurities related to globalization and foreign interventionism which are of concern to many countries in the South. Furthermore, it seems that the broader the measure used to calculate human insecurities, the more difficult meaningful measurement becomes (Owen 2008). Another question that has represented a contention for human security scholars is the kind of threshold that is used to define the limits of security. More specifically how does one put a value on the basic security of life? While this is not the scope of this chapter, it is important to raise such questions when exploring the concept of human security.

In terms of public health, there have been few interesting attempts to use this framework to develop nuanced and context-specific ways of examining the various indicators of health and illness. For example, King & Murray (2002) proposed measuring human security as the "number of years of future life spent outside a state of generalized poverty" (p. 585). Chen & Narasimhan (2004) argued for expanding the focus from threats to human survival and livelihood to threats to human flourishing and dignity. The framework by Leaning et al (2004) defines the psychosocial domains of human security in relation to "home," "community," and "time/sense of future." For Leaning, threats have a historical background and affect the outlook to the future. Darby (2006) linked insecurity with social suffering, arguing for a non-Western perspective of the concept.

All these definitions represent important contributions to the further understanding of the relation between health and human security. While building on these insights and models, we believe that the relevance of human security to public health research, practice, and advocacy in the region is not yet clear. As public health practitioners, we still need to reckon with many questions, such as: What do the different dimensions of this concept mean for public health practice and how do these differ in different contexts? What are the local concerns and threats and how do different communities deal with them? Can the framework be relevant to the conceptualizing of health inequalities and the determinants of ill health in the long term? What are the threats *from* the human security framework itself? By raising these questions we do not try to provide answers, rather we attempt to engage critically to open new paths and directions for public health professionals in the region to rethink the implications of human security to their research and practice.

Human Security in the Arab Regional Context

Although the human security approach might offer an attractive entry to understanding the plight and suffering of people caught in situations of occupation, violent conflicts, and political tension, scholarship on this subject from the Arab world has been quite limited and recent. Prior to the publication of the AHDR 2009 report, most scholarship on the subject in both English and Arabic was limited to newspaper and magazine articles (Chourou 2008; UNDP 2009). Since the publication of the AHDR, reactions to the human security paradigm, mostly in print and electronic media, have been generally dismissive and cynical. Critics saw human security as an imposed construct, attempting to turn a blind eye to the effects of military occupation, distract attention from core Arab matters – such as "unity" and "sovereignty" – and even to give a pretext for military and non-military interventions in the region (Nafaa 2009b). These concerns are not merely as theoretical as the bitter legacy of the selective use and coaptation of the AHDR 2002 to justify the invasion of Iraq by warmongers, such as *New York Times* journalist Thomas Freidman demonstrates:

> "The right reason for this war, as I argued before it started, was to oust Saddam's regime and partner with the Iraqi people to try to implement the Arab Human Development report's prescriptions in the heart of the Arab world. That report said the Arab world is falling off the globe because of a lack of freedom, women's empowerment, and modern education. The right reason for this war was to partner with Arab moderates in a long-term strategy of dehumiliation and redignification" (Friedman 2004).

As a number of "think-tanks" in the West have identified many states in the region as "failed-states" (Bates et al 2003), one wonders whether such "diagnoses" will be used to justify more international interventions. The centrality of the link of the human security debates to military occupation and Western hegemony in the region was clear in the controversy surrounding the release of the AHDR 2009 report. The lead author, Mustapha Kamel Al-Sayyid of Cairo University, withdrew his name from the report in protest over the relegation of "occupation and foreign interventionism" by the UNDP to the last rank of insecurities in the final version (Aljazeera 2009). Similarly in the summary report of "Human Security in the Arab World: Defining A Role for Europe" (Development Policy Forum 2010), occupation and foreign interventionism in the region received little mention while freedom and development "deficits" and "gaps" received the lion's share.

Another concern is how Arab regimes might selectively use and appropriate human security frameworks in service of regime survival. This might happen, for example, by showcasing specific improvements, such as increasing life expectancy, that might reflect positively on human security indicators, without addressing the full spectrum of threats to people, including those from oppressive state institutions. This is again a reminder of the thin line and the ambiguity between the notions of national and human security. In December 2008, the Cairo-based League of Arab States, with support from UN organizations, held a high-profile conference on *Human Security in the Arab Region* that fell short of serious discussions about the responsibilities of Arab states toward their citizens in terms of addressing current threats to human security in the region. It is worth mentioning here that the only centre devoted to human security in the region is the Regional Human Security Centre (RHSC 2010), which is close to the ruling monarchy in Jordan.

Human Security Between Conflict and Structural Threats

While these issues above represent serious concerns, there is no general agreement on what constitutes the main priorities of human security in the Arab world or how the concept of human security can add to the understanding of human conditions in the region. According to Chourou (2008,2009), one of the scholars working on a regional perspective of human security – different priorities exist in the different Arab sub-regions. In the *Mashreq* (or Eastern Mediterranean), the main threats relate to *direct* violence emanating from foreign or state intervention or civil conflict. In the *Maghreb* (or North Africa), *indirect* violence such as deprivation, underdevelopment, and environmental degradation are the main contributors to human insecurity. Health, understood as a broad concept relating to many of these different concerns, is not put forward as a topic for discussion. This was also noted at the 2008 League of Arab States conference – mentioned above – addressing human security in the region. One of the reasons, we believe, is that health is narrowly conceptualized and equated with the provision of health services, instead of being conceptualized as a social construction influenced by political, economic, social, and cultural determinants and a central theme in understanding physical, mental, and social well-being. This broader view of health allows the examination of where people live and work, and the institutions and relations of power that dominate and control people's everyday life in society. This, in turn, situates health as a central theme in relation to different structural threats that form the components of the human security concept.

It is our conviction that health is a political and social construct. Thus, it is our opinion that human security as a concept carries within it the potential to create a crucial debate about the threats that impact people in the Arab world. As a framework, it offers the possibility to situate health at the heart of social and political contexts in our region. What follows illustrates such a context-sensitive application of the human security framework in the OPT.

In 2009, a few months before the publication of the AHDR report, Batniji et al (2009) published an article in *The Lancet* which applied the concept of human security to the examination of the health of Palestinians in the OPT and the understanding of the larger social and political issues that impact the health and well-being of Arab communities under Israeli occupation. The authors used the human security framework developed by Leaning et al (2004) to examine "survival, development, and wellbeing in the context of protracted conflict and occupation in the Palestinian Territory" (Batniji et al p. 1133). Using both quantitative (e.g., mortality data) and qualitative methods (e.g., interviews), the authors reported on a sobering assessment of the dimensions of Palestinian

suffering and demonstrated pervasive threats to their everyday lives. Threats to home included individual and family survival from violence and people's fear for most basic needs such as safety and shelter. Threats to community concerned social relationships, cohesion, and resilience, which have held the Palestinian society together under the long periods of occupation. Threats to the future addressed the hopes of Palestinians for a dignified future. The study concluded that under Israeli occupation, the majority of Palestinians have a compromised "basic security" which adversely affects many health outcomes and indicators.

The use of the human security approach was crucial in dissecting the micro effects of occupation on the everyday lives of ordinary Palestinians. Based on the findings, the research team called for international efforts to alleviate and prevent causes of insecurity in the OPT and to support Palestinian social resilience and institutions. This study clearly demonstrates how a complex human security framework could be deployed successfully and strategically to show the effects of political and military power of an occupying state over a population under siege.

Given the ongoing crises in the region, one can conceive of the utility of this concept in analyzing other settings, for example, in describing the human toll of the large population displacement that followed the invasion and occupation of Iraq by the US-led coalition in 2003. Threats to the everyday lives of individuals and populations can only be understood by paying more attention to the local and social meanings and experiences of threats to health and dignity. A stronger engagement with the social sciences and the humanities is key in exploring the various multi-level connections between the social, the personal, and the medical domains. Ongoing research by Dewachi on Iraqi refugees in Syria, Jordan, and Lebanon provides an illustrative example'.

The term "*mako amān*" (there is no security) has become one of the main mantras of the displaced Iraqi population to express the lack of security at many levels. The use of the term *amān*, which has broader social and personal meaning in Arabic, instead of the word *amn*, which has a more or less institutional connotation related to police and military functions, not only addresses the lack of general security in the country related to threats from roadside bombs, suicide bombing, and killings by the various military and paramilitary forces in the country, but it also addresses the deterioration of the everyday aspects of living, including at the social and economic level. *Amān* incorporates the notion of an internal feeling of safety and security. To have *amān* is to have a certain form of moral and internal integrity. Even though human security is translated in Arabic as "*al-amn al-insani,*" the word "*amn*" does not have the same broader connotation that *amān* has (Dewachi 2011). Hanafi (2008) made the same observation in his attempt to trace the meanings of security in Arab Islamic thought.

The need to examine human security in context is a central challenge for public health research and practice. How we conceptualize health, and consequently health security, is crucial to considering how human security can be employed as a public health tool. Considering health within a human security framework raises issues on different levels of interest to public health in our region. While we recognize that these examples are context-specific, one should further interrogate whether this framework can be used to help analyze the everyday threats in other countries of the region not directly affected by war and conflict. We will try to address this question in the rest of the chapter by attempting to situate human security within a number of public health interests and concerns in our region.

Human Security as a Public Health Problem?

One of the first intersections between human security and public health is the framing of health and illness in terms of the social determinants of the health paradigm. Poverty and the gap between the rich and poor are clear determinants of poor health and inequity in access to health services, as well as to work, food, and housing, all of which represent threats to a secure and dignified life. Whether these threats come from occupation, oppression, exploitation, or global inequalities in access to basic resources for living, they represent forces of underlying social suffering, structural violence, and distress.

Taking such issues into consideration, the human security framework could actually be a powerful tool in examining the social determinants of threats to the integrity of physical, mental, and social well-being. By linking the social, economic, and political processes and their impact on health and health security of both individuals and populations, the human security

framework becomes a useful tool for public health professionals. A security perspective is crucial in understanding the ways in which the state acts both as a provider, and at the same time, as a threat to the health and security of people.

This happened, for example, during the unwarranted slaughtering of swine by the Egyptian government as a preventative measure during the H1N1 campaign in the spring of 2009. While the WHO questioned such a measure as being based on "no scientific bases" the intervention angered many of the swine farmers and garbage collectors – known in Cairo as Zabaleen, who are predominantly members of the Christian Coptic community – who saw in this intervention both the encroaching on their livelihood and the government role in fueling the Muslim – Christian strife in Egypt (Audi Nadim 2009). At the same time the culling of the pigs left Egyptian cities with a serious garbage disposal problem as pigs were used as scavengers going through tons of organic garbage in designated farms and parts of the city, such as *Moqattam* (BBC 2009). Health security here becomes an entry point into understanding the relation between the state and the citizen in the Arab world. The connection between social determinants and human security illustrates how health is at its core a political question. This question becomes central to future public health research in our region.

Secondly, a focus on health security offers another opportunity to challenge the common practice of health care in the region, which is characterized by deteriorating public services, dependency on high technology, over-medicalization, and secondary and tertiary medical care, commonly in unaffordable private care settings, in the context of liberalization and privatization trends since the 1980s (see Chapter 31). If used critically, health security could help bring back the attention to primary health care (Abdullatif 2008). By outlining threats to the everyday lives of individuals, communities, and environments, health security should allow public health advocates to direct policy research and recommendations toward questions of equity, intersectoral collaboration, community mobilization, and participation by addressing the root causes of ill health and key issues in the primary health care agenda that is based on the principles of Alma Ata (Chan 2009). While the Doha Declaration emanating from the November 2008 International Primary Health Care Conference reaffirmed commitment to primary health care (WHO 2008), much work needs to be done to push this commitment further on the ground.

Thirdly, health security can be an effective tool in the hands of public health advocates and social activists to press for greater attention for social policy and more funding for public health programs, and for questioning the health impacts of liberalization reforms that Arab governments have enthusiastically pursued over the past three decades (see also Chapter 2). Like primary health care, weak public health undermines the potential for achieving health security. Broadly defined, health security and public health in the Arab world can, potentially, be mutually reinforcing. Public health can ensure that health security takes a population perspective with a focus on equity rather than a focus on individuals.

These three levels are linked and inter-dependent. Seeing them in their totality determines our abilities to tackle the root causes of ill health, and especially avoidable health inequalities (also referred to as inequities, see Chapter 5). Addressing the root causes of ill health must entail actions inside and outside the health sector: within the health sector, by working to understand inequities in health, to evaluate action, to expand the knowledge base, to develop a workforce that is trained in addressing the social determinants of health, and to raise public awareness about the social determinants of health; and outside the health sector, through long-term investment in social and economic policies including the improvement of daily living conditions of people, and tackling the inequitable distribution of power, money, and resources (CSDH 2008).

At the same time, the turn to health security raises a number of concerns and shortcomings that need to be addressed. One concern relates to how many political and social circles, including the regional and international literature on human security, define health and consequently health security among competing visions (Aldis 2008). The WDR 1994, for example, identifies health security as one of the seven components of security but defines it as the relative freedom from disease and infection, which is narrow-focused when compared with the WHO's definition of health as a state of physical, mental, and social well-being. Failing to represent the broader conceptualization of health relegates health to the realm of disease and care delivery and to the citizen-state dichotomy where the former is accountable for his/her own health and the latter is responsible for service delivery which is largely disease and not health oriented.

Our second concern relates to a rigid application of the human security framework. Although the Cairo conference organized by the WHO in 2002 emphasized the centrality of health as an entry to human security, this approach should be used judiciously and with flexibility depending on the context. It would be disconcerting if different professional groups, including those in public health, argue that insecurities related to their specific discipline (e.g., health security, food security, environmental security) is the only, or better, entry to human security. Selectivity and a narrow disciplinary focus may undermine the comprehensiveness and flexibility of the human security framework as it relates to both health and security in their totality.

Although we believe that health is a key component of human security, it is important to recognize that this framework is not foolproof. We echo the concerns about uses of human security, which can undermine sovereignty and justify foreign intervention. The Western fears of bioterrorism, the profound impact of the HIV/AIDS epidemic, and the emergence of cross-border infections of potential pandemic significance such as SARS, avian flu, and H1N1 have converged to facilitate the emergence of a powerful discourse of securitization of global health (King 2002; Kelle 2007). This is manifested for example in the recently strengthened International Health Regulations requiring member states to report potential threats to global health, and the emergence of the concept of global public health security (WHO 2007). In response to these developments, low and middle-income country researchers have raised justifiable concerns about the potential use of security as a pretext to undermine national sovereignty, serve Northern interests, and push forward neoliberal political and economic agendas. For example, Pereira (2008) warned outright of the risk of militarization and the agendas of hegemonic powers. In addition, global health interventions can undermine the well-being and economic security of particular population groups. Similar to the swine farmers in Egypt, farmers in Vietnam and other parts of Asia lost their livelihoods with large scale slaughtering of poultry as part of the global campaign against avian influenza (Lockerbie & Herring 2009).

The rise of major players in global health, such as the Gates Foundation and major international initiatives (as in the President's Emergency Plan for AIDS Relief-PEPFAR, Global Fund to fight AIDS, Malaria, and Tuberculosis) responding to "global threats," has raised a lot of concerns. While many of these interventions can be seen skewed by Western interests in human and/or national security, these interventions have focused on what Lakoff and Collier calls "Emergency Modality," which do not involve long-term interventions into the social and economic determinants (Lakoff & Collier 2008 p. 17). These developments represent a serious challenge to health advocates in this region in building stronger public health. It further requires them to position themselves critically in relation to addressing such global threats, rather than falling into the trap of this problematic global trend.

Conclusion and Ways Forward

The human security discourse and approach has become the *modus operandi* of many international organizations working on various development and relief projects, especially in conflict areas. Despite the regional critique of the human security framework as a way to justify intervention and occupation in the region, one of the most powerful and competing arguments for its use comes from the contexts of military occupation, specifically in the OPT and Iraq. We have stressed throughout this chapter the need to engage critically with the human security framework, as with other new concepts and frameworks. Rather than swallow it whole as defined by various international groups we need to co-opt the framework and use it to expose a myriad of threats and insecurities in the Arab world. We have argued here that the framework carries enough flexibility (Gasper 2008) to allow its application in different contexts and for the examination of various health and non-health security issues. For example, can arguments for human

security violations be made against a state in relation to its people? Can a human security argument assist in informing national, social, political, and economic policies? What happens when recommendations emanating out of the human security framework contradict the politics of regimes in the region or international interests?

Equally interesting, there is a need for a deeper understanding of what "security" means to people in the Arab world living in different contexts. Are there measures and levels of what constitutes insecurities and threats for people in their daily lives? Can we identify basic human security indicators? Can the concept of human security become people-centered, carrying their voices into the discussion and using it as a tool to struggle for their rights? How would these concepts vary across the Arab world and within different countries? What securities/insecurities would surface as priorities?

Another set of research questions concern building the evidence base of how health inequity and insecurity impact overall human security. For example, research can show how ill health and health expenditures can impoverish families and lead to unemployment and income insecurity. Such research can make the case for strengthening public health efforts and social policy change. Research can also help answer the crucial question of whether framing *certain* social determinants of health as human security threats increases their profile and urgency and the likelihood of policy change.

The debate about and application of the human security framework in the Arab world is in a nascent stage. Answering some of the questions we have raised in this chapter requires multidisciplinary collaboration which can contribute to a better understanding of how human security can contribute to improving health and well-being in the region.

References

Abdullatif AA (2008) Aspiring to build health services and systems led by primary health care in the Eastern Mediterranean Region. *Eastern Mediterranean Health Journal*, 14 (Suppl.): S23–S41

Aldis W (2008) Human security as a public health concept: A critical analysis. *Health Policy & Planning*, 23(6): 369–375

Aljazeera (2009) *Author of Arab development report distances himself from it (18 July, Arabic)*. Available from http://www.aljazeera.net/NR/exeres/E3F9319A-9188–409F-879F-A67AA409AD0F.htm [Accessed 10 September 2010]

Audi Nadim (2009) Culling pigs in flu fight. Egypt angers herders and dismays UN. *The New York Times* (30 April)

Bates HR, Epstein DL, Goldstone JA, et al (2003) *Political instability task force report: Phase IV findings*. McLean, VA: Science Applications International Corporation

Batniji R, Rabaia Y, Nguyen–Gillham V, et al (2009) Health as human security in the Occupied Palestinian territory. *Lancet*, 373: 1133–1143

BBC (2009) *Struggling after Egypt's pig cull* (06 August)

Chan M (2009) Primary health care as a route to health security. *Lancet*, 373: 1586–1587

Chandler D (2004) The responsibility to protect? Imposing the 'liberal peace'. *International Peacekeeping*, 11(1): 59–81

Chen LC, Narasimhan V (2004) Global health and human security. *In*: LC Chen, J Leaning, V Narasimhan (Eds.) *Global health challenges for human security*. (p. 183–189), Cambridge, MA: Harvard University Press

Chourou B (2008) A regional security perspective from and for the Arab World. *In*: HG Brauch, U Oswald Spring, C Mesjasz, et al (Eds.) *Globalization and environmental challenges: Reconceptualizing security in the 21st century*. Hexagon Series on Human and Environmental Security and Peace (vol. 3). Berlin, Germany: Springer-Verlag

Chourou B (2009) Human security in the Arab world: A perspective from the Maghreb. *In*: HG Brauch, U Oswald Spring, J Grin, et al (Eds.) *Facing global environmental change: Environmental, human, energy, food, health and water security concepts*. Hexagon Series on Human and Environmental Security and Peace (vol. 4). New York, NY: Springer-Verlag

CHS (Commission on Human Security) (2003) *Outline of the report of the Commission on Human Security*. Available from http://www.humansecurity-chs.org/finalreport/Outlines/outline.pdf [Accessed 4 September 2010]

Darby P (2006) Security, spaciality and social suffering. *Alternatives*, 31: 453–473

CSDH (Commission on Social Determinants of Health) (2008) *Final report. Closing the gap in a generation. Health equity through action on the social determinants of health*. Geneva, Switzerland: WHO

Development Policy Forum (2010) *Human security in the Arab world: Defining a role for Europe, series of 'future world' debates*. Brussels, Belgium: Friends of Europe

Dewachi O (2011) [Between security, safety and technologies of government]. (in Arabi). *Al-Abhar Newspaper*, suppl. March 24

Duffield M (2001) *Global governance and the new wars: The merging of development and security*. London, UK: Zed Books

Duffield M (2006) Securing humans in a dangerous world. *International Politics*, 43(1): 1–23

Friedman T (2004) *Liberal hawks reconsider the Iraq war: Four reasons to invade Iraq*. Slate.com. Available from http://www.slate.com/id/2093620/entry/2093763/ [Accessed 12 November 2010]

Garrett L (2007) The challenge of global health. *Foreign Affairs, January/February* 2007: 14–38

Gasper D (2008) *The idea of human security*. GARNET working paper: No 28/08. The Hague, the Netherland: Institute for Social Studies

Günter Brauch H (2009) Human security concepts in policy and science. *In*: H Günter Brauch, U Oswald Spring, J Grin, et al (Eds.) *Facing global environmental change: Environmental, human, energy, food, health and water security concepts*. Berlin Heidelberg, Germany: Springer-Verlag

Hanafi H (2008) Security conceptualization in Arab philosophy and ethics and Muslim perspectives. *In*: HG Brauch, U Oswald Spring, C Mesjasz, et al (Eds.) *Globalization and environmental challenges, Reconceptualizing security in the 21st century*. Berlin, Germany: Springer-Verlag

Human Security Report (2009) *The shrinking costs of war*. Canada: The Human Security Report Project

Jolly R, Ray DB (2006) *The human security framework and national human development reports:*

A review of experiences and current debates. UNDP, National Human Development Report Unit, NHDR Occasional paper 5: p. 1

Kaldor M, Martin M, Selchow S (2007) Human security: A new strategic narrative for Europe. *International Affairs*, 83(2): 273–288

Kelle A (2007) Securitization of International public health: Implications for global health governance and the biological weapons prohibition regime. *Global Governance*, 13: 217–235

King G, Murray C (2002) Rethinking human security. *Political Science*, 116(4): 585–610

King NB (2002) Security, disease, commerce: Ideologies of postcolonial global health. *Social Studies of Science*, 32(5/6): 763–789

Lakoff A, Collier SJ (2008) *Biosecurity interventions: Global health and security in question*. New York, NY: Columbia University Press

Leaning J, Arie S, Sites E (2004) Human security in crisis and transition. *Praxis XIX*: 9–10

Lockerbie S, Herring DA (2009) Global panic, local repercussions: Economic and nutritional effects of bird flu in Vietnam. *In*: RA Hahn, MC Inhorn (Eds.) *Anthropology and public health. Bridging differences in culture and society*. Oxford, UK: Oxford University Press

Lonergan S, Gustavson K, Carter B (2000) The index of human insecurity. *AVISO 6*: 1–7

Makaremi C (2010) The utopias of power: From human security to the responsibility to protect. *In*: M Pandolfi, D Fassin, (Eds.) *Contemporary states of emergency*. New York, NY: Zone Books (in print)

Meddings DR (2001) Human security: A prerequisite for health. *British Medical Journal*, 322(7301): 1553

Nafaa H (2009a) *UNDP credibility. Al Ahram Weekly, issue No. 957*. Cairo, Egypt. Available from http://weekly.

ahram.org.eg/2009/957/op1.htm [Accessed 4 February 2011]

Nafaa H (2009b) *Human security revisited. Al Ahram Weekly, issue No. 959*. Cairo, Egypt. Available from http://weekly.ahram.org.eg/2009/959/op5.htm [Accessed 4 February 2011]

Owen T (2008) Measuring human security: Methodological challenges and the importance of geographically referenced determinants. *In*: PH Liotta, DA Mouat, WG Kepner, JM Lancaster (Eds.) *Environmental change and human security: Recognizing and acting on hazard impacts.* Dordrecht, the Netherlands: Springer

Pereira R (2008) Processes of securitization of infectious diseases and western hegemonic power: A historical-political analysis.

Global Health Governance, II(1): 1–15

RHSC (Regional Human Security Centre) (2010) Available from http://www.rhsc.org.jo [Accessed 10 October 2010]

Schütte R, Kübler J (2007) *The responsibility to protect: Concealed power-politics or principled policy?* Marburg: AG Human Security, ad Philipps-Universität Marburg (AG HumSec Occasional Paper 2/2007)

UN (United Nations) General Assembly (2005) *World summit outcome: resolution/adopted by the General Assembly, 24 October 2005, A/RES/60/1.*Available from http://www.unhcr.org/refworld/docid/44168a910.html [Accessed 11 December 2010]

UNDP (United Nations Development Programme) (1994) *Human development report 1994: New*

dimensions of human security. New York, NY: UNDP

UNDP (2009) *Arab human development report 2009: Challenges to human security in the Arab countries.* New York, NY: UNDP

WHO (World Health Organization) (2003) *Cairo consultation on health and human security.* Cairo, Egypt: WHO EMRO (Eastern Mediterranean Region Office)

WHO (2007) *The world health report 2007–A safer future: Global public health security in the 21st century.* Geneva, Switzerland: World Health Organization

WHO (2008) *Doha declaration, health and well-being through health systems based on primary health care.* November, 2008, Doha, Qatar International Primary Health Care Conference, Cairo, Egypt: WHO EMRO

Egypt in Crisis: Politics, Health Care Reform, and Social Mobilization for Health Rights

Alaa Shukrallah and Mohamed Hassan Khalil

"By focusing their gaze only on medicine ... analysts miss the fact that it is not only the practice and institutions of medicine that are in crisis. Other social institutions such as education, welfare, transportation, as well as many political, economic, and ideological institutions, are also ... in crisis ... societal crises are not the mere aggregate of the different sectoral crises; rather the sectoral crises are the sectoral realizations of the overall societal crises"

Vicente Navarro (1968 p. 11).

While we agree with Navarro that one cannot understand sectoral crises in health without understanding the overall societal crises, it is important to add that analyzing such sectoral crises, including health, can give an in-depth understanding of the overall societal crises. Many such crises have their origins in the political systems and power structures. The latter affect health in a myriad of ways that reflect how resources for health are (mis)distributed and result in differential health outcomes. The politics–health links are well outlined in the report of the Commission on Social Determinants of Health (CSDH 2008) and discussed in several chapters in this volume (see for example Chapters 1, 2, 5, and 8).

In this chapter, we examine the politics–health links taking the example of the health care system (HCS) crisis in Egypt. This case study is illustrative because both Egypt and its HCS are in transition with polarization between social forces with alternative visions of diagnoses and remedies for the societal crises; furthermore international forces play an important role (Chiffoleau 2005 p. 213–236; Fintz 2006). After describing the HCS crisis and the solutions proposed by the government of Egypt (GOE), we attempt to identify and analyze some of the major political dimensions and origins of the crisis through a historical review that spans almost two centuries of international influence in Egypt. We then examine the

GOE's most aggressive components of the HCS reform plans and the response of a civil society coalition that has been at the forefront of the fight for defending people's demands for a fair HCS and rights to health care. We conclude with a brief discussion of the lessons of the Egypt case study for understanding the politics-health links and for social mobilization to protect health rights.

The Health System Crisis and Proposals for Reforms

The Current Crisis

In the past decade, a growing public debate has exploded about an HCS crisis manifesting in deteriorating institutions and personnel, low quality of care, lack of accountability, rampant corruption in the public sector, and increasing unaffordability of services in the private sector. A study of citizens' health complaints based on letters to editors in local newspapers in 2006 showed that the major categories of complaints, in order of prevalence, were: increasing cost of care; neglect and bad treatment by doctors, particularly but not solely in the public sector; abuse and corruption; shortage of drugs in the public sector, and overall rising costs of medicines (AHED 2006). The grievance most commonly cited was the unaffordable costs of catastrophic illnesses, leading to severe hardships for families. A government study also documented many complaints about services (Mahmoud et al 2006).

The GOE's response to public discontent took two seemingly conflicting directions. It dismissed critics, lauding its successes in improving general health indicators. It also waged a campaign that emphasized the failings of the HCS, particularly the public sector, and called for large-scale reforms. This coincided with announcements in the media about the GOE's plans to pass a Health Insurance Law in the parliament which was unsuccessfully attempted several times. How do the GOE and international funders view this crisis?

Diagnosing the Ills of the Egyptian Health Care System

The HCS has suffered major problems long before the current crisis has taken its most acute manifestations. Consequently, the GOE launched a series of initiatives, supported by international donors, to "reform" the HCS and redefine the role of different factors including the Ministry of Health and Population (MOHP), and the public and private sectors. The large-scale "Health Sector Reform Program" (HSRP) was launched in 1998, building on two earlier projects: The "Health Profile project" (1977–1987) and the "Cost Recovery for Health Project" (1987–1997). The earlier projects were funded solely by the US Agency for International Development (USAID), whereas the HSRP was additionally supported by the World Bank, the European Commission, and the African Development Bank.

The projects included important studies of the HCS and of the socio-economic and population health situation. Four rounds of national health account (NHA) studies were carried out between 1991 and 2008. Between 1988 and 2008, nine demographic and health surveys (DHS 2010) were carried out. Numerous reports and scholarly publications emanated from these and other studies. The USAID Web site alone (USAID 2010) lists 707 reports for Egypt under "Population, Health and Nutrition." The GOE also released two important studies on the HCS problems and a proposed reform of buying services from the private sector (IDSC 2005a, 2005b).

The studies provide detailed diagnoses of HCS. Their focus is the public sector, including both statal institutions, such as the MOHP, and parastatal institutions, especially the Health Insurance Organization (HIO) that provides services to a large section of the population. The diagnoses (based on MOHP-Egypt, El-Zanaty Associates, & ORC Macro 2003 unless otherwise indicated) can be summarized as follows:

- A free governmental health services to all is not financially sustainable.
- Private expenditures on health are too high. The consecutive NHA studies did not only highlight high levels of out-of-pocket (OOP) health

expenditure but its rise, for example from around 55.3% and 50.3% in the 1991–92 and 1994–95 NHA studies, respectively (Rannan-Eliya 1995; Rannan-Eliya et al 1997) to 60% in the 2007–8 study (MOHP-Egypt & Health Systems 20/20 2010).

- The HCS is highly pluralistic with multiple sources of financing, financing agents and providers (MOHP-Egypt et al 2003) leading to fragmentation, lack of integration between different statal and parastatal providers and between these and private ones. This reflects evolution through various phases leading to a mixed model of public and private financing and delivery.
- There are regional imbalances in the health workforce favoring urban over rural areas and Lower over Upper (poorer) Egypt.
- Budget allocation (46% for curative services, 33% for administrative services, and 21% for prevention and promotion, including primary health care [PHC], family planning and preventive services) favored curative (secondary and tertiary) services over primary services.
- Low-level training of health personnel, particularly PHC doctors and those in the remotest areas.

Strategies for Health Sector Reform Proposed by the GOE and the International Funding Institutions (IFI)

Building on the diagnoses of HCS ills, the GOE launched reforms supported by IFI. For example, the main goal of the Cost Recovery for Health project was "to convert 10 hospitals and 40 polyclinics from entirely government financing to financing shared by government and user payment" (Eltigani & Makinen 1992). In preparation for the HSRP, the World Bank carried out six large studies in 1992–96, which were summarized by McEuen (1997). The recommendations focused on "reforming" the role of the two key public sector actors: the MOHP and HIO. The main recommendations, ad verbatim after McEuen, were:

- "Rationalizing the role of the MOHP in financing curative care by decreasing the proportion of the government's budget, increasing the resources available for preventive and primary health care (PHC)." Proposed strategies include "expanding cost recovery in government hospitals . . . introducing cost

recovery for curative outpatient care in PHC clinics on a pilot basis".
- "...conducting cost-effectiveness analyses to identify a package of essential health services".
- "Reforming the MOHP personnel policy, including ending guaranteed employment for all medical school graduates, reducing the overall number of personnel, redistributing personnel based on needs."
- "Developing the MOHP capacity for national health needs assessment, sectoral strategic planning, and policy development."
- Developing the MOHP role in regulation; accreditation; quality assurance ...; and establishing policies of licensing and continued medical education for physicians."
- "Ensuring the viability of the HIO, transforming it into a purely financing organization, and expanding social health insurance coverage on the long run."

Whatever the stated aims of the HSRP are, the real essence of the proposed strategies can be understood as large scale liberalization of the HCS, continuing the earlier efforts of the Cost Recovery for Health project. For example, we can read, again after McEuen, that with regard to health insurance, the strategies are to "Define and adopt different insurance packages suitable for citizen capabilities," meaning differential services for the poor and the well-off, and "Define the subscription fees upon real cost and use the contributions of the beneficiaries" placing more burden on poor and average Egyptians, the main users of these services. "Reforming" the MOHP and HIO focuses on converting them from service delivery and contracting organizations to financing and regulating bodies and "selling" current facilities (hospitals, polyclinics, and clinics) to the private sector. Considering the sheer size of these institutions, this would represent the largest attempt at privatization in health not just in Egypt and the Arab world but perhaps elsewhere. Regarding HIO workers, no jobs should be guaranteed and advice is given about decreasing their number. The proposed strategies are not far from World Bank prescriptions (see for example Preker and Harding 2003) whereby public hospitals are "reformed" through three stages: "autonomization", "corporatization", and finally "privatization". Fouad (2005) estimated that it would take 15–20 years for full implementation of the HSRP.

The HSRP included pilot activities in several governorates. Gaumer & Rafeh (2005) presented the implementation in Suez governorate between 2002 and 2005. The most significant part of the HSRP came in 2000. We will return to this issue in a later section.

The Antecedents of the Current HCS Crisis

While there is near unanimous agreement on the manifestations of the current HCS crisis, there is limited discussion of its root causes. Conveniently, the reports by the GOE, IFI, and their experts do not discuss the contribution of the practices and policies of the Sadat and Mubarak era in deepening the crisis. To understand the root causes, we argue that it is important to look back in the history of Egypt and its HCS (Shukrallah 2005). The beginning of the nineteenth century is a good place to start for reasons discussed below.

Muhammad Ali and the foundation of modern Egypt

Napoleon's campaign in Egypt (1798–1801) exposed Egyptians to the knowledge and know-how, including medicine, of European powers. Muhammad Ali, who reigned from 1805, built the new modern institutions in Egypt, along the Western model as part of his efforts to develop a powerful state and army. While inviting European expertise, he relied on Egyptians for state-building. Health and education were pivotal to realize these aims (Badran et al 1995 p. 97–85; Kuhnke 1990 p. 3). New medical and nursing schools and a large medical infrastructure were developed. A General Health Council (GHC) was charged with improving public health, and of the district hospitals in the provinces. The Council was the first governmental health organization in modern Egypt. Despite the setbacks it suffered under increasing influence of European powers, the Council could be seen as a nucleus for a future Ministry of Health.

Muhammad Ali's grand plans for a powerful state were undermined after his defeat in Syria and the containment of his regime around 1841. Increasing hegemony of European powers undermined the Egyptian economy and independence and hampered the development of a strong public health. The quarantine procedure to control epidemics became a

479

battleground for competition among such powers and a tool for control and dominance (Kuhnke 1990 p. 3; Badran et al 1995 p. 100–101). European medicine became a tool for colonization and a justification for control and claim to legitimacy. Lyautey, a French leading exponent of military medicine, proclaimed that *"La seule excuse de la colonisation c'est le médecin"* [The sole excuse of colonization is the physician] (Arnold 1988, p. 3). The medical profession became increasingly more subservient to European interests and tied to its ideology and biomedical and entrepreneurial market-oriented framework of health and disease (Chiffoleau (2005 p. 67–75). This would accelerate with the British occupation of Egypt in 1882.

British Colonialism and the Struggle of Egyptian Doctors for the Health Care Market

The British expanded the existing health infrastructure but focused on combating epidemics, important for the colonizers themselves. State public health services receded while private, profit-oriented personal curative services triumphed (Chiffoleau 2005 p. 67). As in other social sectors, the British discouraged state intervention and provision, neglected the need to combat endemic diseases and expand health services to the countryside. Lord Cromer, quoted in Chiffoleau (2005 p. 69), saw that *"The main task of the government is to prevent epidemic diseases and not cure normal diseases."* Policies favored more market-oriented services. In medical education, the British were more inclined to accept students from higher classes who could afford to study later abroad, preferably in Britain, at their own expense. Consequently, the medical profession became more elitist. While the British allowed the more privileged and wealthier Egyptian doctors to join their ranks, they narrowed the door in front of professional successes of most other Egyptian doctors who were assigned poor governmental health posts. This played a role in accumulating social and professional privileges, and resentments, and translated into the formation of a new socio-professional elite which investing its earnings in purchasing landed estates and real estate (Chiffoleau 2005 p. 78–79).

Egyptian doctors participated in the struggle for independence that started after the First World War. But in addition to their nationalist sentiments, they had professional aspirations as well. Feeling marginalized and excluded, they looked forward to affirming their identity, priorities and capacities, to taking a bigger share of the market, and to claiming a more central place in the profession from their foreign colleagues. For example, Egyptian doctors pushed for better control of neglected endemic diseases and expanding health services to the countryside. However, they also pushed for more control over teaching posts in the medical faculty, better share of the urban health market, and improving their knowledge and training. Gradually the Egyptian doctors triumphed and the first Egyptian Dean of the medical faculty was appointed in 1929. These triumphs remained fragile until 1952.

The Nasserite Era and the Development of the Current Health Care System

The 1952 revolution was a movement of army officers against the monarchy and British rule that received immediate popular support. The Nasserite regime adopted many elements of the programs of nationalist and democratic movements of the time including expanding health, education, and social services on a wide scale. The regime also banned independent political action and established an authoritarian one-party system, creating a "patron" state as suggested by Harik (1997). Failing to get aid from the West, Nasser turned to the Eastern bloc, especially the Soviet Union, for help and implemented many "socialist" policies, such as nationalization of vital sectors.

In its first decade, the regime pushed innovative and radical social development policies building on the visions and plans of the Wafd party and Egyptian doctors. For example, Nasser launched an ambitious project to establish 1000 "General Collective Unit" (GCU), each covering 15,000 people in the rural areas that would promote development (Badran et al 1995 p. 240–241). Each unit was to provide health services (including mini-surgery), education, agricultural support, veterinary services, library and sports club for youth. Regional councils in the governorates were to manage GCU as a step towards building a system of local authority and "decentralization". This was a visionary multi-sectoral approach to development. In addition to health services in GCU, vertical programs to combat endemic diseases were developed through extending specialized units to the governorates. To reach the villages and hamlets an ambitious program of semi-mobile clinics provided treatment and health education. The project which started in four governorates covered more than 1000 villages. Public health plans included providing clean drinking water to the whole population within six years.

None of these grand plans were fully implemented, for example only 350 GCU were established by 1962 and many were non-functioning (Badran et al 1995 p. 242). A commonly cited reason is lack of resources, which had to be diverted to war efforts to confront Israel after the Tripartite Aggression in 1956. Other plausible reasons include the autocratic nature of the state which hampered community engagement, crucial for the success of the intersectoral approach, and resistance of the medical profession who fought with social service personnel over administrative control over GCU.

In 1962, the GCU plan was abandoned. A new plan was developed whereby smaller health care units would cover all villages and hamlets, each unit covering around 4000 population and with physical accessibility of only 3–4 kilometers away from populations. Many of the units were established but the major problem was personnel. It was not shortage of physicians as these were actually in abundance but rather their negative attitudes towards serving in poor rural areas (Jan 1968 p. 49–51). This was compounded by the attitudes of the MOH and of medical education which favored private clinical medicine especially in the metropolis. Jan noted that "in most medical schools...the first objective is to ... work in big hospitals, the majority of the medical students take after the model of their professors, with no links or desire to work in the rural areas. Those who are employed in the university hospitals prefer clinical jobs rather than preventive or public health." The main objective of the vast majority of physicians was "to become rich." The positions of the medical establishment, especially its urban elite, would become decisive in shaping the Egyptian HCS and in its future crisis.

During Nasser's 1961 declaration of the "socialist" character of the state, many services were nationalized, including hospitals, particularly those provided by expatriate communities. By 1964, the regime, unable or unwilling to pursue its original plan of a HCS with full state control and free provision, had to compromise. Services based on premiums were established, including the HIO and the "Curative Care Organization" which worked on the basis of cost recovery to provide higher quality service but through contractual agreements with companies and other

institutes or for a fee. Although these institutions were still not-for-profit, they presented a shift from a tax-based financing system to a contractual for-fee services (Badran et al 1995 p. 280–291).

The development of the HCS continued. In addition to primary care, the regime built a strong system of secondary and tertiary care. About 100% of the 125 planned central and district hospitals were built. Tertiary care was offered through five university hospitals and a series of specialized national institutes.

Nasser, the Medical Profession, and the Big Compromise

The medical profession stood with Nasser as long as he helped in their takeover of the health market through nationalizing all expatriate hospitals and restricting the practice of foreigners in Egypt. However, as soon as the "Egyptianization" of the medical profession was achieved, divergent interests within the profession became apparent. To address the unmet needs in rural health, the state proposed that new medical graduates be posted to the countryside for a limited number of years as an obligatory service. The elite took a hard stand to protect its interests (Chiffoleau 2005). As the regime's political base depended heavily on this type of professional, a major compromise took place. The assets of the elite (concentrated mostly in university posts) were left untouched. Professors had reserved slots in medical schools for their children and these did not have to serve in rural areas after graduation. Professors were allowed to hold double employment in private practice in the metropolis and in university hospitals. Increasingly, a clearly demarcated two-tier system developed with university medical staff becoming the major providers of specialized and private practice in the metropolis, while most of the new graduates became the lower echelon, undertaking obligatory service in remote rural areas.

The impact of the compromise was dramatic. Increasingly, the medical staff became an inherited profession, with children of senior doctors taking new available posts. The concept of a full-time university professor was undermined. With dual public-private employment, the university hospitals were used to attract patients to private practice, and public services gradually suffered. Ominously, the medical elite became the base upon which later efforts towards privatization of health services largely depended. The elite could not realize its full potential and exercise its mighty powers until it aligned itself with the national and global liberalization agendas which Sadat started in the 1970s. While Sadat, and later Mubarak, is credited with initiating privatization and market-driven policies, we argue based on this review that, at least with regard to health care institutions and the medical profession, the seeds of these developments were in fact present, albeit in less pronounced forms, during the Nasserite and earlier eras. The same was probably true in other sectors.

From Sadat to Mubarak and the Alignment With the New Global Agenda

The introduction of the "October Policy Paper" in April 1974 represents the first major policy shift under Sadat. The paper called for an "open door" policy to attract Arab and foreign capital investments and encourage the Egyptian private sector to increase its contribution to the economy (El-Issawi 2007 p. 103). Mubarak continued and accelerated the liberalization started by Sadat, who was assassinated in 1981.

Agreements with IFI and international agencies fostered the liberation movement. These agreements were spearheaded by USAID as Egypt became the second favored country to receive US aid in reward for its unilateral peace with Israel. The GOE made agreements with the International Monetary Fund (IMF) and the World Bank in 1991, including the "Economic Reform and Structural Adjustment Program". The IMF pushed for fiscal discipline through removing price control, freeing exchange rates, and cutting government expenditure on services including subsidies for essential goods such as food. The World Bank pushed for reforming internal economic structures and services in the direction of cost recovery and privatization of public firms.

A USAID document exemplifies the influence of international institutions over the Egyptian economy: "As a result of USAID activities, the private sector grew rapidly ... Between 1996 and 1999, the private sector contribution to GDP increased from 63% to 74% as a result of USAID-supported reforms intended to unleash the private sector and the privatization of over 30 firms in 1999, representing more than 10% of all state-owned enterprises. The challenge for the future is to maintain and build upon these outstanding results" (USAID 2001).

The decline of the Nasserite project for building self-sufficiency and a strong economic base based on industrialization was associated with increasing dependency on the West. The growth of the service sector came at the expense of the industrial productive sector and that of the private sector at the expense of the public sector (El-Issawi 2007). Increasing investment in services concerned goods rather than social services such as health care and education (El-Issawi 2007). The liberalization process included concomitant changes: deregulation of external control of the state over trade, internal liberalization of the economy, receding state control and expansion of the private sector (El-Issawi 2007). In most cases, the newly emerging private sector was the result of the marriage between state officials, who had control over the major publicly owned sectors and the decision making processes, and new and old private Egyptian, Arab, and foreign investors willing to do business. A good example of this is Dr. Hatem El-Gabaly who has been both a minister of health and one of the major investors in private health service delivery and private insurance companies.

It was the association of liberalization, deregulation, and privatization with deliberate neglect and misuse of the public sector that proved disastrous for Egypt and its public sector whereby quality of goods and services declined (Ebeid 2004 p. 13–17). Corruption was a major tool in justifying and pushing for the shift from state-controlled to market economy and in, gradually but systematically, dismantling the achievements of the Nasserite era. In the absence of public accountability and transparency, many public resources were misused and wasted to the benefit of building the new business class. For instance, many public firms were sold "for peanuts" to private investors only to be re-introduced in the market some months later at much higher values than what was paid to the state. Selling public assets was so scandalous that it made it to the newspapers despite the risks (Al-Hariri 2008; Harb 2007). The practice of destroying such assets prior to selling them was also thought of as an instrument of privatization in the health sector (Harb 2007). These factors are key to understanding the current crisis of public health services. Speaking out against corruption was punished as happened in 2008 with the famous case of Raouf Hamed, the renowned professor of pharmacology whom the minister of health excluded from national drug oversight committees after pointing out areas of corruption, eliciting widespread condemnation, including by the Association for Freedom of Thought and Expression (AFTE 2008).

Sadat and Mubarak's policies have affected every aspect of Egyptian society, not just the economy. The impact is reflected in health determinants, health-relevant social policies, health sector policies, and ultimately health outcomes. It is beyond our scope to trace this impact across these domains but it is useful to consider a few manifestations.

In the area of policy, perhaps most representative of the policy direction is not official government documents, many containing empty rhetoric, but those of IFI. In a telling statement, the USAID (2001) indicates that it "... *will use the cash transfer program to focus on policy obstacles ... USAID will increase its attention on the legal and regulatory environment which is necessary to attract increased private sector participation and ensure that USAID investments are sustained through cost recovery. The $49 million for population and health will be used to improve the environment for private sector participation in the two sectors, to increase the quality and range of family planning services, to focus public sector service delivery on a more targeted clientele*" (USAID 2001). The Health Insurance Law proposed by the GOE in 2000 is but one translation of this policy.

In the area of social determinants of health, liberalization and various social and economic policies have had profound impact. A growing inequity gap (see also Chapter 5) reflected the shift in the policy of redistributing national wealth through reducing subsidies to foods and basic goods and through readjusting the taxation policy by lowering direct taxes on higher income brackets while widening the base of taxation (El-Issawi 2007). Recent studies confirm the presence of marked inequality of opportunity (Belhaj-Hassine 2010). Vulnerable groups did not benefit from periods of economic growth, modest as it was (El-Laithy et al 2003). As a result, economic insecurity is widespread (Ali 2008). A fifth of Egypt's children today grow up in poverty (UNICEF 2010). Real wages of the vast number of civil servants and public sector employees have declined dramatically. By one estimate the average real wages of civil servants declined 1% annually from 1975 to 2005 (El-Issawi 2007). Educated youth have even greater unemployment: among university graduates, 40% of men and 50% of women are unemployed. Unemployment among those with intermediate education was estimated to be as high as 66.3% in 2004 (El-Issawi 2007). The phenomena of youth fleeing to Europe, through exposing themselves to the risks of drowning at sea and imprisonment, indicate that this segment of the society lost hope in a dignified life. The neoliberal policies led to a "social trap", whereby those born in poorer classes stay there with little hope of upward mobility and decent work and wage and limited access to social protection.

In the health sector, the crisis we described earlier is itself a manifestation of neoliberal "reforms." Another example is the decline of the pharmaceutical industry, once an important driver in the economy and in access to affordable medicines. Within the context of the patent laws, this industry became increasingly unable to compete with foreign companies. A decline in government-sponsored pharmaceutical research compounded the failing. Drug prices soared, especially for new medicines, becoming unaffordable and inaccessible for most of the population (Hamed 2001; Taj Eddine & Hamed 2003). But the GOE had planned for even more HCS liberalization as we discuss next.

Accelerated Governmental Efforts at Neoliberal Health Reforms

The most significant development in the implementation of HSRP came in 2000. The GOE announced through the media that it would discuss a new Health Insurance Law (HIL) in the cabinet on May 13th and present it to the parliament by the weekend. This law was not publicly circulated. It included various liberalization and privatization measures. For example, beneficiary co-payment would become one third of investigations, drugs in outpatient clinics, hospital admissions and surgeries no ceiling for payments. The MOHP would be given the authority to reduce the current health package offered by the HIO. A "basic benefits package" would be offered to all but better packages would be available to those who can pay.

The Minister of Labor and the Workers Syndicate opposed increasing fees and challenged the authority of the MOHP to change the HIO health package. This prevented the transmittal of the HIL to parliament (Al-Ahaly 2000). There was also limited scale popular opposition. Later on, although opposition to the proposed HIL remained weak and fragmented, it seems that, among other factors, the volatile political conditions and the GOE's perception of changing public moods ignited by the second Palestinian uprising of 2000 and later the invasion of Iraq in 2003 froze the introduction of the contested HIL to parliament.

Despite reluctance, the GOE was determined to pursue the planned HCS reform. This was declared in major conferences held by the ruling National Democratic Party (NDP) (see for example NDP 2002). Some opposition members explained NDP's insistence on neoliberal health reforms by the growth of the direct influence of the business sector in the party and its leading committees, which became the major inner "kitchens" for state policy formation. The appointment of Dr. Hatem El-Gabaly, one of the biggest private investors in private health care delivery and health insurance companies, as Minister of Health in 2005 demonstrates this influence.

In the beginning of 2005, the GOE distributed the draft HIL to the parliament. Parliamentarians must have been seen it inappropriate to consider this law in light of the upcoming parliamentary and presidential elections in the summer; passing a law that increases burden on HIO beneficiaries may undermine popular support for the NDP and the President. It was announced that the draft HIL would be presented again in January 2006 to the newly elected parliament.

Along with the attempt to pass the HIL, the GOE adopted other strategies to push *de facto* privatization of public health services as advised by USAID-funded experts. Hassouna & Abou Ali (1996) recommended "issuance of presidential and ministerial decrees or amendments to existing laws" to achieve HSRP objectives. The MOHP's 2003 decree no. 109 to establish the Family Health Fund aimed to pave the way to convert public primary care from a service body to a fund that purchases services from the private sector and see stability through cost recovery from users. The HIO chairman's 2009 decree no. 769 and another joint decree by the Ministers of Health and of Local Administration raised user fees to levels unaffordable by many. But the most blatant decree was the prime ministerial decree no. 637 to change the character of the HIO from a non-for-profit public body to a "Holding Company" run under the principle of profitability. The company would be allowed to outsource its facilities and even sell them to private investors (El-Wakaei El-Masria 2007) to ensure profits. Circumventing the parliament, this decree became another rallying point for an opposition that was gathering strength and momentum and calling for preserving public assets and upholding rights.

Public Opposition and Social Mobilization for Health Rights

In pushing through reforms that would dismantle the current HCS, the GOE misjudged the positions of people. While the public recognized the problems of the public health sector and voiced its dissatisfaction with it, it was not ready to privatize or sell it. Even the GOE's own opinion poll (Mahmoud et al 2006) showed positive views in addition to negative ones. Patient satisfaction was 50–64% in outpatient clinics and drug prescription, not the worst and certainly in the remediable range, while it was 80–89% in surgical procedures, radiology, lab investigations, and rehabilitation. As HIO had, in 2007–8, covered around 45% of the population, one can understand why complaints outweighed praise in the media but also why people need the HIO most to avoid paying OOP for expensive medical services.

After media reports of the proposed HIL in 2000, there was dialogue among different actors including civil society organizations (CSOs) and professional organizations. The Association for Health and Environmental Development (AHED) played a major role in this effort. For example, AHED organized a 2-day conference in 2003 (see conference papers in Khalil 2003) that bought together diverse and prominent participants. It was felt that the HIL would change the current social health insurance into a commercial health insurance (Khalil 2003). Increasing co-payments and creating a two-tier system of benefits would increase health and social inequities. The proposed privatization of the large infrastructure of state and public facilities built with public funds and sacrifices would increase the costs of health care, which would become unaffordable to largest proportion of the population.

A much broader mobilization and participation took place after the announcement of the GOE's intention to pass the HIL in 2005. Again, the proposed law was not publicly published. A media campaign was launched by a small number of CSOs spearheaded by AHED but soon expanded to include nearly all opposition political parties and a wide range of CSOs including syndicates and trade unions. AHED issued a position paper and sent it to all newspapers, famous writers, NGOs, and others. The position paper was re-published in 11 daily and weekly independent and opposition newspapers. Additionally, AHED papers exposed the real motivations behind the HIL and demonstrated that alternative strategies exist to develop a true national social health insurance coverage and that this alternative was within reach of the existing health system (Ebeid & Khalil 2006).

Public opinion started to strongly oppose the proposed law. Popular meetings were held, including

15 in the first four months in five governorates, along with several pickets. The GOE hesitated again to present the HIL to the parliament, announcing it was going to modify the draft and re-present it in the next legislative session (2006–2007). However, continuing social pressure and press campaign, and popular meetings postponed the process.

Amongst the significant milestones of the development of the movement opposing the HIL was engaging civil society actors not traditionally involved. In 2007, the Committee for Defending People's Right to Health was formally launched and included a broad coalition of organizations (the founding statement can be read in Arabic and English at CDPRH [2007]). Since then CDRPH has grown both in number of participating CSOs, opposition parties, and other political and social groups. The Committee called for unifying the statal and para-statal medical infrastructure in a unified not-for-profit structure with integrating the private sector in service provision through transparent contracts. They also called for a comprehensive social health insurance system with a single comprehensive package of services based on premiums only without expensive co-payments.

As part of the committee, six CSOs including the Hisham Mubarak Law Center and the Egyptian Initiative for Personal Rights pushed and succeeded in winning a court case against the prime ministerial decree no. 637 on September 4, 2008, suspending the decree, at least temporarily. The significance of the case was not only in its outcome, but also in the wording of the verdict itself: *"Health care is not a field of investment, bargaining or monopoly. The tendency towards free market economy should not infringe on the right of citizens for health care as a responsibility of the state. Among the principles that the state should not forsake is its duty in the provision of the health and social services or delegating them to economic entities even if it belongs to it, as the aim of such entities is profit."*

As the right to health movement progressed, new forces joined its ranks representing various health workers. Among these the movement of "Doctors without Rights" (2010) struggles for better wages, training, and conditions of work. Although small and informally formed, this group represents the grievances of the increasing number of medical doctors who cannot find a place in the market of health, monopolized by big private health magnates

and corporations and the medical elite. Through the years 2008–2009, nurses carried out dozens of strikes and sit-ins to claim their professional rights. Laboratory technicians were able to form one of the very few independent unions in November 2010. All these groups gathered in a conference held in the Journalist Syndicate in October 2010 and produced the fourth declaration of the movement, adopting the slogans: "Health care is a right not a commodity" and "Right to Health is Right to Life."

Conclusion

The story of the HCS development in Egypt clearly illustrates the interconnectedness of politics and health. The system was a by-product of interactions between local class interests and ideologies and global ones, with the dominant power relations deciding the end results of this interaction. The current HCS crisis is an outcome of this process. Through a historical analysis, we have argued that this crisis is not only due to the policies followed by Sadat and Mubarak but has additional roots in the policies that have shaped the evolution of the HCS and the medical profession.

Any observer of Egypt will recognize that the crisis in the HCS is similar to the crises in other social sectors. In education, a system of low-quality basic education is available for the poor while high-quality education is available for the rich. Indeed, the HCS in Egypt is a witness to and a part of the overall social crisis of development and its hegemonic socio-economic policies. The solutions postulated by the same forces that produced the crises in the first place are in reality pathways to legalizing and structuring inequity. It is these policies that produce the "social trap", whereby those born to poorer classes are destined to stay there without hope for a better future. But we believe in an alternative. By bringing together grassroots activists and representatives of social groups marginalized and excluded by the neoliberal policies of development the Committee for Defending People's Right to Health hopes to contribute to such an alternative. Activists have been successful in halting the main components of the GOE's plans for privatizing the HCS but the battle is not won yet and the struggle must continue.

Afterword

This chapter was written before the eruption of the January 25, 2011, popular revolution that succeeded in toppling the regime of Hosni Mubarak and his ruling oligarchy and corrupt police state. If written today, the chapter would look quite different. However, the description of the current HCS crisis and its historical roots would remain relevant. The revolution validates our findings as the grievances of people about the HCS and the regime's attempts at dismantling its public sector are part of their grievances about the political and social problems under Mubarak. Demands for better health care were voiced by many protesters as part of the demands for wider social justice. In order to understand the root causes of people's grievances leading to the revolution, one has to look at the policies which have dominated the global and local scene during the past few decades, just as this chapter has attempted to do with regard to health care.

We have discussed the very specific manner in which transformation of Egypt has taken place related to the type of the ruling oligarchy with inter-marriage of power and business interests.

A last point to make is that all international agencies who have been key stakeholders in the policies of the Mubarak regime will, undoubtedly, come out now against the corruption of the oligarchy. This would be a welcome position. However, the policies that they have supported and which have produced the current crisis in health, and in the society in general, cannot continue after the revolution. These agencies need to abide to the people's will and adopt a new model. The Egyptian people are now determined to rebuild their HCS on a more equitable basis.

Declaration of Potential Conflict of Interest

The authors are founding members of the Committee for Defending People's Right to Health and are members of the Association for Health and Environmental Development. Both of these organizations are discussed in this chapter.

References

AFTE (Association for Freedom of Thought and Expression) (2008) *A press release about the exclusion of Dr. Raouf Hamed*. Cairo: AFTE (in Arabic)

AHED (Association for Health and Environmental Development) (2006) *A study on citizens' health complaints in newspapers*. Cairo: Association for Health and Environmental Development] (in Arabic)

Al-Hariri A (2008) *[Selling public assets is a crime that started with selling the public sector which will end up in the hands of professional looters]*. Cairo, Egypt: *Al-Youm Al-Sab'ee Daily]* (in Arabic)

Ali AAG (2008) *A note on economic insecurity in the Arab countries*. Kuwait: Arab Planning Institute

Arnold D (1988) *Imperial medicine and indigenous societies*. Manchester: Manchester University Press

Badran IG, Al-Brulusi AW, Salam AM, Al-Roubi AS, Busaila AW, Boulos FS (Eds.) (1995) [History of the scientific movement in modern Egypt: Medical science] *In: Medicine and Health in the 19th and 20th centuries*. Cairo, Egypt: Academy of Scientific Research and Technology (in Arabic)

Belhaj-Hassine N (2010) *Inequality of opportunity in Egypt. Economic Research Forum, Working Paper Series No. 549*. Cairo: Economic Research Forum

Chiffoleau S (2005a) *[Medicine and physicians in Egypt, Building a professional identity and the medical project] (in Arabic)*. Cairo, Egypt: the Higher Institute of Culture. This work is translated into Arabic from: Chiffoleau S (1997) *Médecine et Médecins en Égypte, Construction d'une identité professionnelle et projet médical*. Paris, France: L'Harmattan

Chiffoleau S (2005b) [La réforme du système de santé égyptien: un nouveau type de processus politique entre logique internationale et enjeux nationaux]. *In*: Chiffoleau Sylvia (dir.) *Politique de santé sous influence internationale: Afrique, Moyen-Orient*. Paris, France: Editions du CNRS (in French)

CDPRH (Committee for Defending People's or Citizens' Right to Health) (2007) *Founding Statement*, Cairo, Egypt. Available from: [Accessed 04 October 2010] (in Arabic)

CSDH (Commission on Social Determinants of Health) (2008) *Final report. Closing the gap in a generation*. Geneva: World Health Organization

DHS (Demographic and Health Survey) (2010) Egypt demographic and health surveys. Available from: http://www.mFeasuredhs.com/ [Accessed 04 October 2010]

Doctors Without Rights (2010) *Founding statement*. Cairo, Egypt. Available from http://atebaabelahokook. blogspot.com/ [Accessed 10 November 2010] (in Arabic)

Ebeid AM (2004) *[Towards total socio-economic restructuring of the health care sector in Egypt]*. Cairo, Egypt: *Cairo University*, Faculty of Economics and Political Science,

Public Administration Research & Consultation Center (in Arabic)

Ebeid AM, Khalil MH (2006) *[Health insurance in Egypt].* Cairo, Egypt: Association for Health and Environmental Development & Heinrich Böll Foundation (in Arabic)

El-Issawi I (2007) *[The Egyptian economy in thirty years] An analysis of macroeconomic developments since 1974 and demonstration of their social impact and a vision for an alternative development model.* Cairo, Egypt: The Academic Library (in Arabic)

El-Laithy H, Lokshin M, Banerji A (2003) *Poverty and economic growth in Egypt, 1995–2000. World Bank Policy Research Working Paper No. 3068.* Washington, DC: the World Bank

Eltigani EE, Makinen M (1992) *Beneficiary analysis of five cost recovery for health project facilities. HFS Technical Note No. 14.* Bethesda, MD: Abt Associates

El-Wakaei El-Masria (2007) *Prime Minister Decree No. 637.* Cairo: El-Wakaei El-Masria, issue of 21st March 2007 (in Arabic)

Fintz M (2006) A reform for the poor without them? The fate of the Egyptian health reform programme in 2005. *In:* Kohstall D (dir.), *L'Égypte dans l'année 2005.* Cairo: Centre d'Études et de Documentation Économiques, Juridiques et Sociales (CEDEJ)

Fouad S (2005) *Egypt National Health Accounts 2001–02.* Bethesda, MD: The Partners for Health Reform plus Project, Abt Associates Inc.

Gaumer G, Rafeh N (2005) *Strengthening Egypt's health sector reform program: Pilot activities in Suez.* Bethesda, MD: The Partners for Health Reformplus Project, Abt Associates Inc.

Hamed MR (2001) *[Report on the implementation of GAT agreement and its impact on the pharmaceutical industries and Egyptian Citizens' Health, AHED].* (in Arabic)

Harb S (2007) *[Privatization of health insurance is a danger that threatens Egyptians.* Cairo: Moheet.com. Available from http://www.moheet.com/show_files.aspx?fid=4712. Accessed: 15 November 2010.] (Arabic)

Harik I (1997) *Economic policy reform in Egypt.* Gainesville, FL: University Press of Florida

Hassouna Ali, Abou Ali (1996) *Legal analysis of the health sector policy reform program assistance in Egypt. Technical Report No. 5, Volume IV.* Bethesda, MD: Partnerships for Health Reform Project (PHR), Abt Associates Inc.

IDSC (Information and Decision Support Center) (2005a) *[Challenges facing the Egyptian health care system and policies to overcome it.* Cairo; The Egyptian Cabinet, IDSC] (in Arabic)

IDSC (2005b) *[A study of a proposal for the government to buy health services from the private sector.* Cairo: The Egyptian Cabinet, IDSC.] (in Arabic)

Jan S (1968) *[Men and medicine in the Middle East].* Cairo, Egypt: WHO Eastern Mediterranean Regional Office (in Arabic)

Khalil MH (2003) [Different visions for health insurance philosophy in the era of globalization] *In:* Serag H (Ed.) and Khalil MH. (Reviewer) [Towards comprehensive social health insurance: main issues-current challenges-functions] A report on the Fourth General Conference, 23–24 January 2003, Cairo, Egypt: Association for Health and Environmental Development (in Arabic)

Khalil MH, Ebeid AM (2006) [Health insurance in Egypt] Proceedings of a symposium organized by the Association for Health and Environmental Development in Luxor, 27 January 2006, Cairo, Egypt: Association for Health and Environmental Development (in Arabic)

Kuhnke L (1990) *Lives at risk: Public health in nineteenth-century Egypt.* Berkeley, CA: University of California Press

Mahmoud SM, Sami MC, Shiha NF (2006) *[A poll of citizen's opinions regarding services of the governmental health insurance].* Cairo, Egypt: The Egyptian Cabinet, Information and Decision Support Center (in Arabic)

McEuen M (1997) *Assessing health sector policy reform strategies in Egypt: A summary of PHR analyses, Technical Report No. 5 Vol. VII.* Bethesda, MD: Partnerships for Health Reform Project, Abt Associates Inc.

MOHP-Egypt, El-Zanaty Associates, ORC Macro (2003) *Egypt service provision assessment survey 2002.* Calverton, MD: Ministry of Health and Population, El-Zanaty Associates, and ORC Macro

MOHP- Egypt & Health Systems 20/20 (2010) *National health accounts 2007/2008*: Egypt. Bethesda, MD: Health Systems 20/20 project, Abt Associates Inc

Navarro V (1968) *Crisis, health and medicine.* New York, NY: Tavistok publications

NDP (National Democratic Party) (2002) *[New thought policy papers: Health and population].* Cairo, Egypt: NDP Eighth General Congress, September 2002 (in Arabic)

Preker AS, Harding A (Eds.) (2003) Innovations in health service delivery: The corporatization of public hospitals. Washington, DC: The World Bank

Rannan-Eliya RP (1995) *National health accounts of Egypt. Data for decision making project and Ministry of Public Health of Egypt.* Cambridge, MA: Harvard University

Rannan-Eliya RP, Naka KH, Kamal AM, Ali AI (1997) *Egypt National Health Accounts 1994–1995.*

Partnerships for Health Reform. Bethesda, MD: Abt Associate

Shukrallah A (2005) [Introduction: Historical development of health care in Egypt] *In*: I Yousef, J As-Samra, S Jalal, A Shukrallah, MH Khalil, et al. (Eds.) [*Health status and health services in Egypt. An analytical study of current situation and future outlook*]. Cairo, Egypt: Association for Health and Environmental Development (in Arabic)

Taj Eddine MA, Hamed MR (2003) [*Drug policies in Egypt: Conditions, problems and future*]. *Forum for Public Policies no. 16*. Cairo: Cairo University, Faculty of Economics and Political Science, Public Administration Research and Consultation Centre (in Arabic)

UNICEF (United Nations Children's Fund) (2010) *Child poverty and disparities in Egypt: Building the Social Infrastructure for Egypt's Future*, Cairo, Egypt: UNICEF

USAID (The United States Agency for International Development) (2001) Egypt FY (2001) Program description and activity Data Sheets. Available from http://www.usaid. gov/pubs/bj2001/ane/eg/egypt_ads. html [Accessed 04 October 2010]

USAID (2010) *USAID Documents.* Search filter: Egypt, health. Available from http://dec.usaid. gov/index.cfm?p=search. getSQLResults&q_descrgeo=Egypt [Accessed 15 December 2010]

Chapter

38

Can Action on Health Achieve Political and Social Reform?

Samer Jabbour, Abbas El-Zein, Iman Nuwayhid, and Rita Giacaman

Editors' note: This chapter is an article that appeared in the British Medical Journal (see BMJ 2006; 333;837–839). It is reproduced, with permission from BMJ Publishing Group Ltd., with minor formatting changes. Although the article was published in 2006, we reproduce it here in light of its potential relevance for public health under the dramatic social and political changes that are under way in the Arab world in the winter 2010–2011. The Postscript in this book further elaborates about the implications of these changes for public health and for the role of health professionals.

Public debate about health is rare in Arab countries. But getting the social and political issues underlying health problems onto the agenda could have wider effects on the region's political stagnation.

Arab countries face major challenges, including foreign occupations, deficient liberties, poor governance, squandering of resources, economic regression, inequities, and illiteracy (UNDP 2005). Arab reformists have advocated political, economic, and social change since the late nineteenth century. However, despite decades of local pressure for change, reforms remain elusive. We consider how action on health can contribute to realizing these reforms using examples from Lebanon, Palestine, and Syria.

Health in the Public Sphere

Despite abundant resources, the populations of most Arab countries endure poverty, inequities, and the burden of communicable and maternal and childhood diseases, rising prevalence of non-communicable diseases, and high rates of injury (Akala & El-Saharty 2006). Health indicators vary among Arab countries (WHO EMRO 2006), but they all share common barriers to health (Akala & El-Saharty 2006; Jabbour 2003). The health care systems are weak, unaccountable, and poorly governed, shaped by the political structures in which they are embedded (Jabbour 2003). Although the strong social networks support health, other social norms pose challenges. For example, taboos concerning behaviors and lifestyles such as premarital sex and homosexuality, constrain official policies for prevention and control of HIV infection and other sexually transmitted diseases.

Economic liberalization, which is happening in many Arab countries, presents new health problems. Syria, a signatory to the Framework Convention on Tobacco Control, recently allowed the building of a branch factory of a famous French cigarette maker under the pretext of liberalizing trade and creating jobs. Considering the gravity of the challenges, the lack of public debate on health in Arab countries is remarkable (Fouad & Jabbour 2004). Even when social and political change is discussed, debate on health is largely limited to curative medicine rather than wider health problems (Akala & El-Saharty 2006; Fouad & Jabbour 2004). It is tempting to think that competing public priorities, such as struggle for basic necessities or liberation, are the main factors behind absence of health debates, but other factors are also relevant.

The first is political authoritarianism, which discourages public participation and restricts public debate (Giacaman 1998). However, even in Lebanon, with its tradition of individual liberties and press freedom (Ammar 2003), debate mainly concerns issues of health services and cost rather than rights and policies.

Secondly, health professionals, especially doctors, and their organizations have failed to place health on the public agenda. They have also contributed to medicalizing health systems and policy making so that preventive approaches based on rights and social determinants are excluded. Authoritarian and hierarchical health institutions further discourage public engagement (Fouad & Jabbour 2004).

Thirdly, health is a gendered topic. Although men dominate health policy, management, and medical provision (Riska 2001), health is seen as a softer topic of discussion than employment, war, and political reform (Zuhur 2003). Health is thus devalued and depoliticized.

Opportunities for Change

Although the lack of public debate on health makes it difficult to promote changes in health services, let alone use it as a tool for wider reform, opportunities do exist. Pressing for debate on health builds democracy and supports public health. Health is everyone's business and thus offers a relatively comfortable entrance into public discussion for ordinary citizens including women, disabled people, and minority groups. Many health issues are easier to discuss publicly than subjects such as family law, custody, and inheritance, where religious doctrine and patriarchal traditions have made more definite pronouncements. Arab governments may not view public engagement in health as politically threatening.

The dizzying pace of change in Arab societies creates opportunities for using health for reform.

Globalization, modernity, and post-colonialism directly affect health. The health effects of socio-economic policies, foreign investments, and social doctrines mean that health promotion will have to be linked to work on broader issues. Health practitioners promoting prevention of sexually transmitted diseases, for example, act as agents of change without necessarily pursuing a social reform agenda. Commitment to women's health necessitates expanding the focus from prenatal care and family planning to thornier social issues such as discrimination and domestic violence. Similarly, health practice and policies cannot overlook conflicts, military occupations, and destruction of health infrastructure in Lebanon, Palestine, and Iraq.

Health as a Tool for Reform

We describe two experiences that illustrate interactions between health and wider social and political reform. In the late 1970s, Israeli neglect of health in the Occupied Palestinian Territory and the focus of Palestinian institutions on provision of urban health services created large imbalances between urban and rural areas. The disparity, coupled with imperatives of survival and resistance to occupation, led health practitioners to initiate the Palestinian Social Action

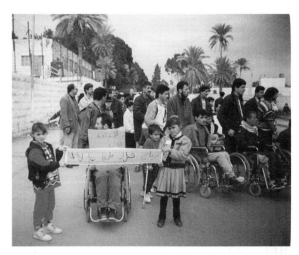

Figure 1. Advocacy march for the rights of disabled people in the Occupied Palestinian Territory.

Movement. By promoting community participation through volunteer work and health committees, the initiative rallied support from different sectors of society and evolved into a genuine grassroots movement. The movement helped overcome problems of access, introduced new concepts and methods in health care provision based on equity, community participation, and intersectoral collaboration, and helped build a primary health care network (Barghouthi & Giacaman 1990). Action was expanded beyond the clinic to include the training and empowerment of (mostly female) community health workers and joint activities with agricultural organizations, women, young people, and disabled people. The movement helped launch the community based rehabilitation network, helping disabled people to organize into a General Union of Disabled Palestinians and to rally support for a law of disability rights, promulgated by the Palestinian Legislative Council in 1999 (Giacaman 2001). Although it is difficult to measure the precise effect of these initiatives on health outcomes, their impact on social reform, exemplified through empowerment of women and disabled people, is undeniable.

The second experience is the Reproductive Health Working Group, an interdisciplinary network of over 50 health and social researchers from Arab countries and Turkey (RHWG 2006). The group advocated a vision of reproductive health based on women's perceptions and priorities. It focused on developing research models to examine issues that receive little local or regional attention, such as reproductive morbidity with emphasis on social determinants (Younis et al 1993). Defining itself as an agent for change from the beginning, the group has had a broad impact. The research broke the "culture of silence," whereby women carry heavy disease burdens silently (Younis et al 1993), and exposed poor medical practice (Choices and Challenges in Changing Childbirth Research Network 2005). It has challenged health ministries and regional programs to prioritize women's health issues and campaigned for doctors and hospitals to adopt women friendly practices and policies. The group is a model for collaboration in a region with limited opportunities for interaction and inadequate space for critical reflection.

Reform Dilemmas

Reformist health professionals face challenging political and social issues, such as corruption, patriarchy, secularism, and religious doctrines. Their responses will affect their abilities to achieve the desired reforms. Commenting on development and patriarchy in the Arab world, Joseph argued that although not every development project can work against patriarchal practices, development efforts should not reinforce them (Joseph 1996). The same argument could be made for health initiatives.

Working with civil health organizations is important in achieving broader reform. However, this is not always straightforward, as shown by Lebanon, where central government is weak and the public health system understaffed and ineffective. The two largest health care networks are the Rafik Hariri Foundation (2006), founded by the assassinated prime minister Rafik Hariri, and the Islamic Health Society (2006), affiliated with Hezbollah. Each of these organizations has developed a network of primary health care centers providing clinical and preventive services to the poor and lower middle classes. Both organizations have used these services to gain support for their political affiliates. Health professionals who disagree with the motivations of either network may find it difficult to engage with them despite the belief that civil participation is essential for social reform.

Syria is in the opposite situation, with dominating state structures and a socialized health system. The government recently introduced important changes, including user fees and private health insurance, without public discussions. Reformist health professionals here must obviously support the development of independent grassroots activities that oversee and monitor state policies, but they also need to engage with state activities. For example, the healthy villages program, adopted in 1996 by the government as a state-village partnership to improve health and social conditions in underserved villages (currently 560), (MOH-Syria 2006) has not had the desired effect on health determinants, services, and outcomes. The program has been limited by governmental bureaucracy and dominance by ruling party loyalists. Health professionals can engage more in the program and push towards making it more transparent, democratic, and, ultimately, more effective.

The Way Forward

Naturally, health professionals are expected to have a central role in promoting reform through actions to improve health. Such a role is fundamentally different from the roles demanded of health professionals in countries that have undergone political reform, such as South Africa and Eastern European countries (McKee & Nolte 2004; Ncayiyana 2004) where the focus has been on monitoring of health effects of democratization. Although priorities for health actions depend on the country and context, health professionals may consider three broad strategies:

Mobilizing health professionals – Acknowledging our current disengagement and historical responsibilities towards the current situation and rallying to the cause of reform are prerequisites to engaging the wider public. This will determine our credibility.

Mobilizing the public – By engaging the public, civil institutions, opposition politicians, and even government agencies in discussions and projects, health professionals will be able to highlight the social and political determinants of health.

Health system actions – We become more effective advocates for reform if we are successful at reforming our hospitals, clinics, and health ministries. Democratizing structures, undoing hierarchies, and advancing transparency and accountability in our institutions will contribute to wider reforms.

Box 1 gives some specific actions corresponding to these strategies. These are not meant to be prescriptive but to stimulate debate. Regional collaborations will prove helpful in advancing the cause of reform through drawing on rich perspectives and experiences from different settings. We need wide contributions and research from countries and regions to inform action leading to change.

491

Box 1. Health Actions That Could Promote Wider Reform

- Convene a regional meeting of health activists to establish an advocacy network
- Collect inspiring local examples of action and disseminate findings to the public
- Raise reform at general meetings of health professional organizations and support representatives who pick up the cause
- Create alliances with global movements of similar interest, such as the People's Health Movement

(www.phmovement.org) and Global Health Watch (www.ghwatch.org)

- Use the media and Internet to make the case to the public
- Identify public figures willing to champion health issues
- Raise funds to support research programs
- Campaign for serious reforms in health sector institutions

References

Ammar W (2003) *Health system and reform in Lebanon*, Beirut, Lebanon: WHO

Akala FA, El-Saharty S (2006) Public health challenges in the Middle East and North Africa. *Lancet*, 367: 961–964

Barghouthi M, Giacaman R (1990) The emergence of an infrastructure of resistance. The case of health, *In*: JR Nassar, R Heacock (Eds.) *Intifada. Palestine at the crossroads* (p. 73–87). New York, NY: Praeger

Choices and Challenges in Changing Childbirth Research Network (2005) Routines in facility based maternity care: Evidence from the Arab World. *British Journal of Obstetrics and Gynecology*, 112: 1270–1276

Fouad FM, Jabbour S (2004) [New concepts in health contradict interests of medical "clergy"] *An-Nahar Daily*, Issue of June 13 (In Arabic)

Giacaman G (1998) In the throes of Oslo: Palestinian society, civil society, and the future. *In*: G Giacaman, D Lonning (Eds.) *After Oslo: New realities, old problems* (p. 1–51). London, UK: Pluto Press

Giacaman R (2001) A community of citizens: Disability rehabilitation in the Palestinian transition to statehood. *Disability and Rehabilitation*, 23: 639–644

Hariri Foundation (2006) *Directorate of Health and Social Services*. Available from www.haririmed.org [Accessed 7 September 2006]

Islamic Health Society (2006). Available from www.hayaa.net [Accessed 23 September 2006]

Jabbour S (2003) Health and development in the Arab world: Which way forward? *British Medical Journal*, 326: 1141–1143.

Joseph S (1996) Patriarchy and development. *Gender and Development*, 4: 14–19

McKee M, Nolte E (2004) Lessons from health during the transition from communism. *British Medical Journal*, 329: 1428–1429

MOH-Syria (Syrian Ministry of Health) (2006) *Healthy villages programme in Syria*. Available from www.moh.gov.sy/arabic/health-services/hvillage.htm [Accessed 1 May 2006]

Ncayiyana DJ (2004) Is democracy good for people's health? A South African perspective. *British Medical Journal*, 329: 1425–1426

RHWG (Reproductive Health Working Group) (2006) *What is the Reproductive Health Working Group?* Available from www.rhwg.org [Accessed 25 September 2006]

Riska E (2001) Towards gender balance: But will women physicians have an impact on medicine? *Social Science and Medicine*, 52: 179–187

UNDP (United Nations Development Programme) (2005) *Arab human development report 2004, towards freedoms in the Arab world*. New York, NY: UNDP

WHO EMRO (World Health Organization Regional Office for the Eastern Mediterranean) (2006) *Country profiles*. Available from www.emro.who.int/emrinfo [Accessed 5 September 2006]

Younis N, Khattab H, Zurayk H, El-Mouelhy M, Main MF, Farag AM (1993) A community study of gynecological and related morbidities in rural Egypt. *Studies in Family Planning*, 24: 175–186

Zuhur S (2003) Women and empowerment in the Arab World. *Arab Studies Quarterly*, 25(4): 17–38

Postscript

In Chapter 18, Afifi et al write that the "health of young people cannot be fully realized without attention to ensuring dignity and the attainment of all human rights". The outcry of Arab youth for political change and the right for self-expression were two of the main themes of the revolts and protests that swept the Arab world in 2011 at the time of submission of the book's manuscript to the press. These events were ignited on December 17, 2010, when Mr. Mohamed Bouazizi from Tunisia self-immolated to protest the indifference of police officers to his situation and the threat to his livelihood and that of his family of eight. Within months, the long-standing political rulers Ben Ali in Tunisia and Mubarak in Egypt stepped down, Gaddafi in Libya has been killed, and the countries of Bahrain, Syria, and Yemen are experiencing unprecedented popular revolts. At the same time, other countries such as Saudi Arabia, Morocco, and Jordan are introducing social and political reforms in anticipation of or in response to popular protest.

The recent developments have raised hope and optimism about political change among people in the region, as well as anxiety and concerns over the prospects for such change, the nature of the emerging political systems if any, the impact of foreign interventions (e.g., NATO in Libya), and the rising number of casualties. Like millions of people in the region, the editors of this book were astonished at the pace of developments and the level of popular mobilization in the face of seemingly absent organization as conventionally conceived, including a fragmented or otherwise unclear political leadership. The unprecedented role of the media (including mass and social media) in the Arab uprisings was also surprising to scholars and lay people alike. A lot can, and will be, learnt from these uprisings and this will form rich material for future multidisciplinary scholarship.

Certainly, these uprisings and protests will lead to some form of political change and social reforms, with important implications for public health.

There are many speculations regarding the root causes of such uprisings and their timing. It is reported that the uprisings were largely steered at least initially by middle class, "detached" youth, with relatively high education and those "fluent" in social media. Further, it is unclear the extent to which job security, food security, the right to health, and access to health services influenced the emergence of these uprisings – even indirectly. Notwithstanding the uniqueness of movements in different Arab countries, these uprisings provide an opportunity to test if relative affluence rather than deprivation or misery seems to be correlated with political action and call for reform as per current scholarly paradigms. Despite this, there are important public health issues surrounding the recent uprisings. For example, little is known how people and health professionals manage the risks of mass gatherings and respond to injuries and other health threats. Nor is it known what proposals for social and health system reforms are emerging, if any, and what the priorities for change are.

We may be living in and observing a new Arab world by the time this book is in print. Indeed, the people of the region are hoping for democratization, good governance and accountability, a brighter future, new opportunities and life with dignity. However, they are also mindful of the political and social complexity facing their countries, the risks of external political and military interventions, and economic pressures which can undermine real change. In the midst of this, public health professionals need to engage with these social and political movements for change until their hopes and those of the peoples in the region are realized.

The editors

Index

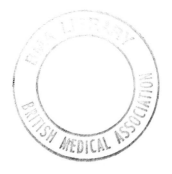